Nursing in Today's World

TRENDS, ISSUES, & MANAGEMENT

Ninth Edition

Janice Rider Ellis, PhD, RN, ANEF
Professor Emeritus and Nursing Education Consultant
Shoreline Community College
Seattle, Washington

Celia Love Hartley, MN, RN, ANEF
Professor Emerita
College of the Desert
Palm Desert, California
Curriculum Consultant
Camano Island, Washington

Illustrations by Tomm Scalera

 Wolters Kluwer | Lippincott Williams & Wilkins
Health

Philadelphia • Baltimore • New York • London
Buenos Aires • Hong Kong • Sydney • Tokyo

Senior Acquisitions Editor: Hilarie Surrena
Senior Managing Editor: Helen Kogut
Editorial Assistant: Elizabeth Harris
Production Project Manager: Cynthia Rudy
Director of Nursing Production: Helen Ewan
Senior Managing Editor / Production: Erika Kors
Design Coordinator: Joan Wendt
Manufacturing Coordinator: Karin Duffield
Production Services / Compositor: Aptara, Inc.

9th edition

9 8 7 6 5 4 3

Printed in China

Library of Congress Cataloging-in-Publication Data

Ellis, Janice Rider.
    Nursing in today's world : trends, issues & management / Janice Rider Ellis, Celia Love Hartley ; illustrations by Tomm Scalera. — 9th ed.
    p. ; cm.
    Includes bibliographical references and index.
    ISBN-13: 978-0-7817-6525-1
    ISBN-10: 0-7817-6525-0
  1. Nursing. 2. Nursing—Practice. 3. Nursing—United States. I. Hartley, Celia Love. II. Title.
    [DNLM: 1. Nursing—trends. 2. Ethics, Nursing. 3. Legislation, Nursing. 4. Nursing Care—organization & administration. 5. Nursing Care—trends. WY 16 E47n 2008]
    RT82.E45 2008
    610.73—dc22

            2007025959

Reviewers

Joanne Bonesteel, MS, RN
Nursing Faculty, ADN Programs
Excelsior College
Albany, New York

Sandy Brannan, MSN, RN
Assistant Professor of Nursing
Lamar University
Beaumont, Texas

Karen K. Cox, MNSc, RN
Assistant Professor
Arkansas Tech University
Russellville, Arkansas

Ellen Davel, RN, MSN, EdD
Coordinator, ADN Program
College of DuPage
Glen Ellyn, Illinois

Doreen DeAngelis, MSN, RN
Professor, School of Nursing
Penn State University, The Eberly Campus
Uniontown, Pennsylvania

Joan Dwyer, MSN, RN
Professor and Program Coordinator, Nursing
St. Louis Community College—Meramec
St. Louis, Missouri

Carol Fanutti, EdD, MS, RN
Professor, Director of Nursing
Trocaire College
Buffalo, New York

Mary Ann Helms, MSN, RN
Assistant Professor, School of Nursing
Tennessee State University
Nashville, Tennessee

Cherry A. Karl, RN, MSN, MA
Associate Professor
Anne Arundel Community College
Arnold, Maryland

Eileen Kaslatas, MSN, RN
Professor, Nursing Faculty
Macomb Community College
Clinton Township, Michigan

Ruth Lindquist, PhD, RN, APRN-BC, FAAN
Professor
University of Minnesota
Minneapolis, Minnesota

Nadine Mason, MSN, CRNP
Assistant Professor
Cedar Crest College
Allentown, Pennsylvania

Tammie McCoy, RN, PhD
Assistant Professor
Baccalaureate Nursing Program
Mississippi University for Women
Columbus, Mississippi

Pamela Moore, RN,C, MSN, CNS
Director, Division of Nursing
Louisiana Tech University
Ruston, Louisiana

Susan M. Mullaney, EdD, MS, RN
Professor of Nursing and Department Chair
Evening Associate Degree Nursing Program
MassBay Community College
Framingham, Massachusetts

Bonnie A. Nelson, MSN, RN, CNS
Director, Instructional Services
Medical College of Ohio, School of Nursing
Toledo, Ohio

Patricia L. Newland, RN, BS, MS
Professor
Broome Community College
Binghamton, New York

Lynda C. Opdyke, RN, MSN
Associate Dean
Mercy School of Nursing
Charlotte, North Carolina

Laurie J. Palmer, RN, MS, AOCN
Associate Professor of Nursing
Monroe Community College
Rochester, New York

Luise Speakman, RN, PhD
Chair, Health Sciences Department
Coordinator, Nursing Program
Cape Cod Community College
West Barnstable, Massachusetts

Linda Wilson, RN, PhD, CPAN, CAPA, BC
Assistant Professor
Drexel University College of Nursing
    and Health Professions
Philadelphia, Pennsylvania

Preface

The ninth edition of *Nursing in Today's World: Trends, Issues, and Management,* like the previous editions of this textbook, focuses on the nonclinical aspects of the professional nursing role. Much of this content is just as critical to practicing safely as is competence in the performance of clinical skills. Nursing continues to experience significant changes as it responds to the transformation occurring in the health care delivery system. As those adjustments and modifications have taken place, we have endeavored to keep the content of this textbook in tune with the times, revising and updating each chapter with the latest information and related Internet resources. Additionally, we have made every effort to be responsive to suggestions provided by our readers and reviewers. Thus, the ninth edition provides increased emphasis on the leadership and management role of the nurse. And we have retained in a concise and readable format the content that is basic to a textbook that has the nursing profession as its focus. Here is what you will find.

TEXT ORGANIZATION

We consistently have attempted to design a textbook that provides a flexible approach to instruction with the intention that each chapter be able to stand alone, with references occurring throughout that will lead the reader to related content appearing in other areas of the book. This goal has been maintained so that content can be reordered if so desired. For example, those of you who prefer a chronologic approach to the advances of the nursing profession are encouraged to adapt your use of the various chapters to match this preference. Thus, you might order your syllabus to present first the text found in Unit II, which explores the development of nursing as a profession, the education of its practitioners, and where the profession may be headed in the future. Similarly, some content areas might be combined or perhaps eliminated if they appear elsewhere in the curriculum of your program.

The textbook is organized into five major units of study.

- Unit I: Economic and Political Aspects of Health Care Delivery

We believe that if students are to gain an appreciation of nursing's place in the health care delivery system, it is best facilitated by gaining an understanding of how the health care delivery system functions and what forces impact its operation. Thus, Chapter 1 begins with an overview of economic and political aspects of health care delivery, including such information as how it got to where it is today, how it operates, how it is financed, and how it is politically influenced. Of particular application to nursing is Chapter 2, which is devoted to the relevance of the political process to nurses, including information describing how one can become informed. It also outlines a variety of ways in which nurses can affect the political process. This chapter also includes a discussion of the many nursing organizations, why so many exist, and the major focus of each. Chapter 3 provides a foundation for understanding nursing's social contract with the community it serves. Included in this chapter is an introduction to alternative and complementary health care and the ways in which they serve the community.

- Unit II: Appreciating the Development of Nursing as a Profession

Chapters 4, 5, and 6 focus on nursing itself. By understanding the origins of nursing and its challenges as a profession, and by exploring the various educational avenues providing entry into the profession of nursing, students will be better prepared to participate in the nonclinical activities and discussions that are part of nursing. Students will learn about the development of the profession and the challenges to its professional standing. The diverse educational paths that prepare graduates for registered nurse licensure are presented. Issues discussed include the controversy that exists regarding the form of educational preparation deemed most appropriate for entry-into-practice, the implementation of differentiated practice, and whether continuing education should be mandatory or voluntary.

- Unit III: Legal and Ethical Responsibility and Accountability for Practice

This area of study comprises four chapters. It begins with a discussion of the credentials found among health care providers, tracing the history of credentialing in the United States, and leads to an exploration of the legal issues facing today's nurses. Also incorporated into this unit is a chapter devoted to ethics that provides a foundation for ethical decision making, including a broad discussion of bioethical issues that impact nursing and nursing practice. The chapter on bioethics will challenge students to consider the many controversial facets of stem cell research, gene therapy, and the human genome project, as well as other topical issues.

- Unit IV: Introduction to Leadership and Management Roles

In response to the requests of our users, this edition provides a greater focus on the nurse as a leader/manager within the health care setting. Leading off the unit is Chapter 11, Understanding the World of Health Care Employment. This material is essential preparation for the next two chapters, which focus on the management role and the importance of working in teams in the modern health care environment. New content related to understanding and developing emotional intelligence will be important to all individuals involved in delivering health care. The final chapter in this unit highlights the process of change, leading within that process, and managing conflict when it occurs.

- Unit V: Career Opportunities and Professional Growth

The final section of *Nursing in Today's World* begins by exploring the employment opportunities available to nurses today and provides valuable information related to seeking, applying for, and resigning from a nursing position. The last chapter examines the challenges of the workplace and includes a discussion of reality shock and burnout in nurses.

PEDAGOGICAL FEATURES

- **Learning Outcomes** introduce each chapter and guide learning efforts.
- **Key Terms** used in the chapter discussion are listed.
- **Critical Thinking Activities** interspersed throughout each chapter help students critically process possible applications of the content.
- **Communication in Action** emphasizes the role of effective communication in every aspect of the nursing role.
- **Examples** provide a vignette of real-life experiences to assist students in understanding difficult concepts presented in the chapter.
- **Key Concepts** summarize each chapter.
- **Relevant Web Sites** related to each chapter's subject matter are presented at the end of the chapters and on thePoint.

SPECIAL FEATURE

The engaging cartoons in the ninth edition of *Nursing in Today's World* provide an eye-catching and provocative interpretation of concepts presented in each chapter. The cartoon feature, always a hallmark of this text, complements the easy reading style and logical approach of this textbook. Over the years, nurses have grown in their ability to find humor in many aspects of the profession. We believe that a little humor keeps us healthier and we hope that you, too, will appreciate this aspect of the text.

STUDENT AND INSTRUCTOR RESOURCES

thePoint (http://thepoint.lww.com), a trademark of Wolters Kluwer Health, is a web-based course and content management system providing every resource that instructors and students need in one easy-to-use site. Advanced technology and superior content combine at thePoint to allow instructors to design and deliver online and offline courses, maintain grade and class rosters, and communicate with students. Students can visit thePoint to access supplemental multimedia resources to enhance their learning experience, check the course syllabus, download content, upload assignments, and join an online study group. thePoint . . . where teaching, learning, and technology click!

YOUR INPUT IS WELCOMED

We continue to appreciate the comments and suggestions of colleagues, friends, and students. We encourage you to review this text critically and to advise us of ways in which we can make it better meet classroom needs. We thank the many educators who continue to select *Nursing in Today's World* as the textbook for their class. In this competitive market, we know there are many texts from which to choose. We appreciate your support and strive to bring to you the book that will continue to best meet your needs.

⊕ SPECIAL ACKNOWLEDGMENTS

We are always appreciative of the help and support that we enjoy from the fine staff at Lippincott Williams & Wilkins, particularly that of our editor Helen Kogut and her editorial assistants, who saw us through a series of changes. We have enjoyed working with Tomm Scalera, who is responsible for capturing our concepts in the colorful illustrations. We continue to value and rely on the ongoing support of our respective husbands, Ivan and Gordon, for their encouragement during the development of another edition of the text. Their good humor about all the crises, both small and large, that occur with any project keeps us grounded. We salute them!

Janice Rider Ellis
Celia Love Hartley

Contents

Contents

UNIT I

Economic and Political Aspects of Health Care Delivery

A significant part of the economic and political life of any nation relates to the health care available to its people. The percentage of a country's gross national product devoted to health helps to demonstrate the values of the society and may also serve to point out those areas where problems exist. Another significant economic indicator is how those finances are distributed across the society in the way of establishing priorities, gaining accessibility, and determining decision-making processes. Concerns about who delivers care—their credentials, knowledge and skills, and availability—are other important aspects of the system. Similarly, there is concern about those who have difficulty obtaining health care because they lack insurance or geographic accessibility.

Because of the importance of this topic, the first unit in this text provides you with a basic overview of the health care delivery system in the United States. Beginning with the part of the system with which you are probably most familiar—those settings that employ nurses—the content expands to include some of those that are lesser known and understood. The specific characteristics of these settings—their roles in health care, the roles of nurses in these settings, the colleagues with whom nurses work, and the financial aspects of the health care delivery system are the focus of the first chapter. Because this topic is much too complex to discuss in detail in a single chapter, an overview must suffice. After gaining an understanding of the various players in the system, you should find it easier to analyze specific issues, such as access, finance, power, and control, as they arise.

Second, the unit moves to a discussion of the political process—how it affects nursing and how nurses can affect it. An understanding of how politics affects the health care delivery system can be relevant to your professional experience.

The unit concludes with a discussion of nursing's role in the community. Whatever their individual practice settings, nurses have an impact on the health of their communities. Moving toward the goals of Healthy People 2010 will require a commitment from all those in the system. Included in this chapter is a discussion on complementary and alternative health care and how that affects the health of both individuals and communities.

1

Understanding the Health Care Environment and Its Financing

LEARNING OUTCOMES

After completing this chapter, you should be able to:

1. Identify the various ways of classifying health care agencies and explain how these classification systems differ in their focus.
2. Compare the approach to the client/resident care between acute care hospitals and long-term care facilities.
3. Describe the roles of the various health care providers and analyze how these roles affect the relationships between providers.
4. Analyze how issues related to education, credentialing, and scope of practice of health care occupations affect individual providers and clients within the health care system.
5. Discuss the various approaches to financing and managing costs in the health care delivery system and how the federal government has influenced this process.
6. Discuss the mechanisms being used to measure and ensure quality in organizations and agencies that are delivering health care.
7. Analyze the use of power by regulatory agencies, payers, providers, and consumers in the health care system.
8. Explain continuing concerns regarding the effective use of health care and concerns about changing the system.
9. Analyze how the nurse could use knowledge of the health care system and its financing when teaching clients and planning for continuity of care.

KEY TERMS

Access	Cost containment	Intensity measures
Accreditation	Diagnosis-related groups (DRGs)	Insurance
Acuity	Disease manager	Key indicators
Capitation	Entitlement	Managed care
Case management	Fee-for-service payment	Medicaid
Case mix	Health maintenance	Medicare
Certification	organization (HMO)	Medicare intermediary (carrier)
Clinical pathway	Independent practice	Medigap insurance
Comorbidity	association (IPO)	Minimum data set

Outcome measures	Proprietary	Skilled nursing facility (SNF)
Point-of-service plan	Prospective payment system	Third-party payer
Power	(PPS)	Vertically integrated systems
Preferred provider	Quality indicators (QI)	Walk-in clinic
organization (PPO)	Resource utilization groups	
Primary care provider (PCP)	(RUGs)	

Health care is an exciting and rewarding field but also a challenging one due to the issues that surround it. The entire health care system reverberates with change. The roles of nurses in this system consistently expand and change. You can function more effectively within this system if you understand the various health care agencies and their services, the roles that nurses perform in those agencies, and the colleagues with whom you work.

CLASSIFICATION OF HEALTH CARE AGENCIES

The health care industry is so large, diverse, and complex that it is difficult to understand. Generally, agencies providing care are classified according to length of stay, ownership, or type of service. These classifications are somewhat arbitrary, and any agency may be placed in more than one classification. With the systemic changes that are occurring, one large entity may exist that includes multiple lengths of stay, types of service, and ownership patterns. Therefore, understanding these categories is useful because they are used to plan for services, to describe institutions, and to allocate funding. Your understanding also can be used to guide clients and families through what sometimes seems a maze of confusion in the health care system (Fig. 1-1).

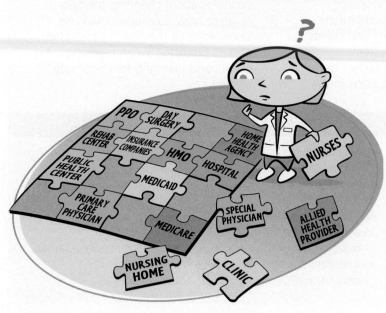

FIGURE 1-1 The many aspects of health care in the United States.

TABLE 1-1	HEALTH CARE INSTITUTIONS CLASSIFIED BY LENGTH OF STAY
LENGTH-OF-STAY	**DESCRIPTION**
In-and-out care	Contact with client is measured in minutes vs. hours. Typical examples are office visits, emergency department visits, and therapy sessions.
Short-stay	Provides care to patients who suffer from acute conditions or require treatments that require less than 24 hours of care and monitoring. Diagnostic tests or minimally invasive surgery are examples.
Acute care	Traditionally occurs in hospitals where patients stay more than 24 hours but less than 30 days. Stays are shortened since the advent of managed care and DRGs.
Long-term care	Provides care to residents for the remainder of their lives; care also includes services to patients with limited recovery needs, functional losses, chronic disease, mental illness, or major rehabilitation, which may range from 30 to 90 days.

Classification According to Length of Stay

One way of classifying inpatient agencies is according to the average *length of stay*, or how long patients remain in the facility. Ambulatory care, short-stay, traditional acute care, and long-term care are terms that reflect the average length of stay in a facility. Table 1-1 outlines the various definitions of care according to length of stay.

Classification According to Ownership

The second method of classifying health care agencies is according to ownership. Agencies may be classified as governmental or public, **proprietary** (private profit-making) or nonprofit. Table 1-2 provides information about the various types of ownership. An important consideration is that all health care agencies, regardless of their ownership, need to have income sufficient to meet the costs of the care provided as well as to maintain and upgrade the equipment and physical facilities that support that care. No agency can continue to exist if it is not adequately funded.

Classification by Type of Care

Health care agencies may also be classified according to *type of care* provided. Many agencies provide more than one type of care. The type of care is based on the **acuity,** the seriousness and rate of change that occurs, of the clients served. Higher acuity signifies that the illness is more

TABLE 1-2	HEALTH CARE INSTITUTIONS CLASSIFIED BY OWNERSHIP
OWNERSHIP	**DESCRIPTION**
Government	Local, county, state, or federal (includes military and veterans facilities)
Nonprofit organization	Religious and philanthropic groups, community organizations
Proprietary corporation	Stockholders own shares and the agency is managed for the benefit of stockholders.
Sole proprietorship	Individual person/family owns and operates the agency

TABLE 1-3	HEALTH CARE INSTITUTIONS CLASSIFIED BY TYPE OF CARE
TYPE OF CARE	**DESCRIPTION**
Acute care inpatient	Illness needing immediate hospitalization and provision of diagnostic tests, treatments, and/or monitoring that require the continuous availability of skilled nursing care. Goals are recovery from illness or injury and restoration to previous level of function.
Long-term acute care	Illness that has stabilized but still needs the ongoing provision of highly skilled care, such as ventilator support or care for major unhealed wounds. Goals are correction of the underlying problem and eventual move to a less skilled level of care.
Subacute care	Care provided after initial recovery from an acute illness needing inpatient care. Skilled care is needed but on a less frequent and intense basis. Goals are to restore function for discharge to home. It is usually provided in a separate unit in an acute care hospital.
Skilled nursing care	Care provided after initial recovery from an acute illness needing inpatient care or following subacute care. Skilled care is still needed but on a less frequent and intense basis. Goals are to restore function for discharge to home. It is usually provided in a nursing home
Custodial care	Care is needed because of functional deficits in activities of daily living rather than due to the illness itself. Care may be provided in an assisted living setting, adult family home (board and care home), or in a nursing home. The goals of care are maintenance of functioning and maximum wellness in the face of disability.
Hospice care	Care provided for the terminally ill in the last 6 months before expected death. May be home care or may be an inpatient hospice. Goals are patient autonomy and relief of symptoms while supporting the patient toward a peaceful death and the family and others in their mourning processes.
Ambulatory care	Care for the person who can come to the health care agency, receive needed health care, and then be discharged to home. It may be a clinic or office. It may also be in hospital departments that provide skilled care for 24 hours or less. Goals are focused on treating a health problem and returning the person to an independent living situation.
Home care	Care providers visit the home to provide some types of care, teach the patient and family how to manage care in the home, and evaluate response to treatment. The goal is effective patient and family self care.

serious and/or changing more rapidly and will demand a greater intensity of services. Other types of care are available to those whose need for services is different. Table 1-3 provides an overview of the different types of care.

Critical Thinking Activity

Recall the last time that you needed health care. Categorize the place where you received care in regard to length of stay, ownership, and type of care provided. Describe those characteristics of the care setting that formed the basis for your decisions regarding classification.

UNDERSTANDING TODAY'S HOSPITAL

The modern hospital is often viewed as the hub or center of the health care delivery system and as central to the health care of a community, although more care is moving into community settings. A primary characteristic of hospital care is its focus on the current problem, rapid assessment, stabilization or treatment, and then discharge to home care or long-term care.

In addition to supplying health care to clients, hospitals also provide education to a wide variety of health care workers and to the community. In many cases, they also serve as centers for research and research dissemination. Hospitals use their status and position in health care to enter into cooperative agreements and alliances with other types of health care providers, insurance companies, and even other hospitals.

The Development of Hospitals in the United States

The history of hospitals in the United States can be traced back to the mid-1700s, when most cities built almshouses, also called poorhouses, at the time. Almshouses provided food and shelter for the homeless poor, and served as homes for the aged, disabled, mentally ill, and orphaned. "Pesthouses" also were built at this time to isolate people with contagious diseases, especially those diseases contracted aboard ship. These facilities housed people suffering from cholera, smallpox, typhus, and yellow fever, and the more common communicable diseases such as scarlet fever. Pesthouses opened and closed as needed.

Neither almshouses nor pesthouses were institutions from which most individuals would want to seek or receive care. They were crowded and unsanitary, with insufficient heat and ventilation. Cross-infection was common, and mortality was high. Those with the financial means were cared for in their homes.

The first **hospital,** founded in what was to become the United States, was started in Philadelphia in 1751, at the urging of Benjamin Franklin. Franklin believed that the public had a duty to provide care to the poor, friendless, sick, and insane. A bill passed that year authorizing the establishment of the Pennsylvania Hospital (Kalisch & Kalisch, 2004). The New York Hospital in New York City was established in 1773, primarily to prevent the spread of infectious diseases brought by sailors and immigrants. Massachusetts General Hospital in Boston opened its doors in 1816, and New Haven Hospital in Connecticut in 1826.

The early hospitals cared for people with acute illnesses and injuries but did not admit the mentally ill. Several separate hospitals were established for this purpose. The first such facility was established as a department of the Pennsylvania Hospital in 1752. The second was founded in Williamsburg, Virginia, in 1773; the third, known as Friends Hospital, was located near Philadelphia in 1817. By 1840, eight hospitals to treat the mentally ill had been established (Kalisch & Kalisch, 2004). The cruel and inhumane treatment of patients in the early mental hospitals is legendary. Dorothea Dix campaigned vigorously for and brought about much reform in the area of mental health treatment. Although never educated as a nurse (she was a schoolteacher), Dix volunteered as a nurse during the Civil War and is included in the Nursing Hall of Fame because of her significant contributions to the profession.

The earliest hospitals left much to be desired. Most were housed in large buildings that had been converted into temporary quarters. Often they were dirty, rank with infection, and poorly ventilated. Linens were used for several patients before being laundered, even though draining, suppurating wounds were common. The stench was overwhelming, and it is said that nurses used snuff to make working conditions more tolerable (Kalisch & Kalisch, 2004). Hospitals constructed during the early 19th century often followed a block plan in their design, and the buildings resembled large barns. In the 1850s, Massachusetts General Hospital constructed a facility divided into wards or pavilions, each one a separate building with high ceilings and good ventilation. The buildings were built of wood because it was believed they would need to be replaced after 20 years because of contamination (Kalisch & Kalisch, 2004, p. 21).

Factors Affecting the Development of Hospitals

Six major forces can be cited as influencing the growth of hospitals throughout the United States. Each played a unique role in the continued development of hospitals and patient care.

Advances in Medical Science

By the end of the colonial period, two medical schools had been established in the United States. Before that time, physicians learned their skills through an apprenticeship with a practicing physician. As medicine became more of a science, advances occurred. One of the most significant was the discovery of anesthesia and the rapid progress in surgery that followed. The germ theory also did much to improve the practice of medicine because it inspired the development of agents or techniques that would sterilize or serve as antiseptics. The growth of hospitals in the United States was a direct result of such progress, which made hospitals safer and more desirable. The discovery of sulfa in the mid-1930s and antibiotics in the mid-1940s heralded even greater changes.

The Development of Medical Technology

The development of specialized medical technology was a natural successor to the advances in medical science. The first hospital laboratory opened in 1889, and x-rays were used in diagnosis in 1896. The electrocardiogram was invented in 1903 and the electroencephalogram in 1929 (Haglund & Dowling, 1993).

Changes in Medical Education

Advances in medical education also had a significant impact on the development of health care in the United States. *The Flexner Report*, a study of medical education, was completed in 1910, and it led to changes in the structure and content of curricula in medical schools. It also expanded the role of hospitals to include education and research and resulted in internships and residencies for medical students.

Growth of the Health Insurance Industry

The growth of the health insurance industry is another factor responsible for the development of hospitals. Although there were some antecedents, most sources indicate that the first hospital insurance plan was initiated at Baylor University Hospital in 1929 to serve the needs of schoolteachers in Dallas, Texas (Raffel, Raffel, & Barsukiewicz, 2001). The approach used there formed the model for Blue Cross plans around the country.

Greater Involvement of the Government

In early times, the government was involved in health care delivery primarily at a local level, building almshouses and facilities for the insane. By 1935, the government was providing grants-in-aid to assist in the establishment of public health and other programs to furnish health assistance to citizens. The Hospital Survey and Construction Act of 1946 (also called the Hill-Burton Act) resulted in the construction of many hospitals and other health facilities. The initiation of **Medicare** (the federal health plan for those on Social Security and their dependents) and **Medicaid** (state health plans for certain low-income individuals paid through a combination of state and federal funds) in 1965 made another significant impact on the health care industry, because the legislation encouraged capital construction and the development of hospitals through the manner in which the system of reimbursement was structured.

The Emergence of Professional Nursing

Another force that significantly influenced the growth of hospitals was the development of professional nursing. Haglund and Dowling (1993, p. 139) cite two ways in which advances in nursing contributed to the growth of hospitals. First, they "increased the efficiency of treatment, cleanliness, nutritious diets, and formal treatment routines" that resulted in patient recovery. Second, they resulted in considerate, skilled patient care that made hospitals acceptable to all people, not just the poor. The role of the nurse and nursing influences the health care delivery system more today than ever before.

Hospital Services for Patients and Families

Two terms used frequently to describe today's modern hospital services are "inpatient care" and "outpatient care." Individuals are termed inpatient when they have been admitted for the purpose of staying 24 hours or longer. The outpatient comes to the hospital for services, but is expected to stay less than 24 hours.

Inpatient units comprise what most people think of when they use the designation "acute care hospital" (Table 1-1). Nurses work in all of these service departments, coordinating the nursing care for individual clients, managing the care environment, delegating and supervising care provided by others, and providing direct skilled care.

In addition to these usual acute care units, hospitals have developed transitional care and rehabilitation units that provide long-term care services, often closing some units and converting them to areas offering these other types of care. A transitional care or rehabilitation unit allows a hospital to discharge an individual from acute, inpatient care in a timely fashion because the next level of services is guaranteed to be available. Reimbursement for the transitional or rehabilitation care is based on long-term care guidelines, and the care must meet long-term care standards for skilled nursing care. Inpatient rehabilitation services may be provided for only a brief period of time, followed by outpatient rehabilitation services.

Many diagnostic and treatment procedures, surgeries, and emergency health needs are treated as outpatient care. The outpatient goes through an admission process, has a procedure performed or care delivered, is determined to be ready for home care, and is discharged. This occurs in less than 24 hours.

The distinction between the categories of inpatient and outpatient is important in regard to both billing and discharge to a nursing home. Both Medicare and Medicaid are billed differently for outpatient care than for inpatient care. Medicare payments for nursing home care after hospitalization require that the person be admitted as an inpatient with a minimum 3-day hospital stay. When these conditions are not met, Medicare payment is denied. Patients and their families may not understand this distinction and how it affects the bills they receive and their eligibility for some types of reimbursement. Nurses must understand that different rules may apply and refer patients and families to appropriate resources for accurate information as they help patients to plan for needed care after discharge.

Hospitals may also be referred to by the mix of traditional inpatient services that are offered (Table 1-4). Not every hospital offers each of the services mentioned earlier, but more are becoming part of a corporate entity that provides all services. The terms most commonly used to describe the mix of services are the "general" or "community" hospital, the "tertiary care" hospital, and the "specialty" hospital.

TABLE 1-4	HOSPITALS CLASSIFIED BY MIX OF SERVICES
TYPE	SERVICES
General or community hospital	Medical, surgical, obstetric, emergency, and diagnostic, plus laboratory services
Tertiary care hospital	Referral centers for clients with complex or unusual health problems such as level 1 trauma, major burns, bone marrow transplant, and research-based oncology, in addition to standard care Part of a large medical center associated with a university. Serves a wide geographic area
Specialty hospital	Offers only a particular type of care (ie, psychiatric, pediatric)

Hospitals may offer a wide variety of other services that are not directed solely at client care. Day procedures and early discharge for inpatient care may present travel difficulties for individuals who live a long distance from a major care center. To facilitate care for these patients and their families, some hospitals have developed hotel-like services, often termed "hospitality units," where the patient scheduled for day surgery may plan to arrive the day before and stay overnight. A family member may also stay in the unit during the individual's hospitalization. After discharge, both the patient and the family member may stay one or more days before traveling home. The cost of staying in a hospitality unit is not covered by insurance, but it is much more convenient than staying in a hotel and typically, the cost is less than in a hotel. Additionally, if an emergency occurs, the patient in a hospitality unit has care immediately available.

Hospitals as Educational Institutions

The education of health care providers is an important function of many hospitals. Although the number of hospital-based schools of nursing offering diplomas has decreased steadily, some are well supported and expect to continue operation. There are also hospital-based programs for respiratory therapy, dietetics, medical laboratory technology, and other health-related occupations.

Many hospitals serve as clinical laboratory sites for individuals enrolled in colleges and universities that provide education for health care professionals. This includes students in nursing, laboratory sciences, nutrition, pharmacy, radiology and imaging, and other disciplines.

Graduate medical education includes all the residency programs for physicians preparing for independent practice. Residents receive a salary from the hospital and are responsible for providing services in return. Residents augment the services of primary physicians, who are often referred to as the attending or staff physicians. Residents often provide the majority of medical services for individuals who are part of the medically underserved in a community, consulting with the staff physician in charge as needed. Part of the funding for graduate medical education comes from money made available through Medicare reimbursement policies.

THE LONG-TERM CARE FACILITY

Long-term care refers to any of the different care settings that involve coordination of the entire multidisciplinary team to provide counseling, nursing care, rehabilitation, nutritional support, social services, and sometimes special education programs over months to years. Managing a positive living environment is as important as managing health problems for long-term care residents. Long-term care facilities include nursing homes, assisted living centers, adult care homes (also called board and care homes), chronic disease hospitals, psychiatric hospitals, and group homes for those with developmental disabilities. The majority of long-term care facilities are nursing homes that care primarily for the elderly.

Nursing Homes

The nursing home is the care facility most often associated with long-term care. Although nursing homes suffer from negative images of the past and not all meet appropriate standards for care, they do offer a far different environment than they did 20 years ago. Nursing homes in the United States provide care and a positive living environment for individuals who have the greatest number of deficits in activities of daily living (ADLs). ADLs include dressing, bathing, eating, toileting, and ambulating. Just as in the acute care hospital, the nursing home is expanding services beyond those traditionally associated with nursing home care. A nursing home that provides skilled care in nursing, physical therapy, and speech therapy is termed a **skilled nursing facility (SNF).**

History of the Nursing Home

Like acute care facilities, the nursing home had a rather harsh beginning. In the 19th century, almshouses sheltered the destitute elderly. These facilities attracted a strange mixture of residents, including those who needed asylum and detention, as well as the poor, the chronically disabled, and the mentally ill. According to the moral perspective that prevailed at the time, poverty and disability were viewed as indications of an undisciplined and wasteful life. A person who was housed in a "county poorhouse" often had no financial resources and no family to provide care and assistance, and endured a certain social stigma. In time, these almshouses became the community dumping grounds for all of society's cast-offs. The early facilities for the country's dependent elderly offered the same grim surroundings as the early hospitals. They were unsanitary, overcrowded, and poorly ventilated. Residents were expected to work to assist with their keep if they were able. Individuals who provided care sought employment there usually as a last resort. Appropriations to manage these facilities were meager because most citizens did not identify with the institutions that housed the poor and the transient, who probably had no history of contributing to the community.

As the United States grew as a society, various groups became concerned about the conditions that existed in the almshouses. Eventually, patients were separated according to their condition, and the mentally and chronically ill were reassigned to different hospitals. An increasing number of churches and fraternal organizations started homes to care for their elderly members. As a result of the Social Security Act of 1935, private (for-profit or proprietary) nursing homes emerged during that decade.

In the postwar period, the Hill-Burton Act of 1946, which supported hospital construction, was expanded to include voluntary (nonprofit) nursing homes, and some states also developed grant programs. Since 1950, government funding for nursing home care has increased steadily and culminated in the 1965 Medicaid program, which by 1991 covered 40% of all nursing home costs (Collopy, Boyle, & Jennings, 1991). Governmental regulation of nursing homes has become increasingly involved and complex.

As changes in funding occurred and as short-term acute care hospitals became increasingly specialized, the role of the nursing home changed. In the 1950s and 1960s, the deinstitutional-ization movement, which saw large numbers of the elderly population discharged from mental hospitals, also affected nursing homes. Nursing homes began to assume the role of providing specialized care for the elderly. By the 1960s, this role was well established, but the nursing home industry was plagued by constant reports of substandard and negligent care and, in some instances, charges of absolute abuse of patients and misuse or embezzlement of their funds. This resulted in even greater scrutiny and regulation by the government.

Today, "nursing home" is a broad term that encompasses a wide spectrum of facilities rang-ing from special units in acute community hospitals to those that are a part of the campus of con-tinuing care retirement centers. Only about 6% have 200 beds or more. The facilities are licensed by the state in which they operate, and each state has its own definitions and requirements. Approximately 85% are certified by Medicare as SNFs (Centers for Disease Control and Pre-vention [CDC], 2002), a necessary qualification if Medicare funds are to pay for the care. Approximately 94% are certified to care for Medicaid patients (CDC, 2002). All facilities receiv-ing federal funds must meet federal as well as state standards. The major reason for admission to a nursing home is functional dependency in terms of basic ADLs and cognitive impairment rather than medical diagnosis.

The Nursing Home Resident

Although most of the elderly live in community settings, many will spend their last years in a nursing home. Approximately two thirds of the residents are women, reflecting the longer life span of women and the greater likelihood that a woman's spouse will precede her in death. The most recent data available from the National Nursing Home Survey (NNHS) indi-cates that the typical nursing home resident of 1999 was less independent and older than the resident of 1977 (CDC, 2002). This may have been due to the increasing number of other options, such as assisted living, for those with greater abilities. Many observers believe that this trend has continued as other types of living environments have become available for those with fewer limitations. Typically, nursing home residents range in age from 65 to older than 100, with an average age of about 84. The NNHSs demonstrate that the age of residents is increasing over time (CDC, 2002.) The NNHS was repeated in 2004, but those data are not yet available.

The number of individuals requiring nursing home care is expected to steadily increase, based on the increasing number of elderly. According to the 2000 census, the number of people ages 80 to 84 increased since the 1990 census by 26%, those 90 to 94 increased by 45%, and those over 100 increased by 35% (U.S. Census Bureau, Statistical Abstract 2004–2005).

Health Services in Nursing Homes

The majority of residents in nursing homes remain there because of major deficits in self-care abilities and the need for ongoing care that is custodial in focus rather than treatment oriented. Maintenance of function, independence, autonomy, and rehabilitation are all goals for nurs-ing home residents. Residents are concerned with the living environment and the health care environment.

Units designed for the cognitively impaired are free of restraints and barriers to mobility. Facility design and alarm systems prevent residents from wandering away. These units provide special approaches to care delivery that decrease stress and reduce the potential for hostile, angry outbursts. Reality orientation is used for those who might benefit from this therapy. Validation therapy and reminiscence also are planned to provide a supportive and rich environment. Staff development assists caregivers in responding appropriately to the special challenges of working with the cognitively impaired.

Some nursing homes have entire wings devoted to individuals receiving post-hospital convalescent care in subacute units where the major focus is rehabilitation. These individuals are admitted with a specific planned stay of 14 to 30 days. During this time, the individual is aided in restoring functional abilities and planning for self or family care. Activities might include physical therapy for the person with a hip replacement or speech therapy after a stroke. The goal is to enable residents to return to independent living in the community. Rehabilitation stays are becoming shorter as reimbursement for inpatient rehabilitation is more restricted to control costs. This trend is expected to continue into the future, as the efforts to contain costs increase (Grabois, 2004).

The level of autonomy expected of nurses employed in nursing homes where physicians visit monthly is often surprising to those who have always worked in acute care hospitals, where physicians visit patients daily and resident physicians are available when needed. In nursing homes, the individual may be a permanent resident and the nurse may be charged with managing both quality of life and quality of care. Additionally, nurses in these settings must manage care conducted by a variety of assistive personnel and work effectively with an interdisciplinary team.

Funding Nursing Home Care

The cost of nursing home care is a concern for many because it often exceeds $5,000 per month, depending on the care needs of the individual and the geographic location of the nursing home. Medicare pays for only a limited number of days for individuals who meet specific criteria regarding hospitalization and who need skilled care or rehabilitation rather than custodial care. Some individuals have long-term care insurance that will pay part of their costs. Although this type of insurance is relatively new, more individuals are purchasing policies, which are available through a number of organizations. The personal financial resources of most individuals may be exhausted by a prolonged nursing home stay. State-administered public assistance in the form of programs such as Medicaid and Medi-Cal (as it is called in California) pays for nursing home care when an individual's personal financial resources have fallen below a certain state-determined level. As the number of elderly individuals requiring nursing home care rise, these costs are becoming a serious budget concern in most states.

Regulation of Nursing Home Care

Nursing homes are among the most regulated of all health care facilities. Because the federal government pays for some of the care, federal regulations affect nursing homes across the country. Starting primarily with the Federal Budget Act of 1987, government regulations mandate specific assessment tools; planning processes; standards of care, including the use of restraints and psychoactive medications; documentation systems used; and evaluation tools. Data are collected according to a standardized minimum data set (MDS). State regulations may place additional requisites on nursing homes. Nursing homes are visited by a survey team that is responsible for ensuring adherence to regulatory standards. The results of nursing home surveys are public documents and must be displayed in each facility in a place accessible to the public and to residents who wish to review them. Nursing home survey results may be seen on the Medicare Web site at *www.medicare.gov/Nhcompare/Home.asp.*

Critical Thinking Activity

Use the Web site *www.medicare.gov/Nhcompare/Home.asp* to investigate a nursing home in your community. Find out its average length of stay, the types of services it offers, and its type of ownership. Analyze the quality of care provided as represented through the nursing home survey. Compare this facility with two other nursing homes in your geographic area.

Assisted-Living Facilities

The **assisted-living facility** provides care for those needing help with up to three ADLs. In an assisted-living arrangement, the resident can maintain maximum independence and use a shared decision-making model to decide when additional help or support is needed. Husbands and wives reside together and may often bring their own furniture and belongings to create a home-like atmosphere. Those who are able to perform any ADLs seek the less costly and more independent and flexible living found here. Assisted-living facilities have been much less regulated than nursing homes. As these facilities admit more impaired individuals, or as individuals living in them want to "age in place," concerns are being raised about the quality of care provided. Increasing regulation is expected. The Joint Commission (formerly known as Joint Commission on Accreditation of Healthcare Organizations [JCAHO]) began a voluntary accrediting process for assisted-living centers (West, 2000).

Care in Assisted-Living Facilities

In an assisted-living facility, all instrumental ADLs such as shopping, cleaning, meal preparation, and laundry are provided. A resident is expected to have some mobility (even though it may require a walker or a cane) and to eat in a dining room except when the person is temporarily ill. Residents also are expected to manage their own medication and health needs, although they may be assisted with remembering to take medications. Assistance is provided with bathing, dressing, and other personal care as needed. Most care is provided by unlicensed assistive personnel. Nurses may be employed in a supervisory capacity and may plan for care. One area of controversy is the level of assistance with medications and health needs that can be provided by unlicensed, unregulated personnel. Some states are authorizing delegation of selected nursing tasks for residents of assisted living, such as giving oral medications, to appropriately trained assistive personnel.

The level of disability that requires a move to a nursing home may vary based on the regulations governing assisted living. In some jurisdictions there is very little regulation, and decisions are made by the agency as to whom they can continue to care for. This sometimes creates difficulties when residents require skilled care and the facility does not have the resources to provide that level of care. For some individuals, the transitions from independent living to assisted living and from assisted living to nursing home care are smooth ones, thus avoiding the transition or relocation stress that affects well-being. This is particularly true when multiple levels of care are available in the same retirement living setting. (See discussion of continuing care retirement communities below.) For others, this change triggers serious stress and is one of the reasons for pressure to allow residents to remain in assisted living settings even when very incapacitated.

Funding Assisted Living

Assisted living is not supported with Medicare funds and therefore does not have to meet the stringent regulatory standards of federal legislation. Public assistance, in the form of Medicaid, Medi-Cal, or other programs, may provide some support for assisted living when the alternative would be expensive nursing home care for which the state would be responsible; however, this is not true in all jurisdictions. Most assisted living is paid for by the individual or family.

Retirement Communities

Retirement communities, which continue to grow, may be self-contained towns, retirement villages, retirement subdivisions, retirement residences, or continuing-care retirement communities. The basic retirement complex is designed to provide the environment for self-care and may support independence longer than would a regular house or apartment. Home care services are provided to those in retirement communities in the same way that they are provided to those in regular homes or apartments.

Continuing care retirement communities provide a variety of levels of independent living and care to residents based on each resident's needs. Most residents enter the community to reside in a retirement apartment or home and then move within the community to an assisted living section and from there to a convalescent or nursing home center if that becomes necessary. Services such as occupational therapy, physical therapy, and dental care also may be available as home care or for those in the convalescent center. The aim is for people to reside in the setting that provides maximum autonomy and independence while ensuring that needs are met. There are data to suggest that residents of continuing care retirement communities maintain better health and require less nursing home care than the general population (Fonda, Clipp, & Maddox, 2002). This may result from living in an environment that supports independence and involvement, or it may be that individuals choosing such a setting are healthier with more resources. A major limiting factor is the cost of such communities to the individual residents.

Rehabilitation Centers

Rehabilitation centers typically focus on a specific health care problem just as rehabilitation units in acute care hospitals do. For example, there are centers for those with spinal cord injuries and other centers focusing on head injuries or cerebral vascular accidents. Although many of these agencies prefer nurses who have taken advanced courses in rehabilitation nursing, many employ nurses with different backgrounds, such as those who have worked in a nursing home focused on rehabilitation principles.

Other Long-Term Care Facilities

Some of the other long-term care facilities available are the group homes for the developmentally disabled and for those with chronic psychiatric illnesses. These smaller residences, most with 12 or fewer residents, strive to create a home-like atmosphere in which individuals can function at their highest capacity. They are often hampered by the lack of stable funding and the difficulty of hiring qualified care providers because of the low wages typically offered.

AMBULATORY CARE SETTINGS

Ambulatory care has long been provided in offices, clinics, and the day-procedure units of hospitals. Some ambulatory care is provided in settings where people work and go to school. Providing care where people routinely spend their days rather than requiring them to go to a different site for health care often results in more effective use of health care services. Some ambulatory care settings rely heavily on the skills of registered nurses (RNs) to provide assessment and teaching, while others focus on medical care provided by physicians, nurse practitioners, and physician assistants with medical assistants for routine tasks.

Physician Offices

One of the major changes in health care has been the decrease in the number of solo practice offices and the growth of group and organizational practices. Many medical practices are owned by health systems that also own hospitals. Within a private-physician practice setting there may be several general practice physicians and many specialists. Advanced practice nurses and physician assistants also are working in many of these group practice settings. Other RNs in these settings may have responsibility for triage, assessment, teaching, and providing direct care. Nursing roles in ambulatory care are expanding as the need for cost-effective use of physician time is modifying practice patterns.

Walk-in Clinics

Walk-in clinics treat clients with emergent conditions that do not require the high-technology resources of the emergency room. Walk-in clinics may be referred to as immediate care facilities, urgent care centers, or emergent care centers and are usually open during extended hours that include evenings and weekends, in addition to the traditional Monday through Friday office hours. Walk-in clinics have grown in popularity as people find it increasingly difficult to gain access to traditional health care settings because of personal time constraints.

Many walk-in clinics have gradually added services such as sports physical examinations for school-age children, pelvic examinations and Pap tests for women, and routine immunizations. Some are beginning to act as primary care providers, advertising the willingness of staff doctors to become family doctors. Walk-in clinics have relatively small nursing staffs, often employing only one RN during a shift; therefore, each nurse must have a wide variety of skills and be able to function with a high degree of autonomy. Some settings do not use RNs in direct care; they are hired in these settings only to supervise other clinic staff members and may oversee more than one facility. Licensed practical nurses (LPNs) may be employed in ambulatory care to collect data, carry out specific treatments, and give medications.

COMMUNITY AGENCIES

Agencies providing care in the community include public health agencies, home care agencies, and home hospice care.

Public Health Agencies

Public health departments are operated as agencies of the government. In general, the focus of health departments has been on broad community issues, communicable diseases, and infant and child health. Public health nurses originally did a great deal of individual family visiting, but today fewer funds are available for visits. As a result, public health nurses now focus on individuals who are high risk and whose health affects the entire community, such as those with tuberculosis. Public health nurses responsible for community health issues are required to have a baccalaureate degree in nursing; however, some agencies operate a variety of clinics (such as immunization clinics) in which RNs with an associate degree or diploma provide teaching and direct care services.

Home Care Agencies

Home care agencies, such as the traditional visiting nurse services and the proprietary home health care companies, provide a broad spectrum of care that may include nursing care, personal care assistance, minor housekeeping, physical therapy, occupational therapy, speech/language therapy, and respiratory therapy for individuals in their homes. Teaching family and caregivers is a large part of the home care professional's responsibility. The focus of home care agencies is broad. It ranges from providing short-term visits for clients who need assistance after a hospital stay or acute illness to assisting clients who will need ongoing home care for years, such as those requiring dialysis or ventilator support in the home. People with these conditions may require nursing care for 8- to 12-hour shifts in the home or episodic visits that last from 15 to 60 minutes.

Hospice Care

The goal of hospice care is to assist the terminally ill individual in living as he or she wishes until death. Hospice care gained momentum as a way to provide maximum quality of life to terminally ill people. Hospice care may be provided in the home with care providers visiting as needed. Some hospices also provide services to individuals living in assisted living or nursing home settings. There are inpatient hospice units for those who do not have family and friends to act as home caregivers or for whom this would be too great a task. Multidisciplinary teams may include physicians, nurses, clergy, occupational and physical therapists, home health aides, social workers, and volunteers. The members of multidisciplinary teams work with both the hospice patient and the family or other caregivers. Nurses provide special skills in symptom management for physical problems, such as pain, nausea, anorexia, and constipation and psychosocial support for end-of-life events and issues. Nurses are usually responsible for the management and coordination of hospice care.

Community Mental Health Centers

Community mental health centers were established to allow individuals with psychiatric problems to remain in their communities and to end the poor care found in large state mental institutions. Services may include individual counseling and therapy, group or family counseling, evaluation, and referral. For those who must be hospitalized, the community mental health center provides follow-up care that facilitates early discharge. These centers usually employ a variety of mental health workers including psychiatrists, clinical psychologists, social workers, marriage and family counselors, psychiatric nurses, and community workers.

Many psychiatric care providers hoped that psychiatric clients who remained in their communities on an outpatient basis, with family and community ties intact, would have more successful treatment outcomes. Another hoped-for advantage of community mental health centers was that people would seek help more readily when it was available in the community. Unfortunately, community mental health centers have not been funded adequately to meet the many and varied needs of individuals with mental health problems. Mentally ill clients often are eligible for care only when they become acutely ill and not for care that can maintain their health. Some people are not eligible for help because of the complex rules and regulations governing funding. Others do not continue with prescribed treatment and experience a relapse; legal constraints do not allow involuntary treatment. Although recognition of the rights of the mentally ill has been important, there also is concern that society expects mentally ill people to make rational decisions about their own best interests when, in fact, they are not mentally capable of understanding the consequences of their actions. The entire area of community mental health has many challenges.

Critical Thinking Activity

Identify an agency in your community that offers home health care. Investigate the services offered by this agency. Compare these with the list of possible services offered by home care agencies mentioned in this chapter. If the lists do not match, analyze the factors in your community that may be responsible for the difference.

Day Care Centers for the Elderly

Elder day care centers provide care for elderly people who cannot safely be alone throughout the day. Each day clients are transported to the center by a family member or a van operated by the center. At the center they receive a variety of social and health services that enable them to continue to live in their own home or a family member's home. Various maintenance and rehabilitative services usually are available, including exercise classes, medication education and supervision, recreational activities, mental health care, and an opportunity to interact with other people. Some centers provide "drop in" or intermittent services for clients who need only one aspect of the program. Other centers provide care each day for clients who need continuing supervision while family members are at work or school. The nursing role in these settings may vary considerably. Some settings have advanced practice nurses who plan care and work with families. Others have RNs who provide medication supervision, assessment for ongoing health problems, and who may lead groups in reminiscence, reality orientation, or validation therapy. LPNs may be hired to give medications and carry out specific treatments.

Ambulatory Care Dialysis Centers

Individuals with chronic renal failure who need ongoing renal dialysis may be managed by home dialysis or by dialysis performed in a dialysis center. A dialysis center provides an environment where the individual who does not have a family care provider or a home dialysis assistant can go two to three times a week for dialysis. Nurses in dialysis centers must have high-level skills, because clients with renal failure who need in-center dialysis usually have the most complex problems and coexisting illnesses. Both LPNs and RNs may be employed in these centers.

COLLEAGUES IN HEALTH CARE

Hundreds of types of health care workers have been identified in the United States. Various providers exist because they all meet the needs of our society in some way. It is not within the scope of this book to discuss each of these occupations individually. Table 1-5 provides an overview of the education and licensure for some of the more common health care providers. The discussion below focuses on some of the issues related to the health care professions.

TABLE 1-5	AN OVERVIEW OF COMMON HEALTH CARE OCCUPATIONS	
OCCUPATION	**EDUCATIONAL REQUIREMENTS**	**ROLE**
Dentistry		
Title: Doctor of Dental Surgery American Dental Association *www.ada.org*	Bachelor's degree followed by 4-year Doctor of Dentistry program Specialty postgraduate programs available	Provide primary care of the teeth and mouth. Prescribe medications related to care of teeth and mouth. Perform some health screening, such as blood pressure monitoring, and examine the mouth and throat for tumors or disease and refer to a physician.
Title: Registered Dental Hygienist American Dental Association	Bachelor's degree or associate degree in dental hygiene.	Provide teaching regarding care of the teeth, clean teeth and apply fluoride and sealants. Take dental x-rays. Perform some health screening such as blood pressure monitoring. In some states have expanded practice to complete simple fillings.
Title: Dental Assistant	Dental assisting vocational program with certificate	Assist the dentist at chair-side. Care for dental equipment and the setting.
Diagnostic Imaging Technology		
Title: Radiologic Technologist American Society of Radiologic Technicians *www.asrt.org*	2-year hospital-based certificate Associate degree or Bachelor's degree in Radiology/Diagnostic Imaging Technology	Perform radiography, radiation therapy, nuclear medicine, sonography, mammography, computed technology, magnetic resonance, dosimetry, and cardiovascular interventional technology.
Title: Sonography Technologist Society of Diagnostic Medical Sonography *www.sdms.org*	1-year certificate programs 2-year associate degree 4-year bachelor's degree	Provide ultrasound technology.
Title: Nuclear Medicine Technologist Society of Nuclear Medicine Technology *www.snm.org*	Post-baccalaureate 1-year certificate programs 2-year associate degree 4-year bachelor's degree	Works with the physician during nuclear medicine procedures.
Nutrition		
Title: Registered Dietitian	Bachelor's degree, plus 6-months to 1-year of internship to become a registered dietitian	Plan for the special dietary needs of client populations. Work with individual clients in planning appropriate diets and teaching nutrition to meet specific needs.

(continued)

TABLE 1-5	AN OVERVIEW OF COMMON HEALTH CARE OCCUPATIONS (*Continued*)

OCCUPATION	EDUCATIONAL REQUIREMENTS	ROLE
Title: Dietetic Technician Registered American Dietetic Association *www.eatright.org*	Associate degree in dietetic technology	Plan menus and adjust diet plans for individuals in institutional settings, under the supervision of the registered dietitian.
Occupational Therapy		
Title: Occupational Therapist Registered	Bachelor's or master's degree in occupational therapy Master's degree required after 2007	Assist the client in restoring fine-motor skills and performing activities of daily living. Perform treatment, including exercise, the making of splints and assistive devices, and identify ways to modify the environment to make the performance of activities of daily living possible.
Title: Occupational Therapy Assistant Assistant American Occupational Therapy Association *www.aota.org*	Associate degree in occupational-therapy assisting	Analyze work environments to determine ergonomic hazards and identify ergonomically sound conditions and practices. Provide diversional activities (such as crafts or games) appropriate to the client's strength, ability, interest, and physical or psychosocial goals. Occupational therapy assistants carry out exercises and treatment plans under the direction of the occupational therapist.
Optometry		
Title: Doctor of Optometry American Optometric Association *www.aoanet.org*	Bachelor's degree, followed by 4 years of optometry school	Examine vision and prescribe eyeglasses and contact lenses, low-vision aids, and vision therapy. Examine, diagnose, treat, and manage diseases and disorders of the visual system, the eyes and associated structures, as well as diagnose-related systemic conditions in states with an expanded scope of practice.
Pharmacy		
Title: Registered Pharmacist American Pharmaceutical Association *www.aphanet.org*	Previously: Bachelor's degree in pharmacy Requirement beginning 2001: Bachelor's degree in science followed by Pharmacy Doctorate program	Dispense drugs, manage drug therapy, consult with physicians, recommend therapy, assist with monitoring therapy, provide consultation for nurses, and teach clients. Perform clinical work in a hospital or other patient care setting.
Title: Pharmacy Assistant	In most states: Associate degree in pharmacy. Some states may allow a certificate program of less than associate degree.	Dispense drugs and manage pharmacy inventory under the direction of a pharmacist.

TABLE 1-5	AN OVERVIEW OF COMMON HEALTH CARE OCCUPATIONS (*Continued*)	
OCCUPATION	**EDUCATIONAL REQUIREMENTS**	**ROLE**
Physical Therapy		
Title: Registered Physical Therapist	Bachelor's degree in any field with specified prerequisites, followed by Master's degree program in physical therapy or doctoral program in physical therapy	Restore normal function of large muscle groups, bones, and joints and perform treatments, including exercise, heat and cold therapy, electrical stimulation, and the use of other physical agents. Teach the client to use crutches, prostheses, and other assistive devices. Also teach individuals about safe exercise, provide direction for exercise fitness, and help individuals with health problems to gain maximum function.
Title: Physical Therapist Assistant American Physical Therapy Association *www.apta.org*	Associate degree in applied science	Carry out treatment plan under direction of physical therapist.
Physician		
Title: Medical Doctor *www.ama.org*	Bachelor's degree followed by 4-year medical school, followed by 1–4 years of medical residency	Diagnose and treat disease, including prescribing medications, providing treatment, and performing surgery; plan and order all diagnostic tests and procedures; refer for therapies by other health care providers; and manage admission and discharge to any health care facility.
Title: Doctor of Osteopathy *www.aoa-net.org*	Bachelor's degree followed by 4-year medical school, followed by 1–4 years of medical residency	Diagnose and treat disease, including prescribing medications, providing treatment, and performing surgery. Plan and order all diagnostic tests and procedures. Refer for therapies by other health care providers. Manage admission and discharge to any health care facility.
Podiatry		
Title: Doctor of Podiatric Medicine American Podiatric Medicine Association *www.apma.org*	Bachelor's degree followed by a 4-year doctor of podiatry medicine program. Two thirds of the states require an additional year of podiatry residency before licensure to practice is allowed.	Care for corns, bunions, and toenails; prescribe and fit corrective shoes and arch supports; perform surgery on the feet, such as correcting deformities and removing bunions and small tumors; and treat wounds of the feet.
Respiratory Therapy		
Title: Registered Respiratory Therapist	Associate degree or baccalaureate degree in respiratory therapy	Provide direct care related to respiratory treatments and the use of respiratory devices, give inhaled medications, and provide client teaching related to respiratory care procedures

(continued)

TABLE 1-5	AN OVERVIEW OF COMMON HEALTH CARE OCCUPATIONS (*Continued*)	
OCCUPATION	**EDUCATIONAL REQUIREMENTS**	**ROLE**
Speech, Language, Hearing Therapy		
Titles: Registered Speech/ Language Pathologist	Bachelor's degree followed by Master's degree in speech/language pathology	Assess and plan treatment for rehabilitation needs in speech and language function and swallowing difficulties, and serve as a consultant to health care team regarding communication strategies and methods to support swallowing.
Title: Speech/Language Pathology Assistant	Associate degree in speech/language pathology	Work with clients to carry out treatment plans and provide speech/ language treatment under the direction of the registered speech/language pathologist.
Title: Audiologist American Speech, Language, and Hearing Association *www.asha.org*	Master's degree in audiology or doctoral degree in audiology	Measure hearing ability; identify hearing disorders; provide rehabilitative services; assess amplification devices and instruct in their care; provide training in speech and reading; and serve as consultants to the education system, the government, and the industry on issues concerning environmental, noise-induced hearing loss.

Roles of Health Care Workers

With the many types of health care workers, some concerns center on how those roles are defined, how education or training is provided, and how the role is regulated. Although the major health occupations provide academic education with legal licensure and a defined scope of practice, many of the allied health workers have much less defined roles. For some health care occupations there are differences in regulations and requirements from state to state. One of the major Pew Reports in the 1990s focused on the need for a more clearly described and uniform regulation of health care professionals across the country (O'Neil, 1993). Unfortunately, there are no data to demonstrate this happening across the various health care professions. This served as added support for the efforts of the National Council of State Boards of Nursing to systematize expectations for both entry level and APNs (advanced practice nurses). While there has been standardization for entry-level RNs for many years, there is still great variation in requirements and in scope of practice for APNs from state to state. National organizations that provide **accreditation** for allied health educational programs serve to provide standardization of some occupations (Display 1-1).

With a shortage of licensed health care workers in areas such as nursing and laboratory sciences, some employers are advocating for short-term training of unlicensed assistive personnel. When shortages of professionals exist, these unlicensed individuals may be used beyond their knowledge and skills.

Even within professions, increasing specialization has sometimes created conflict over expertise and territory (Figure 1-2). Pressure from insurers has mandated a decreased use of specialty physicians and mandated that more care be delivered by the general practice physician. In some

Display 1-1   Organizations Providing Allied Health Accreditation

1. Accreditation Council for Occupational Therapy Education
2. Commission on Accreditation of Allied Health Education Programs (CAAHEP has 17 separate committees on accreditation; each focuses on a different allied health area.)
3. Joint Review Committee on Educational Programs in Nuclear Medicine Technology
4. Joint Review Committee on Education in Radiologic Technology
5. National Accrediting Agency for Clinical Laboratory Sciences

states, clinical psychologists may now obtain authority to prescribe medications, a treatment modality formerly limited to physicians and certain APNs. This eliminates the need for referral to another mental health care provider solely for the prescription of medications to treat psychiatric conditions. Psychiatrists feel that this change decreases the access of clients to the most highly educated person. When nurse anesthetists can be reimbursed independently, more facilities hire those nurse specialists, which decreases the demand for anesthesiologists. Even within hospital units, some facilities eliminated positions for clinical nurse specialists who were prepared at the master's degree level and assigned their duties to less-well-prepared nurses. Those with greater education argue that the patient loses when the provider has a lesser background. The education, regulation, and use of all health care workers will continue to be an issue in the coming years.

Access to Primary Health Care

The health care provider contacted initially by clients who seek health care is considered a **primary care provider (PCP).** The primary health care provider furnishes entry into the health care system. Today the federal government considers general practitioners, family practice specialists,

FIGURE 1-2 Overlapping roles and unclear boundaries between health care occupations can lead to conflict.

pediatricians, internal medicine specialists, obstetricians, physician assistants, and nurse practitioners to be PCPs. The PCP is the mainstay of basic care for most individuals.

All states require licensure of physicians, nurse practitioners, and other providers who are authorized to treat illness and prescribe drugs. The cornerstone of many managed health care plans is an emphasis on the primary health care provider as the gatekeeper for the system. The primary provider implements health maintenance activities that prevent the need for more expensive care. This individual provides referral to more specialized care when it is needed and must often receive permission for referral or for items of higher cost. The belief has been that this would prevent health care consumers from needless focus on higher cost diagnostic tests and specialists. One large managed care company (Aetna) announced in 2001 that beginning in 2002 it would remove this requirement (Coile, 2001). It had identified that there was no significant change in the use of specialists or diagnostic tests with required prior approval for referral and that there was a significant cost to the extensive record-keeping and management necessary to document that this requirement was met.

Lack of access to primary care has been one of the health care problems for individuals residing in rural areas, economically disadvantaged areas in large cities, and those on welfare programs. Often it has resulted in delaying care until the problem is more complex and requires greater resources to resolve. In urban areas, the lack of access to primary care has often resulted in the inappropriate use of emergency room services for routine illnesses. To meet the needs of society, there is pressure to increase the number of professionals who are authorized to deliver primary care.

Interdisciplinary Teamwork

As the health care system grows more complex, it is clear that it is impossible for one individual, educated to a specific role, to manage all aspects of care. This has led to an increasing emphasis on collaborative work that will provide the benefits available through the expertise of different professions. Interdisciplinary teamwork has always been part of hospice care—physicians, nurses, social workers, therapists, home health aides, and pastoral staff all bring their unique insights to the client's care. The current regulations for long-term care require that there be interdisciplinary collaboration in planning for resident care.

In 1995 in a report titled *Critical Challenges: Revitalizing the Health Professions for the Twenty-first Century,* the Pew Health Commission emphasized the importance of interdisciplinary care. Its report further focused on the need for students in health profession programs to begin working in interdisciplinary teams while still students to move effectively into this mode as practitioners. Many nursing programs responded to the Pew report by developing increased opportunities for nursing students to be involved in interdisciplinary health care. Other efforts to act on this recommendation regarding interdisciplinary care came through accreditation. The National League for Nursing Accreditation Commission (NLNAC) standards and criteria for accreditation include the expectation that interdisciplinary functioning will be a part of any nursing program (NLNAC, 2005).

Health Care Worker Supply

There is a short supply of qualified individuals in health occupations such as nursing (National Center for Health Workforce Analysis, 2002) and pharmacy (National Center for Health Workforce Analysis, 2000). There are also geographic shortages, with inner cities and rural areas

FIGURE 1-3 The aging of the nursing workforce will affect the supply of nurses.

experiencing the greatest deficit. Within nursing, the aging work force is contributing to the shortage (Fig. 1-3). Another type of shortage is in regard to the ethnic background of some patient populations (National Center for Health Workforce Analysis, 2004). This poses special difficulties for both the client and the care provider when the two are unable to communicate effectively. To better meet the needs of all clients, many programs have been instituted that strive to increase diversity among health care providers. As the health care work force changes, some clients must alter their perspectives to adapt to a wider diversity in health care providers.

PAYING FOR HEALTH CARE

Throughout the world, the concern over health care has everyone's attention. In most of the industrialized world, with the exception of the United States, health care is seen as a right, or an **entitlement,** of every citizen. Based on this right, health care in most industrialized countries is operated by government systems that provide universal health care coverage. In some countries, such as Sweden (see *www.sweden.se/templates/cs/Print_BasicFactsheet____6856.aspx*) and the Netherlands (see *www.minbuza.nl/default.asp?CMS_ITEM=MBZ426386*), there is strong centralization of financing and control. In other countries, such as Canada (see *www.canadian-healthcare.org*) and Germany (see *www.nchc.org/facts/Germany.pdf*), systems are controlled regionally through provincial authority. These governmental systems are successful in accomplishing overall health outcomes such as low maternal–infant mortality, high immunization rates, and reduction of preventable deaths. The problems found in these systems are related to the high cost of providing health care and subsequent attempts to control those costs. The delay before receiving care may be long, and some care, especially care that is very costly such as dialysis, may be rationed. Because of these situations, private medical care that is paid for by individuals also may be available to those with sufficient income.

In developing nations, health care may be limited or almost nonexistent. Some care may be paid for by the government and some by private means, but there are not enough individual or institutional providers to meet the needs of the population. The available resources may not meet the standards that those in more affluent countries have come to expect. Hospitals may lack adequate safe water and sanitation. Ordinary supplies such as dressing materials and sterile needles may be unavailable. Drugs may be in short supply, and diagnostic and laboratory testing may be nonexistent. Health care outcomes in these countries tend to be poor, especially regarding infant and child mortality. The World Health Organization is most active in these developing nations, trying to improve health outcomes through immunization, sanitation, and other public health programs.

In the United States, health care has not been accepted as a right for the whole society. Therefore, no mechanism exists to build a coordinated health care system. Much of the complexity found in the U.S. health care system relates to the variety of mechanisms for funding and controlling health care. Although the United States has ready access to the most sophisticated medical technology and expertise, deficiencies are seen in some of the key measures of population health. Some individuals have access to the most effective health care in the world, while others have no health care access except in cases of emergency, when hospitals are required by law to provide care.

Financing Health Care for Individuals

Currently, there are many different approaches to financing health care for individuals in the United States. Personal payment, charitable care, **insurance** plans, **health maintenance organizations (HMOs),** and a variety of government programs are all forms of health care financing. Agencies such as insurance companies and government programs that pay providers for health services provided to individuals are termed **third-party payers** (Display 1-2). Increasingly, decisions about an individual's health care are made by a combination of the patient-consumer, the provider, and the payer, rather than by any one of them alone.

Personal Payment

Originally, health care was paid for each time it was provided. Although the payment was usually in cash, in a more rural society payment sometimes extended to barter, with garden produce, chickens, and eggs traded for medical care. Individuals who did not have the means to pay for a doctor or hospital visit often did not receive needed care.

Today most individuals still pay for health care but often in indirect ways that make them less aware of the specific costs. Health insurance premiums may be deducted from a paycheck,

---

Display 1-2   Approaches to Financing Health Care

- Personal payment
- Charitable care
- Health insurance plans
- Health maintenance organizations
- State-administered health plans
- Federal government programs

or an employer may pay premiums directly, considering them part of employee compensation. Most health insurance plans require the subscriber to pay a deductible (a portion of the bill), which may be computed for each service or may be an aggregate for the year. The size of the deductible that is the individual's responsibility is increasing in many insurance plans, giving people greater incentive to use services wisely.

Charitable Care

Charitable care has played a significant role in the history of health care. The earliest hospitals were religious institutions that provided health care as a form of ministry and as a charitable service. Some large charitable groups, such as the Shriner's Children's Hospitals, still provide a great deal of care for people who are unable to pay. Although these hospitals do collect insurance and payment from those who can afford care, they also raise money for the purpose of providing high-level care to children in need.

In 1946, federal funds were made available through the Hill-Burton Act for hospital construction. Hospitals constructed with these funds accepted an obligation to provide some charitable care in their communities. As these obligations expired, concern about what was happening in emergency care led to legislation that requires hospitals to provide emergency care regardless of an individual's ability to pay.

Historically, some money for charitable care was raised through donations. As insurance became more widespread, hospitals often supported charitable care by charging paying clients more than the cost of their care and using the excess income to offset the costs of charitable care. However, as negotiations for lower health care costs for managed care continue and regulations have limited Medicare reimbursement, hospitals are experiencing a decreased ability to provide charitable care without severe financial difficulties. (Medicare is discussed more fully later in this chapter.)

Individual physicians also have provided forms of charitable care. Only rarely did people directly ask physicians for charitable care; rather, the physician sometimes did not pursue the payment of a bill that could not be paid by a family. Physicians and other care providers also have provided charitable care by volunteering their time at free clinics.

Health Insurance Plans

Starting in the 1930s through the 1970s, insurance companies gradually began to pay a larger share of medical fees. The basic framework of insurance coverage is that of shared risk of having high-cost health care needs. Individuals pay for coverage whether or not they incur health care costs; when an insured individual requires health care, the insurance pays for that care. Thus the individual has a stable health care cost without the risk of incurring high costs that are difficult to meet from ordinary income, and the insurance company stays financially solvent because more money is coming in than is going out.

Historically, health insurance was for hospital care and related services only. Outpatient visits, immunizations, costs of drugs, and other such benefits were not covered by insurance policies. One disadvantage of this system was that consumers had no incentive to reduce their use of services; they paid the same regardless of their needs or use of the system. People sought to have care delivered on an inpatient basis to obtain reimbursement. Another disadvantage was that individuals often neglected preventive health care that had to be paid for out-of-pocket. Health insurance policies now cover many preventive services, outpatient costs, and some prescription costs.

At the heart of the process of setting insurance rates and specifying coverage is identifying what will be covered, determining the risk (probability) of health services being needed for different groups of individuals, and projecting the costs of care. It has been found that the more heterogeneous the group, the more likely that the average cost for those in the plan will mirror the population average, thereby keeping insurance costs reasonable for all. Limitations on coverage that eliminate individuals with high probability of needing services (such as the elderly diabetic) protect insurance companies from the risk of excessive costs. When high-risk individuals are excluded from insurance, it lessens the cost for low-risk subscribers within the plan, but leaves those who are most in need of assistance without the benefit of insurance.

Most insurance companies are private profit-making companies owned by stockholders. They provide service to policyholders in return for insurance payments and create profit for stockholders in the company. Aetna is an example of a nationwide for-profit insurance company that primarily provides plans for employers to offer to groups of employees.

Nonprofit insurance companies are established within different legal regulations. They are owned collectively by those who hold insurance policies. All profits from the company are theoretically used to enhance the company or to decrease the cost of the insurance. Additionally, the nonprofit companies have certain benefits in terms of taxes. The "Blues" (Blue Cross and Blue Shield companies) originally were established as not-for-profit organizations.

Legal regulations place restrictions on the rate setting, investments, and general management of nonprofit companies that do not apply to private profit-making companies. This has limited their ability to grow in size and compete for some types of business. In some areas of the country, Blue Cross and Blue Shield have asked regulatory authorities for permission to convert from nonprofit to profit-making status and to sell stock in the company (and have changed their names in the process). In some states, courts have required that these corporations provide remuneration to their communities in return for this change in status. In other states, these changes have occurred without public input.

As the cost of health care has increased, insurance premiums also have increased greatly. An additional public concern is that health insurance is unobtainable for individuals with existing health problems and often economically beyond the means of those who are not insured as part of an employee group. Legislation to require insurance companies to cover everyone has passed in some jurisdictions and is being considered in others. One of the responses by insurance companies to this legislation is to withdraw from selling insurance in the state that requires insurance companies to insure anyone who seeks coverage. The insurance companies argue that individuals do not carry insurance when they are well; when faced with illness, they purchase insurance, receive reimbursement far in excess of any premiums paid, and then drop coverage when they are well.

Although insurance companies originally focused on paying for health care, they now are involved in establishing standards for care, evaluating care, and negotiating charges. They are active participants in all areas of health care and, because of the economic power they wield, have great influence. Insurance companies determine whom they will pay and what procedures they will reimburse. Thus, insurance companies can and do limit health care choices.

All insurance plans have written rules regarding notification, acceptable providers, and precisely when and how reimbursement will occur. Sometimes these rules result in a denial of payment. Many people have expressed concern about the process of reviewing and denying insurance claims (Fig. 1-4). Realistically, the foremost goal of most health insurance plans is to return

FIGURE 1-4   Health care insurance plans are complex and often confusing to the ordinary consumer.

a profit to investors. Providing good health care to an individual is a means to that end and not the focus of effort.

Federal legislation, the Health Insurance Portability and Accountability Act (HIPAA), was passed in 1996. Title 1 of the Act focuses on measures that assist in maintaining health care insurance coverage for those who change or lose their jobs (see *http://aspe.hhs.gov/admn-simp/pl104191.htm* for the full text of the Act). The Centers for Medicare & Medicaid Services (CMS) maintains a Web site (*http://cms.hhs.gov/hipaa*) with consumer information regarding the protections provided by this federal legislation to allow people to maintain coverage when they change jobs. This legislation also has provided tax incentives for those purchasing long-term care insurance. The HIPAA legislation had additional provisions regarding patient health records' privacy that will be discussed in Chapter 8.

Health Maintenance Organizations

HMOs originated as an alternative to traditional insurance plans and were nonprofit in nature. Although traditional insurance plans paid for care when subscribers were ill, HMOs were the first to provide payment for care aimed at preventing illness. HMOs provided well-child care, prenatal care, immunizations, gynecologic examinations, and other preventive services when insurance companies did not.

Because the HMO receives the same income (except for modest co-payments) whether a client requires extensive care or very little care, there is a built-in incentive to emphasize preventive care and avoid costly hospitalization. A flat charge per month covers routine preventive health care; care for illness; hospitalization and, in some instances, prescription costs; outpatient care; and other services. HMO-enrolled individuals are often responsible for a co-payment (meaning the client pays a part of the bill). Co-payments support part of the cost of care and give the consumer an incentive to use services wisely.

HMOs are currently characterized by many differing patterns of finance and governance. Some are operated by insurance companies; some are private profit-making organizations; some are nonprofit organizations; and still others are consumer owned and operated. Many newer HMOs operate as business entities that manage the financial aspects of health care and, through financial management, access to services.

HMOs also are characterized by differing patterns of providing health services. Primary health care providers may be employed by an HMO and receive a fixed salary. In some cases, a group of primary health care providers, termed an **independent practice association,** may contract with an HMO to provide services for a preset fee per individual in the program. HMOs also may employ many other health care workers, including nurses. In some HMOs, clients have a choice of care providers; in others they do not. HMO plans that allow an individual the option of going outside of the plan for services that the plan does not or will not provide are called **point-of-service plans.** Usually the subscriber is eligible for some reimbursement of costs for these outside services, but by a greatly reduced amount.

HMOs were the first type of health plan to provide managed care. **Managed care** refers to any system for "financing and organizing the delivery of health care in which costs are contained by controlling the provision of services" (Taber's, 2005). The concept of managed care has broadened considerably and now includes many types of health plans. Managed care is discussed in detail later in this chapter.

In existence in the United States for more than 50 years, the growth of HMOs was slow until federal legislation in 1972 and 1974 created economic incentives to start new HMOs. Because HMOs traditionally had lower health care costs than conventional fee-for-service systems, the federal government subsidized the creation of new HMOs and encouraged employers to offer HMOs as alternatives to traditional health insurance plans. Federal subsidizing of HMOs also helps to contain costs in all health plans as a result of competition.

People on Medicare also have the option of joining HMOs. Under such circumstances, the person joins the HMO and pays a monthly fee similar to the cost of a supplemental health insurance (Medigap) policy. The individual makes a single payment for each individual Medicare recipient directly to the HMO, and the HMO provides all care. The amount per individual was calculated as an average of the expenses incurred by Medicare recipients for all costs. The original Medicare HMOs advertised "no co-pays" and "full prescription coverage" to attract new members. The HMO is expected to provide this through carefully managed care that would decrease the use of costly services. However, most HMOs in operation today have a co-payment fee and assess some charges for prescriptions.

Beginning in 1998, a crisis occurred in Medicare HMOs. Many plans found that overall costs were greater than anticipated. The savings managed care had successfully demonstrated when caring for a broad range of ages did not materialize when they were working with the older population who tend to have more chronic illnesses and more serious health problems. They could not sustain all the promised benefits within the Medicare payments. These HMOs refused to renew their contracts to provide Medicare-HMO services. This left many elderly individuals with difficult choices to make as they returned to conventional Medicare plus Medigap Supplemental Insurance. Most conventional plans did not provide outpatient pharmacy coverage, thus greatly increasing the costs of health management for the individual. Some HMOs continued coverage with prescription drugs included by increasing rates. Beginning January 2006, Medicare provided an additional Part D for coverage of prescription drugs (to be discussed). The premium for this may be added to the premium for the Medigap policy or HMO contract.

State-Administered Health Plans

States may operate a variety of health care resources for residents. All states manage some type of insurance plan for workers injured on the job. These workers' compensation plans may be managed as a state monopoly or contracted to private insurance companies. Employers are required to pay premiums based on statistical information about covered injuries and hazards in various job categories. An individual injured on the job is assured of receiving care paid for by the workers' compensation plan.

Some states administer health insurance plans on a wider basis. Hawaii ensures universal health care coverage for its residents. Minnesota was a leader in attempting to provide health services for all its residents. The state of Washington developed an insurance plan called the Basic Health Plan for working individuals who earn too much money to be eligible for tax-supported health care, but who do not have incomes high enough to afford regular insurance. Unfortunately, this plan, like many other state plans that are subsidized by tax revenue, cannot accommodate all who are eligible. States with health plans are facing rapidly increasing costs and an inability to cover all those who do not have health plans through their employment. In many states this has become a crisis (Kaiser Family Foundation, 2005).

The federal government also provides funds through the Medicaid programs that are administered by the states and matched with state funds. The costs of health care for families on public assistance and support of nursing home care for those who have exhausted their personal financial resources are included in this funding. In 1999 the federal government provided a mechanism for states to enlarge their Medicaid programs so they could enroll children from low-income families who did not qualify for Medicaid and who would otherwise be without health care coverage. This Children's Health Insurance Plan represents the first time that the United States has supported health care as a right for all children. Not all states have agreed to participate in the plan because it requires their financial contribution and provides for some federal control of the program.

Most states support state mental hospitals and public health services. Additional public health services may be supplied through county and city governments. Hospitals designed to provide care for those who are indigent may be operated by the city (such as New York City hospitals) or by the county (such as Cook County Hospital in Chicago).

Federal Government Programs

The federal government in the United States is deeply involved in health care financing. Federal programs cover the elderly, the poor, federal workers, the military, veterans, and Native Americans and Native Alaskans. Some individuals are concerned about government involvement in our health care system. When all of these programs and agencies are considered together, it is clear that, for good or ill, the federal government already controls many aspects of health care.

Medicare and Medicaid. In 1965, after years of effort and testimony by many health-related groups (including the American Nurses Association [ANA]), and with widespread public support, an amendment to the Social Security Act was passed. Title XVIII of the Act, which was termed Medicare, provided payment for hospitalization (Part A) and insurance that could be purchased to meet physicians' fees and outpatient costs (Part B) for people over age 65 and certain others who were receiving Social Security payments. In 2004, Medicare Part D, which covers prescription drugs was approved; it took effect in 2006.

Participation in Medicare Part A is automatic for those on Social Security, whereas participation in Medicare Part B is optional and a premium is deducted from the Social Security check to pay for Part B. Medicare Part A pays only for acute hospitalization and a limited amount of rehabilitative care that may occur in a nursing home. Medicare does not pay for any long-term or custodial care in a nursing home. Part B reimburses for physician care and outpatient services based on a fixed schedule of payments. Medicare is administered through CMS (center for medicare/medicaid services), formerly called the Health Care Financing Administration, which uses contracted insurance companies termed **Medicare carriers** or **Medicare intermediaries** to process claims (*www.cms.gov*). Payments from Medicare do not cover the entire cost of the care provided. The amount authorized is determined by CMS. Medicare then pays a fixed percentage of that authorized amount. The individual pays the remaining percentage of the authorized amount. If the provider charges more than the authorized amount, that portion of the fee is not recoverable from either Medicare or from the patient. Many individuals who receive Medicare also pay for supplemental insurance to cover the part of the health care bill for which Medicare Parts A and B do not pay. This is commonly referred to as "Medigap" insurance and is available from many different insurance companies, such as Blue Cross and Blue Shield.

The newest part of Medicare, Plan D for prescription drug coverage, is administered through insurance plans and requires the payment of an insurance premium that may be subsidized for low-income individuals. The cost of prescriptions under Part D is subsidized by Medicare by payments to the insurance company. The drug plan will pay part of a person's drug costs up to approximately $2,600. Then there is no coverage until the person enters the category of costs over $3,600 per year. When this amount is reached, the plan usually will pay 90% of costs. Plans differ in cost and have different benefits and requirements, such as co-pays, deductibles, coverage of different generic and brand name drugs, and additional coverage in the "gap" or "doughnut hole" (that area of costs between $2,600 and $3,600) that is built into the general plan. Each plan is free to establish its own formulary of drugs that are covered and may change that formulary once a month. Participants must investigate each plan to determine whether the drugs they currently take are covered. If new drugs are prescribed, the provider will need to check on the plan to learn what therapeutic equivalent drugs may be covered by that particular plan. Participants may change plans once each year. Individuals who belong to Medicare managed care plans have their Part D integrated into that plan. The prediction is that these drug plans will significantly increase the cost of Medicare. Details are available on the CMS Web site at *www.medicare.gov/medicarereform/drugbenefit.asp*.

Title IX of the Social Security Act, which was termed Medicaid, provides funds for health care for those dependent on public assistance and certain other low-income individuals. Costs for Medicaid are shared between the federal government and each state. Very low-income individuals who are eligible for Medicare may be covered by Medicaid in the same way that those who can pay are covered by Medigap policies. This often is referred to as being "dual-eligible." Each state is responsible for administering Medicaid: The state determines eligibility and level of coverage. Payments from the federal government to the states are administered by CMS. Benefits vary greatly among states. California's plan, called Medi-Cal, historically has been one of the most comprehensive. As health care costs rise, there has been great pressure to cut this program. To avoid federal control, a few states have not participated in the Medicaid program. Some states, such as Oregon, have requested waivers from CMS's usual regulations governing Medicaid to allow experimentation with different plans that might help to control costs.

The complexity of filing claims with Medicare and also with an insurance company designed to supplement Medicare coverage (the Medigap policy) is problematic for many people because the insurance company will not pay until Medicare has determined coverage and paid its share. If there are many different health claims, the sending and receiving of the various claims requires careful record keeping. Even when claims are filed by the provider, they may be denied payment if they do not conform to specific rules and regulations. Often elderly people accept an initial denial of payment for the claim as the final decision and do not pursue the matter further. There is a high rate of reconsideration when denials are appealed; therefore, it is often wise to encourage clients to appeal a denial of payment.

Medicare and Medicaid are important health care resources, but they have not been without problems. Costs have been much greater and have been rising faster than anticipated. There has been a great deal of publicity about instances of abuse, and even fraud, associated with these two programs. The goals of providing cost-effective health care to the elderly and the indigent through these programs have yet to be achieved.

The Medicare bill contains many provisions that have made a significant impact on nursing. The definition of skilled nursing care in the original bill was narrow and excluded many important aspects of care necessary to maintaining the health of clients. Through later efforts and testimony, nursing organizations were instrumental in convincing legislators to recognize that the definition of skilled nursing was critical. As a result, a Senate subcommittee asked the ANA to study skilled nursing care to provide background data for the Senate. Amendments to the Medicare/Medicaid Act of 1972 encouraged study of alternative ways of providing health care to contain costs. These alternatives included the use of nurses in expanded roles and the use of HMOs.

Amendments to the Medicare/Medicaid Act were also responsible for mandating review and evaluation of health care. This was done in the interests of cost control or containment. Institutions must review records of Medicare/Medicaid clients and compare them with specific criteria for care. Many insurance companies have followed this pattern and required review and evaluation of care of their clients.

In 1982, the 97th Congress revised Medicare to prevent the serious financial deficits in the system that escalating costs could potentially create. The revisions increased the premium for Part B of Medicare (the optional portion that provides for out-of-hospital and physician care) and also increased the deductible that the individual must pay for covered service. The system of payment was changed to prospective payment based on diagnosis-related groups (DRGs). The planners who revised Medicare also included a new mechanism for reimbursing hospice care.

In 1993, more changes, restrictions, and controls were instituted in the Medicare system: the payroll deduction for Medicare (paid by all employed individuals regardless of income level or age) was increased; the length of stay was shortened; and rehabilitation and convalescent services moved from acute care environments to newly created subacute units in long-term care facilities and in hospitals. Many procedures that previously required an inpatient stay became outpatient services.

The growing number of elderly; the rising costs of medications, supplies, and wages; and the widespread use of costly, highly technical diagnostic tools and therapies all have contributed to escalating health care costs. As the baby boom generation moves into retirement years, this will further strain the financial resources of the system. Despite these concerns, Medicare and Medicaid have provided health care dollars and services to many people who would otherwise have done without.

Critical Thinking Activity

What changes are occurring in the health care systems in your community? Are some hospitals growing or merging? Are some facilities changing their focus? Have any health care providers had economic difficulties or even closed? Have new providers established facilities? Analyze how these changes may affect nursing practice.

Military Health Care. The military branches of the Defense Department operate hospitals and clinics and also finance health care through civilian health providers in an extensive program known as TRICARE (*www.tricare.osd.mil*). This program has three options for those under age 65. TRICARE Prime is a managed care plan (the required plan for active duty military personnel), TRICARE Extra is a preferred provider plan, and TRICARE Standard is a fee-for-service option that costs the individual more but allows for greater choices. TRICARE for Life is a program coordinated with Medicare for retired military personnel and their dependents.

Other Federal Health Care Programs. The U.S. Department of Health and Human Services (DHHS) provides direct health care services to identified underserved populations. Through the Health Resources and Services Administration, it provides community and migrant health centers and primary care programs for the homeless and residents of public housing (DHHS, 2004). Another agency, the Indian Health Service, operates hospitals, health centers, school health centers, health stations and urban Indian health centers (DHHS, 2004).

The Department of Veterans' Affairs operates many clinics, hospitals, and nursing homes for veterans. These are found across the country. For those who are eligible for care from the Veterans' Administration (VA), benefits are comprehensive. The VA is engaged in a major effort to improve services to veterans. Information on the VA's Strategic Plan 2000–2006 is available at *www.va.gov.*

Patterns of Payment

Understanding the various methods of paying for health care services can help you understand what is happening in the organizations and agencies involved in the health care system. The following discussion covers those most commonly used methods of paying for health care services.

Fee-For-Service Payment

Fee-for-service payment means that each time a service is provided a fee is generated and then billed to the care recipient. The more services provided, the more fees charged. This was the traditional method of charging for health care in the United States. Initially, private individuals paid almost all fees. When insurance companies began assisting with payment, the bill was sent to the insurance company and to the client. The insurance company then paid the amount established in the policy (eg, 80%), and the client was required to pay the rest.

As costs rose, insurance companies began setting a standard for reimbursement. Under this system, if a policy stated that a company reimbursed at 80%, this meant 80% of a fee that the insurance company determined was reasonable. If the provider charged more than what was considered reasonable, the client was responsible for the excess, in addition to 20% of the "reasonable" fee. Insurance companies usually set these fees based on statistical analysis of prevailing fees in a geographic area. In a time of rapid inflation, providers complained that there was often a serious discrepancy between the fee used for calculating benefits and the actual fees being charged. This standard fee still provided for paying a fee for each service rendered.

Prospective Payment

A **prospective payment** is a fixed reimbursement amount for all the care required for a particular surgical procedure, an illness, or an acuity category. This reimbursement amount is determined in advance of the provision of service. The predetermined amount is paid without regard to actual services required or the costs of those services in individual situations. Thus, the same payment is made whether the person is healthy and has an uncomplicated hospital stay or whether the person is in poor health and has complications that increase the cost of care or the length of the hospital stay.

Prospective payment is designed to provide an incentive for hospitals to control costs. Prospective payment has accomplished this as hospitals began to monitor the use of high-cost testing and pharmaceutical products and to limit the length of stay. Another advantage to payers in a prospective payment system is that costs are predictable. The system transfers the burden of risk (the probability that an individual may require extraordinary services) from the payer to the provider. Several specific types of prospective payment are in operation that have particular significance for nurses. These are DRGs and Resource Utilization Groups (RUGs).

Diagnosis-Related Groups. The first major change in the method of payment for health care services began October 1, 1983, when the federal government stopped using a fee-for-service reimbursement system for Medicare, and introduced a prospective payment system using **diagnosis-related groups (DRGs)** to determine the payment for each Medicare client admitted to the hospital. This change was designed to stop the spiraling costs of Medicare and to correct inequities that made the costs of care in one facility very different from those in another facility.

The method of determining the rates to be paid in the Medicare prospective payment system— the creation of DRGs—resulted from a computerized analysis of costs that had been billed for hospitalized individuals in the past and a determination of an average length of stay. This analysis led to the formation of categories of medical diagnoses that require similar treatment and for which costs are similar. Each category (or DRG) has a name and number; for example, DRG 236 is "fracture of the hip and pelvis." In addition, a decision was made to increase the payment for care when another illness or condition is present. This second condition is termed a **comorbidity.** Thus, a person with heart failure whose basic DRG is "fractured hip" is designated "fractured hip with congestive heart failure." A hospital receives greater reimbursement for providing service to this person because care is more complex and costs are higher. Hospitals also receive additional amounts for cases that are determined to be "outliers." An outlier is a case in which the client's length of stay significantly exceeds the average. The number of days needed to qualify a case as an outlier is predetermined. For example, the average length of stay for DRG 236, "Fractured hip and pelvis," is 6.2 days, but the stay must reach 29 days for the case to be considered an outlier. Pressure is placed on all providers to ensure that the patient is discharged within the average length of stay on which payment is based.

Most hospital costs are included in the DRG reimbursement. The actual DRG reimbursement amount is calculated each year by CMS through a complex formula that considers the area of the country in which the care was provided (eg, Northwest, Southeast), the urbanization of the area (eg, rural, suburban), and the type of care required. Some hospital costs still are reimbursed separately. In the past, the separate reimbursements included costs for medical education of resident physicians and research conducted by the hospital. These were reimbursed because the federal government supports the need for research and medical education and also acknowledges that the resident physicians provide care to Medicare and Medicaid recipients. However, pressure is mounting to stop this as a separate payment. Private physicians bill and are paid independently, but some suggest that when these services relate to hospital care, they should be included in a single rate for the entire hospitalization and care. The American Medical Association has vigorously opposed this.

Most of the controversy surrounding the implementation of DRGs has not been concerned with the incentives for cost control, or the prospective reimbursement system itself, but rather how the payment amounts are determined and how the system is being administered. A concern continues that clients reportedly are discharged after much shorter stays, when they are still in need of care (the "quicker and sicker" concern—clients are discharged quicker and feeling sicker). Because the method of calculation of payments was based on costs before the system was implemented, providers in some areas of the country receive significantly higher payments for the same DRG than do others. For example, payments in the Southeast are greater than those in the Northwest. Providers in the areas with lower reimbursement express concern that they cannot continue to provide care and remain economically viable with the current reimbursement.

Hospitals with a large population of extra-high-risk clients (eg, the very elderly or poor) have expressed concern that discharging a client for convalescence in a home with a caring family, good food, and a clean environment is much different from discharging a client to an impoverished environment. Many believe the individual situation should be considered when determining regulations for length of stay. The proponents of shortened stays point out that shortened stays are effective cost-containment measures. They argue further that a client's lack of a support system is a social problem and that hospitalization cannot be used to solve social problems. Alterations and modifications of the system will continue, but the basic prospective plan is not expected to change.

Resource Utilization Groups. Resource utilization groups (RUGs) are the categories used to determine prospective payment for nursing home clients. Each RUG represents a group of residents who require a similar amount of care and thus will be similar in the cost to support that care each day. Unlike the hospital prospective payment, which is a flat amount for the entire hospital stay, the prospective payment for nursing home care is a fixed daily rate. This daily rate must include all the services, including medications and treatments, that a resident needs. The actual daily rate of reimbursement to the nursing home is the average of the RUGs for all residents. This is often referred to as the **case mix.**

The basis for determining to which RUG a nursing home resident will be assigned for reimbursement purposes is the comprehensive **minimum data set (MDS)** prepared by the registered nurse. This assessment must be transmitted electronically to the appropriate center for review and payment categorization. If the assessments are not completed accurately or are not submitted in a timely manner, the resident automatically is assigned to the lowest reimbursement RUG category. The facility is then unable to recover the difference between the lowest RUG and the actual RUG to which the resident is eventually assigned. Reassessments are required at specified intervals. These reassessments are used to reassign the resident to a RUG.

The use of a **prospective payment system (PPS)** for long-term care—that is, a fixed reimbursement for all the care provided—was phased in over 2 years, beginning in 1997 with the first pilot groups. The PPS has created great consternation throughout the nursing home industry because payments to nursing homes have dropped precipitously since its implementation.

The nursing home industry is lobbying for changes in the reimbursement plan because it believes that low reimbursement is undermining its ability to provide appropriate care. The costs of compliance are high, the reimbursements are lower, and there are more restrictions on such items as the provision of therapy services. Many nursing homes have reduced staff, changed practice patterns, and made other adjustments to adapt to the decrease in reimbursement. One unintended result of the move to PPS for the nursing home has been the refusal of nursing homes to admit high-cost residents. For example, an individual with an extensive wound that requires intensive wound care with expensive products might cost more per day for care than the highest RUG category allows. In the past, it was possible to bill separately for the expensive dressings and topical agents used. When this is not possible, the facility may refuse to admit the patient. This actually may increase costs for the payer, because patients remain in the high-cost hospital if no long-term care facility will admit them.

Other Prospective Payment Systems. In addition to Medicare and Medicaid, many states are adopting systems similar to DRGs, and some private insurance carriers are now using these basic concepts in their cost-control efforts through prospective payment. These prospective payments are often the result of negotiations between health care agencies and the insurance companies. Although the specific amounts and the totals of what is included may differ, some of the same concerns regarding the adequacy of payments remain.

Capitation

Capitation is yet another way of determining payment within the health care system. In a capitated system, a fee is paid to a provider organization for each person (each "head," thus the term) signed up for the plan whether or not that person uses any health care services. Global capitation refers to the inclusion of all services, both inpatient and outpatient, including physician costs in the capitated amount. Capitation may also be limited and only include outpatient and physician costs.

Capitation shifts an even greater share of the risk of providing costly health care from the third-party payer to the provider organization. Providers in a capitated system have an incentive to guide individuals to low-cost outpatient services or other care environments rather than to the acute care hospital. A goal of this payment system is to encourage preventive services that may make high-cost interventions unnecessary. Thus, in a capitated system you may find that services such as mammograms, immunizations, stop-smoking clinics, and back-injury classes do not have any co-payments attached, or the co-payments may be quite low. HMOs were the original capitated systems.

A criticism of a capitated system is that when the provider is at risk for providing care, there may be an unconscious (or even deliberate) attempt to deny medically necessary care to keep costs down. In some capitated systems, consumers have complained that they were unable to obtain services they believed were medically necessary.

COST CONTROL IN HEALTH CARE

Because health care costs continue to rise, cost control is a major focus of the health care system of today. Many factors contribute to the rising costs of health, and many strategies have been used to attempt to limit the rate of increase.

Understanding Increasing Costs

Many factors contribute to the rising costs of health care (Display 1-3).

High Technology and New Facilities

One important factor in cost increase is the price of new technology. New, more sophisticated diagnostic and treatment devices are developed each year. The rising cost of technology affects every area of the health care field, from the cardiac care unit to the laboratory. Companies that manufacture health-related devices and drugs reportedly have some of the highest profits in any industry. These companies justify their profits as appropriate relative to the risk and cost involved in research and development; however, some critics believe these companies take advantage of the public's dependence on their products. For example, recent evidence indicates that drug companies spend as much on advertising as they do on research. For those health insurance plans and HMOs providing prescription coverage, the costs of prescription drugs are cited as a key reason for premium increases. The public has expressed concern that drug companies sell identical drugs in other countries for far less money than what they charge consumers in the United States.

Display 1-3   Contributing Factors in Rising Health Care Costs

- Price of new technology
- Construction of new facilities
- Higher survival rates, leading to greater need for costly intensive or long-term care
- Growing population of elderly adults requiring health care
- Rise in salaries for health care workers
- High costs of drugs and health-related equipment

Drug companies contend that high costs in the United States are essential to support continued drug research, which is very costly. One of the realities contributing to this situation is that other countries place price controls on drugs and the United States does not.

An increasing population needs a greater number of facilities, and the construction of new care facilities also contributes to rising costs. In addition, existing facilities often require modifications. More space is needed for new technologies both at the bedside and in many hospital departments. Computer systems are used more often for documentation of care. Bedside computers that enable documentation to be done at the point of care decrease the amount of time required for paperwork. More offices and conference rooms are needed. The regulations governing hospital construction also have become more stringent, requiring more fire-safety and infection-control measures and protection against environmental hazards. These factors combine to make the per-bed cost of new hospital construction or remodeling increasingly expensive. Additionally, decreases in the length of hospital stay and the move to outpatient services have left many hospital beds unused on a fluctuating basis. Unoccupied hospital beds create a major drain on organizations, because large sums of capital investment are tied up and not returning any income.

Changing Patient Profile

The average length of hospital stay for standard diagnoses has decreased steadily. The typical client in today's hospital is discharged rapidly to convalesce at home or in a long-term care facility, leaving behind only the acutely ill. Many clients who would have died quickly in earlier years live through a crisis but require long and intensive care. All of these factors make the acuity level of a client today much greater. This in turn requires more intensive observation and care and the use of more specialized equipment.

The population of the United States as a whole is growing older and, statistically, the elderly have an increased incidence of all chronic illnesses. A greater percentage of that population requires health care on a regular basis and may depend on medications, treatments, and therapies for continued functioning.

Uncompensated Care

Health plans in the United States are primarily linked to employment, except for those eligible for Medicare and Medicaid, because the cost of independent plans is prohibitive. Individuals and families whose incomes are marginal may be unable to purchase insurance because of the high cost of individual policies. Nationwide, annual premiums averaged $2,268 for single coverage and $4,424 for a family plan in 2004 (American Health Insurance Plans, 2005). For the family headed by a worker earning $10 per hour, this is more than 20% of the gross income going toward health insurance. According to the Kaiser Family Foundation, in 2004 69% of families without insurance had at least one full-time employed worker (Kaiser Family Foundation, 2004). Small businesses are finding it increasingly difficult to provide health insurance, and even large corporations find the cost of health care to be a major problem. As more people fall into the categories of those without coverage, the amount of uncompensated care continues to rise. Private providers steer patients to public providers such as county clinics and hospitals. According to the National Association of Counties (2003), 100% of those counties with populations of 500,000 to 1 million report increased costs related to uncompensated care. For smaller counties the rise is less apparent, so that 61% of all counties report increased costs related to uncompensated care.

Many health care providers are struggling with the financial problem of uncompensated care. Uncompensated care is a particular concern for hospitals. Individuals arrive at emergency rooms and laws require that they be assessed before they leave. If an acute problem is found, they must be treated. If the patient has no insurance and is not able to pay privately (which is the common case for those without insurance), the provider is never compensated for the care given. For hospitals with trauma centers and busy emergency rooms, these cases may be ones that require extensive resources lasting over months. Research by the Institute of Medicine has shown that uncompensated care harms not only the individuals without insurance and the immediate providers, but the entire community by reducing access to emergency services and trauma care, access to specialists, and availability of hospital-based services (Kellerman, 2003). Uncompensated care may threaten the viability of institutions in their communities. While this problem grows, there is no national plan to address it.

Other Factors Affecting Costs

Until recently, the salaries of health care workers (except for physicians) were far below those of the general society. To remedy this, for a time, salaries of health care workers rose more rapidly than the general inflation rate. Physicians also had an increase in income greater than the relative inflation rate, until the mid 1990s, when changes in the system began to affect income levels for physicians.

Lack of competition in the health care field is one factor that may contribute to higher costs. Although physicians continue to be primary gatekeepers in the system, the advent of other primary care providers, such as nurse practitioners and nurse midwives, offers alternative and less costly care for many routine problems and normal life processes such as pregnancy and childbirth. However, there is opposition to allowing these practitioners to operate in collaborative rather than dependent or subsidiary roles. Display 1-3 provides an overview of the factors contributing to rising health care costs.

Critical Thinking Activity

Choose a patient you currently care for. Make a list of all the therapies, medications, diagnostic tests, and surgeries or procedures that this patient has received. Research the cost of these therapies and the daily rate for hospital care in your area for one day. Research the DRG reimbursement for that diagnostic group. Compare the reimbursement with the costs being incurred for this individual patient. Identify ways that nurses could reduce the costs involved in this patient's care.

Strategies for Cost Control

As health care costs continue to rise, third-party payers have used several methods to control costs, including changing patterns of payment and controlling the actions of providers. These strategies are often referred to as **cost containment** actions.

Limiting Hospital Costs

With the changes in payment, hospitals have developed many mechanisms to limit costs. Because federal regulations limit the reimbursement to hospitals, physicians are asked to judge carefully the necessity of diagnostic studies and costly procedures for hospitalized patients.

Physicians sometimes are asked to consult with a pharmacist before prescribing certain high-cost drugs to determine whether a low-cost therapeutic alternative exists. For example, although the latest aminoglycoside antibiotic might be effective, an inexpensive first-generation cephalosporin antibiotic also might be effective, while costing 90% less. There is great pressure on physicians to discharge patients by the average length of stay to ensure that costs remain within the established prospective payment amount. Physician practices are monitored and they have even been threatened with denial of hospital privileges if their patients consistently stay beyond the expected length of stay. Many physicians are upset about these cost-containment measures because they may interfere with the physician's independent decision making about what care is needed and when.

To add new high-cost equipment or additional client care facilities, a health care institution may be required to apply for a certificate of need from the state. This establishes that there will not be unnecessary duplication of services in an area and that a need for them exists. For example, if every hospital purchased magnetic resonance imaging equipment that was used to only one fourth or one third of its capacity, the cost per use would have to be higher to cover the investment and maintenance costs than if the device were used to capacity.

In many states, nonprofit hospitals must apply for rate increases. In their applications, they must document all the factors contributing to the need for an increase. Hearings are held, and permission for rate increases is given only when the evidence indicates that all possible economies are being observed. Private profit-making hospitals are not held to these rules.

Preferred Providers Contracts

In an attempt to contain costs, third-party payers such as insurance companies, HMOs, and managed care organizations sometimes negotiate with providers of health care to supply certain kinds of care at an agreed-upon, usually lower, price. The third-party payers then provide incentives for clients to use these preferred providers. These incentives may include the waiver of all or part of co-payments by the insured or coverage of additional conditions or situations.

Preferred provider organizations (PPOs) include hospitals, nursing homes, corporations employing care providers, or groups of care providers who have cooperated to negotiate more successfully with third-party payers for these special contracts. The advantage to the provider is the ensured number of clients and the guaranteed income. In a time of competition in health care, this may be a significant advantage. Each PPO operates independently without government regulation; therefore, the exact structure and contractual arrangements are independently determined.

Managed Care

As previously noted, managed care refers to any system for "financing and organizing the delivery of health care in which costs are contained by controlling the provision of services." Taber's, 2005 identifies managed care more specifically as "a system to control the cost of health care by using a select group of providers who have agreed to a predetermined payment, with the clinical interventions being managed via utilization and/or a case management process." A managed care plan may be controlled by the payer (eg, an insurance company), include both payers and providers, or be a business entity that serves only as a go-between. HMOs always have acted as managed care systems. Many of the current health plans referred to as HMOs are in reality managed care systems that do not focus on health maintenance at all.

In a managed care system, there is always someone assigned to the role of gatekeeper. This person monitors and restricts the use of services by the client. In most managed care plans the primary physician is expected to serve as the gatekeeper. The physician sees the client first and then determines whether referral or diagnostic services are needed. In some managed care systems, the primary physician has decision-making authority. However, in many managed care systems, the actual gatekeeper is a plan manager who must be consulted regarding the use of services. A written request may be required before the client receives permission for a referral. This may result in delay or denial of needed care and is one source of consumer dissatisfaction with some managed care plans.

Many managed care decisions about individual clients are made based on a set of predetermined protocols for treatment. The original protocols were developed by physicians, based on broad statistical patterns. Thus the protocol may not be responsive to individual differences. These protocols often are administered by plan employees who are not health care providers. Some physicians express dismay over a mechanism that allows a nonphysician who has never seen a client to make critical decisions about the care needed and to deny any individualization of the plan.

Managed care usually requires that care be authorized or approved for payment before it is provided. Clients identify the required approval of any type of care as a major problem. A managed care plan may not approve or pay for care that it considers nonessential. If a health care provider and a plan consultant disagree about which type of treatment is appropriate, the client often feels caught in the middle. This situation frequently occurs in emergency care. Even when approval is granted, the process may have been long and frustrating for the client and physician involved.

In some managed care plans, a subscriber who needs emergency care and is outside the appropriate service area is subject to what is called the standard of the "prudent consumer." This means that if a prudent layperson would consider the symptoms an emergency, the plan will pay for care. Thus, if a person with chest pain goes to an emergency room, the plan pays even if the chest pain turns out to be esophageal reflux. Some plans created a standard related to the final medical diagnosis. A plan with this standard would pay for an individual who visited the emergency room with chest pain only if the final diagnosis were myocardial infarction, but would not pay if the final diagnosis were esophageal reflux. This approach caused such public consternation that legislation was enacted in some areas that required any kind of health plan to cover emergency care based on the prudent consumer model.

Some plans require that an individual travel to a designated hospital when an emergency is not life-threatening. Thus, one consumer was denied payment for a fractured ankle sustained while skiing because it was not life-threatening and because the injury was treated in the skiing community rather than back home in the consumer's designated hospital.

Managed care controls extend to such matters as the medications that can be prescribed. A managed care company may have a specific formulary or list of drugs that are allowed to be prescribed. The company usually negotiates for drug purchases at lower prices than paid by the general public. For many conditions, there are clear therapeutic equivalents and medication restrictions are not a concern. For the person with a chronic health condition who has been stabilized on specific medications, however, moving into a managed care plan can pose a real threat to health maintenance if the plan will not approve the client's current drugs.

All of these actions are designed to hold down costs. Managed care plans that originally focused on health maintenance and keeping healthy people well showed great promise for controlling health care costs. However, as managed care has encompassed people with serious chronic illnesses, controlling costs has become more difficult.

Case Management

Case management is a technique used to efficiently move an individual requiring major health services through the system. This results in more effective use of services and lessens cost. According to the Case Management Society of America (CMSA), case management is

> a collaborative process which assesses, plans, implements, coordinates, monitors, and evaluates options and services to meet an individual's health needs through communication and available resources to promote quality cost-effective outcomes (CMSA, 2007).

Case managers most commonly are assigned to high-risk clients, such as those with chronic illnesses or major traumas, who will require rehabilitation. In some settings, the case manager specializes in a particular group of high-risk clients, such as those with diabetes, and is referred to as a **disease manager.**

The case manager is an experienced health professional with knowledge of available resources who oversees or monitors a case to ensure that necessary care is instituted promptly and is provided in the most cost-effective setting. Nurses have often assumed the role of case manager. In this role, the nurse monitors the care as it is provided, ensuring that appropriate referrals are made, changes in the plan of care are instituted appropriately, and the care follows established standards. Because of their understanding of the whole person, both physiologically and psychosocially, and their understanding of how the system works, nurses are particularly well suited to this role. The CMSA provides a system for certifying professional case managers.

Case managers may operate within only one part of the system (eg, managing cases from admission through discharge in a nursing home or hospital). These managers are often referred to as internal case managers. Some may manage cases across all phases of care from outpatient through hospitalization, rehabilitation, and back to outpatient. These individuals are termed external case managers. At their best, case management systems ensure that delays in patient transfer or breaks in communication do not occur, and that costs are minimized through efficiency. Case managers often act as advocates for clients in the system. Physicians sometimes object to what they see as the interference of the case manager in a decision-making process that previously included only the client and the physician.

Vertically Integrated Health Care Systems

Organizations contracting to provide managed care also are expanding their own control through the development of **vertically integrated systems,** that is, those that provide every level of health care service. A vertically integrated system may have contracted physicians, laboratories, a hospital, a subacute facility, a rehabilitation facility, and a home care agency. This allows the contracting organization to offer managed care corporations a package that provides care at all levels for each enrolled member of the managed care plan for a capitated fee. The contracting organization then has an incentive to control costs by decreasing the use of high-cost services and more effectively using low-cost alternatives. It is also in a better position to negotiate with the managed care system about reimbursement. As large systems develop in this manner, hospitals become a cost center rather than a revenue center. This merging of systems is resulting in the closure of hospitals in many communities.

Using Acuity Measures to Determine Costs

Health care providers who negotiate contracts and plan care need accurate data regarding the specific cost of each service. One way of trying to understand and control these costs is through the development of acuity measures. Acuity in this context refers to the severity of illness and the rapidity of change in the client, and thus the intensity of medical and nursing care and other therapies required.

There are various ways of measuring acuity in both acute and long-term care settings. Most systems use categories that reflect the different types of care needed. Each category is assigned a numerical value (eg, a scale of 1 to 4). All applicable category values are summed and compared with a standard. For example, an acuity measuring system might have one category reflecting the need for assistance in personal hygiene. As a person needs more assistance, more points are assigned. Another category might reflect the amount of time needed for monitoring vital signs: The more time required, the more points assigned. Each category is assigned an appropriate number of points, and the total is computed. The points identified for an individual client are then compared with a standard, and the client is assigned an acuity level. Clients with the fewest points are level 1 and require the least care. Those with the most points are level 4 and require the most care. Each system in use has its own scale for determining acuity. Acuity values are sometimes called **intensity measures** because they reflect the intensity of care needed.

In some settings, acuity levels or intensity measures are used as a mechanism for determining the staffing needs of a client care unit. Acuity levels also are used as a means of billing for the level of nursing care needed, and are reflected in a variable, rather than flat, charge for the nursing portion of a client's room charge. It also has been suggested that prospective reimbursement might be based on acuity level rather than on medical diagnosis because acuity levels reflect the real impact on resources more accurately than do medical diagnoses. The RUGs developed for prospective reimbursement in long-term care are essentially an acuity measure based on the nursing assessment.

Increasing the Availability of Mid-Level Providers

Because physicians are the most costly health care providers, increasing the use of nonphysician primary care providers, PCPs, (such as nurse practitioners and physician assistants), often referred to as mid-level providers, has been used to decrease health care costs. The use of nonphysician providers relies on the ability to obtain reimbursement for the care these individuals deliver.

One attempt to increase the availability of nonphysician care has been the movement to obtain legislation requiring that government agencies and third-party payers pay the nonphysician who provides primary care service. The traditional pattern required that payment always be made to a physician, who in turn paid the nonphysician provider. Progress has been made in regard to third-party reimbursement for nurses in primary care; however, this continues to be a problem and a major thrust of political pressure by nurses.

Changing Fee Structures

In addition to reducing payments through prospective payment systems, the federal government has sought to control costs for Medicare and Medicaid by establishing higher deductibles (the portions that individual clients must pay) and by limiting the fees that the government will pay. Because the elderly and the poor are often unable to pay these deductible amounts, they become liabilities for health care providers, who cover these costs by collecting higher fees from those who do pay their bills. Hospitals, physicians, and pharmacies argue that as more limits have been imposed, the limited reimbursement no longer covers the actual costs of care. This jeopardizes the entire system. Medicaid costs also have been contained by tightening eligibility requirements, which shuts more people out of the health care system. Many employer plans are also requiring more cost sharing by employees both to reduce the cost to the employer and as an incentive for the employee to use health care wisely.

Controlling Fraud and Abuse

As Medicare and Medicaid have become a larger part of the financing for the health care system, fraud also has become a larger problem. HIPAA created a federal Health Care Fraud and Abuse Control Program. This program coordinates federal, state, and local law enforcement activities in fighting health care fraud and abuse. Information on preventing Medicare fraud is available at the Medicare Web site *www.medicare.gov/fraudabuse/overview.asp*.

Other Cost-Containment Measures

In medical facilities, personnel now are asked to be more cost conscious. Nursing personnel must be aware of the tremendous cost of any complication or prolonged length of stay. Preventing complications and getting clients ready for early discharge have become a major focus of care. Care pathways specify care and identify outcomes for each day of hospitalization with the goal of ensuring that resources are used wisely. Cost consciousness also involves such ordinary measures as being conservative with telephone use, canceling meal trays when clients are discharged, and using expensive supplies with care.

All of these efforts at reducing costs affect the health care system in areas other than cost containment. They affect decision-making processes, power structures, the kinds of care provided, and the ways that individual health care providers practice. Concerns about cost continue to exert pressure for change in the system.

Critical Thinking Activity

What cost-control measures have you seen in places where you have had clinical practice? Analyze the effects of these cost-control measures on client care.

ACCESS TO HEALTH CARE

Access to health care refers to the individual's ability to obtain and use needed services. Access can be an economic, a geographic, or a sociocultural issue. Creating access requires a broad approach that encompasses not only access to health providers and hospitalization, but that also addresses other factors that affect health. In addition to providing a family with a prescription, for example, a provider must determine whether there is a way to fill that prescription. It is not enough to prescribe a special diet without learning whether that the individual has the necessary knowledge and resources to follow that diet.

Economic Access

The problem of economic access to health care was discussed from a system perspective when the various methods of paying for health care were presented. Economic access is often dependent on having a health plan or being eligible for one of the government programs. Some of the decisions made for purposes of cost containment may have unforeseen consequences in terms of economic access. Although giving people an incentive to use services wisely is the stated goal of raising deductibles and co-payments, the result for lower-income families may be the delay or avoidance of timely care.

Some individuals are unable to obtain health insurance because of preexisting illnesses. These are often the people who are most in need of health care services. Another group concerned about being denied insurance coverage are those with the potential for serious health problems. As genetic testing for potential health problems becomes more widespread and the information gleaned from it more exact, insurance companies may use the results of these tests as a basis for denying coverage to healthy individuals. As more tests become available, this issue is a cause for growing concern, especially as it relates to access to health care (see Chapter 10).

Some groups, such as minorities and the elderly, that experience disparities in health care access, are heavily affected by the co-existence of poverty in these groups. Even those eligible for Medicaid-financed care may not be able to find a PCP willing to care for them. The low reimbursement rates and the need to cope with the complex governmental system lead many private providers to opt out of such care.

Geographic Access

Geographic access to health care is a special concern for those in rural areas. As changes occur in the health care system, small rural hospitals have found themselves unable to compete or to manage financially. This has led to the closure of some of those hospitals. When a rural hospital closes, area residents lose emergency room care, hospital access, and diagnostic services. The need to travel to receive health care especially affects the elderly and poor (Rosenthal & Fox, 2000).

Communities without hospitals find it more difficult to recruit physicians and other primary care providers. Historically, most health care providers have preferred not to work in areas that lack hospitals available to provide diagnostic and treatment services; consequently, rural communities find it difficult to recruit health care providers. Many medical schools, with the support of both federal and state funds, developed programs to encourage medical students and residents to consider family practice as a specialty and practice in a rural location. Although successful in increasing the number of physicians entering rural practice, in some states that number couldn't make up for how many physicians were leaving rural practice.

Geographic access may be a concern for those in urban areas as well. Economically depressed areas of large cities have fewer health care providers, thus forcing the residents of those areas to travel long distances, often using inconvenient public transportation, to receive health care.

Access to health care also is affected by whether all services are available in one location. It is common for individuals to be required to visit several geographically separate locations to receive all needed health care. Some organizations now offer all health services in one geographic location. A single health care site makes it unnecessary for an individual to go to one location to see a primary provider, a second to see a specialist, a third for diagnostic tests, and yet another for procedures. This makes efficient use of the client's time, increases the likelihood that the client will follow through with recommended procedures, and simplifies communication between providers.

Sociocultural Access

Sociocultural differences also affect access. When individuals feel uncomfortable in a setting because of their socioeconomic status or because their cultural background and beliefs are not respected, they are reluctant to use the services provided. Making care culturally accessible may mean having available in the care setting translation services, materials in multiple languages, and care providers who understand and are sensitive to cultural differences.

EVALUATION AND ACCREDITATION OF HEALTH CARE AGENCIES

Evaluation takes many forms in health care. The most universal is some type of evaluation against standards. A variety of standards and processes to enforce those standards have been established. Meeting the standards of a state governmental agency is termed approval or **certification.** Meeting the standards of a nongovernment agency is usually designated as accreditation. Health care institutions are often both certified by a government body and accredited by a non-government agency. In some instances, government bodies accept accreditation as the equivalent of government standards and do not require an additional approval process. Approval by a specific organization may be required for an agency to receive some types of third-party payment. Therefore, accreditation is important for the agencies involved. Some evaluation processes involve evaluating client outcomes as well as the processes of care.

Government Approval

Institutions and agencies providing health care usually must be approved by the governmental agency, often a department of health, in the state where they are located. Approval may take the form of state licensing, which usually focuses on maintaining minimum standards to safeguard public health. For some agencies, this meets their needs.

Medicare/Medicaid Certification

Those agencies that seek Medicare or Medicaid funding must meet specific federal standards and be Medicare certified in addition to meeting the basic state standards. For example, Medicare certifies nursing homes as meeting Medicare standards. The Medicare standards relate to many aspects of care. By designating those to whom payment will be given, Medicare effectively exerts control. Because the costs of private care are so high, most people choose to receive care where it can be reimbursed. When care is not reimbursable, individuals may make other choices.

Health care institutions and agencies also may seek accreditation from nongovernment bodies that set standards for high quality and provide guidelines to assist in developing policies and procedures. Medicare and Medicaid have granted several of these nongovernment agencies what is called "deemed status." This means that the standards of the agency are considered equal to or exceeding the Medicare standard. Therefore, a health care agency that has been accredited by the voluntary process may be deemed as meeting the standards set by Medicare and Medicaid and not required to pursue an additional Medicare certification process.

The Joint Commission

Hospitals, nursing homes, and related organizations may seek accreditation from The Joint Commission. This nonprofit, voluntary organization originally was established by the American

College of Surgeons and the American Society of Internal Medicine to set standards for hospital care. Today's organization has a board of directors with members from many health care and public occupations. The standards of the organization are comprehensive and involve evaluating the structural aspects of institutions, policies and procedures, and the outcomes of care provided. It has deemed status for federal programs. In the past, assisted living settings have not had a standard accreditation, and, in many states, little regulation. The Joint Commission began providing accreditation for assisted living facilities in 2001.

During surveys, The Joint Commission investigates all aspects of an organization, including the physical plant, the entire delivery of care process, and the evaluation and quality improvement plans being used. It has the power to demand change in order for accreditation to continue. In most instances, however, problems that are not of serious danger to patients are noted for remediation and the facility is asked to report on the changes made.

Community Health Accreditation Program

The Community Health Accreditation Program (CHAP) was established to provide a voluntary accreditation system for community health and home health agencies. This is a peer-reviewed process governed entirely by community health agencies with public representation. Medicare and Medicaid do not require a separate Medicare certification for an organization that has CHAP accreditation.

National Committee for Quality Assurance

The National Committee for Quality Assurance (NCQA) reviews and evaluates HMOs. It is a relatively new, independent nonprofit organization developed by the HMO industry. NCQA has established a set of statistical measures called Health Plan Employer Data and Information Set (HEDIS). This information is available from its Web site, *www.ncqa.org*. These data provide a standard set of information that both employers and consumers can use to compare and evaluate HMOs. Included in the HEDIS data set are nine indicators of quality, seven of which are related to processes and two that are related to outcomes. Most of these data relate to prevention and not to the effective diagnosis and treatment of illness.

Peer Review and Quality Assurance

The first systematic evaluation of health care services was established through the Professional Standards Review Organization set up by Medicare and Medicaid. As part of the 1982 revisions of Medicare, the evaluation process was altered to require that hospitals contract with an external medical review organization, called a Utilization and Quality Control Peer Review Organization (PRO). These organizations were established through competitive bidding for contracts awarded by the Secretary of HHS. Most of the PROs are statewide in scope and are required to have a substantial number of physicians represented in the organization to set standards and review care effectively.

Evaluation may include pre-admission, pre-procedure, concurrent, or retrospective (after discharge) reviews. The purpose of the reviews is to determine whether care given was necessary and whether it was given in the appropriate manner. For example, the reviews have resulted in an increase in the number of outpatient surgeries (day procedures) performed, and a subsequent decrease in the number of inpatient surgeries. These changes have resulted in significant economic savings. The PRO also is required to evaluate outcomes of care to ensure that the changes made do not jeopardize clients.

Display 1-4   Outcomes From *Healthy People 2010*

A. Health and Disease Outcomes
1. General physical well-being
2. Infant mortality
3. Death rates from preventable causes
4. Disability-free survivorship
5. Self-reported health status
6. Sexually transmitted diseases
7. HIV
8. Cancer
9. Low birth weight
10. Cardiovascular disease (CVD)
11. Asthma or chronic obstructive pulmonary disease (COPD)
12. Hip fractures or osteoporosis
13. Injury
14. Diabetes
15. Disability days

B. Preventive Health Behaviors
1. Unintended pregnancies
2. Immunizations
3. Tobacco use
4. Physical activity
5. Alcohol use
6. Substance abuse
7. Appropriate body weight
8. Nutrition

C. Mental Health
1. Psychological status

D. Health System Access
1. Physical accessibility
2. Poverty
3. Health literacy
4. Education levels

E. Ecologic
1. Air quality
2. Iatrogenesis
3. Firearm death and injury rates
4. Violence
5. Homelessness
6. Motor vehicle accident death and injury rates

Outcome Measures

Outcome measures refer to actual health results in the clients and communities served. Outcomes now are measured in relationship to hospitals, long-term care facilities, and the population as a whole. Some outcomes have been designated **key indicators,** also termed **quality indicators (QIs),** which are specific, measurable aspects of health care that show the effectiveness of the system as a whole and indicate whether access to services is available. These are major factors in changes health care institutions are undertaking. Some of the outcome measures are based in the outcomes identified by Healthy People 2010. See Display 1-4.

Hospital Health Care Outcomes

The federal government compiles statistics related to hospital health care outcomes. These include infection rates and morbidity and mortality rates associated with specific hospitals and procedures. In 1995, the federal government began releasing these figures to the public. These government statistics may be helpful in evaluating some aspects of care. One result of outcome studies has been the recommendation that only hospitals that perform a specified number of highly technical surgeries (eg, cardiac surgeries) each year should offer those procedures. Hospitals that perform fewer procedures per year have higher complication and mortality rates.

The Agency for Health Care Research and Quality (AHRQ) has identified a set of items that could be used as indicators of quality of care and community access to care. It identified three groups of QIs: prevention QIs, inpatient QIs, and patient safety QIs. Since their beginning in the early 1990s, these QIs have been refined through the use of extensive data banks maintained by the HHS.

The prevention QIs consist of "ambulatory care sensitive conditions," hospital admissions that evidence suggests could have been avoided through high-quality outpatient care or that reflect conditions that could be less severe, if treated early and appropriately (AHRQ, 2004a). The inpatient QIs reflect

> quality of care inside hospitals and include inpatient mortality; utilization of procedures (such as hysterectomy) for which there are questions of overuse, under use, or misuse; and volume of procedures (such as cardiac catheterization) for which there is evidence that a higher volume of procedures is associated with lower mortality (AHRQ, 2006a).

The patient safety indicators are adverse outcomes for hospitalized patients that reflect an adverse event that is preventable such as falls and nosocomial (originating in the health care system) infections (AHRQ, 2006b). Programs to facilitate the collection and aggregation of data in relationship to these QIs are now available on-line.

Many health care agencies are constructing their documentation systems to collect data that demonstrates performance in relationship to these quality indicators. This is enlarging the purpose of documentation from a focus on the individual client to a focus that includes system concerns.

Institutional Outcomes Measurement

Individual institutions also are establishing ways to measure the outcomes of the care they provide. Outcomes here refers to data such as the number of clients admitted with a fractured hip who had uncomplicated recoveries leading to effective rehabilitation and the number of clients who had complications or did not recover. Knowledge of outcomes is essential for planning and, increasingly, for effective marketing. Often data have been collected but are scattered among many different records and are difficult to retrieve. Because data only become valuable for planning when they are organized in a useful framework for analysis, health care agencies have moved rapidly to the computerization of data and the implementation of standardized protocols for data collection.

One of the standardized tools hospitals use to monitor outcomes is called the **clinical pathway.** This is also referred to as a critical path, a care map, or an anticipated recovery path. The clinical pathway describes the optimum progression through the system of the individual with a particular health problem. By establishing the desired outcome for day 2 of the postoperative client with a fractured hip, it is possible to determine when an individual client is not meeting the desired outcome. The advantage for the client is that care can be modified immediately to address the problem. The advantage for the system is the ability to aggregate data across all clients and examine what is working well and what needs to be changed.

Long-Term Care Quality Indicators

QIs also are used in long-term care as part of the regulatory process. CMS has identified 11 areas of care containing 24 QIs. It states that these 24 indicators represent common conditions and items that are important to residents. These QIs serve as the focus for the state surveyors. Long-term care facilities track these indicators themselves and use them as a focus of improvement.

Home Care Quality Indicators

The Home Care Quality Indicators provide tools for measuring quality in home care (Fries & Geron, n.d.). They are based in assessments using the Minimum Data Set for Home Care. These 22 indicators can be monitored to evaluate the performance of a home care agency. Examples of indicators are "prevalence of weight loss in individuals who are not palliative care clients" and "prevalence of decrease in ability to dress one's upper body." One area of concern in comparing agencies based on these indicators is that the population served by the agency affects the outcomes of care. Those agencies caring for a greater percentage of the poor and disadvantaged face challenges in meeting the same outcome standards (Hirdes et al., 2004).

National Health Indicators

In 1992, HHS and the Public Health Service published *Healthy People 2000, National Health Promotion and Disease Prevention Objectives*. The purpose of this document was to establish national goals to serve as a focus for health promotion and disease prevention activities by individuals, organizations, and the federal government. Achievement of these benchmarks could indicate the overall health status of the population being served. Unfortunately, achievement of these benchmarks has been a far more difficult task than originally envisioned.

In an effort to continue moving forward, the Healthy People 2010 project was developed. Five sets of indicators of the overall health of the population of the United States have been developed. These include health and disease outcomes (such as the incidence of specific preventable diseases), preventive health behaviors (such as the percentage of individuals who smoke), mental health indicators (such as psychological status), health system access (such as physical accessibility of health resources), and ecological indicators (such as firearms injuries and deaths). The specific indicators and measurable criteria for tracking the nation's progress are being refined through consultation with many interested groups (Display 1-4).

POWER IN THE HEALTH CARE SYSTEM

Part of trying to understand any system involves examining some of the unique sources of power and authority within it. If we define **power** as the capability of doing or accomplishing something, then understanding how power is distributed and used in the health care system can help us to function more effectively. Sources of power unique to the health care system are the authority to decide who may enter and leave the system, who may practice in it, and how funding is controlled. An understanding of power in the health care system provides a foundation for nurses to accomplish their goals for patients and their families. Without this understanding, nurses may find themselves without power and thus unable to accomplish desired goals.

Regulatory Power

The primary regulatory agencies in health care are government bodies. These agencies administer licensing laws that govern who is allowed to practice and which institutions are allowed to provide care. Other agencies approve or accredit institutions that educate personnel for health care and licensing, or approve those that provide services. Through regulation, these agencies have a profound effect on how institutions operate.

The accrediting bodies (eg, The Joint Commission, CHAP, and NCQA) all have power to stimulate change in the system. If you have the opportunity to be in an institution when accreditation visitors are present, you will note that every aspect of the physical plant, the policies and procedures, and the competence of staff are examined. Preparing for an accreditation visit stimulates the agency to self-evaluate and correct any deficiencies.

Third-Party Payer Power

Because they represent the financial interests of large groups of people and control payments for services, third-party payers have the power to demand changes in the health care system. When they were first established, these agencies did not see their role in health care as anything beyond a financial relationship. As health care costs rose, these agencies began looking for ways of controlling costs to maintain their competitive place in the insurance market. They have set increasingly rigid criteria for payment for services. The standard rates set for payment for procedures tend to place some restraints on charges (although actual fees often are slightly ahead of payment schedules). By determining whom they will pay for services, insurance companies reduce the choices available to those who carry insurance—and subscribers usually must select from the choices available if they wish to be reimbursed. Third-party payers therefore exert a more powerful influence over institutions and care providers than do individual subscribers.

Physician Power

Physicians historically had almost unlimited power within the health care system. They determined who entered the system and when. They decided whether and when other services and personnel would be used, and they determined when clients would leave the system. As other agencies and professionals in the health care system have obtained some power and independence, the overall power of the physician has diminished.

As a group, physicians have opposed changes that would disperse power in the system, arguing that they are the most educated and knowledgeable of all health care providers and that their professional judgment should be accepted. Those favoring increased distribution of power have argued that more competition, more choice for consumers, and input from a greater variety of health care providers and from consumers will make the system more balanced and more responsive. Despite changes, physicians are still powerful in the health care system.

Consumer Power

The sources of power previously discussed present problems because the client is excluded. Clearly, the client is involved in only the most basic aspect of entry into the system: determining that he or she needs care. The client cannot enter any institution without the express approval of a physician. The client has no control over who becomes a primary care provider, and, with the advent of HMOs and PPOs, may have limited choice in selecting providers. Funding usually is controlled by third-party payers, and the client is often powerless to determine who will be paid, how much will be paid, and when payments will be made.

Consumers do have rights in the health care system. These are stated in different ways by different institutions and groups, but all revolve around the recognition of the health care consumer as an individual with the ability and right to be self-determining. As a general rule, consumers are not aware of their rights, and even when they are aware, they may be reluctant to take advantage of them. Consumers are in a particularly vulnerable position in the health care system. Because they put their lives in the hands of those in the system, they are often reluctant to complain or request changes for fear of offending those on whom they depend. In addition, when consumers try to exert power in the system, they may meet with resistance. Consumers are most often effective in exerting power in the system by working in groups and through established committees and agencies.

A health care consumer bill of rights was passed by the U.S. House of Representatives in 2001 and forwarded to the Senate. It did not pass, and no legislation has been considered since that time. According to the Kaiser Family Foundation, support for such legislation has decreased (Kaiser Family Foundation, 2006). In 2003 the American Hospital Association published "The Patient Care Partnership: Understanding Expectations, Rights, and Responsibilities". This document, which emphasizes that responsibilities accompany rights, is further discussed in Chapter 9.

Nurse Power

Nurses have had limited power in the health care system, a situation that has its roots in many of the traditional aspects of nursing discussed in Chapter 4. Change may not occur as rapidly as desired, and nurses often are frustrated because of their inability to influence the system. Many new graduates are especially distressed to learn that, as individuals, they cannot affect the system. Somehow they expect that if they speak with a voice of reason and act in the best interest of their clients, others will respond positively. But this may not happen. Nevertheless, things are changing in nursing. Nursing organizations are working to provide nurses with a voice at higher decision-making levels in health care. By understanding the political realities and the ways in which decisions are made, and by working together to speak with a united voice, nurses can increase their power in the system (see Chapter 3). Nursing education programs increasingly try to educate nurses to act as client advocates and agents of change (see Chapters 6 and 14). Collective bargaining and shared governance have provided nurses with mechanisms for demanding recognition of the importance of their role within the system (see Chapter 11).

There are a variety of implications for nurses in the current cost-control environment. The availability and accuracy of documents that reflect the acuity level and multiple problems of a client when records are audited for compliance is essential (determination of acuity level is discussed earlier in this chapter).

Critical Thinking Activity

Nurses are actively seeking power in the health care system. Consider the roles of nurses in the facilities with which you are familiar. How might nurses in these settings increase their power?

IMPLICATIONS FOR NURSES

Nurses have continuing interest and concern in the direction in which health care moves. They are most concerned about client well-being in the midst of a powerful system. As pressures to change increase, nurses continue to speak out for consumers. Who will help consumers cope with their health problems and those of their families? Who will assist them in negotiating the various parts of the health care system? Will the individual identities and unique needs of consumers be addressed, or will each person be treated as the mythical "standard client"? Nurses in home health agencies and long-term care facilities are caring for clients with complex nursing needs. A major concern is whether the reimbursement system provides adequate funds for quality nursing care to be delivered.

Another important concern of nurses is whether that aspect of health care that we call nursing, with its focus on the individual, will be maintained. Will the pressures for demonstrating cost-effectiveness result in a loss of caring because it is not always quantifiable? Will the system recognize the critical thinking skills and abilities of nurses as well as their technical skills? Will many educated and skilled nurses be replaced by unlicensed assistive personnel? The future poses many as yet unanswered questions.

There are ongoing concerns in the health care system relating to the actual use of health care services by the public and to the structure of the system itself. The impetus for change continues to grow. Several states already have instituted efforts to create a more coordinated health care system for their citizens. In the 1990s, the U.S. Congress considered several bills for health care reform, but none passed. After that time the pressure for health care reform at the federal level decreased as the party in power did not support it. No one can predict the details of the future system with certainty, but we have tried to point out the major changes now occurring and the directions in which the new health care system is moving. Nurses need to remain knowledgeable and involved in the political processes involved as changes are proposed in the health care system.

Critical Thinking Activity

Identify clients you have encountered from a variety of social, cultural, and economic backgrounds. Given these clients' needs and backgrounds, what type of practitioner would best meet their needs for primary care? What barriers might they meet in trying to gain access to primary care? What might you do to assist these individuals?

Key Concepts

- The various types of health care services are differentiated by the needs of the client being served and range from specific specialized services to skilled care to custodial care.
- Many different types of agencies provide health care services, including long-term care settings, acute care hospitals, ambulatory care centers, home care agencies, and health care businesses. There are a wide variety of nursing roles in these different settings. Health care agencies are classified according to length of stay, mix of services provided, and ownership of the agency.
- Acute care facilities center around the work of the traditional hospital, which has become a hub for health care in most communities.
- Long-term care facilities provide many types of care. Nursing homes provide care for those without the ability to manage ADLs and who need ongoing care. Assisted-living centers provide fewer services. Rehabilitation centers assist the individual in returning to a maximum level of independence.
- Ambulatory care settings provide care on an outpatient basis. This care may range from simple office calls for common illnesses and health promotion activities such as immunizations to the performance of ambulatory surgery.

- Home health agencies offer a wide variety of care services that may include traditional public health services, high-intensity skilled care in the home, and rehabilitation services. Home care agencies offer services within the home that assist individuals in avoiding institutional care settings when they are unable to complete their own ADLs.
- Changes in the health care delivery system are creating many problems that affect health care workers. Among these are issues related to primary care, accreditation of health professional education programs, and the future of health professional education and licensure.
- The financing of health care is complex and involves personal payment, insurance companies, HMOs, preferred providers, and governmental systems, each of which operates differently.
- Through control of financing, third-party payers exert control over all aspects of health care.
- Cost increases have created stress in the health care system. Understanding the basis of these increases is essential for planning to contain costs.
- Mechanisms for controlling costs and improving patterns of care have been instituted. These have included changing methods of payment, controlling health care providers, and managing care. The federal government has played a major role in the development and implementation of these mechanisms.
- Access to health care must be considered in terms of economic, geographic, and sociocultural access. A major concern in the system is those who do not have access.
- Quality of care is maintained by a wide variety of mechanisms. Institutions and agencies providing care receive oversight in the form of governmental approval and accreditation by certifying organizations.
- Quality is evaluated through peer review and the use of outcome measures, including key indicators and individual patient outcome standards.
- Power is exerted in the health care system by those who control finances, those who control access, and those with special knowledge. Traditionally, nurses and consumers have experienced little power in the system. Both are working to gain recognition and to affect more significantly the way the system functions.
- There are many implications for nurses in the financing and control of health care, including cost control, the well-being of the client, the effective use of health care resources, and changing the health care system.

Relevant Web Sites

Agency for Health Care Quality and Research (AHCQR): *www.ahcpr.gov*
Agency for Healthcare Research and Quality (AHRQ): *www.ahrq.gov*
American Pain Society: *www.ampainsoc.org*
Center for Medicare & Medicaid Services (CMS): *www.cms.hhs.gov*
Department of Health and Human Services (HHS): *www.hhs.gov/agencies*
Department of Veteran's Affairs (VA): *www.va.gov*
Foundation for Accountability (FACCT): *www.facct.org*
Healthy People 2010: *www.healthypeople.gov*
The Joint Commission: *www.jointcommission.org*
Medicare Information for the Consumer: *www.medicare.gov*

Medicare Part D Drug Benefit: *www.medicare.gov/medicarereform/drugbenefit.asp*
National Committee for Quality Assurance (NCQA): *www.ncqa.org*
National Guideline Clearinghouse: *www.guideline.gov*
National League for Nursing Accrediting Commission (NLNAC): *www.nlnac.org*
National Library of Medicine, MEDLINE database search through PubMed:
     www.pubmed.gov
TRICARE, Health Care for Military and their Dependents: *www.tricare.osd.mil*

References

American Health Insurance Plans Center for Policy and Research. (2005). Individual health insurance: A comprehensive survey of affordability, access, and benefits. Americas Health Insurance Plans [On-line] *www.ahipresearch.com/pdfs/ Individual_Insurance_Survey_Report8-26-2005.pdf*. Accessed February 26, 2006.

Agency for Health Care Research and Quality. (2006a). Inpatient quality indicators [On-line]. *www.qualityindicators.ahrq.gov/ iqi_download.htm*. Accessed February 22, 2006.

Agency for Health Care Research and Quality. (2006b). Patient safety indicators [On-line]. *www.qualityindicators.ahrq.gov/ psi_download.htm*. Accessed February 24, 2006.

Agency for Health Care Research and Quality. (2004a). Prevention Quality Indicators [On-line] *www.qualityindicators.ahrq. gov/pqi_download.htm*. Accessed February 24, 2006.

Agency for Health Care Research and Quality. (2004b). General questions about the AHRQ QIs. Rockville, MD: Agency for Healthcare Research and Quality [On-line]. *www.qualityindicators.ahrq.gov/general_faq.htm*. Accessed March 17, 2006.

Case Management Society of America (CMSA). *www.cmsa.org/ Aboutus/*. Accessed May 17, 2007.

Centers for Disease Control and Prevention, National Center for Health Statistics. (2002). National nursing home survey: 1999 summary. Vital and health statistics series 13 number 152 [On-line]. *www.cdc.gov/nchs/data/series/sr_13/sr13_152.pdf*. Accessed February 23, 2006.

Coile, R. C. (2001). Competing in a "consumer choice" market. *Journal of Healthcare Management 46*(5), 297–301.

Collopy, B., Boyle, P., & Jennings, B. (1991). New directions in nursing home ethics (A Hastings Center Report Special Supplement, March–April). *Hastings Center Report 21*(2), 1–16.

Decker, F. H. (2005). Nursing homes 1977–1999: What has changed, what has not: Data from the National Nursing Home Survey, Hyattsville, MD: National Center for Health Statistics [On-line]. *www.cdc.gov/nchs/data/nnhsd/NursingHomes 1977_99.pdf*. Accessed February 24, 2006.

Department of Health and Human Services. (1990). Healthy people 2010, Washington, DC: U.S. Government Printing Office [On-line]. *www.healthypeople.gov/document*. Accessed February 24, 2006.

Department of Health and Human Services. Health insurance and portability act [On-line]. *http://cms.hhs.gov/hipaa*. Accessed February 24, 2006.

Department of Health and Human Services. (2004). HHS agencies [On-line]. *www.hhs.gov/agencies*. Accessed February 24, 2006.

Dower, C., O'Neil, E., Hough, H. (2001). Profiling the professions: A model for evaluating emerging health professions, Center for the Health Professions, University of California [On-line]. *www.futurehealth.ucsf.ed/pd_files/Model2.pdf*. Accessed February 24, 2006

Fonda, S. J., Clipp, E. C., & Maddox, G. L. (2002). Patterns in functioning among residents in affordable assisted living housing facility. *Gerontologist 42*(2), 178–187.

Fries, B. E., & Geron, S. M. (n.d.). Home care quality indicators [On-line].   *www.ahrq.gov/news/ulp/stateltc/stateltc9.htm*. Accessed February 22, 2006.

Grabois, M. (2004). Health care reform: The looming battle and impact on rehabilitation medicine [On-line]. *www.aapmr. org/zdocs/assembly/handouts/C187_1.pdf*. Accessed February 22, 2006.

Haglund, C. L., & Dowling, W. L. (1993). The hospital. In S. J. Williams & P. R. Torrens, *Introduction to health service* (4th ed., pp. 135–176). New York: Delmar Publishers, Inc.

Health Insurance Portability and Accountability Act of 1996 *http://aspe.hhs.gov/admnsimp/pl104191.htm*. Accessed February 22, 2006.

Healthcare demand soars. (October 3, 2001). *The Herald*, p. A9, Everett, WA.

Hirdes J. P., Fries, B. E., Morris, J. N., Ikegami, N., Zimmerman, D., Dalby, D. M., et al. (2004). Home care quality indicators (HCQIs) based on the MDS-HC. *Gerontologist, 44*(5), 665– 679.

Inner turmoil. (2002). *Scientific American, 287*(1), 25–26.

Kaiser Family Foundation. (2004). State health facts [On-line]. *www.statehealthfacts.org/cgi-bin/healthfacts.cgi*. Accessed February 24, 2006.

Kaiser Family Foundation. (2005). State health policy [On-line]. *www.kff.org/statepolicy/index.cfm*. Accessed February 24, 2006.

Kaiser Family Foundation. (2006). The public, managed care, and consumer protection. Kaiser public opinion spotlight [On-line]. *www.kff.org/spotlight/managedcare/index.cfm*. Accessed February 24, 2006.

Kalisch, P. A., & Kalisch, B. J. (2004). *American nursing: A history* (4th ed.) Philadelphia: Lippincott Williams & Wilkins.

Kellerman, A. L. (2003). A shared destiny: The effects of the uninsured on individuals, families, and communities, A statement on behalf of the Committee on the Consequences of Uninsurance of the Institute of Medicine before the Subcommittee on Labor, Health and Human Services, and Education, Committee on Appropriations U.S. Senate [On-line]. *www7.nationalacademies.org/ocga/testimony/Health_Care_Access_Affordability.asp*. Accessed February 24, 2006.

Kirchheimer, B. (1999). Cutting the docs loose. *Modern Healthcare, 29*(36), 2.

National Association of Counties. (2003). Revisiting uncompensated care expenses: A report [On-line]. *www.house.gov/commerce_democrats/medicaidblockgrant/naco-report.pdf*. Accessed February 24, 2006.

National Center for Health Workforce Analysis. (December, 2000). The pharmacist workforce: A study of the supply and demand for pharmacists, U.S. Department of Health and Human Services, Health Resources and Services Administration, Bureau of Health Professions [On-line]. *http://bhpr.hrsa.gov/healthworkforce/reports/pharmacist.htm*. Accessed February 22, 2006.

National Center for Health Workforce Analysis. (July 2002). Projected supply, demand, and shortages of registered nurses: 2000-2020, U.S. Department of Health and Human Services, Health Resources and Services Administration, Bureau of Health Professions [On-line]. *http://bhpr.hrsa.gov/healthworkforce/reports/rnproject/report.htm*. Accessed February 22, 2006.

National Center for Health Workforce Analysis. (2004). State health workforce profiles, highlights from the 2000 profiles U.S. Department of Health and Human Services, Health Resources and Services Administration, Bureau of Health Professions [On-line]. *http://bhpr.hrsa.gov/healthworkforce/reports/profiles/*. Accessed February 22, 2006.

National League for Nursing Accrediting Commission. (2005). *Accreditation manual with interpretive guidelines by program type* (2005 ed.). New York: NLNAC.

O'Neil, E. H. (1993). Health professions education for the future: Schools in service to the nation. San Francisco, CA: Pew Health Professions Commission.

Owens, C. (1995). *Managed care organizations*. New York: McGraw-Hill.

Pew Health Profession Commission. (1995). *Critical challenges: Revitalizing the health professions for the twenty-first century*. San Francisco, CA: UCSF Center for the Health Professions.

Raffel, M. W., Raffel, N. K., & Barsukiewicz, C. K., (2001). *The U.S. health system: Origins and functions* (5th ed.). Clifton Park, NY: Thompson Delmar Learning.

Rosenthal, T. C., & Fox, C. (2000). Access to health care for the rural elderly. *Journal of the American Medical Association, 284*, 2034–2036.

Taber's cyclopedic medical dictionary (20th ed.). (2005). Philadelphia: F.A. Davis Co.

U.S. Census Bureau. (2004). U.S. interim projections by age, sex, race, and hispanic origin [On-line]. *www.census.gov/ipc/www/usinterimproj/*. Accessed March 17, 2006.

West, B. (2000). Assisted living gains accreditation option. *Provider, 26*(11), 53–54.

2

The Political Process in Society and in Nursing Organizations

LEARNING OUTCOMES

After completing this chapter, you should be able to:

1. Explain why it is important for nurses to be knowledgeable about and involved in the political process.
2. Discuss seven ways you might influence the political process.
3. Describe ways in which the current U.S. federal government is involved in health care.
4. Discuss common state legislative concerns.
5. Discuss common local political concerns.
6. Explain why there are so many nursing organizations.
7. Identify the major purpose of each nursing organization presented in the chapter.
8. Analyze the ways that nursing organizations seek to affect the health care delivery system and the political processes that control it.
9. Explain how politics is relevant to your participation in organizations.

KEY TERMS

Accreditation
Allocation of resources
Appropriations act
Authorization act
Conditions of participation
Department of Health and Human Services (HHS)

Hatch Act
Lobbying
Nurse Practice Act
Nurses Strategic Action Team (N-STAT)
Occupational Safety and Health Act (OSHA)

Omnibus Budget Reconciliation Act (OBRA)
Political action committees (PACs)
Politics
Tricouncil for Nursing
Whistleblower

Politics is the way in which people in any society try to influence decision making and the **allocation of resources** (money, time, and personnel). Because resources are limited, it is necessary to make choices regarding their use. There is no perfect process for making optimum choices, because whenever one valuable option is chosen, some other option must be left out. Politics is a part of every organization and a part of government at every level. In a democratic society, all individuals can choose to be involved at some level in this decision-making process. This chapter presents the political process, discusses some of the current issues regarding political decisions, and describes how nurses can play a role in the political arena and in nursing organizations.

RELEVANCE OF THE POLITICAL PROCESS FOR NURSES

Nurses always have been involved in politics. Florence Nightingale used her contacts with powerful men in government to obtain supplies and the personnel she needed to care for wounded soldiers in Crimea (Woodham-Smith, 1983). Hannah Ropes was able to fight incompetence and obtain decent care for wounded Civil War soldiers because she understood who was influential in Washington and who would be receptive to her efforts on the soldiers' behalf (Lienhard, 2002). Isabel Hampton used the buildup and excitement of the World's Fair and Columbian Exposition to bring together nurse leaders to form the first nursing organization (ANA, 1996).

Modern times are no different. With many voices competing to be heard in the decision-making circles of any nation, the person who understands power and politics is the one most likely to obtain the resources needed to accomplish desired ends.

In addition, health care is costly, and public dollars can be spent in many ways. What part of the federal budget should be allocated to health care? What part of the state budget? The local governmental budget? Of the money allocated, what part should be used for preventive health programs? What part for research? What part for care and treatment? What part for education? What diseases or conditions should be targeted for investigation? Who should receive those dollars? Where can more dollars be obtained? These questions are answered by legislation and by administrative decisions of governmental agencies.

Decisions also must be made at the level of the health care agency. What positions will be funded? What equipment purchased? What programs should be adopted and which of the current programs should be dropped? These questions are answered by committees, managers, and governing boards.

Nursing organizations are confronted with similar questions. What is the role of the organization? Should resources be spent on benefits for members? On activities relevant to the nursing profession as a whole? On activities related to general health care? In the political arena? How can nurses affect decision making? What is the individual's role as a nurse in the organization? These questions may be answered by representative assemblies, committees and commissions, and elected officers.

Your practice as a nurse is controlled by a wide variety of governmental decisions. One of the most basic is the **Nurse Practice Act** of your state or province. In that document, nursing is defined legally, and the scope of nursing practice is outlined. This document affects what you do each day that you practice. All of the philosophic discussions about the role of the nurse must return to the reality of the nurse's role as legally defined in the state's practice act. Do you care what that role is now or what changes are made in it? Does it make any difference to you what education that law requires, or if that law requires continuing education? Answering "yes" to any of these questions emphasizes the relevance of the political process for you.

Many decisions are made in the various nurses' organizations. These organizations speak for nurses in many settings. Are you happy with the way they are spending funds paid in dues? Do you agree with all of the public statements they make or position papers they publish? Do you support their mechanisms for decision making? Are you happy with the image of nurses and nursing the public receives from these organizations? Do you care what these organizations do with their resources? The political process is an important part of their functioning, too.

Knowing where the decision making occurs, who makes the decision, and being familiar with how you can influence that process is critical. Each governmental entity, agency, and organization has its own mechanism for operating. However, they share many similarities that can help you plan your activities.

Critical Thinking Activity

Identify a current health care issue in your state or province. Investigate that issue and form a position that you can support with data. Examine your position for personal biases.

INFLUENCING THE POLITICAL PROCESS

You can have an effect on such things as what health care legislation is submitted, the content of the legislation, and what legislation is passed. However, this does not happen without effort and action. Historically, women have been less active in politics than men. This has been the result of a variety of societal factors. Gradually, women are assuming a more active role in politics: More are being appointed the high offices within the government, more are running for and being elected to office, more work with policy-making bodies, and more vote. Because more than 94% of nurses are women, this changing social climate is important to nursing (Health Resources and Services Administration [HRSA], 2004). All women, and nurses in particular, have demonstrated increasing political awareness.

Each person must determine his or her own level of personal involvement, but there is, in the broad realm of the political process, room for everyone to find a suitable role. Some of these ways are outlined here and in Display 2-1.

Becoming Informed

To become informed about legislation and health care, you need to learn about the sources of information available. Each source of information is valuable to you but should be weighed based on its known biases. Even the most objective-sounding report can be biased, not only in

---

 Display 2-1   Influencing the Political Process

- Become informed through a variety of sources.
- Vote for candidates or ballot issues that reflect your concerns.
- Vote for officers within professional or political organizations.
- Express your opinions through letters or in public forums.
- Communicate directly with legislators and public officials.
- Work for or contribute to nonlobbying nursing organizations or political action committees.
- Work for or contribute to candidates who represent your views.
- Testify before decision-making bodies.

what is reported, but also in what is not reported. Identifying the groups that support or oppose a particular viewpoint might help you to recognize bias. Typically, do those groups take a liberal or a conservative stand on issues? Determine whether a group and its members would tend to gain or lose personally by the passage of proposed legislation. Are special interest groups voicing an opinion? When biases are evident, it is advisable to obtain information from groups with divergent viewpoints. Decisions based on firm factual data are more likely to benefit the entire group, organization, or society as a whole.

Once you are informed about the current issues in legislation or in an organization, you are better prepared to form personal opinions about them and to try to influence the outcome of the political process. A wide variety of resources are available.

News Media

Your daily newspaper or weekly news magazine can be an excellent source of information about significant legislation being proposed, when an issue is controversial, or when an issue has attracted widespread interest. When you rely on the newspaper for information, however, you sometimes learn of legislation only after it has already been passed.

Television and radio news reports are usually quite brief and give only an overview of a particular piece of legislation being introduced. This overview may be helpful in alerting you to something that you will want to study more intensively. Many radio commentators clearly speak from a particular viewpoint or bias. Remember to weigh information in light of that viewpoint and seek information more broadly. Some television programs, such as those on public television, do discuss issues in depth with commentators who hold different positions on an issue. In an attempt to meet the Federal Communications Commission rules regarding equal time, these programs usually make an attempt to present both sides of any issue.

Specialized Publications

Professional journals usually devote some space to current legislative issues. This is done routinely in *American Journal of Nursing* and *The American Nurse* in the United States and in *Canadian Nurse* in Canada. When major issues are being debated, other nursing periodicals often contain articles of interest. The journals of other health care professions also may carry information regarding current nursing issues. Newsletters and journals of organizations that have a political focus provide information on what they see as current issues. These organizations include consumer groups such as Common Cause, political groups such as the Young Democrats of America and Young Republicans, and nonpartisan groups such as the League of Women Voters. Magazines directed to special interest groups such as *AARP The Magazine* for those over the age of 50, carry articles related to political issues that would be of particular interest to that group.

Copies of legislation are usually available through your congressional representatives (for federal matters) and your state or provincial representatives (for state/provincial matters). Along with copies of the legislation, a legislator may send other informational material. Government agencies affected by proposed legislation also may provide information about the legislation's potential effects, although they are not allowed to try to influence legislation. You will find it helpful to understand the process of how a bill becomes a law to recognize where and when communication with a legislator might influence the process (Display 2-2).

Display 2-2 How a Bill Becomes a Law

House	Constituent	Senate
Representative introduces bill. Clerk of the House refers it to appropriate committee.	Start with your letter-writing campaign urging representatives and senators to cosponsor the legislation.	Senator introduces bill. Clerk of the Senate refers it to appropriate committee.
Committee chair refers bill to a subcommittee, which holds hearings to examine arguments for or against the bill.	Write to each subcommittee member. Place special emphasis on members from your state.	Committee chair refers it to a subcommittee, which holds hearings to examine arguments for or against the bill.
Subcommittee holds a 'mark-up' session to discuss and vote on the bill. A majority vote in favor moves the bill to full committee.	Request that your local paper print an article you've written. Meet with the paper's editorial board to urge its support.	Subcommittee holds a 'mark-up' session to discuss and vote on the bill. A majority vote in favor moves the bill to full committee.
Full committee reviews subcommittee hearing record and may hold additional hearings. A mark-up session is held and if the bill is approved it is reported to the full House.	Meet with your representative and senators in their home district offices. Send a copy of your paper's editorial to every member of the full committee.	Full committee reviews subcommittee record and may hold additional hearings. A mark-up session is held and if the bill is approved, it is reported to the full Senate.
Prior to the House vote, the Rules Committee sets the rules on length of debate and whether amendments are allowed.	Keep up your media campaign with letters to the editor, and call congress members' Washington offices to check their voting plans. Urge your friends to do the same.	Prior to the Senate vote, senators must unanimously agree to a time limit. There are seldom-used parliamentary maneuvers to get around this.
The bill passes if a majority approves it. / A bill can be expedited under 'suspension of the rules.' Suspension bills bypass Rules Committee, require a two-thirds vote for passage, and cannot be amended.	Let conference committee members know whether you prefer the House or the Senate version. Ask your representative and senators to lobby the conference committee.	The bill passes if a Senate majority approve it.
	Differences in House and Senate versions of bills are resolved in a conference committee comprised of senators and representatives from the bill's original committee.	
House votes on conference report.		Senate votes on conference report.
	When conference report is approved by both House and Senate, the bill goes to the President. If President vetoes, a two-thirds vote of both House and Senate is required to override.	

Internet Web Sites

Internet Web sites are an increasingly useful source of information. Federal legislation can be found at *http://thomas.loc.gov/*, a site maintained in the public interest by Congress. In most states, the text of bills being introduced is available on a governmental Web site, where you can read the bill on the computer or print the document to read. You can access state sites by going to *www.loc.gov/rr/news/stategov/stategov.html*. Nursing and health care organizations that maintain Web sites often have a site devoted to political issues affecting members of the organization or relevant issues that affect health care. The American Nurses Association (ANA), for example, maintains a legislative Web site at *http://nursingworld.org/gova/*. Many news organizations (television stations, newspapers, and magazines) maintain Web sites with information on current issues. Any of these sites may provide links to still more sites that provide useful information.

Organizational Meetings

Nursing organizations and other health-related organizations, as well as community groups, sometimes hold open meetings to present and discuss legislative issues. Often, knowledgeable speakers can help you to understand what is being proposed and the potential effects of a proposal. These organizations also may sponsor e-mail networks to get out information on important pending legislation. Nursing organizations can be excellent sources of information because they often are in touch with legislators and legislative staff.

EXAMPLE

Seeking Information About a Political Concern

Jeff Whitmore was a registered nurse (RN) in a long-term care facility. One day another nurse asked, "Do you know what this new change in the Medicare regulations will mean for us?" He replied, "I am not even sure what those changes are. I'll have to check on it." Once home, he went onto the Internet and began searching. He looked at the Web site for Medicare to see whether there was an announcement of changes in regulations. After reading the section on "Spotlight" that gave an overview of the changes, he then began looking for articles and other people's views of what was happening. He checked *http://nursingworld.org* to see what the ANA had to say. He thought about it for awhile and then decided that the organizations associated with nursing homes and long-term care might have information of value. After spending an hour researching the new regulations he felt that he understood them enough to discuss them with his colleague and began to form an opinion on what it might mean for their facility.

Voting

Your individual vote on a ballot issue is significant. Recent major elections in the United States have demonstrated how important every vote can be. One of the unfortunate statistics in the United States is that only 62% of citizens eligible to vote actually do so (McDonald, 2005). Many others are not eligible due to failure to register to vote. Nurses, as a group, vote in higher percentages than the general population. When legislators hear statistics such as "1 in 17 women voters is a nurse," or "1 in every 44 voters is a nurse" (Grieschar-Billiard, 2000 p. 6.), they pay attention to the opinions of nurses. Although you cannot vote directly on legislative issues, you can vote for candidates whose positions you support on initiatives and referendums and who share your values. Absentee ballots are always available for those who cannot be present at their polling place on the day of an election. These ballots must be requested well in advance of the election, however.

Voting for officers in organizations may be ignored by a large majority of members. They look at the ballot, cannot identify those running for office, and therefore do not vote. Most organizations do make an attempt to introduce members to the various candidates. If you do not know the candidates, you can seek information about them by reading their prepared statements of position and learning about their previous activities. Those elected to office usually determine the direction and priorities of an organization. If you are contributing your dues dollars, you want to have a voice in choosing those who are entrusted with making the decisions.

Shaping Public Opinion

Public opinion does influence the actions of legislators and regulatory bodies. As an RN, you can help to shape public opinion; your judgment about matters that affect health care can help others make their own decisions. Share the knowledge you have gained through your personal experience and research. Do not be afraid to state your own position, although you must be prepared to support your position with evidence if you want to be considered a thoughtful health care professional. Certainly, you will not want to make every social occasion an opportunity to share political positions, but do take advantage of opportunities that arise to present your concerns to others (Fig. 2-1).

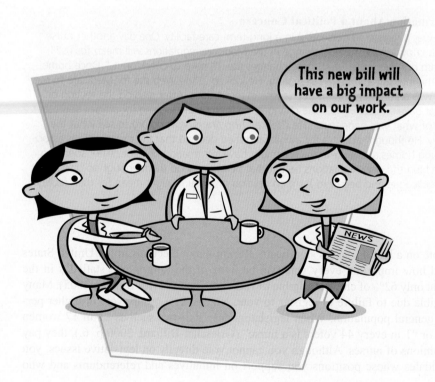

This new bill will have a big impact on our work.

FIGURE 2-1 Sharing your opinions is one avenue of political involvement.

■■ COMMUNICATION IN *ACTION*
■■

> Ed Johnson, a nurse in a long-term care facility, is in a group discussing events of the day. The issue of government regulation of nursing homes arises. One member of the group states, "The government ought to get out of everybody's way and let the professionals doing the work make the decisions. Legislators and bureaucrats have no idea of how to manage a nursing home." Ed responds, "From my perspective as a nurse in a nursing home, I view regulations differently than you appear to. The regulations have, for the most part, made nursing homes more accountable to patients and families and more focused on the quality of care. While the regulations are sometimes difficult to meet, for the most part they focus on important concerns. The movement toward restraint-free environments, for example, has been supported by regulations limiting the use of restraints."

Another means of shaping public opinion is by writing a letter to the editor of a newspaper or news magazine. Editorial letters are read by many people. The suggestions in Display 2-3 will maximize your chances of appearing in print.

Within an organization, you may also influence opinion and action by clearly presenting reasoned arguments. You can discuss issues with other members and present your opinion at meetings. Remember that a viewpoint supported by strong, reasoned judgment and rationale will be better received than a simple statement of opinion.

Communicating With Legislators and Officials

Legislators are affected by the views of their constituents. The legislator's staff reviews incoming letters, tabulates views, and directs letters with significant opinions or information to the legislator for individual consideration. Although some groups encourage members to sign form letters or postcards, personal letters have a greater impact.

Concern regarding the rules and regulations of a specific department of government can be addressed to the officials of that department. It is possible for officials to become insulated from the effects of their decision making. Communication from concerned citizens can be as important

---

Display 2-3   Writing Letters to the Editor

- Carefully follow the instructions provided by the publication for letters to the editor. These usually will refer to length, signature, address, and telephone number. Typically, letters should be short and to the point, about 200 to 300 words.
- Clearly present your opinion with well-reasoned arguments. Make only one point per letter.
- Including personal experiences that illustrate health care concerns can be useful; however, be careful that health care examples do not violate the confidentiality of clients or divulge confidential information regarding your employer.
- Use a direct but respectful tone. Avoid personal attacks on others.
- Include your name, address, and phone number as well as your nursing credentials after your name.
- If responding to a particular article, give the title of the article and include the date of publication in parentheses.

to them as it is to legislators. To be most effective, letters addressed to officials should reflect the same care and professional viewpoint as those addressed to legislators.

A carefully written personal letter reflecting thoughtful and informed opinions on an issue will receive the most attention from any governmental person or department. As an RN, your expertise can provide a valuable viewpoint. Identify yourself as an RN in your letter and outline why you are concerned about the issue in question. Legislators often appreciate personal anecdotes from your practice (with identities concealed, of course) that underscore your point. The names and addresses of your congressional representatives are available on the Senate and House Web sites. Go to *www.firstgov.gov* and link to the House or Senate. These sites also explain who serves on which committees. Canada maintains a similar site at *http://canada.gc.ca/main_e.html*. The names and contact information for your individual state representatives also are linked online from the ANA Government Affairs page *http://nursingworld.org/gova*. Additional information about effective communication with legislators also is provided by the ANA from this same Web site. The Canadian Nurses Association maintains a similar Web site at *www.cna-nurses.ca/CNA/issues/matters/default_e.aspx*. Information about provincial officials is available on the Web site of each individual province.

Many governmental agencies, both legislative and regulatory, accept letters in the form of e-mail. E-mail has the advantage of being extremely timely. However, be aware of the rules for Internet usage at your facility. Although you may have e-mail access at your place of work, your employer may not allow you to use it for political activity. If you are employed by a government entity, such as a public health department, the law prohibits you from using governmental resources such as e-mail for political activity.

An e-mail message should be composed as carefully as a letter. One important point is to include your full name and home address in your message. Staff members review the address, forwarding only those messages that are personally identifiable and noting those from a congressperson's district. Do remember that e-mail is public. Do not state things in an e-mail that would make you feel uncomfortable to present in public. See Display 2-4 for an example.

You may make a telephone call to a legislator's office. Staff members keep a record of all calls, and the positions of callers are noted. To call a member of Congress, contact the U.S. Capitol Switchboard at (202) 224-3121 and ask for the individual's office. In some states, a toll-free number is maintained for calls to state legislators during the legislative session. You will be asked to leave a message. Be sure to identify yourself fully, including both your name and address. State the bill or issue about which you are calling and clearly state your position.

Visiting congressional or state representatives also is an effective means of expressing your concerns. One of the best ways to arrange to speak with congressional representatives and senators is to contact their local offices. Through these offices you may receive assistance in arranging your visit. Staff members may help you to arrange other interesting and valuable activities, such as attending committee hearings, taking tours, and observing Congress in session. Make appointments well in advance, as representatives and senators have busy schedules. If your time is limited, you may have to modify your expectations and meet with a staff member who will relay your concerns. Plan carefully for your visit; it is helpful to write out concerns and questions. Be sure to leave time for answers to the questions that you pose. Even when you disagree with the position taken by your legislator, be polite and present your concerns calmly. Rudeness could result in the legislator's unwillingness to listen to what you have to say.

Some legislators hold public meetings (often referred to as "town hall" meetings) in their legislative districts for the purpose of hearing from their constituents. These meetings can be

Display 2-4   A Carefully Written E-mail

Re: House Bill 1458 Safe Patient Handling

Dear Representative Smith:

As a registered nurse constituent in your legislative district, I urge you to support passage of this important legislation. As a nurse in a hospital, I am familiar with the care needs of dependent individuals. Unfortunately, the current solution to care has been to urge care providers to lift and move patients, resulting in injuries, lost work, and even lost careers for the caregivers. I personally know two registered nurses who have become unable to work as nurses after sustaining back injuries in moving incapacitated patients. In addition to the human cost, the community cannot sustain the loss of needed registered nurses when there is such a shortage. There are now many effective lifting and transfer devices available for purchase. This legislation will provide the impetus for health care agencies to purchase them and implement their use. Thank you for your attention to this important matter.

Mary K. Winslow, RN
2314 12th Ave.
Seattle, WA 98201
Phone: (206) 981-1234

both an opportunity to learn about issues and the legislator's current position and to give input regarding issues of concern to you. If you bring written materials to support your viewpoint, these may be given to the legislator and further reinforce your position.

These same activities may be useful in working within an organization. Those elected to office do not know the views of members unless communication occurs. For communication to be effective, you must know when and where boards meet, how to get information to board members, and the names of those responsible for specific aspects of the organization's operations.

Critical Thinking Activity

Identify a current political issue about which you feel strongly. Write a letter or an e-mail to a governmental official that provides a sound rationale in support of your position. Ask someone else to review it for you and then send it.

Group Action

The political process in the nursing profession takes many forms. Nurses can be involved as individuals, but they are far more effective when they work in groups. Because nursing is the largest single health care occupation, nurses have many votes. For this reason, legislators pay attention to positions held by groups of nurses.

Nonlobbying Nursing Organization Efforts

Most traditional nursing organizations are nonprofit groups and therefore are limited in their political activity. The major role of nonprofit groups in politics involves testifying to facts, organizational positions, and concerns in the health care arena. The ANA has an office in Washington, DC, and tries to keep the nursing profession informed about legislative matters of importance in health care. The ANA also provides experts in the nursing profession who testify before congressional and regulatory groups about proposed legislation.

The **Tricouncil for Nursing** is a collaborative effort of the ANA, the National League for Nursing (NLN), the American Organization of Nurse Executives (AONE), and the American Association of Colleges of Nursing (AACN). It represents the interests of nursing practice, research, and education. By working collaboratively, these organizations have strengthened the voice of nursing and its visibility in Washington, DC. This coalition has become the trusted representation for nursing. Legislators rely on the information it provides and recognize it as a united voice for the nursing profession.

The ANA organized the **Nurses Strategic Action Team (N-STAT)** to provide nurses with a means to mobilize quickly to influence legislative policy. This organization promotes grassroots involvement in legislative issues, meets with members of Congress, and organizes letter-writing and telephone campaigns. Interested nurses can sign up to be a part of N-STAT on the *http://nursingworld.org* Web site. Those registered with N-STAT receive a message about an issue of importance along with information and resources on how to contact legislators. N-STAT includes thousands of nurses. You can imagine that receiving thousands of letters about a single topic might get the attention of a legislator.

Another effort by the ANA to inform nurses about legislative issues is *Capitol Update*, a legislative newsletter for nurses found at *www.capitolupdate.org/newsletter*. This publication brings the latest in legislative concerns to your attention on a regular basis throughout the year.

Many specialty nursing organizations have a political action interest as well. Their Web sites and publications often provide information about issues of concern, and the organization may provide expert testimony for legislators.

Most state and district nurses' associations have legislative committees that monitor legislative and regulatory actions in their areas. They may provide educational events for nurses regarding current issues and testify at hearings concerning health-related issues. They also may seek to mobilize letter-writing or telephone campaigns.

Political Action Committees

Lobbying is the process of attempting to influence legislators to take a particular action. The law differentiates lobbying from providing general information and places restrictions on who can lobby. Nonprofit groups such as the ANA can provide information but cannot take direct action on behalf of specific candidates or partisan issues. To take a more active role in seeking the passage of desired legislation, the defeat of undesired measures, and the election of particular candidates, groups form organizations called political action committees (PACs). These organizations are registered as political action groups and are free to try to affect the political process. They are not considered nonprofit organizations because their funds are used for political purposes; therefore, donations to them are not tax deductible (Fig. 2-2).

The ANA political action organization is titled the ANA-Political Action Committee (ANA-PAC). ANA-PAC actually lobbies for the passage or defeat of bills and supports candidates for public office.

FIGURE 2-2 Nurses may lobby to get desired legislation passed by visiting legislators, by presenting information and arguments about the bill, and by writing letters.

Since the 1976 federal elections, ANA-PAC has raised funds to support candidates for the Senate and the House of Representatives based on their expressed and demonstrated stands on key health issues, such as health care reform proposals, funding for nursing and biomedical research, funding for nursing education, and third-party reimbursement for nurses. Not all candidates endorsed by ANA-PAC were supported financially because of the limited funds available. Candidates' successes are attributable to many factors, but the effect of nursing support has been demonstrated. Many state nursing associations also have political action organizations. These groups serve the same function on the state level as ANA-PAC does on the national level. Many candidates actively seek the endorsement of nursing organizations that are perceived as influential with voters.

Although these nursing political action groups have not grown rapidly, they have grown steadily. In addition, nurses are gaining more sophistication in their approach to the political process. Through their combined financial contributions, nurses can significantly help a candidate or issue. All of these factors have resulted in nurses gaining increased power in the political sphere. There is still a long way to go before nurses have the same kind of power that is wielded by those in labor, education, and medicine, but change is occurring.

Critical Thinking Activity

Locate your state nurses' association Web site. Identify the issues that the organization believes are important to nurses in the state. Investigate those issues and identify ways you could support one of the issues presented.

Other Politically Important Groups

Many organizations, in addition to those specifically related to nursing, are concerned about health and social issues. Some are official lobbying groups; others provide information resources. Groups such as Common Cause (a consumer lobbying group), AARP (formerly the American Association of Retired Persons), the League of Women Voters, and even church organizations often act to affect the political process. You may support these groups by donating money for their needs or by being actively involved in their work.

Testifying for Decision-Making Bodies

Many decisions affecting nursing and health care are made by committees and commissions at various levels of government. These decision-making bodies often hold hearings to gather information before decisions are made. As a nurse, your testimony may have particular value in certain areas of health care. A nurse may testify either as an official representative of an organization or as an independent individual.

You may learn of opportunities to testify through announcements in the newspaper and professional publications. In general, you must register in advance to testify. In some instances, there is registration at the door before a meeting begins, but for more formal situations, you will need to notify the committee in advance that you wish to testify. Increasingly, you can sign up online to testify.

If you have an opportunity to testify, be sure to make your position clear so that the decision makers know whether you speak for yourself or for a larger group. Keep your testimony brief and concise. Prepare your testimony ahead of time (with copies for committee members), but do not simply read a statement. A less-formal presentation is usually more interesting for the listener. Be prepared with sources for any facts or figures you present and explain any technical terms you use. Find out whether there is a time limit for each testimony. If you are given a time limit, make sure that you present your most important arguments and facts first. Most committees will accept written testimony if you cannot be there in person, but the personal presentation is usually more effective.

Individual Support for Legislation and Candidates

You may choose to personally support a specific piece of legislation by contributing money for publicity and campaigning, posting political signs, visiting door-to-door, sponsoring coffee hours, or working on a committee that is striving for the passage of a proposal. Both time and money are valuable to every candidate. Funds are needed for newspaper ads, television and radio announcements, and printing and distributing literature. Workers may be needed to perform secretarial tasks, contact people in a door-to-door campaign, and speak on behalf of the issue.

Supporting a candidate for public office is accomplished in the same way. In our political system, the reality is that those who have actively supported a candidate during an election campaign are listened to more closely when decisions are being made. Working for a candidate is one way to make your view known. It is also an excellent way to gain firsthand knowledge of the political process.

EXAMPLE

Working in a Political Campaign

Inge Helgeson was an RN working in a community health center that provided health care on a sliding scale fee for homeless, unemployed, and low-income residents of their service area. She was distressed when she learned that one of the two candidates for county executive had announced that there was really no need for such health services and they should be cut back as a budgetary reduction. The opposing candidate, however, made a strong proposal for strengthening the role of the community health clinics. Inge decided to call the candidate who was supporting community health and volunteer to work on the campaign. She spent one evening a week on a phone bank. She called residents, explained the issues, and asked for their vote for her candidate. When it was time for the election, she said to a colleague at work, "For the first time I feel as if I am really doing something about the problem, not just watching while others do all the work."

Working in Policy-Making Agencies

Nurses have been appointed to major administrative positions in state and federal health agencies and to the staffs of several senators and representatives. In these roles, they have major policy-making responsibilities. Knowledgeable nurses may be appointed to task forces that study health care concerns and recommend regulatory or legislative action. The Robert Wood Johnson Foundation has provided 1-year fellowships for nurses to study policy in Washington, DC. Nurses who complete these fellowships have the skills and abilities to be effective in influencing health care policy. All of this points to nurses having a promising future in the health policy arena.

Seeking Election to an Office

Those elected or appointed to an office, whether in a local nursing organization or the U.S. Congress, have the power to affect outcomes considerably. Leaders in nursing organizations help to shape the direction and efforts of those organizations. Legislators have power to affect significant regulations and spending plans. Nurses in several states have been effective in shaping health policy by being elected to office as members of their state legislatures. Eddie Bernice Johnson, elected as a congresswoman from Texas in 1994, was the first nurse to hold an elective federal office and still serves in that role. As women in general become more politically visible, nursing as a whole feels the impact. Each year more nurses are elected to political office.

Limitations on Your Political Activity

If you are an employee of any government agency, such as a public health department or the Veterans Administration, your political activity is subject to restrictions that do not apply to the general public. Restrictions applying to federal government employees are defined in the **Hatch Act** (5 USCA 7324) revision of 1993 (Hatch Act, 1993). Prohibited activities are mainly those that have to do with supporting a particular political party by being an officer or party spokesperson. The Hatch Act also prohibits any political activity on the part of a government employee, on behalf of a party or in support of legislation, that could be construed as representing his or her government agency.

The Hatch Act does not interfere with a private citizen's right to support parties and candidates financially, to join political parties, to work for or against measures that will appear on a ballot, or to participate in nonpartisan (ie, not connected with a political party) elections as a candidate.

Each state has its own version of the Hatch Act. If you are employed by a government agency of any kind, investigate the limitations that your employment may place on your political activity.

THE FEDERAL GOVERNMENT'S ROLE IN HEALTH CARE

Federal legislation affects nursing and health care in important ways. If you understand key concepts of the federal government's involvement in health care and how federal legislation affects health care delivery, you will be more effective in the political arena.

Federal Agencies Related to Health Care

The federal government operates in the health care field in complex ways. Literally dozens of federal agencies are involved with health care in some way. The **Department of Health and Human Services (HHS)** is a cabinet-level administrative unit of the federal government with four major service divisions (Display 2-5).

The Public Health Service, which includes the Centers for Disease Control and Prevention (CDC), is one agency with which you should already be familiar. The National Institutes of Health (NIH), the Food and Drug Administration, the Health Resources Administration, and the Center for Medical & Medicare Services (CMS) are all part of HHS. This agency has tremendous impact through its rules and regulations and the projects it funds.

The Federal Budget Process

Because funding is a driving force in all decision making, you will find it useful to understand something of the federal budget process. The availability of government funding for each federal program depends on two legislative actions. The first action is the **authorization act**. This is a bill, passed by both the House of Representatives (where any revenue bill must originate) and the Senate that describes a program and outlines the rules under which funds for the program can be expended. It also sets a ceiling on the amount of money that can be provided. It is under these authorization acts (often referred to by the title of the section of the authorizing act) that funds are dispensed for all the health-related activities described in this chapter.

Display 2-5   Major Service Divisions of the Department of Health and Human Services

Office of Human Development Services
Administration on Aging
Administration for Child, Youth, and Families
Administration for Native Americans
Administration for Public Service

Public Health Service
Centers for Disease Control and Prevention
Food and Drug Administration
Health Resources Administration
Health Services Administration
National Institutes of Health
Alcohol, Drug Abuse, and Mental Health
   Administration

Social Security Administration
Systems
Governmental Affairs
Family Assistance
Hearings and Appeals
Operational Policy and Procedure Assessment

Health Care Financing Administration
Health Standards and Quality Bureau
Bureau of Quality Control
Bureau of Program Operations
Bureau of Program Policy
Bureau of Support Services
Office of Child Support Enforcement

The second necessary legislative action is the **appropriations act**. The appropriations process establishes the federal budget and the specific amounts of money appropriated for actual spending for each previously authorized program. Both the House and the Senate pass a budget appropriations act. Then a joint House and Senate committee meets to achieve a compromise that both will accept. The final result is called the **Omnibus Budget Reconciliation Act (OBRA)**, and it includes the compromises the budget committee has worked out between the House and Senate versions of the budget. Each budget act—for example, OBRA 2004—is identified by the year in the title. This is sometimes confusing because two monetary amounts, the authorized amount and the final budgeted (or appropriated) amount, may be reported in connection with the same act.

The budget act also may place restrictions on the people and organizations receiving federal funds. It is under this authority that the federal government sets standards for nursing homes that receive reimbursement through Medicaid and Medicare. The rules and regulations for nursing homes, called the **conditions of participation (COPs)**, included in OBRA 1987, were extensive and included such issues as restraint reduction, nursing assistant training, and resident privacy. These rules and regulations did not take effect until October 1, 1990. This allowed the affected organizations to begin the process of change to meet the new requirements.

COPs for Medicare continue to have great effects on health care systems as they are revised. For example, in 2001 when the COPs were being revised to delete nurse anesthetists from payment unless overseen by an anesthesiologist, there was consternation in many places where nurse anesthetists are the primary anesthesia providers. The COPs were then modified to allow for states to opt out of this provision through state legislation determining it is in the best interests of the state's citizens to not follow this requirement. In 2005, the COPs were revised to allow dispensers for alcohol-based hand cleaners to be placed in hallways (they had previously been prohibited in that location as a fire safety measure) (CMS, n.d. Spotlight).

Historically, a third factor has affected the amount of money available for a specific federal program: the participation of the executive branch of government in decisions regarding how and when available funds will be spent. If money that has been authorized and appropriated has not been spent by the end of a budget period, it is lost. This money then must be reauthorized and re-appropriated. The executive branch has used this mechanism to withdraw support for programs it opposes.

Funding for Nursing Education and Research

Beginning in 1964, the federal government provided funding to support nursing education through the Nurse Training Act, later called the Nurse Education Act, signed by President Bush in 2002 as the Nurse Reinvestment Act. In the 1960s and early 1970s, the funding was generous and included money for buildings, classroom renovation, equipment, faculty education and development, and student scholarships and traineeships. As the shortage of nurses abated and priorities changed in Washington, DC, the amount of funding declined. The current nurse shortage has once again resulted in political pressure by nursing organizations for the designation of funds for nursing education.

Every 2 years, when the biennial budget is passed, nurses try to rally congressional support for additional funding for nursing education. With the current nursing shortage, more groups are supporting nursing efforts to increase support for nursing education. Legislators are more open to discussions of the major needs of nursing. However, budget deficits at all levels of government arrived at the same time that the need for funds for nursing has increased.

A major advance for nursing research in the 1980s was the addition of a National Institute for Nursing Research (NINR) to the other major divisions of the NIH. Nurses and nursing organizations lobbied long and hard for legislative authorization for this institute. It is now a major financial source of nursing research dollars. Nursing groups continue to lobby for increases in the appropriation for the NINR. However, even the existence of the NINR is not guaranteed. Proposals for reorganizing the work and research conducted in all areas of health care have included the elimination of many specialty institutes and a different method of focusing research. Many nurses view this proposal with alarm because nursing research does not claim the high profile of disease-specific research.

Occupational Safety and Health

The **Occupational Safety and Health Act (OSHA)** mandates actions and prescribes safety equipment to improve the health and safety of the working environment. Many people think the rules and regulations created by OSHA are too cumbersome. Nevertheless, concern for the safety of the working person is of considerable importance to nurses. Occupational injuries create major health problems for the adult population. They are costly not only in terms of health and personal loss but also in terms of lost productivity. Nurses also are affected by the provisions of OSHA in their own work environments. They, too, are subject to injury and accident on the job. The safety concerns of nurses in the workplace are discussed in Chapter 15.

Nurses in occupational health nursing are involved in OSHA through educating workers about job safety. In some situations, using safety precautions may be time-consuming and physically uncomfortable, and workers may be tempted to ignore them. Nurses may be able to curb this by helping workers understand the importance of following health and safety regulations. Occupational health nurses also assist management in planning to make the environment safe and in establishing appropriate procedures for treating injuries.

OSHA regulations have required health care employers to provide the equipment, supplies, immunizations, and education to enable the implementation of CDC recommendations for universal precautions. The antiregulatory stance of Congress since 1994 has been reflected in the failure of OSHA to upgrade infection-control requirements to the CDC recommendation for Standard Precautions.

More recently, OSHA has been investigating the effects of repetitive strain injuries, among which are back injuries in health care workers. Funds for National Academy of Sciences research related to the link between repetitive motions and workplace injuries were included in the 1999 fiscal year (FY) appropriation, but have not been renewed since that time. OSHA regulations regarding prevention of this type of injury were developed, but they were not implemented during the Clinton presidency. These regulations were rescinded by the new Congress after President G. W. Bush took office. In 2003, the ANA launched Handle With Care, a campaign focusing on solutions to the problem of musculoskeletal injuries among caregivers. Since that time, some states have passed legislation regarding safe patient handling in hospitals and nursing homes. Manufacturers are providing a greater variety of lifting and moving equipment, and many facilities are developing policies that promote greater safety in patient handling. The ANA supports these efforts with information and resources for nurses and associations addressing this issue (ANA, 2005, *http://nursingworld.org/handlewithcare*).

However, there is a "general duty" clause in the OSHA regulations that states that employers "must provide each employee a place of employment which is free from recognized hazards that are causing or likely to cause death or serious physical harm to his employees" (OSHA, Section 5A, 2004). Under this clause, if the hazard is recognized, if it can cause serious harm, and if there are reasonable methods to avoid that hazard, the employer may be cited for failure to maintain safety. This general duty clause is now being directed toward health care workplace concerns such as infection and repetitive strain injuries.

Another occupational concern to nurses is needlestick injuries. OSHA has mandated that all health care agencies have in place a blood-borne pathogens prevention program. This includes training for both behaviors of staff and what are termed "engineering" controls. Engineering controls are the use of safe equipment that does not rely solely on the action of the individual to maintain protection. The FY 1999 appropriations bill included a requirement that employers record all injuries from potentially contaminated needles and other sharp instruments. The CDC, in November 1999, changed its recommendation to include the use of safe needles (National Institutes for Occupational Safety and Health, 1999, *www.cdc.gov/niosh*). In 2000, the federal Needlestick Safety and Prevention Act was passed. This requires that hospitals provide safer devices to prevent needlestick injury. Several states have introduced needle safety legislation, and the prevention of needlestick injuries continues to be a focus of concern (Nelson, 2004.)

Another safety concern of health care workers is violence in the workplace. Nurses in psychiatric settings have long recognized the hazards they face in working with aggressive, violent, and sometimes out-of-control clients. Emergency rooms are sites where the violence of society spills over into the health care setting. Even obstetric units may encounter violence by family members. Nurses are asking that OSHA mandate health care workplaces to provide safety from violence. See Chapter 11 for a further discussion of violence in the workplace.

■■ COMMUNICATION IN *ACTION*
■ ■

Mobilizing Support for Safety Measures in the Workplace

Irma Gunderson was an RN in the emergency room of a large urban hospital. There had been several instances when friends of patients had become belligerent and threatening to the staff, but there were no plans in place for managing staff safety. Irma began talking with her nurse manager. She said, "I was here the two evenings when those visitors threatened doctors, nurses, and others on the staff. I believe that we need to develop policies of how to manage such instances." Her manager replied, "What is the problem? I wasn't here those evenings, but I think the staff did fine—no one was hurt and the patient was cared for." Irma then said, "I was really afraid, and it is affecting my work. I have talked to some of the others on the evening shift and some of them even have nightmares. Millie the receptionist said she is going to ask for a transfer because she doesn't want to be here the next time it happens. We don't have a clear plan of how to call security, what people are supposed to do, and what our rights are in terms of protecting ourselves." The manager said, "No one else has said anything." Irma said, "I think they believe that nothing can be done. I have done some reading and I have learned that other hospitals have extensive plans in place. Could we get a committee together to investigate some of those and make some recommendations?" The manager said, "I appreciate your talking with me. I will talk with the management team tomorrow and maybe we can get something started here." By speaking directly to the person in charge who had the authority to initiate change, by having specific instances and concerns, Irma had facilitated improving the workplace climate.

Nursing Home Regulations

OBRA 1987 contained regulations that for the first time mandated a national standard for quality of care in nursing homes receiving federal money through Medicare or Medicaid. Although the provisions of this act were set to take effect in October 1990, there were delays because of legal challenges to the requirements and because of the extra time that was needed to establish monitoring mechanisms. This is not unusual when legislation requires difficult and costly implementation. Therefore, some of the provisions of OBRA 1987 took effect as late as 1994. Despite earlier concerns, it is now clear that these regulations have positively affected the care environment in nursing homes. The use of restraints has decreased, resident rights are more effectively supported, and basic care needs are identified and met. More recently, the budget bill for 1999 established a prospective payment system for skilled nursing facilities that resulted in decreased payments from Medicare and Medicaid.

THE STATE GOVERNMENT'S ROLE IN HEALTH CARE

Many issues that vitally affect the health care arena are decided at the state level. Because the health care issues in each state are different, only some general areas of concern are outlined here.

State Agencies and Health Care

State institutions range from those that care for the mentally retarded and the mentally ill to penal systems and institutions of higher education. Health care is a consideration in all of these settings. When budgets are planned, topics as diverse as immunization and contraception may be part of the debate. Nurses often can advocate for those who are unable to speak for themselves about their own health care needs. Sometimes nurses who work in these settings are unable to deliver quality care because of severe budgetary deficiencies. All nurses can support efforts to provide quality health care in such settings.

Nurse Practice Acts

Nurse practice acts are being discussed and revised in many states. This process is long and difficult and requires intense political effort by nurses to avoid creating problems for the profession. One current concern about placing the act before a state legislature for change is that the legislature might lessen the standards or allow unlicensed assistive personnel to perform more nursing tasks because of the nursing shortage. Another concern is the implementation of multistate licensure. See Chapter 7 for further discussion of licensure laws.

State Legislative Concerns

Some of the major workplace concerns of nurses are emerging as topics of state legislation. The ANA has identified nine major state-level legislative issues of importance to nurses (see Display 2-6). In some states legislation has already been passed regarding some of these issues. Concerns about the nurse's vulnerability when unsafe care is part of an institution's practice have led to efforts toward achieving whistleblower protection. A **whistleblower** is a person who reports to authorities the wrongdoing of individuals in their own work setting or the organizations in which they are employed. The state of New Jersey was the first to pass legislation that protects from retaliation health care employees who refuse to participate in or who report unsafe practices. The federal government encourages whistleblowing to reveal fraud in the Medicare and Medicaid programs and posts information on how to report fraud on its Web site (CMS, n.d.).

Many of the state-level issues, such as prohibition of mandatory overtime, nursing staffing systems and ratios, and safety in the workplace, relate to increasing workplace satisfaction. Improving working conditions is an important aspect of addressing the nursing shortage. These issues will be discussed in greater detail in Chapter 11.

Display 2-6   State-Level Legislative Concerns Identified by ANA

- Prohibition of mandatory overtime
- Nurse staffing systems and ratios
- Nursing workforce data collection
- Nursing education incentives
- Ergonomics
- Needlestick injury prevention
- Nursing quality indicators
- Violence in the workplace
- Whistleblower protection

LOCAL POLITICAL CONCERNS

The budgetary process seems to be at the root of most political and legislative concerns. Because only a limited amount of money is available, budgets always are developed through a series of compromises. To gain one objective, it is sometimes necessary to recognize that funds will not be available for achieving another. In most communities, budgets for public health departments, school nurses, and so forth are developed over a period of several months. Hearings are often held, at which members of the public may ask questions and address issues. Nurses often have found that involvement at this planning stage is most rewarding. Determining priorities for health care is essential, and nurses can speak with authority on these matters. Nurses actually employed in a public department undergoing review may be limited in making their views known because of regulations governing their action in the political sphere. For this reason, it is significant that nurses outside of government institutions recognize the importance of community health. It is not only the practice of the public health nurse that is affected by the priorities of the agency. For example, a nurse who is employed in a hospital may wish to refer a discharged patient to a public health nurse for follow-up, only to find that, owing to changes in the ordering of priorities, home visits for the identified purpose are no longer being made.

In many communities, decisions about the allocation of federal money are made at the local level. Recent congressional actions have leaned toward enhancing state and local control through creating large block grants where priorities would be decided locally. Support for alternative health care centers, blood pressure screening, and senior citizen centers may depend on whether those who are knowledgeable about the benefits of these services are willing to voice their advocacy in local decision-making bodies.

HEALTH CARE REFORM

Financing health care for all citizens has been the focus of many efforts for health care reform. Again and again the failure of the U.S. health care system to provide care for all individuals is highlighted. As the number of people without insurance rises and the cost of insurance for those who have it continues to escalate, common questions recur:

- Do people have a right to health care?
- If there is such a right, what level of health care can people expect to receive? Routine preventive services? Surgery and hospitalization for all conditions? Or treatment only for serious, life-threatening conditions?

- Should catastrophic illnesses, transplantation, and experimental treatments and medications be included?
- What about fertility-enhancing services? Should contraceptive costs be covered? Should abortion services be included?
- How can health care be transformed into an effective, coordinated system?
- How will changes in the health care system be financed?

These are difficult philosophic and ethical questions, and there are no simple answers.

Nursing's Agenda for the Future

The ANA, the NLN, and 60 other nursing organizations cooperated in developing Nursing's Agenda for the Future, which addresses the nation's need for nursing care. Ten areas of concern are addressed in this document (see Display 2-7). For each of these areas, the agenda contains objectives and strategies to move toward those objectives. The current focus is on action plans developed by nursing organizations and groups that will implement the strategies. In addition to combating the current nursing shortage, these action plans will move the profession forward, creating a desired future for nursing within the health care system. See the ANA Web site for complete text of Nursing's Agenda for the Future: *http://nursingworld.org/naf/*.

Critical Thinking Activity

Identify an aspect of health care reform that concerns you. Analyze the various proposals currently before Congress or your state legislature regarding that specific concern. Rank the proposals in order of your preference, providing rationales for your decision making. In a small group, hold a discussion in which you share your analysis of the various proposals.

NURSING ORGANIZATIONS

A student once said that it seems that every time nurses identify a problem, their first action is to form a new organization. Although this may be something of an exaggeration, it contains a bit of truth. When you first learn about the great number of nursing and nursing-related organizations, it all seems confusing and their purposes and functions may seem duplicative.

Display 2-7   Nursing's Agenda for the Future: Areas of Concern

- Leadership and planning
- Delivery systems/nursing models
- Legislation/regulation/policy
- Professional/nursing culture
- Recruitment and retention
- Economic value
- Work environment
- Public relations/communications
- Education
- Diversity

THE DEVELOPMENT OF NURSING ORGANIZATIONS

Understanding the genesis of nursing organizations can help you to understand their current focus and activities. By the end of the 19th century, changes were accomplished most effectively through organizations. Nursing pioneers saw this as an opportunity to bring about transformation in nursing practice and nursing education and began forming nursing organizations.

Nursing Organizations in England

In England, the establishment of an organization for nursing was driven by the energies of Mrs. Bedford Fenwick (Ethel Gordon Manson), a prominent leader who, in 1887, campaigned for nurse registration. She believed that standards were necessary to improve nursing. Although her ideas for nurse registration were not well accepted, she founded the British Nurses' Association in 1888. It grew rapidly to 1,000 members by the end of the first year. It later became the Royal British Nurses' Association.

The American Society of Superintendents of Training Schools for Nurses

In 1893, the World's Fair and Columbian Exposition was held in Chicago to celebrate the 400th anniversary of Columbus' arrival in the United States. The Fair provided the meeting place for many professions and artisans. The first nurses' meeting was held in the Hall of Columbus June 15–17, 1893, as part of the International Congress of Charities, Corrections, and Philanthropy. The nursing meeting was chaired by Isabel Hampton and was attended by American and Canadian nurses. Attendees included such individuals as Lavinia Dock—suffragist, nurse activist, historian, and educator—who spoke about the relation of training schools to hospitals. An address sent by Florence Nightingale was presented to the group. The papers presented were later compiled in a publication, *Nursing the Sick, 1893*. The day after the meeting, Isabel Hampton arranged a meeting of a small group of leaders to discuss the possibility of starting a nursing organization. This meeting resulted in the formation in 1896 of the American Society of Superintendents of Training Schools for Nurses, so named because most of the attendees were directors of nursing schools and the membership was restricted to those nurses associated with nurse training. Concern for the standards of nursing education was primary, and a committee to study nursing education was quickly appointed. In 1907, the Canadian members formed their own organization, the Canadian Society of Superintendents of Training Schools. The American organization changed its name in 1912 to the National League for Nursing Education (Donahue, 1996, p. 326).

In 1952, the National League for Nursing Education became the NLN when six organizations merged into one. The organizations involved in the merger were the National Organization for Public Health Nursing (est. 1912), the Association of Collegiate Schools of Nursing (est. 1933), the Joint Committee on Practical Nurses and Auxiliary Workers in Nursing Services (est. 1945), the Joint Committee on Careers in Nursing (est. 1946), the National Committee for the Improvement of Nursing Services (est. 1949), and the National Nursing Accrediting Service (est. 1949).

Nurses' Associated Alumnae of the United States and Canada

As the number of nurses increased throughout the United States and hospitals formed individual alumnae groups, the need arose for an organization of trained nurses. At the third meeting of the American Society of Superintendents of Training Schools in 1896, a committee prepared a constitution and bylaws for such an organization with the delegates representing the various alumnae associations. The constitution was accepted a year later, and the Nurses' Associated Alumnae of the United States and Canada was formed. The first president was Isabel Hampton Robb. The group had three purposes:

1. To establish and maintain a code of ethics
2. To elevate the standards of nursing education
3. To promote the usefulness and honor, the financial and other interests of the nursing profession (ANA, 1996, p. 2)

When it was discovered that New York law would not permit foreign membership in an incorporated association, the words "and Canada" were dropped from the title in 1901 and Canadian participation was prohibited. In 1911, the name of the organization in the United States became the American Nurses Association.

The Provisional Organization of the Canadian National Association of Trained Nurses was formed in 1908, and renamed the Canadian Nurses Association in 1924. This group also had as its primary concerns the education of nursing students, the improvement of nursing care, the amelioration of conditions for nurses, and state registration of nurses to protect the public.

NURSING ORGANIZATIONS OF TODAY

The existence of a large number of diverse organizations for nurses is, in many ways, a reflection of nursing itself. The profession offers a wide variety of employment opportunities to its members, with distinct and varied contributions and interests in health care. When nurses become committed to a particular specialty group, they have a tendency to want to advance the purposes and interests of the people working in that area. For example, operating room nurses have more in common with other operating room nurses, in terms of interests and concerns, than they have with nurses working in hospice care. Likewise, nurses involved in hospice care would probably prefer to share concerns with one another than to discuss them with critical care nurses. With more than 2.9 million nurses in the United States (HRSA, 2004), it is understandable that there are many different areas of nursing interest, and therefore many different nursing organizations.

The formation of so many nursing organizations has resulted in concern regarding the overlapping of function and interrelationships among some of the organizations. Unfortunately, there has been a spirit of competition rather than cooperation among these groups in the past. Because nurses traditionally have not had high incomes, joining more than one organization has not been a desirable option for economic as well as philosophic reasons. Different nursing organizations can be found listed on the World Wide Web at *http://nursingworld.org/rnindex*. The links provided at this Web site can help you to research individual organizations that may be of interest to you. As you review that list, you can understand why some critics suggest that nursing has too many organizations working in too many different directions.

Nursing organizations recently have made a concerted effort to promote cooperation. Nurses are better informed about the various organizations and receive better salaries than in the past. However, these facts have not resulted in significantly greater participation by professional nurses in their organizations. Some people specifically do not join because of philosophic differences, but many nurses seem to be apathetic and do not recognize the importance of nurses acting together. Some, because they are combining a job with family and home responsibilities, feel they do not have the time or energy to become involved. Nurses need to recognize the potential for power that they possess as a group. As the nation moves toward health care reform, this has never been a more critical issue.

The International Council of Nurses

The International Council of Nurses, the oldest of all international nursing organizations, was formed in 1899. Founded by Mrs. Bedford Fenwick, it held its first meeting in Buffalo, New York, at the World Exposition in 1901. Mrs. Fenwick was the first president of the organization. The membership originally was composed of self-governing national nurses' associations rather than individual members, although, until 1904, individual members could belong because few countries had organized nursing associations. Its purpose was to encourage communication among nurses of all nations and to provide opportunities for nurses from all over the world to meet and discuss concerns about the profession and about patient care. At the present time, the International Council of Nurses meets every 4 years.

The International Council of Nurses (ICN) is the international organization for professional nursing, with membership consisting of national nursing organizations. The ANA, as a constituent member of the ICN, sends delegates to its convention and participates in its activities. The ICN is interested in health care in general and nursing care in particular throughout the world. It works with the United Nations, when appropriate, and with other international health-related groups, such as the International Red Cross.

The ICN concerns itself with such issues as the social and economic welfare of nurses, the role of the nurse in health care, and the roles of national nursing organizations throughout the world and their relationships to their governing bodies. The primary governing body of the organization is the Council of National Representatives, which meets biennially.

The ICN has representatives from more than 120 national nurses' organizations. The Council of National Representatives governs the organization, which consists of all the presidents of the member organizations. Activities of the organization are carried out by its Board of Directors, the officers, volunteer nurse members of constituent organizations, and employed staff, including an executive director. The ICN maintains headquarters in Geneva, Switzerland.

Every 4 years a quadrennial congress is held. This meeting is open to all nurses and to delegates from the national organizations. Concerns addressed at recent congresses focused on such issues as career ladders, educational standards, research, human rights, and nursing's role in the planning of a national health policy. Current major efforts lie in the areas of international nurse migration, nursing regulation, and an innovations database. Information about all of these efforts may be found on the ICN Web site *www.icn.ch*.

American Nurses Association

The ANA has been identified as the professional organization for all RNs. As such, it has always had as its primary interest the concerns of the nurses it represents. Throughout history, the organization has been active in issues relating to licensure (see Chapter 7), collective bargaining (see Chapter 11), nursing education (see Chapter 5), and a host of other concerns facing nurses and nursing. The ANA is referred to many times throughout this book. As a professional association, it has been involved in all the issues that nursing has confronted.

Membership

The ANA membership comprises the 50 state nurses' associations and the three territorial constituent units. State nurses' associations comprise the district nurses' associations. In most cases, the individual nurse belongs to the ANA through the SNA. Since the organization has been restructured, individuals may now join the ANA directly. There are also opportunities for affiliate memberships.

While the reported supply of registered nurses is 2.9 million (HRSA, 2004), the membership in the constituent associations of the ANA is less than half of that (*http://nursingworld.org*). Those who do participate are often the leaders in the nursing profession. Individuals who do not join give a variety of reasons, such as cost, a lack of time to participate in activities, and a lack of interest in the issues put forth. Some nurses do not join because they do not agree with the position of the ANA on major issues such as collective bargaining, nursing education, and political involvement.

In 1995, the California Nurses Association (CNA) experienced a great deal of internal turmoil because of a perceived lack of support from the ANA regarding the massive changes being created by health care reform (Costello, 1995). As a result, the CNA delegate assembly voted to withdraw from the ANA and to establish itself as an independent international organization. This enabled the CNA to keep all of the dues in the state for its own purposes, but it also deprived CNA members of a voice and opportunities at the national level. Some nurses who did not support the separation of the CNA from the ANA joined ANA affiliate organizations in bordering states during the dispute. The ANA tried to resolve the problems but was unsuccessful; instead, it subsequently established another organization called ANA-California. ANA is encouraging nurses in California who are interested in being part of the national organization and its efforts to join this new organization. In 2001, a similar situation arose in Massachusetts, resulting in the withdrawal of the Massachusetts Nurses Association from the ANA.

Activities and Services

The ANA currently focuses its efforts on five core initiatives: the nursing shortage, workplace rights, patient safety/advocacy, appropriate staffing, and workplace health and safety. These initiatives are put forward through a variety of activities.

Advancement of the Profession. The ANA supports work on policies related to the profession as a whole, such as the Code of Ethics for Nurses (ANA, 2001). The ANA also supports research on topics related to the profession itself, such as historical patterns of licensure. By serving as the coordinating body for the various affiliate organizations, the ANA helps to ensure its ongoing effectiveness.

In its efforts to support the profession of nursing, the ANA has developed the Bill of Rights for Registered Nurses. This tool addresses the workplace environment needed for effective nursing practice. While not a legal document, this Bill of Rights serves as a guide to nurses as they seek to influence policy in organizations where they are employed (see Display 2-8). A discussion of how this Bill of Rights might be used and the foundations underlying the rights are found in a special supplement to the *American Nurse* (September/October 2006).

Legislative Activity. The ANA is extensively involved in legislative activity. The organization often represents the profession in testimony before Congress on numerous issues affecting nursing. The need to be geographically closer to legislators to have greater participation in legislative efforts

Display 2-8   American Nurses Association's Bill of Rights for Registered Nurses

1. Nurses have the right to practice in a manner that fulfills their obligations to society and to those who receive nursing care.
2. Nurses have the right to practice in environments that allow them to act in accordance with professional standards and legally authorized scopes of practice.
3. Nurses have the right to a work environment that supports and facilitates ethical practice, in accordance with the *Code of Ethics for Nurses with Interpretive Statements.*
4. Nurses have the right to freely and openly advocate for themselves and their patients, without fear of retribution.
5. Nurses have the right to fair compensation for their work, consistent with their knowledge, experience and professional responsibilities.
6. Nurses have the right to a work environment that is safe for themselves and for their patients.
7. Nurses have the right to negotiate the conditions of their employment, either as individuals or collectively, in all practice settings.

Adopted by the ANA Board of Directors June 26, 2001. *http://nursingworld.org/ajn/2001/nov/issues.htm*

was the major reason for the relocation of the ANA offices to Washington, DC, in 1992. The organization provides testimony for or against legislation that will affect the profession, either directly or indirectly; legislative topics include funds for nursing education, collective bargaining issues, concerns for higher education, and human rights issues. It also testifies on health-related issues affecting the general public, such as the quality of care in nursing homes and health care reform. A newsletter, *Capitol Update*, is published monthly and provides information to the reader about issues currently being addressed in the Capitol. Capitol Update is available on the ANA Web site, *www.capitolupdate.org/newsletter*.

Other Resources and Services. In addition to its activities, the ANA provides direct services to members. These services include access to a group professional liability insurance plan and group insurance for health, disability, and accident coverage. From time to time, the ANA also provides access to group travel arrangements and purchasing discounts.

Through its educational services, the ANA produces and distributes a wide variety of nursing educational materials, such as films, as well as a biennial report entitled *Facts About Nursing*. This report provides basic statistical information that is used by many organizations and individuals. Reports of committees and commissions and special studies supported by the ANA also are published.

The American Nurse is the official publication of the ANA; official announcements of ANA business are published in this paper. The paper also contains current news relevant to nursing and health care, editorials, letters, and classified advertisements. The *American Journal of Nursing* is the official journal of the organization. It is published monthly and contains some current news, but its major focus is on professional articles. It is published by Lippincott Williams & Wilkins, but the ANA retains autonomy over its own content.

The ANA also publishes many pamphlets and informational resources of value to nurses. A complete list of publications is available at the ANA Web site and in print from the organization. The ANA Web site continues to expand the content available and now includes the *Online Journal of Nursing*, continuing education programs, and the many documents and position statements produced by the ANA.

American Nurses Credentialing Center

The ANA in collaboration with specialty nursing organization established the American Nurses Credentialing Center (ANCC) as an autonomous organization to manage the process of specialty credentialing. The ANCC also operates the magnet hospital recognition program for hospitals that demonstrate excellence in nursing practice and the environment for nursing. The ANCC remains an affiliated organization for the ANA.

American Nurses Foundation

In 1955, the ANA established the American Nurses Foundation (ANF), an affiliate of the ANA, as a tax-exempt, nonprofit corporation for the purpose of supporting research related to nursing. It is independently financed and self-governing. Its board of trustees is composed of members of the board of directors of the ANA, other nurse members, and non-nurse members from other health-related fields and from the public. To accomplish its varied objectives, the ANF solicits gifts and contributions from individuals and organizations. These gifts are tax deductible.

The ANF maintains a three-pronged approach to supporting research. The first objective is to conduct policy analyses to provide nursing leaders and public-policy makers with the information they need for decision making. The second objective is related to developing nurse scholars, individuals who engage in study of such areas as journalism and public policy. Support is directed toward independent study, research, and doctoral and postdoctoral work for these nurse scholars. The third objective is to facilitate the research and educational activities of ANA. This includes providing consultation and funding for groups in the ANA that wish to initiate projects.

American Academy of Nursing

The ANA established the American Academy of Nursing (AAN) in 1973 as an honorary association in the ANA. The ANA's board of directors chose the original members. The AAN is now an independent organization that is an affiliate of ANA, and new members are selected by those currently in the AAN. Those elected to the AAN are considered fellows and may use the title Fellow of the American Academy of Nursing. The purpose of this organization is to recognize nurses who have made significant contributions to the profession of nursing.

United American Nurses

The United American Nurses (UAN) is the union for RNs established by the ANA in 1999 with the sole purpose of representing RNs. To this end, the UAN represents nurses in workplace issues such as mandatory overtime and safe staffing and provides a forum for collective bargaining (see Chapter 12 for information related to collective bargaining). While most collective bargaining is done on the state level, the national UAN is able to provide collective bargaining where state-level organizations are unable to do this. The UAN functions as an independent organization, although still related to the ANA as its collective bargaining arm. Affiliation with the American

Federation of Labor-Congress of Industrial Organizations places the UAN within the larger labor movement in the United States.

Center for American Nurses

Established in 2003, the Center for American Nurses focuses on supporting nurses in being their own best advocates in the workplace. The Center includes research, continuing education, and sharing of information that will help nurses to improve their practice environments, meet their personal and professional goals, and promote excellence in patient care. As an ANA affiliate, it particularly targets nurses who do not have collective bargaining and therefore need other resources to help them in their places of employment.

National League for Nursing

The mission for the NLN states, "The National League for Nursing advances quality nursing education that prepares the nursing workforce to meet the needs of diverse populations in an ever-changing healthcare environment" (NLN, 2005). The goals of the organization focus on five areas: (1) nursing education development and improvement, (2) faculty development, (3) nursing education research, (4) data collection, and (5) assessment and evaluation.

Membership

The NLN offers membership to individuals and agencies. It is unique among nursing organizations in that it also offers membership and participation to consumers, non-nursing members of health care teams, and institutions concerned with nursing service and nursing education.

Activities and Services

The NLN works in a complementary, rather than competitive, manner with the ANA. Whereas the ANA speaks as the official voice of nurses, the NLN seeks to unite the interests of nursing with those of the community in support of excellence in nursing education.

Assessment and Evaluation Services. Until 1982, the NLN produced the licensing examination for the state boards of nursing. Although it no longer has this responsibility, it does have a large testing service that produces standardized assessment tests to be used in the nursing program admission process, achievement tests for various levels in a program that can be used by a program for evaluation, the NLN mobility examinations (which are used to provide advanced placement credit), and diagnostic examinations for those preparing for the National Council Licensure Examination, or NCLEX.

Program and Professional Development. The NLN sponsors continuing education workshops and conferences throughout the country, often repeating a workshop in different locations to spare participants the expense of travel. Subjects are determined in consultation with members and are geared to current needs and interests. Curriculum, research, accreditation, testing and evaluation, student recruitment and retention, political awareness and health care legislation, and a nurse executive series are regular subjects for continuing education. The constituent leagues, which are grouped by regional assemblies, also offer workshops designed to meet the interests of particular areas of the country.

Division of Research. When any group needs figures on nursing education, it cites data gathered by NLN's Division of Research. The Division is a primary provider of statistics on nursing education, and each year surveys all schools of registered and practical nursing for enrollments, admissions, and graduations. It also conducts a yearly survey of newly RNs regarding the characteristics of their employment. Every 2 years, the nurse-faculty census is taken; every 3 years, data are gathered on men and minorities in schools of nursing.

Career Information and Publications. The career information service answers thousands of inquiries about nursing education that arrive each year by mail and telephone. The NLN Web site contains information for individuals interested in exploring nursing careers.

Through its journal, *Nursing Education Perspectives*, and a newsletter, *NLN Update* (both available on the Web), members are kept informed about current issues. Sometimes NLN spokespersons offer testimony on legislation or rulings significant to the organization. The NLN publishes many texts and references about curriculum, ethics, public policy, nursing administration, long-term care, and other topics of interest to nursing. It also produces educational videos.

National League for Nursing Accrediting Commission

Many students are aware of **accreditation** that provides standards and criteria against which nursing programs can be evaluated. The National League for Nursing Accrediting Commission (NLNAC) accredits nursing programs of all types: practical nursing, diploma nursing, associate degree nursing, and baccalaureate-and-higher degree programs. Initially, nursing accreditation was performed by the National Nursing Accrediting Service, which merged in 1952 with other groups to form the NLN. After the merger, the NLN provided accreditation of nursing programs. In the 1990s, the Department of Education (DOE), which provides approval for accrediting bodies, required the NLN to develop a new structure that clearly separated the accreditation process from the rest of the organization. Beginning in 1997, the separate-but-related organization, the NLNAC, assumed accrediting responsibilities formerly carried out by the NLN (Fig. 2-3).

American Association of Colleges of Nursing

The AACN was formed to assist collegiate schools of nursing in working cooperatively to improve higher education for professional nursing. Membership is limited to deans and directors of programs that offer a baccalaureate degree in nursing, with an upper-division nursing major, and that are part of a regionally accredited college or university. The AACN focuses on the quality of nursing education in baccalaureate and higher degree programs and support and assistance to deans and programs in providing excellence in education. The organization also provides data regarding these programs and is active in public advocacy for nursing and nursing education.

Commission on Collegiate Nursing Education

Another organization that provides accreditation of baccalaureate-and-higher degree programs is the Commission on Collegiate Nursing Education (CCNE), which was formed by the AACN in 1996 and began accrediting activities in 1999. Thus, there are now two specialized accreditation organizations for baccalaureate-and-higher degree nursing programs. This organization provides a set of standards and key elements of those standards upon which to base evaluation. The evaluation processes used by both accrediting agencies are quite similar, with both requiring a self-study report related to the standards, a visit by evaluators, and a decision by a national body. Both organizations are approved by the DOE as accrediting bodies. The development of two organizations for accreditation of these programs has created concerns in some areas of nursing that point to competition rather than cooperative efforts for excellence in nursing education.

FIGURE 2-3   Accreditation is designed to help ensure that the desired outcomes of education are achieved.

National Council of State Boards of Nursing

Although it is not a nursing organization like those previously discussed, our discussion would not be complete without mention of the National Council of State Boards of Nursing, Inc. (NCSBN). This organization was formed in 1978 to replace the Council of State Boards that had been part of the ANA. The purpose of this organization is to provide a forum for the legal regulatory bodies (whatever their particular state titles might be) of all states, the District of Columbia, and U.S. territories to act together in the regulation of nursing practice for the protection of the public. There is one delegate to this council from each state agency. The actions of this council are particularly important because its membership represents the legal authority for the control of nursing education and nursing practice.

Although each state agency must operate within its own laws, it does have authority to establish many specific rules and regulations. Working together, the state boards hope to promote uniform standards for the nursing profession. One of the agenda items they have addressed is the development of a Model Nurse Practice Act, which serves to guide states as they work on licensure laws. Much energy has gone into the development, validation, and establishment of computerized testing for the licensing examination for both registered and practical nursing. Currently the organization is studying the methods used to approve and license advanced practice nurses and the concerns associated with multistate practice.

Organizations Representing Licensed Practical Nurses

Two nursing organizations are concerned primarily with advancing the interests of licensed practical (vocational) nurses (LPN). These two organizations are the National Federation of Licensed Practical Nurses (NFLPN) and the National Association for Practical Nurse Education and Service (NAPNES).

The NFLPN is the professional organization for LPNs. Founded in 1949, its membership is limited to LPNs and students in practical nursing programs. This organization has developed a set of practice standards for the LPN and provides a liaison with Educational Resources Inc. that administers two certification examinations for LPNs, one in gerontology and one in intravenous therapy. State and local groups of the NFLPN are active in educational issues affecting the LPN and have supported the associate degree as the appropriate educational preparation for the responsibilities of the LPN in the current health care system. Further information is available on the NFLPN Web site, *http://nflpn.org*.

The NAPNES was organized as the Association of Practical Nurse Schools in 1941. Its purpose was to address the needs of practical nursing education. The name was changed in 1942 to the National Association for Practical Nurse Education; in 1959, it added "and Service" to that title. The official publication of the organization is *The Journal of Practical Nursing*, which has been published since 1951. It also publishes a newsletter, *NAPNES Forum*, that keeps members alert to activities of the organization. Membership is open to LPNs, practical/vocational nursing students, faculty, directors, and others interested in promoting the purposes of the organization. It was the first organization to provide accreditation for practical nursing programs, although that role now rests with the NLNAC. See *www.napnes.org*.

NANDA-I

The NANDA-International (NANDA–I), originally the North American Nursing Diagnosis Association, was first established in 1982, and is open to individuals as well as group members. The purpose of this group is to work toward uniform terminology and definitions to be used in nursing diagnosis and to share ideas and information regarding this topic. The general outline of the taxonomy (classification system) was established by a group of nursing theorists and then accepted by the organization. NANDA-I is now using Taxonomy II, a revision of the original classification system. Members identify and research problems nurses manage, prepare documentation, and submit these to NANDA-I to be included in the consideration process. Committees then review the problems. Those that meet the basic criteria for nursing diagnoses are submitted to the membership. For each problem, defining characteristics are identified, conditions that form the etiology or are related to the development of the diagnosis are identified, and a place in the classification is established. An international convention held every 2 years is the final forum for the debate and discussion of proposed new nursing diagnoses. Two publications—*The International Journal of Nursing Terminologies and Classification* and *Nursing Diagnoses and Classifications*—are used to disseminate the work of the organization. See the Web site at *www.nanda.org*. More recently, this organization is coordinating its work with those working on the Nursing Interventions Classification and the Nursing Outcomes Classification to fulfill the goal of a coordinated system of nursing terminology.

American Organization of Nurse Executives

According to their Web site, AONE is the "national professional organization for nurses who design, facilitate, and manage care" (*www.aha.org/resources/AboutAone.html*). This organization provides the forum for nurses with managerial and executive responsibility to work collaboratively both with other nurses in similar roles and through the organization with other organizations. AONE is one of the members of the Tricouncil for Nursing, which serves as an information resource for legislative and governmental personnel.

Sigma Theta Tau

Sigma Theta Tau is an international organization established in collegiate schools of nursing to recognize those with superior ability and leadership potential, and those who have made important contributions to nursing. Candidates may be asked to join during the senior year of a baccalaureate program, or any time thereafter. Sigma Theta Tau has established a nursing library at its headquarters in Indianapolis that has reference abilities to support advanced scholarship; the organization also provides two print journals *Journal of Nursing Scholarship* and *Reflections on Nursing Leadership* (which is also available online). Local chapters may maintain funds to support individual research projects, hold research conferences, and recognize those who have made significant contributions to nursing.

Clinical Organizations

Some of the earliest specialty organizations were related to specific clinical practice areas of nursing. A major focus of these organizations now is continuing education related to a particular nursing specialty. Most groups also have some mechanisms, such as certification, for recognizing achievement in the field. One of the earliest specialty organizations, founded in 1941, was the American Association of Nurse Anesthetists, a group of approximately 34,000 members. Of those who work full time, approximately 49% are men (American Association of Nurse Anesthetists, 2006).

Specialty organizations also include groups that began as auxiliaries to specialty physicians' organizations, such as the Association of Women's Health, Obstetric and Neonatal Nurses. This organization was started for nurses affiliated with physicians who were "fellows" of the American College of Obstetricians and Gynecologists. As more members joined and nurses became more active, groups such as this one became autonomous.

The overlapping purpose and actions of the Councils on Practice of the ANA and the corresponding specialty organizations have caused some concern. One attempt to promote a more cooperative effort was the creation of the Nursing Organization Liaison Forum, which operates as a forum in the ANA.

One of the newest nursing organizations is the National Alliance of Nurse Practitioners, organized in 1986. Its purpose is to promote the health care of the nation by promoting the visibility, viability, and unity of nurse practitioners. Its activities focus on advancing the role of the nurse practitioner in the health care delivery system. Issues related to the reimbursement of nurse practitioners are of major concern to this organization.

Groups Related to Ethnic Origin

As the movement for self-determination and preservation of identity arose within ethnic groups in the United States, nurses within various ethnic groups began to unite to achieve a greater voice in health care. Some ethnic groups are nationally organized; others are organized on a more local level. As these groups have become stronger and more organized, their interests have included the recruitment and support of nursing students from the particular ethnic groups they represent.

These ethnic groups also encourage their members to become more politically involved in nursing and nursing leadership.

Religious Organizations

The National Council of Catholic Nurses and the Nurses' Christian Fellowship (primarily a non-denominational Protestant group) were organized to assist nurses in sharing concerns and integrating their work and their religious beliefs. These two organizations place special emphasis on meeting a patient's spiritual needs and on dealing with ethical issues.

National Student Nurses' Association

The National Student Nurses' Association (NSNA), started in 1952, is a professional organization for students in schools of nursing. Although it works with the ANA, it is a fully independent organization, run and financed by nursing students. It sponsors its own annual convention.

Although the NSNA is an autonomous organization, it has close ties with the ANA. Members of the NSNA serve on selected committees in the ANA, speak to the House of Delegates at the ANA convention to provide a student viewpoint, and work together with the ANA regarding current issues.

Each state has a nursing student association that operates in the same relationship to the state professional organization as the NSNA does to the ANA. State conventions and workshops are held in many states. State issues are addressed by the state association in the same way that national issues are addressed by the NSNA. Local nursing student organizations may or may not exist in individual schools of nursing. These local organizations may be closely tied to the state and national groups, or they may be independent. It is possible for an individual student to join the state and national student nurses' organizations even if no local counterpart exists.

A major project of the NSNA is "Breakthrough into Nursing," organized in 1965. This project is designed to recruit and maintain the enrollment of minorities in schools of nursing through mentoring and to create a respect for the differences and similarities between people. The project has enlisted nursing students to speak to minority teenagers to interest them in nursing early in their scholastic careers, and to act as preceptors and tutors to increase the retention of minority students when they enroll in schools of nursing.

The NSNA often is asked to testify before congressional committees when issues relevant to nursing education are being considered. In this role, the organization becomes the public voice for all nursing students.

In 1975, the NSNA developed a Student Bill of Rights. This document, which was updated in 1991, supports the view of students as competent adults who are engaged in an educational program. The rights that are outlined relate to educational programs, to the rules and policies of an institution, and to freedom in personal life and decision making. In 1999, the NSNA adopted a Code of Professional Conduct that was structured as a pledge. The NSNA expanded this work in 2001 by passing a Code of Academic and Clinical Conduct for nursing students that speaks to the responsibilities of nursing students in both these settings. These documents are all available from the NSNA Web site (*http://nsna.org/pubs/index.asp*).

Educational Organizations

Since the 1960s, there has been a great deal of change and development in nursing education as it has moved from the hospital into the educational setting. During this time, there has been an increased emphasis on educational methods, curriculum development, and research.

In several major geographic regions of the United States, education organizations extending membership to schools of nursing, members of the state boards of nursing, and other interested individuals were developed to promote interstate and interinstitutional cooperation in seeking ways to improve nursing education and scholarship. These organizations are the Western Institute of Nursing, the Council on Collegiate Education for Nursing of the Southern Regional Education Board, the New England Organization for Nursing, the Midwest Alliance in Nursing, and the Mid-Atlantic Regional Nursing Association.

The National Organization for the Advancement of Associate Degree Nursing has four purposes: to speak for associate degree nursing education and practice, reinforce the value of associate degree nursing education and practice, maintain endorsement of RN licensure from state to state for the associate degree nurse, and retain the RN licensure examination for graduates of associate degree nursing programs. Membership is open to individuals, states, agencies, and organizations.

Miscellaneous Organizations

The American Assembly for Men in Nursing was formed by those who believed that, as a minority in the profession, men needed to speak about issues with a united voice. The membership has expanded to include women who are concerned about gender issues in nursing. The organization has addressed the issue of discrimination toward men in nursing and seeks to present nursing as a profession in which both men and women can contribute and excel. In March 2006, *Men in Nursing*, the first journal to address issues and concerns facing the growing number of men who have chosen nursing as a career, was published.

Nurses House, Inc. provides assistance for nurses in need. It originated from a bequest in 1922 from Emily Bourne, who donated $300,000 to establish a country home where nurses might find needed rest. As the need for this residence decreased, supporters of this endeavor sold the estate and invested the proceeds. Income from the investment and funds donated by nurses (and friends of nurses) are used to provide guidance and counseling for nurses with emotional and chemical dependency problems, encouragement to homebound nurses, and temporary financial assistance to nurses who are ill, convalescing, or unemployed. Nurses House seeks members and donations to assist in continuing these activities.

The Gay Nurses' Alliance was an outgrowth of the movement of homosexual individuals to be accepted without having to disguise their sexual orientation. This group primarily has focused on the issue of gay rights. They also provide a forum for gay individuals to address the difficulties they may face in the nursing profession.

Critical Thinking Activity

As a new graduate, assume you have $400 per year to spend on membership in a nursing organization. In trying to decide which organization to join, how would you go about learning the focus of several groups that have attracted your interest? What process could you use to ensure that you are joining the group that best serves your needs? Which organization would you join? Provide a clear rationale based on both economic and professional reasons for your choice.

**Key
Concepts**

- Because scarce resources are allocated through the political process, nurses will find that understanding this process is essential to influencing the health care system.
- Each nurse has many opportunities to affect the political process. This can be done simply by keeping informed, voting, or trying to shape public opinion. Communicating with legislators and officials can be done individually or as part of a group. Testifying presents issues of importance, and individual support can be given to those running for office. You may even decide to run for a public office.
- The federal government is active in health care through many existing agencies in the HHS and in other branches of government. The federal budget process affects the health care services available through the many legislative acts affecting health care such as Medicare, for the elderly and certain disabled individuals, and Medicaid, for the poor.
- A political process is part of any large organization, and nursing organizations are no exception. Understanding the political process can help you participate more effectively in a large organization.
- The variety of organizations in nursing is often confusing to the new nursing graduate and to the public. These organizations represent the nursing profession as a whole, as well as special interest groups within nursing.
- The ANA, whose membership is open to RNs only through their state constituencies, provides the voice of professional nursing. Actions of the ANA are directed toward nursing practice issues, economic welfare of nurses, and broader issues of health care.
- Another major nursing organization is the NLN, which, historically, has championed better nursing education. Membership is open to individuals and agencies interested in nursing.
- The NLNAC, which is related to the NLN, provides for the accreditation of all types of nursing programs throughout the United States. The CCNE, which is related to the AACN, is another organization providing accreditation for baccalaureate and higher degree programs.
- The NCSBN coordinates the development of the licensure examinations used for both practical nurses and RNs. It also coordinates and supports the development of common licensure standards, licensure agreements between states, and an examination for certifying nursing assistants.
- Two nursing organizations exist expressly to serve the needs of LPNs. These groups are the NFLPN and the NAPNES.
- Organizations also exist that represent specialty groups in nursing. Members usually are drawn together by their common interests and concerns. The organizations provide continuing education and, in some instances, certification.
- Some organizations, such as Sigma Theta Tau, are honorary in their focus. These groups strive to bring recognition to nurses and nursing.
- The NSNA addresses the interests and needs of nursing students. As a fully autonomous organization, NSNA membership is open to nursing students only.
- A wide variety of other organizations meet the special needs of their membership. This may relate to social interests, ethnic background, or other common denominators. A very active and prominent organization is the AONE.

Relevant Web Sites

American Association for History of Nursing (AAHN): *www.aahn.org*

American Journal of Nursing, Lippincott Williams & Wilkins: *www.nursingcenter.com*

American Nurses Association (ANA) home page: *http://nursingworld.org*; *Capitol Update* legislative newsletter: *www.capitolupdate.org/newsletter*; Government/legislative information: *http://nursingworld.org/gova*; Nursing's Agenda for the Future: *http://nursingworld.org/naf*; Nursing Organizations List and Links: *http://nursingworld.org/rnindex*; Safe Patient Handling: *http://nursingworld.org/handlewithcare*

Canadian Government Access: *http://canada.gc.ca/main_e.html*

Canadian Nurses Association: *www.cna-nurses.ca/CNA/issues/matters/default_e.aspx*

Centers for Disease Control and Prevention (CDC): *www.cdc.gov*

International Council of Nurses (ICN): *www.icn.ch*

Library of Congress: Access to current legislation in the "Spirit of Thomas Jefferson": *http://thomas.loc.gov*

National Federation of Licensed Practical Nurses (NFLPN): *http://nflpn.org*

National League for Nursing (NLN): *www.nln.org*

National League for Nursing Accrediting Commission (NLNAC): *www.nlnac.org*

National Student Nurses' Association (NSNA): *www.nsna.org*; Publications: *http://nsna.org/pubs/index.asp*

North American Nursing Diagnosis Association-International (NANDA-I): *www.nanda.org*

Sigma Theta Tau International: *www.nursingsociety.org*

State and local government information links on the Web: *www.loc.gov/rr/news/stategov/stategov.html*

United States government gateway, First Gov: *www.firstgov.gov*

References

American Association for History of Nursing. Hannah A. Ropes [On-line]. *www.aahn.org/gravesites/ropes.html.* Accessed March 10, 2006.

American Association of Nurse Anesthetists. (2006). Nurse anesthetists at a glance. Certified registered nurse anesthetists [On-line]. *www.aana.com.* Accessed March 6, 2006.

American Nurses Association. (1996). In the beginning [On-line]. *http://nursingworld.org/centenn/centbegn.htm.* Accessed March 10, 2006.

American Nurses Association. (2001). Code of ethics for nurses with interpretive statements. Washington, DC: ANA Publications [On-line]. *http://nursingworld.org/ethics/code/protected_nwcoe303.htm.* Accessed March 13, 2006.

American Nurses Association. (2002). Hill basics: Communications tips [On-line]. *http://nursingworld.org/gova/federal/politic/hill/gcomtips.htm.* Accessed March 9, 2006.

American Nurses Association. (2002). Nursing's agenda for the future [On-line]. *http://nursingworld.org/naf/Plan.pdf.* Accessed March 12, 2006.

American Nurses Association. (2005). Handle with care [On-line]. *http://nursingworld.org/handlewithcare.* Accessed March 13, 2006.

Bill of Rights for Registered Nurses. (2006). *The American Nurse.* 38(5) Special Cover Feature. September/October, 2006.

Centers for Medicare & Medicaid Services. (n.d.). Fraud reporting [On-line]. *www.cms.hhs.gov/FraudAbuseforConsumers/02_How_to_Report_Suspected_Fraud.* Accessed March 13, 2006.

Centers for Medicare & Medicaid Services. (n.d.). Spotlight [On-line]. *www.cms.hhs.gov/CFCsAndCoPs/02_Spotlight.asp#TopOfPage.* Accessed February 25, 2006.

Costello, K. (1995). ANA weak on protecting nursing practice. *California Nurse, 91*(8): 4, 16.

Donahue, M. P. (1996). *Nursing: The finest art* (2nd ed.). St. Louis, MO: CV Mosby.

Grieschar-Billiard, J. E. (2000). Nurse power! Using the internet to influence the political process. University of Kansas Medical Center [On-line]. *www.continuingeducation.com/nursing/nursepower/nursepower.pdf*. Accessed March 14, 2006.

Hatch Act. (1993). [On-line]. *www.osc.gov/ha_fed.htm*. Accessed February 24, 2006.

Health Resources and Services Administration (HRSA). (March, 2004). National sample survey of registered nurses, March 2004: Preliminary findings [On-line]. *http://bhpr.hrsa.gov/healthworkforce/reports/rnpopulation/preliminaryfindings.htm*. Accessed March 10, 2006.

Lienhard, J. H. (2002). Engines of our ingenuity: Episode 867-Hannah Ropes [On-line]. *www.uh.edu/engines/epi867.htm*. Accessed March 14, 2006.

McDonald, M. (2005). United States election project: 2004 voting-age and voting-eligible population estimates and voter turnout [On-line]. *http://elections.gmu.edu/Voter_Turnout_2004.htm*. Accessed March 15, 2006.

National Center for Health Workforce Analysis. (July 2002). Projected supply, demand, and shortages of registered nurses: 2000–2020, U.S. Department of Health and Human Services, Health Resources and Services Administration, Bureau of Health Professions [On-line]. *www.ahca.org/research/rnsupply_demand.pdf* Accessed February 24, 2006.

National Institutes for Occupational Safety and Health. (1999). NIOSH alert: preventing needlestick injuries in health care settings. Pub #2000-108 [On-line]. *www.cdc.gov/niosh/2000-108.html*. Accessed March 13, 2006.

National League for Nursing. (2005). Our mission [On-line]. *www.nln.org/aboutnln/ourmission.htm*. Accessed March 14, 2006.

Nelson, R. (2004). Needlestick injuries: Going but not gone? *American Journal of Nursing, 104*(11): 25.

Occupational Health and Safety Act. (n.d.). Public law 91-596, 84 STAT. 1590, 91st Congress, S.2193, December 29, 1970, as amended through January 1, 2004 [On-line]. *www.osha.gov/pls/oshaweb/owadisp.show_document?p_table=OSHACT&p_id=2743*. Accessed March 13, 2006.

The Upright Fight. (2002). Washington watch. *American Journal of Nursing, 102*(7): 24.

Woodham-Smith, C. (1983). *Florence Nightingale*. New York: Atheneum. (1983 reprint of 1951 edition).

See the following regular publications for current information:

American Journal of Nursing, Washington Watch (a monthly column)

The American Nurse. Kansas City, MO: American Nurses Association (a monthly newspaper)

See also the official publication of your state nurses association.

3

The Nursing Profession and the Community

LEARNING OUTCOMES

After completing this chapter, you should be able to:

1. Discuss the social contract between the community and the nursing profession.
2. Describe the philosophy behind community-based care.
3. Explain approaches to patient/client empowerment.
4. Differentiate primary, secondary, and tertiary prevention and how these concepts can be applied in different nursing settings.
5. Outline the various components of disease management and how those provide for health promotion.
6. Discuss how Healthy People 2010 priority areas and leading health

indicators relate to the goals of Healthy People 2010.
7. Explain the nurse's role in disaster response in the community.
8. List the major categories of complementary/alternative health care medicine.
9. Identify major issues that surround the use of complementary/alternative medicine.
10. Describe ways in which you could use your knowledge of complementary/alternative therapies when working with clients.

KEY TERMS

Alternative health care
Biologically-based practices
Continuity of care
Community-based nursing
Complementary health care
Complementary therapy
Disaster management
Disease management
Energy medicine

Health disparities
Health-related quality of life
Healthy People 2010
Herbal medicine
Homeopathy
Integrative medicine
Manipulative and body-based
    practices
Medication reconciliation

Mind–body medicine
Naturopathy
Primary prevention
Secondary prevention
Therapeutic touch
Tertiary prevention
Transition planning
Transitions
Triage

The nursing profession's relationship with its community has long been explained in terms of a social contract. In a social contract, two or more parties in society agree to reciprocal obligations. Professional nursing arose to meet many health care needs, starting with the need for skilled individuals in hospitals, then moving out to homes and the wider community. In return for the nursing profession's commitment to the well-being of the community through acquiring and using the knowledge and skills to meet health needs, the community has granted the nursing profession unique privileges that include a trusted relationship, access to individuals at their most vulnerable, and a legal status as a profession.

As the community's needs change, the nursing profession has an obligation to expand its knowledge base for practice, enlarge its repertoire of skills and abilities, and commit to meeting newly identified needs in innovative and creative ways. Over the past few years, health care has moved toward a promotion/prevention model that requires nurses to broaden their focus. They have met that requirement by better understanding community-based nursing, health promotion and prevention, transition planning, and alternative and complementary care that individuals in the community choose for their health care.

UNDERSTANDING COMMUNITY-BASED NURSING

The emphasis in health care has increasingly moved out of the institutional setting and into the community. **Community-based nursing** refers to the wide variety of settings other than institutions in which nursing is practiced. It includes public health, home health, ambulatory care, occupational health, and school nursing.

From the inception of modern nursing, community-based care has been part of the nursing profession. Graduate nurses of the first hospital training schools worked in homes nursing the sick. In the early part of the twentieth century, the public health nurses working in settlement houses in the immigrant neighborhoods of New York and other large cities brought health education, direct care, and advocacy skills to bear on the many health problems confronting the community. As more aspects of health care moved into hospitals and other institutional settings, more nursing took place in those environments. However, public health and home care continued the long tradition of nursing in the community.

In today's world, community-based nursing encompasses more than traditional home care and public health nursing. It occurs wherever people have health needs. In addition to the home and public health arenas, nurses provide care in schools, places of work, traditional medical offices and clinics, nurse-run clinics, homeless shelters, senior centers, high-rise apartment neighborhoods, church parishes, and within support groups. The key in all of these settings is that the patient/client is in charge. The client decides to work with the nurse, to accept or reject advice and suggestions, and to enter and leave care. The nurse serves as an educator, a guide, a resource person, and an advocate, but health action is taken by the client and family.

Care in the community is cost-effective and often more acceptable to the client because it causes less disruption in life. New opportunities arise as the understanding of care in the community enlarges. The principles of community-based care include an emphasis on advocating for patients, promoting self-care, focusing on health promotion and disease prevention, and recognizing the importance of family, culture, and the community. Community-based care requires effective communication and collaboration.

In addition to those who see themselves as working in a community-based setting, all nurses need to be aware of the community in which the client resides and be able to provide care that fits within the scope of the person's life rather than simply an unrelated "episode" of illness. Care must be family-centered and culturally competent. Nurses working in community environments must be aware of public health services, knowledgeable about availability and accessibility of services and supplies, and familiar with the location and specialty of health care providers. As all nurses become more community-focused, the boundaries between the institutional nurse and the community-based nurse blur. All need an understanding of how the client functions in each setting; and each setting must adapt to facilitate transitions from one care environment to another.

CLIENT EMPOWERMENT

A community-based philosophy rests on a fundamental belief in the right of the client to control his or her life, including situations related to health care. Giving over control to clients removes health care professionals from a position of power over others and requires instead that they participate by recognizing support power as their legitimate field.

Support power, or empowerment, is based on possessing sufficient knowledge to be aware of the alternatives available, the ability to make decisions based on that knowledge, and the skills to carry out those decisions. Teaching people to manage their own health, giving them the information necessary to make choices within their lives, and helping them to carry out those choices empowers them.

Clients are often fearful of making health care decisions because so much is unknown. Part of support power is ensuring that clients have the information they need to make informed decisions. However, not everyone has the same interest in decision making. In a study of the treatment decisions made by patients with advanced, non-curable cancer, it was noted that while some patients want to make decisions and need the information to do that, others do not want the burden of decision making (Gaston & Mitchell, 2005). Nurses must navigate these difficult situations and recognize that a decision to not have information or to not be burdened with certain types of judgments also represents the patient's autonomy. In such situations, determining what type of information and the depth of information a client wishes to receive is an important aspect of providing care.

Empowerment supports patients/clients in remaining who they are, not in remaking them into some ideal of a person. The elderly woman who asks that her son make decisions for her is empowered when caregivers respect her enough to allow her to live her life as she chooses. Trying to persuade this woman to change who she is and become the model of an independent person does a disservice to her and increases the distance between her and her caregivers when she most needs to be able to trust in them (Fig. 3-1).

HEALTH PROMOTION AND DISEASE PREVENTION SERVICES

Health promotion and disease prevention have long been the major focus of public health nurses, who concentrate on entire populations. This same focus on health promotion and disease prevention is now expanding to nursing in every setting. By recognizing that the determinants of

FIGURE 3-1 Teaching people to manage their own health, giving them the information to make choices within their lives, and helping them to carry out those choices empowers them.

health lie outside of the institution in the community, nurses in the acute care setting enlarge their practice to make it more community-based in philosophy. The various levels of prevention can be addressed wherever the nurse practices.

Primary Prevention

Primary prevention involves the efforts to prevent disease from ever occurring. Primary prevention can be aimed at stopping the cause of disease. On a community-wide level, water treatment and sanitation prevent the spread of communicable diseases by eliminating their sources for the entire population. Helping individuals to be more successful in resisting disease and maintaining health forms another aim of primary prevention. Generalized efforts to educate regarding healthy diet, such as the publicity over the new food pyramid, are aimed at this type of primary prevention. Some efforts involve the individual client and family as the primary focus, although they may benefit the entire community. Immunizations prevent disease not only in the people immunized but also in others by lowering the overall existence of communicable disease throughout the community. Smoking cessation campaigns are aimed at primary prevention and help the individual who quits smoking, but also benefit those who might otherwise be subject to second-hand smoke.

Primary prevention can be a focus of nurses in acute and long-term care settings as well as those who work in the community. Nurses need to think in terms of life span development and identify the common preventable diseases and disorders that occur at any point in life. For example, when the patient must stop smoking to have surgery and remain in the hospital, the impetus may exist to stop smoking for good. Nurses may help patients to examine their options, consult with physicians for medications to manage withdrawal, point out available smoking cessation programs, and in other ways help the patient to quit smoking. Some facilities focus on each contact with a patient as an opportunity to review immunization history and encourage updating of immunizations before leaving the hospital. This is particularly important in ensuring that the elderly have pneumococcal pneumonia immunization or flu vaccine. When planning for discharge, nurses can build in teaching regarding better dietary practices and help patients understand how those will help in long-term health as well as recovery from the current episode of illness.

Long-term care environments have steadily increased their emphasis on health promotion for even the most disabled individuals. Immunizations, fall prevention through strengthening and balance exercises, and activity programs to prevent social isolation and the depression that often accompanies social isolation serve as primary prevention interventions. Nurses are typically the professionals championing these programs, teaching clients and their families, and increasing public awareness of the concerns.

Secondary Prevention

Secondary prevention involves early identification of health problems through screening and the prevention of complications and adverse consequences of illness. Nurses in ambulatory settings help clients to identify screening tests that are important and facilitate scheduling those tests. When admission histories are obtained, the nurse in the acute care setting can attend to information about screenings that are needed and encourage the patient to value that activity. To do this effectively, the nurse must understand the current recommendation for screening in specific groups within the population. Asking about screening emphasizes its importance to clients and reinforces other information they may have. It may also create an opportunity for clients to gather further information. Similarly, in the long-term setting, it is important that nurses continue their focus on prevention activities among the residents. Screening of the elderly population includes different priorities based on the incidence of problems in that age group and the potential years left.

Complications of illness greatly increase morbidity and mortality. Nurses in both acute and long-term care focus on preventing complications as a consistent part of their practice. Careful assessment and timely nursing intervention can prevent the formation of pressure ulcers, falls, and hypostatic pneumonia. These are only a sample of the many secondary prevention actions taken in the institutional care environment.

Tertiary Prevention

Tertiary prevention focuses on preventing long-term disability and restoring functional capacity. Rehabilitation efforts have often been singled out as the major place where tertiary prevention occurs. However, long-term care has a regulatory mandate to prevent deterioration of elderly individuals. Although some argue that decreased functional status is a realistic process that happens at the end of life, the increased emphasis on maintenance of function has revealed that even the extremely debilitated elderly may be helped to avoid the complications of dependency and to maintain functional independence in the face of disability longer than was previously thought.

Disease Management

One approach to increasingly sophisticated and targeted prevention services is found in disease management programs. **Disease management** focuses on providing the best evidence-based care for an individual with a specific chronic illness, such as diabetes. These programs are often instituted by health plans or clinics that recognize that failure to manage chronic illnesses well results in increased rates of hospitalization, increased demand on the system for high-cost care, and increased incidence of potentially life-altering complications.

By targeting high-impact diseases such as diabetes for special attention, the aim is for both secondary and tertiary prevention. The person with diabetes who is enrolled in such a program receives comprehensive nutrition education, teaching regarding the management of blood glucose through medication and activity, and regular diagnostic evaluations that include hemoglobin A1c and blood glucose measurements to identify glucose management over time, urine analysis to identify renal function, regular eye examinations to prevent retinal complications, and regular foot exams to prevent lesions that might progress to gangrene and amputation. While the intensive involvement in prevention services is costly, the process saves money overall through the lowered incidence of hospitalization, blindness, renal failure, and amputations, not to mention the cost of human suffering.

Computerized documentation systems facilitate the activities of nurses who are charged with tracking individuals enrolled in a disease management program. They alert the nurse to contact the person through telephone calls, e-mails, or letters when screening services are needed. This same nurse meets with the person to discuss test results. By providing a consistent contact person, the patient feels more comfortable asking questions and is more motivated to maintain needed health practices and lifestyle changes.

HEALTHY PEOPLE 2010

Healthy People 2010 is "a set of health objectives for the Nation to achieve over the first decade of the new century" (U.S.DHHS, 2000, p. 7). These objectives are used in schools, in health agencies, and for the general public to guide efforts aimed at promoting a higher quality of life over a longer period of life.

Goals of Healthy People 2010

The two main goals of Healthy People 2010 are shown in Display 3-1. For each major goal, specific objectives have been formulated. Healthy people can only exist in healthy communities; therefore, some of the objectives relate to improving communities.

Goal 1 relates to increasing the years of healthy life. Life expectancy is a relatively easy part of Goal 1 by which to measure progress. Statistics regarding birthdates and deaths are kept by all states. Because there are substantial differences in life expectancy among different groups of people within

Display 3-1   Healthy People 2010 Goals

Goal 1: Increase quality and years of healthy life
Goal 2: Eliminate health disparities

U.S.DHHS, Healthy People 2010

the United States, efforts toward Goal 1—increasing life expectancy—are focused on groups most at risk. This focus also has led to analysis of the reasons for shortened life span and actions aimed at primary prevention whenever possible. The second part of this goal focuses on quality of life for those extended years: "**Health-related quality of life** reflects a personal sense of physical and mental health and the ability to react to factors in the physical and social environments" (U.S.DHHS, 2000, p. 10). Because quality of life is subjective, attempts to measure it have been challenging.

Goal 2 focuses on the health disparities that are found in the United States. **Health disparities** refer to differences in health outcomes achieved by identifiable groups within the population. Racial and ethnic minorities and the poor all show disparities in their health states when compared with the majority population. Part of the effort of Healthy People 2010 is to study these disparities and determine their origins. For example, inaccessibility of ongoing preventive services is a barrier to health for many groups. Improved access must be achieved in order for health objectives to be achieved. In the course of improving access, one barrier identified has been the lack of minorities in the health provider work force. Therefore, an objective in the health profession to improve access is to "increase the proportion of all degrees awarded to members of under-represented racial and ethnic groups" (U.S.DHHS, pp. 1–8).

Achieving the goals of Healthy People 2010 requires that individuals become aware of their own responsibility for their health. They need to be knowledgeable about what promotes health and what interferes with health. They must make informed choices that lead toward greater health. In addition to health professionals' roles in teaching, they must recognize the role of motivation in taking action to improve health. Exploring motivation and the structures that support positive health behaviors will facilitate people's engagement in health promotion activities.

Priority Areas of Healthy People 2010

The priority areas for action under the Healthy People 2010 plan include promotion of healthy behaviors, promotion of a healthy and safe community, improvement in the systems for personal and public health, and the prevention or reduction of major diseases and disorders that account for a large proportion of the health care problems in society (Display 3-2). All of these areas for action will help to achieve the two overall goals.

Healthy behaviors are easy to identify and hard to put into practice. These include adding physical activity to life, managing nutrition well, avoiding overweight and obesity, ceasing tobacco use, practicing safe sexual behaviors, and being judicious in the use of alcohol. These are primary prevention behaviors that nurses in all settings can address. The challenges of behavioral change on a large scale have led to increased use of media, such as television advertisements, to impart to individuals information regarding healthy behavior. However, behavioral change is a complex phenomenon and whether these broad strategies are effective is not clear.

Promoting safe communities has long been considered the province of public health departments. As our understanding of safe communities broadens, the role of domestic violence as a health problem has become more prominent. Many agencies promote awareness of what constitutes domestic violence through posters in public rest rooms, through television spots that highlight resources for help for those facing this problem, and by adding routine assessment for abuse to health histories.

Addressing individual behavior is only successful when the systems of the community support it. Access to health services is essential for people to obtain the screenings and preventive care they need. For example, family planning services contribute to the health of

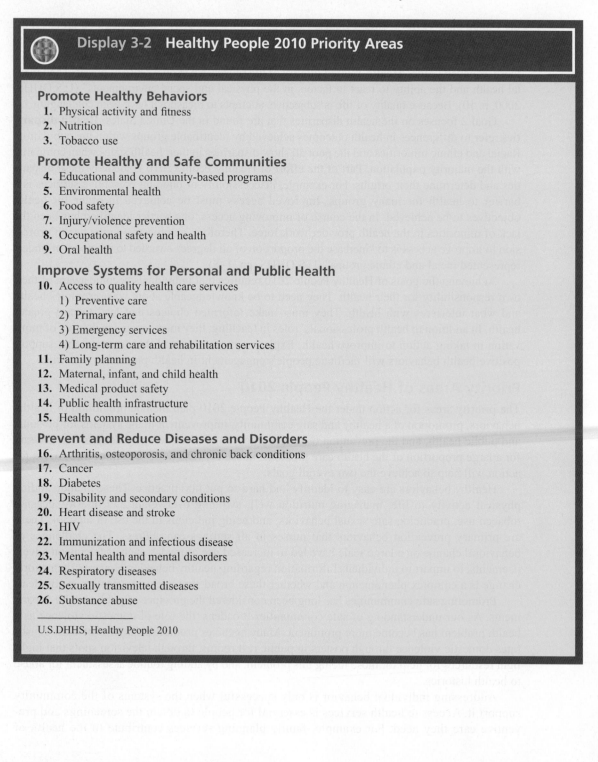

Display 3-2   Healthy People 2010 Priority Areas

Promote Healthy Behaviors
1. Physical activity and fitness
2. Nutrition
3. Tobacco use

Promote Healthy and Safe Communities
4. Educational and community-based programs
5. Environmental health
6. Food safety
7. Injury/violence prevention
8. Occupational safety and health
9. Oral health

Improve Systems for Personal and Public Health
10. Access to quality health care services
    1) Preventive care
    2) Primary care
    3) Emergency services
    4) Long-term care and rehabilitation services
11. Family planning
12. Maternal, infant, and child health
13. Medical product safety
14. Public health infrastructure
15. Health communication

Prevent and Reduce Diseases and Disorders
16. Arthritis, osteoporosis, and chronic back conditions
17. Cancer
18. Diabetes
19. Disability and secondary conditions
20. Heart disease and stroke
21. HIV
22. Immunization and infectious disease
23. Mental health and mental disorders
24. Respiratory diseases
25. Sexually transmitted diseases
26. Substance abuse

U.S.DHHS, Healthy People 2010

both mothers and infants. Medical products must be safe and a public health infrastructure must be in place to support a healthy community. Nurses recognize that many individuals never visit a dentist and that assessment of oral health can be part of physical assessment done in other settings, with referral to dental professionals when obvious problems are identified.

While the number of different diseases and conditions fills volumes of books, there are a limited number of conditions that account for the majority of illness and disability. The successful identification and treatment of these diseases creates a substantial move toward greater health and quality of life for millions.

Leading Health Indicators for Healthy People 2010

Leading health indicators are classifications for measurement to determine the success of Healthy People 2010 (Display 3-3). Measures for each category have been devised and are being tracked to determine trends and to evaluate specific strategies for targeted groups. For example, access to health care is being measured through determining the increase in the proportion of persons with health insurance, the increase in the proportion of persons who have a specific source of ongoing care, and the increase in the proportion of pregnant women who begin prenatal care during the first trimester of pregnancy. While these are not the only things that might indicate increased access, they are representative of the various characteristics of access.

Nurses' Roles in Supporting Healthy Communities

While many nurses work professionally in the community, all nurses can support personally the health of their communities. One personal role is as a supporter and advocate for political measures that would improve the health of the community. This might include contacting representatives at local, state, or national levels and advocating for passage of important health-related laws or projects. Strategies for this were discussed in Chapter 2.

 Display 3-3   The Leading Health Indicators

- Physical activity
- Overweight and obesity
- Tobacco use
- Substance abuse
- Responsible sexual behavior

- Mental health
- Injury and violence
- Environmental quality
- Immunization
- Access to health care

U.S.DHHS, Healthy People 2010

Another personal role includes being active as a community service volunteer in a homeless shelter, school, or other community agency. Blood drives, blood pressure screening events, and educational programs may all seek the services of nurses as community volunteers. Within a neighborhood, church, or other setting, nurses are often asked to be a resource person for health-related questions. While nurses need to be careful not to give medical advice or make recommendations without adequate information, they can teach people about their medications, advise healthy behaviors, help identify that a problem exists, suggest seeing a health care provider for a problem presented, help them to understand the directions given them by their physician, or suggest health-related screening. Some have suggested that nurses can also be role models of healthy lifestyles for those around them. Although many nurses reject the idea that their lives should be lived with this in mind, others recognize that actions often speak to others much louder than words. The nurse who persists in smoking has less credibility when suggesting healthy lifestyle behaviors to others. Some nurses have used this situation to illustrate their understanding of the difficulty of undertaking lifestyle changes and have entered into groups that work together on healthier living.

■■ ■ COMMUNICATION IN *ACTION*
■ ■■

Talking With a Neighbor about Health Concerns

Joe Reynolds is a nurse who works on the surgical unit of a local community hospital. While he works in his yard, a neighbor approaches him and begins to chat. After a few minutes of talking about yard maintenance, the neighbor says, "Uh—Joe, do you know much about these PSA tests?" Joe replies, "A bit. Do you have a question about them?" "Well, I went in to see my doctor. He did some tests and said my PSA is too high and I should go see a urologist. What the heck is it anyway and why should I see another doctor?" Joe asks, "What explanation did the doctor give you?" The neighbor replies, "Well, he said something about cancer and then I don't remember what else he said." Knowing that even hearing the word cancer can cause enough stress that a person might not hear additional explanation, Joe decides to do some simple teaching. He explains, "Well, the test means that something is going on in your prostate. It is an important test, but the results can be positive even when you don't have cancer; other things can cause it to be high. However, it really should be checked out so that you get the proper treatment. A urologist specializes in this kind of problem and will do more tests to find out exactly what is going on and then talk to you about whether you need treatment." The neighbor says, "Thanks, Joe. Guess I should make that appointment." Joe replies, "Yes, I think you should. Let me know if there is anything else I can help with."

⊕ MAINTAINING CONTINUITY OF CARE

Continuity of care for the individual means that there is an uninterrupted process across settings in which a person seeks care. In an ideal world, there would never be a duplicated test, a failure to account for medications currently prescribed, or a lack of information upon which the care provider could make decisions. However, the current system is far from ideal. When a mother with young children goes to the emergency room and does not have immunization information, this may affect the care provided. When a person leaves the hospital and does not understand the discharge instructions, that person's health is compromised. When an elderly resident moves from the nursing home to the hospital and information on medications for chronic illnesses does not accompany that person, serious complications may result. The Joint Commission requires that the institutions it accredits study this problem and establish effective policies and procedures to ensure continuity of care.

Transition Planning

Transitions are the movement of the patient from one care environment to another, such as from home care to hospital, from hospital to nursing home, or from one unit in a hospital (such as the intensive care unit [ICU]) to another (such as the general medical unit) as needs for care change. **Transition planning** refers to the process that takes place before a patient changes care environments, through the change itself, and as that person integrates into the new environment.

The transition to a new care environment has been identified as a time in which the potential for error rises. Medications may be missed or duplicated. Problems that were identified but not resolved may be overlooked. Whether moving from home to an outpatient setting or between units in the same facility, transition planning is critical to effective care. While physicians usually have the authority to prescribe the move, the nurses are the ones who usually serve as the coordinators of transitions.

Discharge Planning

Planning for a transition often begins when a decision is made for the patient's care to be moved to another setting. Some transitions can be predicted before the decision about timing is made. For most patients, discharge from a hospital is an expected event; therefore, teaching for discharge begins immediately upon admission, if possible. Upon admission to a hospital, a projected timeline for care may contain specific outcomes to be met along a care pathway. The nurse assumes responsibility for ensuring that medical orders and nursing plans move with the patient to the next location. Written materials that document these orders and plans are essential for accuracy. When discharge is to a nursing home or rehabilitation setting, the goal is that the receiving setting is prepared to provide the care needed. When the person is going home, the nurse is often responsible for ensuring that needed referrals have been arranged and for providing discharge teaching. Patients going home also need written materials to refer to in relationship to self care. Family members, when available, are integrated into the planning for discharge. The nurse in the institutional setting may follow up with the patient after discharge to ensure that the patient's health care needs are being met in the new environment and that communication has been clear. Appropriate documentation of this process is essential.

Transfers Within an Institution

When an individual moves from one unit within an institution to another, a careful plan is still needed. While some transfers occur because of sudden changes in a patient's condition or because the demand for ICU beds has accelerated transfers out to other units, most are part of the ongoing therapeutic plan. For a patient admitted for surgery, this might include an admitting unit, the surgical suite, the post-anesthesia care unit, the surgical unit, and then discharge to home or a rehabilitation setting. Many facilities now have a separate transfer form that is initiated by the nurse in the unit where the patient's care begins. This form identifies all the key transition information. When the patient is moved, the receiving nurse can quickly review the key information, assess the patient, and enter the receiving assessment and acknowledgment of the information on the form. The advantage of this process is that the receiving nurse does not need to spend a lengthy time trying to find the most important information in a voluminous medical record. Both nurses are accountable for ensuring that the key information is identified and acted upon.

Medication Reconciliation

One of the major areas of concern for patient safety at the time of any transition is the continuity of medications that the patient has been taking for the successful management of health problems. The recognition of the importance of this with regard to patient safety has resulted in the process called **medication reconciliation**, which occurs after a person is admitted to a care facility. This process is the result of recommendations by The Joint Commission Patient Safety Goals and the Institute for Safe Medication Practices (JCAHO, 2005).

Medication reconciliation at admission involves carefully documenting all the medications and their dosages, including prescribed medications, over-the-counter medications, vitamin/mineral supplements, and herbal products the person was taking before admission to the care setting. These are then compared to what has been ordered for current care. Any differences are brought to the attention of the medical care provider in order for the best care decision to be made.

This same process is used at all times of transition. Medications change when a person leaves an ICU. Nurses on a surgical unit must be aware of the medications a patient received while in the operating room. When a patient is admitted through an emergency room, the medication given there will affect ongoing care. If additional medications are ordered in that setting, the nurses must know whether they were given or must still be given after the patient comes to the care unit.

Facilities develop a standardized form on which medication reconciliation is documented. These records become part of the patient record and are also used to document quality improvement in maintaining safe medication administration by ensuring appropriate continuity of medication orders across transitions.

Critical Thinking Activity

A charge nurse in a nursing home is planning for the transfer to the hospital of an 87-year-old resident who fell and fractured her hip. This resident has a history of congestive heart failure, osteoarthritis, and osteoporosis, but had been ambulatory using a cane and cognitively intact before the fall. What concerns should be addressed before the transfer occurs? What are the issues that will be of concern during the transfer? What information will the receiving nursing unit need in order to provide effective care?

Care-Continuity Records

Medical records for any individual may be scattered among the various offices of a primary care physician, a number of specialty physicians, one or more pharmacies, a physical therapist's office, and a hospital. If an individual has geographically moved more than once, these health care record sites are multiplied by the number of cities or areas in which the person lived. This may result in discontinuity in care. Clients may not remember exactly what tests were done or their exact results. They may find it difficult to pinpoint whether a particular episode of symptoms occurred three or five years ago. Although everyone is encouraged to keep a current list of prescription medications and their dosages with them, how many actually carry through with this? When seeking past records is too cumbersome, tests may be redone; there may be no baseline against which to compare results, or significant problems may be overlooked.

The hurricanes of 2005 that saw tens of thousands of individuals displaced from the Gulf Coast region of the United States brought these concerns to the forefront. Cancer patients were evacuated but needed to continue treatment; however, their records remained in flooded hospitals. Individuals with chronic illnesses ran out of prescriptions and were unable to get needed medications. These and many other problems occurred because health records were no longer accessible.

Several groups are calling for the systematization of all health care records. The American Association of Family Physicians has launched a national initiative called Project Continuity of Care. They envision an environment in which each patient has a computerized health record that can be carried on some type of computer memory (such as a USB flash drive). This Care-Continuity Record would be downloadable into any document system, and it would contain summary information about allergies, diagnoses, test results, medications, and other data essential to effective care (Darves, 2005). While this plan may seem impossible to carry out, more health care institutions are converting to computerized documentation. And the technology to create such a computerized document is available (Fig. 3-2).

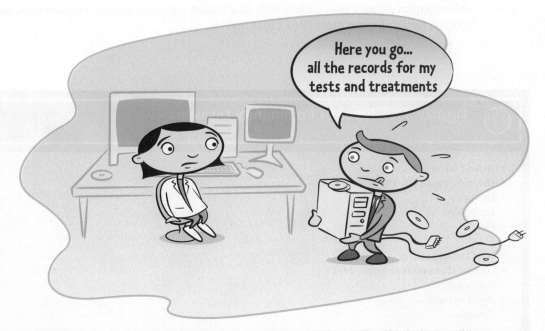

FIGURE 3-2   In an ideal health care system every person would have a "Care Continuity Record."

🌐 DISASTER RESPONSE IN THE COMMUNITY

Potential disasters have always been a concern in communities, but they have become a greater focus of attention since the 9/11 collapse of the Twin Towers in New York City. Display 3-4 lists the 11 major causes of community disasters. Some disasters, such as a fire, may occur in any community; others, such as an earthquake or a hurricane, occur more frequently in one part of the country than in another. **Disaster management** refers to the plans that are in place designating the community's reponse to a disaster.

Volunteers in Disaster Response

Many communities have plans in place to mobilize volunteers for some roles in a disaster. For example, in areas with earthquake potential, community planning focuses at the neighborhood level, with volunteers responding to neighbors. Basic first aid and management of food, water, and shelter cannot wait for professional rescuers to arrive in the event of widespread damage to roads, power, and other infrastructure. Nurses might take a leadership role in their own neighborhoods because they understand issues of both public health and disease management. Their ability to respond to people's emotional needs as well as physical concerns provides a foundation for effective leadership.

Disaster response volunteers may include Red Cross workers. The Red Cross is designated by the federal government as the key disaster response voluntary agency. Although there is a central paid staff, the majority of Red Cross workers are volunteers. The Red Cross provides training and organization for both health care professionals and others who are willing to respond to disasters. It manages shelters and serves as a conduit for donated funds and services to help those who are victims of disaster. They have also produced, in conjunction with Federal Emergency Management Agency, publications with information regarding disaster preparedness, such as the one on family disaster plans (Red Cross, 1991).

🌐 Display 3-4   Types of Community Disasters

- Acts of terror
- Disease—especially epidemic disease
- Drought
- Earthquake
- Fire
- Flood
- Food contamination
- Hazmat (hazardous material spill)
- Hurricane
- Power outages
- Tornado

Other voluntary and nonprofit organizations also respond to disasters. One of the largest and most widely known is the Salvation Army, a Christian group that provides a wide array of social services at all times. During disasters, Salvation Army workers are active in setting up shelters, providing meals, and helping affected individuals to rebuild their lives. Other religious and disaster response organizations may also be mobilized depending on the size of the disaster.

Institution and Agency Disaster Response

Firefighters, police officers, ambulance drivers, and health professionals are all part of response plans. Most of these individuals are trained for disaster response by their employers.

Firefighters are often the frontline responders to those injured in a disaster. They provide the rescue and emergency medical response skills to save lives. As first responders, firefighters risk the potential for serious injury, smoke or dust inhalation, carbon monoxide poisoning, and heat-related illness from the wearing of protective gear in hot environments. Nurses working in triage must be cognizant of this risk to emergency workers.

Hospitals often serve a pivotal role in managing injuries or illness related to a disaster. Each hospital has plans in place for both internal disasters (such as a fire in one wing of the hospital) and external disasters (such as a tornado in the community). In communities with multiple hospitals, coordination in disaster planning and preparation is essential. Based on their locations and services, each might be designated for a different role.

Learning about their agency's disaster plans should be part of the orientation of all employees. Nurses in hospitals have major roles in responding to disasters. Current patients will be discharged as quickly as possible to open up beds for disaster victims. Units will be reorganized to enable the acceptance and treatment of multiple victims. Nurses may be asked to move to emergency departments to be part of teams that will provide triage. **Triage** involves the initial screening of victims for the purpose of prioritizing treatment and making the most effective and efficient use of both human and material resources. When major triage is no longer needed, nurses may then return to units for patient care.

Part of a disaster plan for any agency is a call-in system. This system is a planned process for notifying staff not on duty that there is a disaster and they should report for work. Building such a call-in list is usually the responsibility of the manager of each unit. There may be a telephone tree with people designated to call others within their neighborhood or geographic area, in order for everyone to be notified more quickly. Health care professionals sometimes face an ethical dilemma regarding being called in for a disaster. Their own families and neighborhoods may need them, but the hospital is treating the most seriously injured or ill and needs everyone.

Specific Disaster Concerns

Hurricane Katrina on the Gulf Coast pointed out the tremendous challenges of managing a widespread disaster when the local resources for response are also destroyed. Without hospitals, fire departments, and other agencies, all help had to come from outside the community. Transportation and communication were identified as major problems. Moving large numbers of people, arranging for shelters, and communicating among those trying to provide emergency help all became more than the system was prepared to manage. The total resulting effect on people's lives and health is still not known. As a consequence of this situation, communities are looking more closely at their disaster planning and requesting that both the federal and state governments develop better contingency plans. The federal government operates a Web site that is an entry point for learning about the federal government's disaster information and services (*www.disasterhelp.gov/portal/jhtml/index.jhtml*).

Avian influenza, or "bird flu," while still found only in birds and those people and other animals that have direct contact with birds, continues to have the potential for becoming a disease that can be transmitted from person to person (Centers for Disease Control and Prevention, 2006). The world has not had a true influenza pandemic (worldwide epidemic) since 1918, when a strain of influenza moved around the world at the close of World War I, causing the deaths of 20 to 50 million people worldwide (Billings, 2005). Nurses need to become knowledgeable about transmission methods for communicable diseases and be prepared to give accurate information to those who express concerns. They also need to understand their role in any institutional plan for response to an infectious disease disaster.

Terrorism, while not visible in the United States since 9/11, remains a concern. The subway and bus bombings in London in 2005 demonstrated the vulnerability of large cities to the concerted efforts of a few terrorists (Cable News Network, 2005). A great deal of the federal government's support for disaster planning is focused on terrorism. Part of the disaster planning of every urban community relates to terrorism response. Whole communities may be involved in disaster response drills, and people may be recruited to play the part of victims. A simulated disaster is staged, and all the plans of the various community agencies are activated. A disaster drill provides a mechanism to find out what works and to plan more effectively.

COMPLEMENTARY AND ALTERNATIVE HEALTH CARE

The National Center for Complementary and Alternative Medicine (NCCAM, 2002) has defined this field as "a group of diverse medical and health care systems, practices, and products that are not presently considered to be part of conventional medicine" (*http://nccam.nih.gov/health/whatiscam*, 2006). Conventional medicine may also be referred to as allopathy, Western, mainstream, orthodox, regular medicine, and biomedicine. This definition of complementary and alternative medicine (CAM) focuses more on what alternative care is *not* than what it *is*, because of the broad range of health care practices included in this category. Common among these practices are acupuncture, homeopathy, naturopathy, music therapy, and herbal medicine. NCCAM includes prayer for health reasons as a therapy practice. The list of health care practices considered complementary and alternative shifts constantly as some are proven safe and effective, others are proven of little value or even harmful and fade from use, and still others emerge. According to recent surveys, 36% of adults in the United States use some form of CAM. When megavitamin therapy and prayer specifically for health reasons are included in the definition of CAM, that number rises to 62%. Overall, CAM use is greater among women, people with higher education levels, people who have been hospitalized in the past year, and former smokers (compared with current smokers or those who have never smoked). Survey results indicated that CAM is most often used to treat and/or prevent musculoskeletal conditions or other conditions that involve chronic or recurring pain (*http://nccam.nih.gov/news/camsurvey_fs1.htm*, 2004). The increasing numbers of individuals who seek non-allopathic health care usually pay out of pocket for the services because few of the practices are covered by private or government insurance plans.

These health care approaches are considered *alternative* when they are used in place of conventional medical care. The same approaches are considered *complementary* when they are used along with conventional medicine. **Integrative medicine**, as defined by NCCAM, "combines mainstream medical therapies and CAM therapies for which there is some high-quality scientific evidence of safety and effectiveness" (NCCAM, 2006). Thus, integrative medicine supports the higher standard of research evidence for effectiveness. NCCAM provides training for researchers in the area of CAM, funds grants for research into the effectiveness of all types of alternative care, and disseminates research findings about CAM to both professionals and the public. The National Library of Medicine maintains a database, CAM on PUBMED, which allows for research in relationship to specific diseases, conditions, and therapies. (See end of chapter Web sites.)

CAM takes place almost entirely within the community, and the client often serves as its primary controlling factor, as opposed to conventional medicine, in which the official health care provider controls access to care through ordering diagnostics, prescribing treatments, and determining admission to and discharge from a care facility. As **complementary** and **alternative health care** practices remain popular with the public, health care providers are challenged to understand these diverse approaches and to work effectively with clients who choose those resources. There is also a need to assist in client education so that choices are made wisely and with sound information. This has become so important for nurses that the NCLEX-RN examination now includes questions related to the nurse's role in assisting clients who use CAM (Helms, 2006). Accreditation agencies are stimulating those nursing programs that have not already begun discussing CAM to add this information to their curriculum (Helms, 2006).

Major Types of Complementary and Alternative Medicine

As of 2002, NCCAM had categorized CAM into five domains for the purpose of discussion and study. These domains include whole medical systems, mind–body medicine, biologically-based practices, manipulative and body-based practices, and energy medicine (Tables 3-1 and 3-2).

Specific alternative care providers may use more than one type of treatment in their practice. Additionally, there are many areas of overlap between conventional medical practice and CAM. The major types of alternative care available are described briefly in the following sections.

TABLE 3-1   ALTERNATIVE WHOLE MEDICAL SYSTEMS

SYSTEM	EXAMPLES
Traditional indigenous systems	Traditional Oriental medicine Qi gong Acupuncture Herbal medicine Oriental massage Ayurvedic medicine Native American medicine Other folk medicine systems (Mexican, South American, etc.)
Unconventional Western systems	Homeopathy Naturopathy

TABLE 3-2	TYPES OF COMPLEMENTARY AND ALTERNATIVE PRACTICES
CLASSIFICATIONS	**SPECIFIC THERAPIES**
Mind–body medicine	Relaxation exercises Hypnosis Meditation Dance Prayer Visualization Biofeedback
Biologically based practices	Herbal medicines Special diets Food supplements Vitamin therapy Biologic substances, such as bovine and shark cartilage
Manipulative and body-based practices	Chiropractic Massage therapy Reflexology
Energy medicine	Bioelectromagnetic applications to the body Radiofrequency hyperthermia Radiofrequency diathermy Magnets Nerve stimulators Biofields—Manipulations of energy fields originating within the body: Reiki, therapeutic touch

Whole Medical Systems

Whole medical systems represent complete systems of theory and practice that approach health care differently than the traditional Western biomedical approach. NCCAM has identified two approaches to entire systems of health care that differ from Western medicine: traditional indigenous systems and unconventional Western systems of medicine (NCCAM, 2006). Each system uses a variety of specific therapies.

Traditional Indigenous Systems. In indigenous medicine, there are complete systems of explanation for health and illness, and therapies are chosen based on these theoretic systems of belief.

Some indigenous systems are quite formal in approach, with individuals studying and serving apprenticeships before practice. These include traditional Asian medicine and Ayurvedic medicine from India. Traditional Asian medicine may include the use of qi gong (a form of energy therapy), oriental massage, acupuncture, and herbs. Ayurvedic medicine, a traditional system from India, has existed for more than 5,000 years and has a specific theoretic and therapeutic focus on imbalance in the individual's consciousness. Lifestyle interventions are the major form of Ayurvedic preventive and therapeutic treatment. Currently there is only one Ayurvedic hospital in North America.

Informal approaches are often termed *folk medicine*; these traditions usually are handed down by word of mouth and are used by individuals and families to treat common health problems. Indigenous medicine practitioners use a variety of approaches to health care, often combining herbs, food, and traditional ceremonies. Little is understood about many of the herbs used, but some have demonstrated therapeutic effects while others may be questionable.

In a given ethnic group, certain people may be designated as healers or as having special knowledge and ability regarding illness. They may have had a period of apprenticeship, but it is informal in nature and not mandated by any outside authority. The advice of the indigenous healer may be sought instead of the advice of a physician. Native American cultures may use a *shaman*, or medicine man/woman. Mexican-Americans may use the services of a *curandero*, or healer. A system of understanding hot and cold disorders and foods that help to balance heat and cold in the body is part of many of these folk traditions. NCCAM points out that "other traditional medical systems have been developed by Native American, Australian Aboriginal, African, Middle Eastern, Tibetan, Central and South American cultures" (NCCAM, 2006). To work most effectively with a client who uses folk medicine, you need to learn about the specific beliefs and resources that the client is using.

Unconventional Western Systems of Medicine. Unconventional Western systems of medicine originated in Western society but did not find general support. Some individuals continue to practice in the theoretic precepts of these systems and have re-emerged as the public looks for alternatives to conventional medical care.

Perhaps the most common of these unconventional Western systems is homeopathy. **Homeopathy** is based on the belief that exposure to extremely small quantities of either the substance causing an illness or a related substance will stimulate a cure. Of course, this principle is also the basis for immunization and allergy desensitization. The application of this principle to other diseases, however, has not been accepted by the medical community. The dilutions used in many homeopathic remedies are so great that a dosage may contain only a few molecules of a substance. Homeopathy was popular in the early twentieth century but fell into disrepute as standard medical research advanced. There is currently a resurgence of interest in this approach to therapy, and new research is being done. Homeopathic practitioners once again are offering an alternative to standard medical care.

Naturopathy. Naturopathy gets its name from the natural agents used in treating disease, such as food, exercise, air, water, and sunshine. The naturopathic physician treats people by recommending changes in lifestyle, diet, and exercise, and promoting the use of vitamins and herbs. For many, lifestyle and dietary changes are a successful form of treatment. Naturopathic physicians follow a prescribed course of study that includes clinical experiences with clients and results in the doctor of naturopathy degree. Naturopathy is licensed in 13 states; however, questions have been raised about the use of naturopathic physicians in primary care, especially regarding the adequacy of their training in the recognition and treatment of more serious illnesses and the concern that many of the herbal remedies prescribed by naturopathic physicians are untested and unregulated.

Mind–Body Medicine

Mind–body medicine seeks to control physical processes through the mind's capacities. In addition, it treats emotional concerns. When prayer is included in this catagory, mind–body medicine is the most commonly used domain (53%). When it is not included, biologically based practices (22%) are more popular than mind–body medicine (17%) (*http://nccam.nih.gov/news/camsurvey_fs1.htm*, 2004). Increasingly, mind–body interventions are being incorporated into standard health care practice. Traditional psychotherapy, a well-established part of standard health care, is a mind–body approach to health. The use of prayer, support groups, yoga, meditation, relaxation, biofeedback, and visualization are all mind–body therapies.

Relaxation exercises, hypnosis, and meditation are examples of controlling physiologic stress responses through mental processes. Relaxation exercises, breathing techniques, meditation, and visualization are used to reduce anxiety, reduce blood pressure, and lessen the body's response to stressors. These techniques also are designed to prevent stress-related problems from developing; for many people, they are part of a plan to increase health and well-being. These techniques also are suggested for the management of specific health problems and may be used in conjunction with traditional medical treatment.

Every major religion of the world responds in particular ways to those who are ill. A well-established way for supporting an ill person is through the prayers of others who care. Nurses recognize that spiritual distress has a significant impact on a client's ability to move toward wellness. Supporting the individual's quest for spiritual solace and healing has been a part of the mission of many health care agencies that were established by religious bodies. The separation of prayer and spiritual care from other health care is a modern phenomenon.

Visualization may be used to help children manage painful medical procedures. Suggestions regarding healing and postoperative recovery are used in the operating room by some anesthesiologists and surgeons. The anesthesiologist may talk to the patient who is still anesthetized, suggesting that pain will be minimal, nausea will not occur, and recovery will be rapid. This is similar to posthypnotic suggestion. Hypnosis has been used in other illnesses for symptom relief (Fig. 3-3).

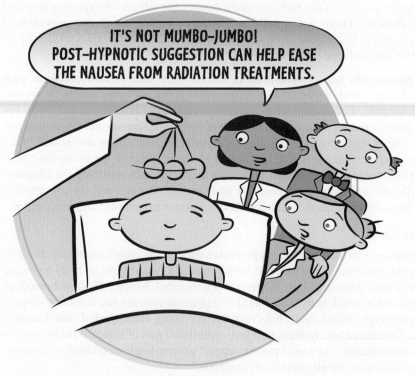

IT'S NOT MUMBO-JUMBO! POST-HYPNOTIC SUGGESTION CAN HELP EASE THE NAUSEA FROM RADIATION TREATMENTS.

FIGURE 3-3. Alternative health care is moving more and more into mainstream practice.

Biofeedback is a specific mechanism used to assist individuals by altering physiologic responses through mental processes. The machines used for biofeedback provide visual or auditory feedback of physiologic parameters such as blood pressure or galvanic skin response. By observing these parameters, the individual learns to change the underlying physiologic process. Some individuals with migraine headaches use biofeedback control over circulation to abort migraine attacks rather than take medications. Biofeedback is recognized as effective for a variety of processes that are under autonomic nervous system control.

Mind–body interventions in general allow people to participate actively in their own care. People often are changed emotionally and psychologically in the process of treating illness or disease. A big advantage of the mind–body therapies is that they are safe and economical and can be used easily in conjunction with other therapies.

Biologically-based Practices

Biologically-based practices include **herbal medicine**, special diets, food supplements, vitamins, and specific biologic substances such as bovine and shark cartilage.

Herbal medicines are plant products that are used to treat almost all illnesses. We know that plants often have active ingredients that affect the human body. Digitalis, for example, was originally a dried leaf of the foxglove plant (digitalis drugs, such as digoxin, are now synthesized in the laboratory). It was indeed a potent and effective medication when used as an herb, but dosage was not accurate and little scientific information existed regarding its effects. As research into plant products continues, our understanding of the efficacy of herbs increases. Many in the United States who describe themselves as herbalists received their training in herbs during an apprenticeship with an experienced herbalist. There are educational programs for herbalists, but they are not regulated in every state.

These products all have the potential to interact with medications prescribed, and many may cause adverse effects. When nurses interview patients regarding their medication history, asking specific questions about vitamins, herbs, supplements, and other therapeutic agents is critical. Patients may not consider these to be "medication" and so may not provide information about these substances being taken. The result may be that the source of an adverse response is missed or a harmful interaction with prescribed medications occurs.

It is wise to recognize the potential problems as well as the potential benefits of the use of herbal medicines. These problems include dosage and bioavailability, safety and efficacy, and interactions with prescribed medications.

The bioavailability of various herbal preparations may vary widely, making it difficult to stabilize dosage. And because plants grow under different circumstances and with different soil and other conditions, the proportion of active ingredient within the plant may vary considerably. This makes accurate and stable dosage of herbs difficult.

While herbal products are available in tablet form with doses listed on the label, at present, there are no laws regulating the potency or purity of herbs sold in the United States. Many herbs are imported from around the world. Rules and regulations regarding accurate labeling and content purity may not be as strict in some developing countries as they are in the United States. And because herbs are not considered drugs, there are no regulations regarding testing for efficacy or safety, as there are with drugs that must be approved by the Food and Drug Administration (FDA). This means that some herbs that are sold may contain contaminants. Serious illnesses and even deaths have been traced to contaminants in herbal medicines (Warren & Devine, 2004).

Sometimes the active ingredient in an herb may have potent side effects. For example, many individuals have used herbs that contain ephedra. Ephedra acts as a stimulant, dilates bronchioles, and decreases appetite. Therefore, it has been used for the herbal treatment of fatigue, asthma, and obesity. It also raises blood pressure, increases pulse rate, and creates feelings of tension and anxiety. These side effects have been severe enough to precipitate stroke and cardiac problems in some individuals (FDA, 2003).

Herbs may also interact with prescription and over-the-counter medications, altering the effect or increasing side effects. For example, some herbal preparations exacerbate the anticoagulant effect of warfarin and thus increase potential for bleeding; and individuals on prescribed dosages of immunosuppressants cannot drink green tea because green tea stimulates the immune system.

Some countries, such as Germany, have regulated herbal medications for many years. Canada has a system of regulating "natural health products" that includes regulations for herbal and homeopathic remedies. The Canadian system is based on a phased-in process that addresses products with the highest risk potential first (Natural Health Products Directorate, 2004).

Clients taking herbal medicines should be encouraged to share this information with their health care provider. They also should be encouraged to question carefully the sources of the herbs that they take. These actions might help clients avoid potentially harmful interactions with prescribed medications or other adverse effects.

■■ COMMUNICATION IN *ACTION*
■■

Assisting With Complete Reporting

Maggie Wilson works in an ambulatory clinic. She is reviewing Mabel Wilson's written new patient information. As she speaks with Mrs. Wilson, she says, "I see that you wrote here that you take supplements. Would you please tell me exactly what supplements you are taking?" Mrs. Wilson says, "Oh, I figured those didn't make any difference; they aren't like real medicine or anything, just like food." Maggie replies, "Supplements need to be considered along with medicines because they all have some effect. Sometimes that is a benefit to you, but sometimes they interfere with certain drugs that might be prescribed. Whenever you see a doctor, you need to be sure to let the doctor know all the prescribed medicines, over-the-counter medicines, and supplements that you use. Please tell me what you take so I can add them to your record."

Biologic treatments include a variety of substances not approved as medical treatment by the FDA. These products have been developed by individuals and organizations and are often sold as food supplements rather than as medicines. Cartilage products from sharks, cattle, sheep, and chickens are being used to treat both cancer and arthritis. Peptide fractions derived from human blood and urine, called antineoplastons, are being used to treat cancer. Coley's toxins are killed cultures of bacteria that have been used for treating cancer. Apitherapy is the use of honeybee venom to treat rheumatic diseases, dermatologic conditions, chronic pain, and cancer. Research on the efficacy of these treatments is costly, and sponsors willing to bear that cost are hard to find. Some small studies are being funded with federal grants.

The health food movement in the United States is extraordinarily popular. Countless books are written and innumerable products are produced for this market. One of the appeals of this approach to health care is that it focuses on everyday, natural resources as opposed to science and technology. Poor dietary practices are common in the United States, with many individuals eating far more fat than is recommended while neglecting fruits, vegetables, and whole grains. Many people achieve better health by paying attention to good nutrition.

Medical research is beginning to identify some benefits of using food and vitamins in therapeutic ways. We have long known that many individuals who develop type 2 diabetes may be able to manage their blood sugar through dietary control. The role of antioxidants in decreasing cell damage and the effect of certain phytochemicals contained in cruciferous vegetables in preventing bowel cancer are just two examples of the theoretic benefits of nutrients. Some parents have used strict dietary regulation as a management tool for children with attention deficit hyperactivity disorder.

There are hazards in this approach to health care, however. Megadoses of vitamins may prove toxic. Some nutrients interact with medications, decreasing their effectiveness. Individuals who choose to avoid all traditional medical care and rely on unsubstantiated claims about the therapeutic effects of nutrients may suffer deterioration in health.

All health care professionals need to support and encourage healthy dietary practices. Often it is possible to assist clients who rely on the use of nutrients for health care by becoming knowledgeable about the research regarding nutrition, accepting what clients believe helps them (as long as it is not detrimental to their well-being), and keeping an open mind. When we are willing to acknowledge the validity of some aspects of their preferred approach to health care, these clients may be willing to combine more conventional medical care along with their nutritional approaches.

Manipulative and Body-Based Practices

Manipulative and body-based practices include the physical manipulation of the body to achieve health goals. Some authors refer to these as "manual healing." Manipulative therapy is found in massage therapy and reflexology. Massage therapy uses both fixed and movable pressure and holding by the hands and sometimes the forearms, elbows, or feet. There is evidence that these techniques affect the musculoskeletal, circulatory–lymphatic, and nervous systems. Reflexology is massage of the feet to activate points on the feet that correspond to other body parts or systems.

Perhaps the most commonly known type of manipulative practice is chiropractic. Chiropractic care is based on the theory that disease is caused by interference with nerve function. It uses manipulation of the body joints, especially the spinal vertebrae, in seeking to restore normal function. The chiropractor also may use other treatments commonly associated with physical therapy, such as massage and exercise. There are definite differences among chiropractors. Some state that there are illnesses that cannot be treated through manual healing and do recommend that certain clients seek conventional medical care. Others believe that all illnesses may be treated by chiropractic methods and do not refer clients for conventional medical care. A major concern is that some clients may have more serious illnesses that may be missed altogether or not recognized in time to be given optimal medical attention. Another problem with chiropractic care is the use of chiropractic treatments on infants and young children in place of immunizations and other well-child services.

Many people with joint and muscle strain and tension find that chiropractic treatments relieve discomfort and support effective functioning. In 1994, the Agency for Health Care

Research and Quality (AHRQ) recommended chiropractic treatment as a useful option in specific circumstances for relieving pain and discomfort in acute back pain in their clinical guideline (AHRQ, 1994). While this document is no longer the definitive guideline for acute low back pain, it brought chiropractic care into the range of options that were considered validated for use.

Energy Medicine

The use of **energy medicine** (sometimes referred to bioelectromagnetic [BEM] therapies) is based on the understanding that electrical phenomena are found in all living organisms. There are magnetic fields that extend from the body, which can be measured and may be affected by external forces. The mechanisms by which the electromagnetic fields occur in the body, how these can be changed, and the effects of such changes are under study. Many modalities have been used for years without clear studies of their effectiveness. Some believe that BEM may be a unifying theory explaining why such widely diverse therapies as acupuncture and homeopathy produce results.

Some energy medicine is based on applying external energy to the body. There are thermal applications of BEM therapy in the form of radiofrequency hyperthermia and radiofrequency diathermy. Nonthermal applications include magnets and nerve stimulation. One common application is the use of magnets to relieve musculoskeletal problems. Magnetic insoles for shoes and magnets to be worn on the body are widely available.

There are also methods used to manipulate the interior biofields of the individual. These include **therapeutic touch** and reiki. Both of these practices are based on a system of changing the energy fields without applying external energy forces to the body. In therapeutic touch, the practitioner moves hands above the body or touches lightly, perceives energy fields, and modifies them through hand movements. Dr. Dolores Krieger integrated work in therapeutic touch in nursing (Krieger, 1993) and believes that her studies validate its effectiveness. Others studying therapeutic touch have not been able to discern either the energy fields or methods of change. Therapeutic touch has found acceptance by some within the nursing community, and a nursing diagnosis titled "energy field disturbance" has been included in the NANDA-I taxonomy. This is a matter of controversy, and there are strong objections by some to its inclusion without replicable research support. Nurses interested in therapeutic touch should research it further.

Understanding the Use of Complementary and Alternative Health Care

According to a recent study (Tindle, Davis, Phillips, & Eisenberg, 2005), the number of people using CAM has remained stable since it was last studied in 1997, with approximately 72 million Americans using alternative and complementary therapies. For many clients with chronic conditions, mainstream medical care offers few options. Long-term treatments with medications often produce their own iatrogenic (treatment-caused) health problems, some of which are as troubling to the individual as the original disease process. A common response of conventional medicine to these problems has been to add more medications and more treatments, each with its own potential adverse effects. Mainstream health care providers often give little attention to the problems of daily living that are of greatest concern to the individual. Stress and anxiety also add to the burden of these clients. For clients with acute health conditions, certain treatments or medications may produce unpleasant or harmful side effects. Clients often are looking for alternative treatment methods that do not appear to have the same potential for harm.

Some alternative therapies have been available for many years, and there are people who believe that they have been helped significantly by these approaches. Unfortunately, traditional health care providers often have dismissed these therapies without investigating them thoroughly. On the other hand, few alternative therapies have been formally researched, and proponents often rely on undocumented reports of effectiveness.

Research into alternative therapies now is supported by the federal government but only in a small way compared to other research. The federal government has an Office of Alternative Health Care, the NCCAM, and a Web page of references (see list of Web sites). More attention is being paid to the responses of individuals. Concern about the role of stress in illness has prompted an increased openness to nonmedical methods of managing stress. The possibility of alternative care practices working in a complementary fashion with traditional medical care is gaining wider acceptance. Often these complementary therapies are used to address the whole person and not simply the disease.

Part of the appeal of alternative health care is the caring and personalized response that clients often receive. People who have been intimidated by businesslike clinics and made to feel unimportant by impersonal professionals may find that the warm, concerned, accepting atmosphere of the nonconventional setting meets many personal needs. The fact that stress and anxiety play a major role in any health problem may help explain why many people are helped by therapies that may not be based on sound scientific knowledge. Nurses are in a unique position to relate with people about the issues that surround alternative and complementary therapy because of the trust placed in them. A recent Gallup poll has identified nurses as the most trusted professionals when ethics are considered (Gallup Poll, 2004),

To learn more about any specific therapy, or to research alternative and complementary therapies for any condition, use the CAM Citation Index found on the Web site of the NCCAM (see references). You may also search MEDLINE, the database of the National Library of Medicine, through the free PubMed Web site (*www.nlm.nih.gov/nccam/camonpubmed.html*) to research various therapies.

Assisting Clients Who Choose Alternative Health Care

Many people who support conventional methods of health care have long ignored or repudiated the value of unorthodox health care traditions. We must recognize that complementary and alternative health care practices persist because people find them to be valuable. Acknowledging health care alternatives and working cooperatively with them is usually much more productive than trying to oppose them.

NCCAM suggests a five-step process for the consumer considering a particular complementary or alternative therapy. This process has a heavy emphasis on careful information gathering.

Assess Safety and Effectiveness

The first step is for the individual to assess the safety and effectiveness of the therapy in relationship to his or her own condition. One of the difficulties is finding accurate safety and efficacy data. Web sites and other sources of information require close scrutiny to determine the qualifications and bias of the sponsoring individual or group. The NCCAM Web site (*www.nccam.nih.gov*) contains Fact Sheets regarding specific therapies and additional links to research reports and scientific papers. Research reports may also be found through PubMed, the National Library of Medicine's online access (*www.ncbi.nlm.nih.gov/PubMed*). All complementary and alternative therapies are classified there under the Medical Subject Heading of "complementary therapies." The University of Pittsburgh Health Sciences Library System maintains an Alternative Medicine Homepage (*www.pitt.edu/~cbw/altm.html*) that provides links to additional information sites on the Web.

Examine the Expertise of the Therapy Practitioner

The second step is to examine the expertise of any therapy practitioner. Whether this person is a physician or another type of provider, determine whether there is appropriate education and licensing if that is required. Consumers should be encouraged to ask directly about education and credentials for practice. Some consumer organizations will direct individuals to reliable practitioners in the community. Clients who may be reluctant to ask directly about credentials can check whether credentials are available on a Web site or in printed information from the practitioner.

The client might also want to talk with others who have had experience with the practitioner in question. The Center for the Health Professions at the University of California, San Francisco, published a template by Dower, O'Neil, and Hough (2001) for asking questions about an alternative health care provider.

Investigate Service Delivery

Service delivery is the third aspect the client should investigate. How many patients are seen per day? Where is the therapy available and what barriers does that pose? Are standards for safety, privacy, and confidentiality in place? Remember that alternative providers are not included in the federal Health Insurance Portability and Accountability Act of 1996 legislation that mandates confidentiality in conventional health care settings unless they are eligible for reimbursement through Medicare or Medicaid. Most alternative providers are responsible for establishing their own standards and policies without outside oversight.

Investigate the Cost of Therapy

A fourth consideration is the cost of the therapy. Part of this is investigating what coverage may be obtained from an insurance carrier or whether any is available. Are the costs clear? How are payments made? Some unscrupulous practitioners collect large sums of money before any service and then may not provide what was promised. Some types of alternative care (for example, chiropractic care for an acute back injury) may be reimbursable under a traditional health plan.

Discuss the Treatment With Your Regular Health Care Provider

The fifth step is to discuss this proposed treatment with a regular health care provider. The interaction of any traditional treatment and a complementary or alternative treatment may or may not pose a problem. Many health care providers support the use of various complementary therapies.

Things that the health care provider must also consider are such issues as client choice, informed consent, and the ethical principles of beneficence and nonmaleficence (see Chapter 9).

As complementary and alternative therapies move into the mainstream, greater accountability to the public is essential.

Critical Thinking Activity

Identify a specific form of complementary or alternative therapy. Do a literature search regarding this therapy. Review the information available in other sources. Analyze the information to determine whether the data supporting the use of this therapy are weak, moderate, or strong. Provide a rationale for your determination.

Key Concepts

- Community-based nursing emphasizes advocating for patients, promoting self-care, focusing on health promotion and disease prevention, and recognizing the importance of family, culture, and the community.
- Health promotion and prevention of illness and disease are a part of nursing practice in all settings.
- Client empowerment through teaching, explaining options, and supporting decision making is a foundation for community-based care.
- Primary prevention focuses on preventing disease; secondary prevention focuses on early diagnosis through screening and preventing complications; tertiary prevention focuses on preventing long-term disability and restoring functional capacity.
- Disease management strives to promote health through effective treatment of targeted diseases and health conditions.
- Healthy People 2010 is a federal effort that includes overall goals, priority areas, and leading indicators to measure progress in developing healthier communities.
- Maintaining continuity of care requires transition planning, with special emphasis on reconciling medication records from one setting to another.
- Ensuring that health care records are available wherever the client seeks care is becoming a possibility through computerization of medical records and the development of the care continuity record.
- Alternative health care encompasses those types of care outside of conventional Western medicine and includes alternative whole medical systems, mind–body medicine, biologically based practices, manipulative and body-based practices, and energy medicine.
- Alternative care therapies are considered complementary therapies when used along with traditional medical care. Integrative medicine involves the deliberative planning for using both traditional medical care and alternative care in a coordinated manner.
- Understanding the different types of alternative health care services, why people choose alternative health care, and how nurses may assist people who seek this care will form a foundation for more effective relationships with clients.
- Alternative and complementary therapies can be evaluated based on a five-step process that includes safety and effectiveness of the therapy, credentials of the provider, service delivery, cost of services, and consultation with the regular health care provider.

Relevant Web Sites

Alternative Medicine: Health Information Resources for Patients, Their Families, Friends, and Health Care Workers. McMaster University: *http://hsl.mcmaster.ca/tomflem/altmed.html*

Alternative Medicine Home Page. Folk Library of the Health Sciences, University of Pittsburgh provides links to Internet information regarding alternative health care: *www.pitt.edu/~cbw/altm.html*

American Holistic Nurses Association: *www.ahna.org*

American Music Therapy Association: *www.musictherapy.org*

CAM on PubMed: An entry point to PubMed with assistance in using PubMed to search the National Library of Medicine for relevant research: *www.nlm.nih.gov/nccam/camonpubmed.html*

Center for the Health Professions, University of California at San Francisco. Focuses on the study of the health care work force and its challenges in the modern health care system: *www.futurehealth.ucsf.edu*

Disaster Help: The President's Disaster Management Egov Initiative: *www.disasterhelp.gov/portal/jhtml/index.jhtml*

Food and Drug Administration. (n.d.) Dietary Supplements: Warnings and Safety Information. U.S. Food and Drug Administration:*www.cfsan.fda.gov/%7Edms/ds-warn.html*

National Association for Holistic Aromatherapy: *www.naha.org*

NCCAM: Federal Government database of scientific articles and abstracts: *www.nccam.nih.gov*

The Friends of Alternative and Complementary Therapies Society: *www.thefacts.org*

NCCAM: Federal Government Introductory Web Site for information on CAM: *http://nccam.nih.gov/health/*

Whole Health MD, Resource site for Integrative Medicine approaches to CAM, provides references to research, expert opinions, and resources for care. *www.wholehealthmd.com*

References

Agency for Healthcare Research and Quality. (1994). Acute low back problems in adults. AHCPR Publication No. 95-0642 [On-line]. Available: *www.ahrq.gov/clinic/cpgarchv.htm*. Accessed November 15, 2005.

Billings, M. (2005). The influenza pandemic of 1918. Stanford University [On-line]. *www.stanford.edu/group/virus/uda/*. Accessed March 15, 2006.

Centers for Disease Control and Prevention. (2006). Key facts about avian influenza (bird flu) and avian influenza A (H5N1) virus [On-line]. *www.cdc.gov/flu/avian/gen-info/facts.htm*. Accessed March 14, 2006.

Cable News Network. (2005). Investigators pick through London carnage. July 8, 2005 [On-line]. *www.cnn.com/2005/WORLD/europe/07/07/london.tube/index.html*. Accessed March 15, 2006.

Darves, B. (2005). AAFP calls for universal adoption of care-continuity record. Medscape Medical News [On-line]. *www.medscape. com/viewarticle/514049*. Accessed November 12, 2005.

Dower, C., O'Neil, E., & Hough, H. (2001). Profiling the professions: A model for evaluating emerging health professions, Center for the Health Professions, University of California [On-line]. *www.futurehealth.ucsf.edu/pdf_files/Model2.pdf*. Accessed November 12, 2005.

Food and Drug Administration. (2003). FDA fact sheet. HHS acts to reduce safety concerns associated with dietary supplements containing ephedra [On-line]. *www.fda.gov/bbs/topics/NEWS/ ephedra/factsheet.html*. Accessed March 13, 2006.

Gallup Poll. (2004). Honesty and ethical standards of professions survey, 2004 [On-line]. *http://poll.gallup.com/*. Accessed March 18, 2006.

Gaston, C. M., & Mitchell, G. (2005). Information giving and decision-making in patients with advanced cancer: A systematic review, *Social Science & Medicine 61*(10): 2252–2264.

Helms, J. E. (2006). Complementary and alternative therapies: A new frontier for nursing education, *Journal of Nursing Education 45*(3): 117–123.

Joint Commission on Accreditation of Healthcare Organizations. (2005). Medication reconciliation: An organizational approach to improving patient safety outcomes, Chicago: Author [On-line]. *www.jcrinc.com/education.asp?durki=10078&site=5 &return=8386*. Accessed November 12, 2005.

Krieger, D. (1993*).* Accepting your power to heal: The personal practice of therapeutic touch. Santa Fe, NM: Bear & Co.

National Center for Complementary and Alternative Medicine. (2002). What is complementary and alternative medicine? [On-line]. *http://nccam.nih.gov/health/whatiscam/* Accessed October 15, 2005.

National Center for Complementary and Alternative Medicine. (2006). The use of complementary and alternative medicine in the United States [On-line]. Available: *http://nccam.nih.gov/news/camsurvey_fs1.htm*. Accessed March 24, 2006.

Natural Health Products Directorate. (2004). Natural health products compliance guide. Health Canada [Online]. *www.hc-sc.gc.ca/dhp-mps/prodnatur/legislation/pol/compli-conform/complian-conform_guide_e.html#1*. Accessed Nov. 11, 2005.

Red Cross. (1991). Your family disaster plan [On-line]. *www.redcross.org/static/file_cont36_lang0_23.pdf*. Accessed March 15, 2006.

Tindle, H. A., Davis, R. B., Phillips, R. S., & Eisenberg, D. M. (2005). Trends in use of complementary and alternative medicine by US adults: 1997-2002, *Alternative Therapies in Health and Medicine, 11*(1): 42–49.

U.S. Department of Health and Human Services. (November 2000). Healthy people 2010: Understanding and improving health. 2nd ed. Washington, DC: U.S. Government Printing Office [On-line]. *www.healthypeople.gov/document/*. Accessed November 19, 2005.

Warren, B. S. & Devine, C. M. (2004). Herbal medicines and breast cancer risk. Fact Sheet #3, Cornell program on breast cancer and environmental risk, Cornell University [On-line]. *http://envirocancer.cornell.edu/factsheet/diet/fs53.herbal.cfm*. Accessed November 20, 2005.

UNIT II

Appreciating the Development of Nursing as a Profession

The purpose of Unit II is to provide an understanding of the events that resulted in nursing developing into the profession it is today. Gaining knowledge about the history and development of nursing helps the individual who is just starting a caring career to better understand and interpret the things that occur now and, thereby, move into the future more comfortably. Learning about the history and development of the profession can help you to appreciate the heritage of the discipline and the events that resulted in nursing offering the opportunities and challenges that it provides today. This unit begins with a history of nursing that describes its growth from early times to an era when preparation for nursing existed as apprentice-type training to a profession that now encompasses doctoral and postdoctoral education.

Many believe that nursing is a young profession. Some note that nursing has always existed in some form, while others question whether nursing should be considered a profession at all. These debates are considered in this unit. Some of the studies that were conducted about nursing and their impact on the development of the profession are described.

The educational processes by which we prepare nurses continue to experience change, modification, and refinement in response to changes that occur in the health care delivery system. The various routes to educational preparation for a nursing career, including a history of the different avenues, are discussed. You will learn about some of the individuals who made significant contributions to the profession. The unit concludes with a discussion of the future of nursing education.

4

Exploring the Growth of Nursing as a Profession

Development of Nursing

LEARNING OUTCOMES

After completing this chapter, you should be able to:

1. Discuss early historical influences on the development of nursing.
2. Describe Florence Nightingale's contribution to nursing and to the development of nursing education.
3. Analyze the impact wars have had on the development of nursing and nursing education.
4. Discuss the development and characteristics of the early nursing schools.
5. Analyze the challenges of defining nursing and formulate a personal definition of nursing.
6. Explain the ways in which nursing differs from medicine.
7. Identify the seven characteristics against which social scientists have evaluated professions and how these have been applied to nursing.
8. Compare and contrast the terms "profession" and "professional" and relate the terms to the image others hold of nursing.

9. Describe some of the traditions in nursing and explain why they were adopted.
10. Discuss the history of the image of nursing in the United States and why it is important for nursing to have a positive image within society.
11. Analyze areas of nursing about which studies have been conducted and explain why each is important.
12. Explain how a universal language for nursing that includes the North American Nursing Diagnosis Association International (NANDA-I), Nursing Outcomes Classification (NOC), and Nursing Interventions Classification (NIC) systems of nursing classification support the growth of nursing as a profession.
13. Describe how specific documentation systems such as the OMAHA system affect nursing practice.

KEY TERMS

Characteristics of a profession
Classification systems
Folk image
Florence Nightingale

International Classification for Nursing Practice Project (ICNPP)
Military influence

Minimum Data Set for Nursing Home Resident Assessment and Care Screening (MDS)

National Information and Data Set Evaluation Center (NIDSEC)	Nursing Interventions Classification (NIC)	Profession
		Professional
	Nursing nomenclatures	Servant image
North American Nursing Diagnosis Association- International (NANDA-I)	Nursing Outcomes Classification (NOC)	Religious image
		Taxonomy
	Omaha System	

What is nursing? Is it an art or a science? Are hunches, gut feelings, and intuition useful in a world of practicality constructed on scientific rationale and evidence-based practice, steeped in protocol, and immersed in critical thinking and clinical pathways? Should nursing be considered a profession or an occupation? Does nursing possess a unique body of knowledge? Is the nurse a professional? If so, what educational background qualifies the nurse for professional standing? How will the skills of graduates from various programs be differentiated in practice? What is the status of the nurse in relation to other members of the health care team? What is the language of nursing? Is a single language adequate? How has its history affected the image of nursing today? These and other questions are the foundation of our need to understand the historical progress of nursing as a profession.

There is no particular date or time period when nursing came into being. While nursing as we know it today may go back less than 150 years, the early origins of nursing, like those of medicine, are intertwined with the ancient civilizations and cultures of the world. Little written reference to nursing is found in the earliest history from 500 B.C. to 476 A.D. (Kalisch & Kalisch, 2004). Our best speculations regarding the origins of nursing are tied to our knowledge of the varied cultures that existed in the past, and to the contributions that these cultures left for future generations. They reflected the events and developments that characterized each period in history. Let us review some of the various cultures and historical events that have contributed to the development of nursing as a profession.

HEALTH CARE IN ANCIENT CULTURES

Primitive societies and ancient cultures were nomadic out of necessity. Well-defined groups, built around the nucleus of family relationships, wandered in search of food, warmth, and an environment that supported life. Solidarity among these scattered groups, organized for the convenient management of human affairs, existed for purposes of mutual protection. Anthropologists believe that primitive groups originated in Africa and migrated across the world. Ice ages in the northern latitudes may have driven these groups back to the warmer climates found around the Mediterranean Sea, in India, and in China, where civilizations developed.

In early human history, the regions around the Mediterranean Sea were thought to occupy the center of the earth, with all areas to the east known as "eastern" and all those to the west known as "western" (Donahue, 1996, p. 28). The sophistication of health care practices varied considerably from one culture to another, and was based largely on the ingenuity of the group. Consistent among most of the groups were strong beliefs in the power of gods, with sickness and

TABLE 4-1	SUMMARY OF HEALTH CARE PRACTICES OF SELECTED EARLY CIVILIZATIONS*
SOCIETY & APPROXIMATE TIME PERIOD	**CHARACTERISTICS AND CONTRIBUTIONS**
Egypt 3000 B.C.	Provided the earliest medical records, dating back as far as 3000 B.C., which included more than 700 classified drugs Developed a system of community planning that helped avoid public health problems Established strict rules regarding cleanliness, food, drink exercise, and sexual relations Was credited with being one of the healthiest of the ancient civilizations
Ancient Israel 1900 B.C.	Developed the Mosaic Code under the leadership of Moses, which included an organized method of disease prevention Isolated people with communicable diseases, differentiated clean from unclean, and established rules that forbade eating meat past the 3rd day after slaughter, monitored by priest-physicians who functioned as health inspectors Shared knowledge with other cultures
Babylonia 2100 B.C.	Credited with being skilled mathematicians and astrologers: Many beliefs were based on study of nature, beliefs in the potency of numbers, and observations of the movement of stars and planets Believed illness was a punishment for sin and used incantations and herbs for purification; surgery was more advanced than internal medicine Developed Code of Hammurabi, which perhaps represents the first sliding scale for payment based on class
Assyria 745–635 B.C.	A group with strong instruments of war, had severe laws, and made frequent use of mutilation and death as punishments Believed in good and evil spirits, magic and superstition, and in many gods; ill health was viewed as a punishment for sin
Persia 600 B.C.–300 B.C.	An extensive empire whose people followed the preaching of Zoroaster, who introduced the concept of two creators: one good, one evil Adopted many of the medical practices of the lands they conquered Established early schools for priest-physicians, from which evolved three types of physicians: those who healed by the knife, those who healed with herbs, and those who healed through exorcism
Greece 800 B.C.–300 B.C.	Society with beliefs in the power of a wide array of gods who had human characteristics Divination of the future and animal sacrifice to seek healing were common Placed much emphasis on healthy bodies; founded the Olympic games Built exquisite temples where learning and healing occurred Built institutions to care for sick and injured called *xendochium; iatrion* were built to offer ambulatory care The home of Hippocrates, born about 400 B.C., who became known as the Father of Modern Medicine Hippocrates stressed natural causes for disease, a patient-centered approach; and the necessity of accurate observations and record keeping
Rome 800 B.C.–476 A.D.	Borrowed medical practices from the countries they conquered; physicians were often slaves Had a pantheon of gods similar to the Greeks with different names Used both sacrifice and herbs when faced with illness Practiced advanced hygiene and sanitation with emphasis on bathing Society divided into two classes: the patricians (the upper class) and the plebeians (the common people); women enjoyed more independence than in other comparable societies

TABLE 4-1	SUMMARY OF HEALTH CARE PRACTICES OF SELECTED EARLY CIVILIZATIONS* (*Continued*)
SOCIETY & APPROXIMATE TIME PERIOD	**CHARACTERISTICS AND CONTRIBUTIONS**
India (3000–1500 B.C.)	Early civilizations highly developed, with systems of sanitation, bathrooms, public baths, and other amenities Vedic age (1500 B.C.) characterized by worship of Brahma (Brahmanism or Hinduism), which resulted in segregation of society into four castes and sacrifice to satisfy gods Sacred book, the Vedas, a source of information about health practices and considered some of the oldest known written material Emphasized hygiene and prevention of sickness and described major and minor surgery, children's diseases, and diseases of the nervous and urinary system
500 B.C.	Buddhism emerged about 500 B.C.; and during this period an advanced understanding of disease prevention, hygiene and sanitation, medicine, and surgery was developed Prenatal care was emphasized for mothers and public hospitals were constructed which were staffed with nurses (mostly men)
China 3000 B.C.–249 B.C.	Followed the teachings of Confucius emphasizing the value of knowledge Patriarchal rule dominated with emphasis on whole family; women considered vastly inferior to men Developed concept of yin and yang and had elaborate material medica, using many drugs still used today Developed acupuncture skills still in practice today, studied circulation, and developed approach to examination: look, listen, ask, feel Baths used for reduction of fever, bloodletting to release evil spirits from the body
Arabia 570 A.D.	Populated by nomadic people who lived a difficult life in the hot, dry desert Muhammad, born about 570 A.D., developed the religion of Islam that worshipped the god Allah; his teachings established strict rules of living, dictating habits of cleanliness, eating, and human interaction
The Americas Mayan and Aztec civilizations 2000–1000 B.C.	Civilization may have begun 10,000 to 20,000 years ago, with nomadic early inhabitants coming from Central Asia The great civilizations that created cities and far-flung empires were in Central and South America Sun god of particular significance; health viewed as a balance between man, nature, and the supernatural Rites, ceremonies, herbal treatments, charms, and perhaps human sacrifice contributed to healing practices Medicine men (known first as shamans and later as priests) were responsible for curing ills of body and mind

*Compiled from Donahue, 1996.

suffering attributed to the presence of evil spirits. These evil spirits were dealt with in many ways, including performing noisy incantations and dances, making offerings and sacrifices, and working with medicine men who performed magic to drive away the demons (Kalisch & Kalisch, 2004). A sound theory of disease was absent from most early cultures. The health care practices of some of the early cultures are summarized in Table 4-1.

Critical Thinking Activity

After studying Table 4-1, how would you characterize the early societies? Given the lack of organized nursing, how do you believe the people of the early cultures received care? Who do you think provided that care? How did they know what to do? From whom did they learn the skills they used? What was the quality of that care?

HISTORIC PERSPECTIVES OF NURSING

Although ancient cultures developed medicine as a science and a profession, writings about early health care make little or no mention of nursing or nurses. One might assume that a family member, particularly the wife or mother, provided needed care. The possible exceptions to this were the male attendants in early Buddhist hospitals in India and midwives who had an established role in several cultures. It was not until the early Christian period that nursing as we think of it today began to develop.

EARLY IMAGES OF NURSES

Nursing has carried forward three heritages from the past that some believe impeded the development of nursing as a profession. They are the **folk image** of the nurse brought forward from primitive times, the **religious image** of the nurse inherited from the medieval period, and the **servant image** of the nurse created by the Protestant-capitalist ethic from the 16th to 19th century. Whether they hampered progress, these concepts of the nurse have certainly had an impact. A summary of these images is provided in Table 4-2.

TABLE 4-2	NURSING HERITAGES FROM THE PAST
The folk image of the nurse	Primary responsibilities focused on nourishing and nurturing children, caring for the elderly, and caring for aging family members. Skills were learned through trial and error and passed from one generation to another. This image presents the nurse as a "caring" person who uses common sense to help the sick individual.
The religious image of the nurse	Groups were organized in conjunction with the establishment of churches in the Christian era with their primary concern focused on care for the sick, the poor, orphans, widows, the aged, slaves, and prisoners. These groups included the deaconesses of the Eastern Christian Church, the Order of Widows and the Order of Virgins, and monastic orders including the Benedictines, which still exist. The first hospitals were also developed at this time, being located close to monasteries. The Crusades, (1096–1291) witnessed the founding of military nursing orders, such as the Knights Hospitallers of St. John, the Knights Templars, and the Knights of the Teutonic Order.
The servant image of the nurse	The Reformation, which began in Germany in 1517, brought with it a change in the role of women, limiting it to the confines of the home. Duties were those of bearing children and caring for the home. Hospital care was relegated to uncommon women, a group comprising prisoners, prostitutes, and drunks (Fig. 4-1). This began what may be called the "Dark Ages" of nursing reflected in Charles Dickens's (1936) description of Sairey Gamp and Betsy Prig in his book *Martin Chuzzlewit*. This image may have greatly influenced the development of nursing as a profession as many capable and desirable persons were unwilling to enter nursing while it had this image.

FIGURE 4-1   From the Middle Ages to the 19th century, nursing was often left to "uncommon women."

THE BEGINNING OF CHANGE

During the 17th century, social reform began in Europe. Several nursing groups were organized. These groups gave money, time, and service to the sick and the poor, visiting them in their homes and ministering to their needs. One such group founded in Paris in 1633 was the Sisters of Charity, a religious nursing order with a widespread mission toward the poor and sick. They developed an educational program for the intelligent young women they recruited that included experience in a hospital as well as visits to the home. Receiving help, counsel, and encouragement from St. Vincent de Paul, the Sisters of Charity expanded its services to include caring for abandoned children. In 1640, St. Vincent established the Hospital for Foundlings in Paris. Later, in 1809, the Sisters of Charity established a nursing order in the United States under the direction of Elizabeth Bayley Seton.

Those countries in Europe that remained Roman Catholic escaped some of the disorganization of the groups providing social services that was caused by the Reformation. During the 1500s, the Spanish and the Portuguese began traveling to the Americas. Early colonists to the area included members of Catholic religious orders, who became the doctors, nurses, and teachers of the new land. In 1524, the first hospital on the American continent, the Hospital of Immaculate Conception (Hospital de Nuestra Senora O Limpia Concepçion), was built in Mexico City. Mission colleges were founded. The first medical school in America was founded in 1578 at the University of Mexico, the second at the University of Lima before 1600.

In 1639, three Augustinian nuns arrived in Quebec, Canada, to staff the Hôtel–Dieu de Quebec, a hospital that opened that year. The Ursuline Sisters, an order of teaching nuns who accompanied the Augustinians from France, are credited with attempting to organize the first training for nurses on the North American continent. They taught the native women of the area to care for their sick during a smallpox epidemic.

In Europe, outstanding men of medicine made vital and valuable contributions to medical knowledge. Among laypersons influencing social change during this time was a young minister in Kaiserwerth, Germany, Theodore Fliedner (1800–1864). With the assistance of his first wife, Friederike, Fliedner revived the Christian deaconess movement by establishing a training institute for deaconesses at Kaiserwerth in 1836. The duties of the deaconesses at Kaiserwerth included care of the sick, visitations and work in the parish, and teaching. A course in nursing was developed that included lectures by physicians.

In 1849, Pastor Fliedner traveled to the United States, where he helped to establish the first Motherhouse of Kaiserwerth Deaconesses in Pittsburgh, Pennsylvania. With the help of four deaconesses, the Motherhouse of Kaiserwerth Deaconesses assumed responsibility for the Pittsburgh Infirmary, which was the first Protestant hospital in the United States. The hospital is now called Passavant Hospital.

In England, at about the same time, Elizabeth Fry (1780–1845) organized the Institute of Nursing Sisters, a secular group often called the Fry Sisters. Two other groups followed shortly: the Sisters of Mercy, a Roman Catholic group formed by Catherine McAuley (1787–1841), and another Catholic group called the Irish Sisters of Charity, formed by Mary Aikenhead (1787–1858).

Critical Thinking Activity

Knowing what you do about the history and early image of nursing, how will you, as a nurse of the future, advance the image of nursing? What aspects of the role are most critical? Who are the people who most need to be influenced? How do you think they can best be encouraged to select nursing as a career?

THE NIGHTINGALE INFLUENCE

In the latter half of the 18th century, one woman dramatically changed the form and direction of nursing and succeeded in establishing it as a respected field of endeavor. This outstanding woman was **Florence Nightingale**.

Born May 12, 1820, the second daughter of a wealthy family, she was named after the city in which she was born—Florence, Italy. Because of her family's high social and economic standing, she was cultured, well traveled, and educated. By the age of 17, as the result of tutoring from her father, she had mastered several languages and mathematics and was extremely well read. This was very unusual for a woman of her time, as she was expected to select a desirable husband from the influential people she met, marry, and assume her place in society.

Florence Nightingale had other ideas, however. She wanted to become a nurse, but this aspiration was unthinkable to her family because of the terrible conditions of the hospitals at that time. She continued to travel with her family and their friends and, in the course of these travels, met Sidney Herbert and his wife, who were interested in hospital reform. Inspired, she began collecting information on public health and hospitals and soon became recognized as an important authority on the subject.

Through friends, she learned about Pastor Fliedner's institute at Kaiserwerth and visited it in 1850. Because it was a religious institution under the auspices of the church, her parents would permit her to go there, although she could not go to English hospitals. In 1851, she spent three months studying at Kaiserwerth. She never returned to her parents' home to live after this time.

In 1853, she began working with a committee that supervised an "Establishment for Gentlewomen During Illness." She eventually was appointed superintendent of the establishment, a position she held from August 1853 to October 1854. As her knowledge of hospitals and nursing reform grew, she was consulted by reformers and physicians who were beginning to see the need for trained nurses.

After the Crimean War began in March 1854, war correspondents wrote about the abominable manner in which the British Army cared for sick and wounded soldiers. Florence Nightingale, by then a recognized authority on hospital care, wrote to her friend Sir Sidney Herbert, who was then Secretary of War, and offered to take a group of 38 nurses to the Crimea. (At the same time, he had written a letter proposing that she assume direction of all nursing operations at the war front. Their letters crossed in the mail.) Her tireless efforts in the Crimea resulted in greatly reduced mortality rates among the sick and wounded. There is a museum in her honor in the barracks where she worked in what is now part of Istanbul, Turkey.

When the war ended in 1856, Florence Nightingale returned to England as a national heroine but with her health broken. Much has been written of her "illness," some suggesting that it was brucellosis; others stating that it was, to a large degree, a neurosis; and more recently some declaring that it was posttraumatic stress disorder. She retreated to her bedroom, and for the next 43 years conducted her extensive involvement in health care from her secluded apartment. She helped to reform health care for all the British military forces and moved from there to the health of the entire nation.

Throughout her lifetime, Florence Nightingale wrote extensively about hospitals, sanitation, health, and health statistics (creating the first pie chart), and especially about nursing and nursing education. Among her most popular books is *Notes on Nursing*, published in 1859. She crusaded for and brought about great reform in nursing education.

In 1860, she devoted her efforts to the creation of a school of nursing at St. Thomas' Hospital in London, financed by the Nightingale Fund. The basic principles on which Miss Nightingale established her school included the following:

- Nurses would be trained in teaching hospitals associated with medical schools and organized for that purpose.
- Nurses would be selected carefully and would reside in nurses' houses designed to encourage discipline and form character.
- The school matron would have final authority over the curriculum, living arrangements, and all other aspects of the school.
- The curriculum would include both theoretic material and practical experience.
- Teachers would be paid for their instruction.
- Records would be kept on the students, who would be required to attend lectures, take quizzes, write papers, and keep diaries.

In many other ways, Florence Nightingale advanced nursing as a profession. She believed that nurses should spend their time caring for patients, not cleaning; that nurses must continue learning throughout their lifetime and not become "stagnant;" that nurses should be intelligent

Display 4-1   Ways in Which Florence Nightingale Influenced Health Care

- Believed outcomes of care should be monitored and reported systematically
- Developed a hospital statistical system that compared outcomes, mortality, and morbidity
- Implemented systems of total patient care
- Believed childbirth was a normal physiologic occurrence and not an illness
- Recognized that noise, colors, light, and music affect the success of patient care
- Promoted the concept of delegation of responsibilities
- Used statistics to understand and make recommendations regarding care
- Believed nurse's role was to help people maintain their health as well as help the sick get well
- Encouraged the concept of networking

Compiled from Ulrich (2005).

and use that intelligence to improve conditions for the patient; and that nursing leaders should have social standing. She had a vision of what nursing could and should be. Display 4-1 outlines some of ways she influenced nursing and health care. Further discussion of Florence Nightingale's definition of nursing occurs later in this chapter.

Florence Nightingale received many honors from foreign governments, and in 1907 she was recognized by the Queen of England, who awarded her the British Order of Merit. It was the first time it was given to a woman.

Florence Nightingale died in her sleep at the age of 90 on August 13, 1910. The week during which she was born is now honored as National Nurses Week. The enthusiastic student is encouraged to learn more about this fascinating woman in Cecil Woodham-Smith's biography *Florence Nightingale*, or by pursuing the topic of Florence Nightingale through the Internet.

THE MILITARY INFLUENCE

Through her experience in the Crimean War, Florence Nightingale first brought attention to nursing as a career and profession and to needed changes in health care delivery. Similarly, other wars have brought advances in how care is provided. Likewise, in war after war, nurses have provided care, expanded the role of nursing, and created new nursing techniques. In the following section, we will highlight some of those areas of **military influence**; however, it is impossible, in the context of this book, to provide more than just an overview.

The American Revolution

All of the English colonies scattered along the Atlantic Coast of the United States were involved in the American Revolution. The hastily organized army existed without the benefit of a medical corps or trained nurses. The nuns of the Catholic Church, who also cared for those who were ill with epidemic diseases, such as scarlet fever, dysentery, and smallpox, nursed wounded soldiers. Women who had followed their husbands to the battlefield often nursed soldiers. Homes and barns near the battles were turned into hospitals. Other women contributed to the cause by making clothing and bandages or by helping to feed the soldiers from their own pantries.

When the war ended, the usual type of poverty existed, with invalids and the disabled who needed care. However, the colonies were not sufficiently developed to have such services available. In response, a new type of institution evolved, which is perhaps the forerunner of today's clinic or hospital outpatient department. In 1786, the Philadelphia Dispensary was established, and volunteer physicians treated those needing care at no charge. These dispensaries later became a major site for controlling disease. Vaccination against smallpox was one of the earliest preventive treatments offered there.

The Civil War

The Civil War broke out in the United States in 1861. Although social reform was on the rise, the nursing profession was still in an embryonic, unorganized stage. There was neither an army nurse corps nor an organized medical corps. There were no ambulance services or hospital units. Responding to the nursing needs created by the war, in which it is estimated that 618,000 men died (Donahue, 1996, p. 247), many men and women volunteered to help. After a brief training course, they performed nursing duties on behalf of the Union. The poet Walt Whitman is one of the better known individuals who became nurses during this time. Many religious orders also volunteered and provided service. A steamer, captured from the Confederates, was converted into a floating hospital and anchored near Vicksburg, Mississippi. Considered the first Navy hospital ship, the *Red Rover* was staffed through the volunteer efforts of the Catholic Sisters of Mercy, who became the first Navy nurses. An account of some of the contributions of nurses during the Civil War and afterward is found in Table 4-3. The serious need for trained nurses created by the Civil War was undoubtedly a significant factor in the development of nursing in the United States.

The Spanish-American War and the Boer War

These two conflicts occurred at about the same time in history. The United States entered the Spanish-American War in 1898, and the British went to war against the Boers of South Africa in late 1899. By this time, the Red Cross, founded by Clara Barton, a New England schoolteacher, had organized, and the United States, Canada, and Great Britain all had nursing schools to prepare young women for nursing roles.

In the early days of the Spanish-American War, little attention was given to the selection of nurses to care for the wounded. Volunteers, both men and women, included nurses with training, those partly trained, and the untrained. The entire system lacked organization; needed supplies were seriously deficient. These conditions attracted the attention of both the government and the people. Among groups addressing the concern was the Nurses' Associated Alumnae of the United States and Canada, who offered to develop a process through which better skilled nurses might be secured. The management of the chosen nurses was given over to the Red Cross, which retained this role throughout the war.

Nursing occurred in the military camps, where problems such as inadequate water facilities, lack of laundry and laundry services, and inadequate medical supplies were encountered. Many nurses became ill with typhoid fever. A memorial in Arlington National Cemetery honors the memory of the women who gave their lives as Army nurses in the Spanish-American War. It was erected by the Society of Spanish-American War Nurses.

TABLE 4-3   NURSES OF THE CIVIL WAR AND THEIR CONTRIBUTIONS*

NURSE	CONTRIBUTION
Sojourner Truth (1797–1883)	Born into slavery and named Isabella, this African-American was sold three times by the time she was 13, the last time for $300. She married an older slave and bore him 5 children, some of whom were also sold into slavery. In 1843 she changed her name to Sojourner Truth. She nursed Union soldiers, worked for improvement in sanitary facilities, and sought contributions of food and clothing for black volunteer regiments. She supported her travel from sales of her *Narrative* of *Sojourner Truth: A Northern Slave* (1850), dictated to Olive Gilbert because she was illiterate. She continued her work as a nurse/counselor for the Freedmen's Relief Association after the war (Whitman, 1985, pp. 814–816).
Dorothea Lynde Dix (1802–1881)	A Boston schoolteacher already known for her humanitarian efforts on behalf of the mentally ill, she was commissioned as Superintendent of Women Nurses for All Military Hospitals during the Civil War when she was over 60 years of age. Her authority was often challenged by the physicians.
Mary Ann Ball Bickerdyke (1817–1901)	Called "Mother" Bickerdyke by the troops, this Illinois woman challenged the work of lazy, corrupt medical officers. She served under fire in 19 battles. Her efforts were recognized by the government in the launching of the hospital ship, the *SS Mary A. Bickerdyke* in 1943.
Walt Whitman (1819–1892)	A well-respected poet, who worked as a volunteer in hospital wards after searching for a brother who had been wounded. Dressed wounds, wrote letters, read to soldiers, brought gifts and food. Later wrote about the war and suffering of soldiers.
Harriet Ross Tubman (1820–1913)	An abolitionist sometimes called "Conductor of the Underground Railroad" this black nurse was commended for caring for the sick and wounded without regard for color.
Mary Livermore (1820–1905)	Another untrained nurse of the Civil War, she later became a suffragist and advocated education for all women. Addressing the 6th annual convention of the Nurses' Associated Alumnae, she described the activities of the Civil War nurses.
Clara Barton (1821–1912)	Served as a Volunteer with the Sixth Massachusetts Regiment. Independently operated a large-scale relief operation. Was instrumental in founding the American Red Cross in 1882. Called "little lone lady in black silk" (Donahue 1996, p. 255).
Kate Cummings (1828–1909)	A volunteer in the Southern army, her diaries chronicled the work of the "matrons" who served in the Confederate hospitals.
Louisa May Alcott (1832–1888)	Served as a volunteer nurse during the Civil War. From these experiences she wrote a small book entitled *Hospital Sketches,* which described the work of the volunteer nurses of the Civil War. The nurse character of the book was Miss Tribulation Periwinkle.
Jane Stuart Woolsey (1830–1891)	One of three sisters from a cultivated and elite northeastern family with colonial ancestry, Jane served the Union Army as supervisor of the nursing and cooking department. She provided much narrative to describe the conditions of the day, authoring a book entitled *Hospital Days.* Later she served as the directress of the Presbyterian Hospital in New York.
Abby Howland Woolsey (1828–1893)	A sister of Jane, she too served as a volunteer nurse for the Union Army and fought diligently for the abolition of slavery. Helped found the Bellevue Hospital Training School for Nurses and wrote one of the first books on the organization of nursing schools—*A Century of Nursing with Hints Toward the Organization of a Training School* (1876) (Whitman, 1985, pp. 904–906).
Georgeanna Muirson Woolsey (1833–1906)	Another Woolsey sister involved in war efforts, she benefited from a month-long nursing training experience in New York when selected by the Woman's Central Association of Relief as one of a group of 100 for leadership potential. She wrote of her war experiences in a book entitled *Three Weeks at Gettysburg.* She later helped found the Connecticut Training School for Nursing in New Haven, enjoying the support of her husband, Dr. Francis Bacon (Whitman, 1985, pp. 903–906).
Susie King Taylor (1848–1901)	Born into slavery, as a young girl she secretly learned to read and write. While serving as a volunteer nurse for the Union Army, she also worked as a teacher.

*Compiled from Kalisch & Kalisch, 2004, except as otherwise noted.

When the war ended, nurse leaders exerted pressure to secure legislation to ensure an efficient army nursing service. A bill establishing the Army Nurse Corps was passed in 1901, and in 1908 the Navy Nurse Corps was established. At about this time, the Red Cross began a complete reorganization, and William Howard Taft served as its president for 8 years. He also became president of the United States during this time.

In South Africa, the situation was much the same as in the United States—the need for more efficient and educationally prepared nurses was apparent. The British Army Nursing Service, organized in 1881 as a result of the Crimean experience, recruited nurse volunteers who functioned in army hospitals but not at army lines. Britain soon learned that it needed a group of nurses who could be called upon in an emergency, and, in March 1902, the Queen Alexandra's Imperial Military Nursing Service became the permanent military nursing service, replacing its predecessor the British Army Nursing Service (The National Archives, 2004).

World War I

In 1914, Austria declared war on Serbia; Germany invaded Belgium and France; and England became involved in the conflict. The United States joined them on April 6, 1917. Through Queen Alexandra's Imperial Military Nursing Service, England was prepared to meet the emergency needs for care. Navy and Air Force branches were added to that of the Army, and an organized Voluntary Aid Detachment composed of laypersons was organized. When the United States joined the conflict, nurses from the Army and Navy Nurse Corps were ready to provide care to the wounded; other experienced nurses were recruited and enlisted. Despite continuous efforts to provide an adequate supply of nurses in both civilian and army hospitals, the lack of qualified nurses became more marked as time went on. The influenza epidemic of 1918 was of major proportions; pneumonia and typhus also claimed many lives, including those of doctors and nurses. In this time of great national need, the Army Nursing Corps finally agreed to admit black nurses, although the war had ended before they began their service. Recognizing the demand for a long-term supply of military nurses, the Army School of Nursing was organized in 1918. In 1938, a statue sculpted by Francis Rich from Tennessee marble, titled "Spirit of Nursing," was erected at Arlington National Cemetery among the graves of nurses who had served their country. The only one of its kind to honor nurses in all the services, it was rededicated in 1971 (Klein, 1997).

The experiences of the war also pointed to the serious need for uniformity in methods of nursing education. In response, England founded the Royal College of Nursing in 1916. Inspection and accreditation of schools became one of this group's major concerns.

World War II

In response to Germany's invasion of Austria and Poland, England declared war against Germany and Italy in September 1939. The United States entered the war after Japan attacked Pearl Harbor on December 7, 1941. Thus began a conflict that was to be known as a "total war" because it affected every nation in the world. In the United States, the National Nursing Council for War Service was organized in July 1940 to help meet the increasing need for individuals at all levels of preparation who could care for the sick and wounded. The U.S. Cadet Nurse Corps was established under the Bolton Act, which was authorized in June 1943 and lasted until 1948. Under this program, almost 124,065 women graduated from the Cadet Nurse Corps (PHS-The Cadet Nurse Corps, 1943–48, 2004). It provided funds for tuition, a monthly allowance, uniforms, and other expenses for women who would enter nursing and, upon completion of their education, serve in

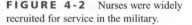

U.S. PUBLIC HEALTH SERVICE

become a Nurse
YOUR COUNTRY NEEDS YOU
Write Nursing Information Bureau , 1790 Broadway , New York City

FIGURE 4-2   Nurses were widely recruited for service in the military.

the military service (Fig. 4-2). Volunteer nurse aides were given short, intensive training so that they might assist nurses in hospitals.

In World War II, nurses were given commissions as officers and had military rank, something that had not been true previously. This gave them a level of status and authority that supported their work. Nurses who were assigned to war zones, as opposed to working in military hospitals, often found themselves facing a serious dilemma. The Army had done nothing to prepare them for battlefield medicine or for life in the field. Wounded men were treated in field hospitals close to battle lines with supplies and equipment that might be inadequate, while bombs dropped around them. Although they were in the Army, the nurses considered themselves healers, not soldiers. Elizabeth Norman (1999) poignantly describes the situation in her book *We Band of Angels*:

> Then the shooting started, and they found themselves confronting as much danger and deprivation as any dogface in the field. The men who worked with them—doctors, medics, orderlies and attendants—were no longer "colleagues" and "staff," they were comrades in arms now, and "the girls," as so many referred to them, were no longer anomalies in the ranks, they were a military unit in the middle of battle. They were women at war. (p. 39)

(Note: "dogface" was a slang term for the ordinary soldier.)

During this time, flight nursing came into existence, as nurses were taught to assist with the air evacuation of sick and wounded soldiers and at ground medical installations. Nurses in these roles worked under extremely dangerous circumstances because the planes used to transport patients also were used to transport cargo. Because of this dual activity, the planes were not marked with the Geneva Red Cross or other insignia, and they remained fair targets for enemy fighters.

Meanwhile, the United States experienced an industrial boom as defense plants mushroomed in response to military needs. Public health nurses moved into industry to carry out preventive health education and programs. Industrial nursing evolved on a national scale, with nurses employed in all types of manufacturing plants.

All of these activities left the country desperate for nurses. Serious shortages were felt in civilian hospitals and military situations. Nursing students began to carry much of the workload in hospitals that had nursing education programs.

The Korean and Vietnam Conflicts

On June 25, 1950, the Korean Conflict broke out. Once again nurses were called into military service. Learning from the experiences of World War II, treatment centers located close to the front lines were established—the Mobile Army Surgical Hospital (MASH). Triage care evolved, made more effective by advances in antibiotics and medical technology. Flight nursing saw a significant resurgence, as the need for air evacuation of the wounded reached new heights.

The American commitment to the Vietnamese government began about the same time as the Korean conflict, with a 35-man advisory team sent by President Truman to aid the French in their fight against the North Vietnamese. By 1963, approximately 15,000 military advisers were in South Vietnam working with Vietnamese troops in their battles against the Viet Cong troops. The first 13 nurses were placed on the staff at the Eighth Field Hospital in Nha Trang in March 1962 (Kalisch & Kalisch, 2004). Recruitment of nurses was once again a major activity; extraordinary incentives were offered because of widespread lack of support for the Vietnam conflict. Due to the guerrilla tactics of the Viet Cong, no military front existed. The country was partitioned into separate field zones, and semipermanent, air-conditioned hospitals were constructed. Fixed installations were assigned to area-support missions, with ground evacuation of the wounded almost impossible. Terrain and climate were tremendous obstacles. Advances in medical technology, however, permitted far better care than during any other combat situation. The contribution of nurses during this conflict was recognized publicly in a sculpture, designed by Glenna Goodacre, of three nurses and a wounded soldier erected near the Vietnam Memorial in Washington, DC, in 1993.

On October 18, 1997, the Women in Military Service for America memorial was dedicated at the Arlington National Cemetery. This marble, stone, and glass memorial is located at the gateway to the cemetery. The dedication included a special nurses' ceremony in which wreaths were placed at the "Spirit of Nursing" statue (Klein, 1997).

The Gulf War

The Iraqi Republican Guard invaded Kuwait on August 2, 1990, and seized control of that country. In an effort to protect Kuwait and deter any invasion of Saudi Arabia, Kuwait's oil-rich neighbor, the United States mounted Operation Desert Shield, the code name of the military action to eject the Iraqi army from Kuwait. When no withdrawal occurred, as mandated in a United Nations ultimatum, a U.S.-led coalition launched air and ground attacks against Iraqi targets, thus initiating the first Gulf War.

Again, nurses were deployed to the area of battle, setting up MASH units in conditions quite different from anything they previously had experienced. Often equipped with protective gas masks to combat any chemical warfare that might have been present, these nurses endured rocket attacks, the cold rains, hot winds, and dust and sand storms of the Arabian desert. Operating from tents, they mobilized triage areas, assisted with surgery, treated shrapnel wounds, and cared for the innocent Iraqi victims of war, many of whom were women and children, as well as wounded soldiers. As in other war situations, a major challenge was found in improvising equipment and techniques to handle emergency situations. If you are interested in learning more about nurses and the Gulf War, an extensive bibliography of articles related to the topic is available at *www.gulflink.osd.mil/gwv_bib/nursing.html*.

The Iraq Conflict

When the conflict began in Iraq in 2003, nurses were again playing critical roles in helping care for soldiers and civilians. In field hospitals housed in tents and placed close to the front, rapid trauma care was required along with better bandages and ways to stem uncontrolled bleeding. The need to speedily airlift seriously injured soldiers from aero-medical staging facilities in Iraq to military field hospitals in Germany and then to other countries became critical. Nurses played important roles in air force hospitals preparing patients for aero-medical evacuation from Iraq, assessing conditions before and during transport in what were sometimes referred to as flying intensive care units. Working in expanded roles as nurse practitioners and anesthetists, nurses provided care to American and coalition armed services, merchant marines, Iraqi nationals (including women and children), and Iraqi enemy prisoners of war on the navy hospital ship *USNS Comfort* as a part of Operation Iraqi Freedom and Operation Enduring Freedom missions.

⊕ THE TERRORIST ATTACKS AND NATURAL DISASTERS

Some of the most devastating events calling for skilled nursing actions and leadership behavior occur at times other than wartime. Such events as the terrorist attacks on the World Trade Center or the destruction, damage, and illness that occur as the result of hurricanes, floods, and earthquakes are examples. Being able to respond quickly and decisively in times of national crisis requires preparedness, collaboration, and formalized deployment roles. Human, financial, and technical resources must be maximized.

Critical Thinking Activity

In which of the wartime conflicts described do you believe nurses' roles were most critical? Provide the rationale for your choice, focusing on the factors that resulted in your choosing this conflict.

⊕ THE BEGINNING OF NURSING EDUCATION IN THE UNITED STATES

After the establishment of the Nightingale School in England, nursing programs flourished and the Nightingale system spread to other countries. In the United States, much of the push for nursing education occurred shortly after the Civil War, during which the lack of trained nurses presented a serious concern.

The Establishment of Early Schools

As with many other significant events that have evolved from a variety of influences, it is difficult to pinpoint the first nursing program in the United States. As early as 1798, a pioneer physician, Dr. Valentine Seaman, is said to have initiated the first system of instruction for nurses at New York Hospital (Donahue, 1996, p. 235). A society was formed in 1839 under Quaker influence, called the Nurse Society of Philadelphia, and a combined Home and School were opened. Historical records show that before 1850, some intermittent preparation was provided to individuals who cared for the sick. A plan of instruction also had been developed for women who would supply maternity service in the home, under the guidance of Dr. Joseph Warrington, who was the obstetric physician for the Philadelphia Dispensary for the Medical Relief of the Poor.

In 1850, a commission of the Massachusetts legislature recommended that institutions be formed to educate nurses. A plan for educating nurses was included in the formation of the *New England Female Medical College*, and a few nurses were educated through this institution. Other hospitals operated training programs, although the course of studies lasted only 6 months. The *Woman's Hospital of Philadelphia*, which operated under the direction of two female physicians, opened a training school in 1861, but it made little progress until it was endowed in 1872. Despite these efforts, the nursing services provided by most hospitals during the 1860s were disorganized and inadequate. In many cases, nursing care was provided by women who had been recruited from among the poor who were sheltered in almshouses or from those who had been arrested for drunkenness or disorderly conduct and who were serving out 10-day sentences. The better hospitals benefited from the work of Catholic sisters or Protestant deaconesses, although most of them also were untrained (Kalisch & Kalisch, 2004, p. 60–61).

In 1869, responding to the impetus given nursing during the Civil War, the American Medical Association established a committee to study the issue of training for nurses. The committee, chaired by Dr. Samuel D. Gross (1805–1884), was charged with identifying the best possible method to organize and manage institutions for training nurses. Its report concluded that every large hospital should have a nursing school, emphasized that the union between religious exercises and nursing would be conducive to the welfare of the sick, and recommended that schools be placed under the guardianship of county medical societies (Donahue, 1996, p. 265).

The *New England Hospital for Women and Children* is often credited with being the first hospital to establish a formal 1-year program to train nurses in 1872. It operated under the guidance of a female physician, Susan Dimock, who had received her medical education in Europe and had some knowledge of the work of Florence Nightingale. Five probationers started the program on September 1. It was from this school that Melinda Ann (Linda) Richards graduated in 1873, to become America's first trained nurse. This school was also the alma mater for the first black nurse graduate, Mary Eliza Mahoney, in 1879.

By 1873, three additional schools had opened: the *Bellevue Training School* in New York City, the *Connecticut Training School* in New Haven, and the *Boston Training School*. Typically, these schools did not admit men. In 1888, the *Mills School of Nursing* at Bellevue Hospital opened to train male nurses for patient care. Separate schools to educate black nurses also opened; among them *Spelman Seminary* in Atlanta in 1886, *Hampton Institute* in Virginia and *Providence Hospital* in Chicago in 1891, and *Tuskegee Institute* in Alabama in1892 (Kalisch & Kalisch, 2004). Table 4-4 identifies some of the early schools.

TABLE 4-4	EARLY NORTH AMERICAN TRAINING SCHOOLS FOR NURSES*	
DATE	**NAME AND PLACE**	**COMMENTS**
1798	New York Hospital—New York	Dr. Valentine Seaman initiated a system of instruction for nurses. His lectures covered the topics of anatomy, physiology, maternal nursing, and care of children.
1839	Philadelphia Dispensary—Philadelphia	Dr. Joseph Warrington provided obstetric training to a group of women who would work with families who would otherwise not receive care. The Nurse Society of Philadelphia grew out of this training.
1861	Bellevue Hospital—New York	Dr. Elizabeth Blackwell converted Bellevue Hospital into a training center for nurses. About 100 women were trained to provide care during the Civil War in an intensive 4-week course.
1861–1862	Woman's Hospital of Philadelphia—Philadelphia	Opened a training school, but it progressed slowly until 1872, when it became endowed—the first endowed school of nursing in America. Organized and conducted by two female physicians.
1862	New England Hospital for Women and Children—Boston	Dr. Marie Zakrzewska, a colleague of Dr. Blackwell's, offered a 6-month program to nurses.
1872	New England Training School—Boston	An expansion of the New England Hospital Program was identified as the first formal school for nurses, directed by Dr. Susan Dimock. The first graduate was Linda Ann Richards. Mary Mahoney, the first black nurse, also graduated here.
1873–May	Bellevue Training School—New York	First of a trio of schools modeled after the Nightingale model–Lavinia Dock was one of the early graduates.
1873–October	Connecticut Training School—New Haven	Second of the trio of schools started in 1873—introduced first textbook, *New Haven Manual of Nursing*, written by a committee of nurses and physicians.
1873–November	Boston Training School—Boston (attached to Massachusetts General)	Third of the trio—Linda Richards became superintendent of nurses in November 1894. Idea for school initiated by the Woman's Educational Association. Medical staff did not support initiation of the school.
1874	St. Catharine's General and Marine Hospital—Ontario, Canada—later called the Mack Training School	Patterned after the Nightingale schools, this program included instruction in the art of nursing, chemistry, sanitary science, physiology, and anatomy.
1877	Training School of the New York Hospital—New York	Offered an 18-month course to prepare graduates for nursing.
1878	Boston City Hospital Training School—Boston	Required graduates to complete a 2-year program of study.
1884	Toronto General Hospital—Toronto, Canada	Mary Agnes Snively became superintendent of this school, which had early beginnings in 1877.
1884–1885	Farrand Training School for Nurses—Harper Hospital, Detroit	Considered one of the better schools, students had two annual series of lectures, approximately 20 hours total.
1886	Spelman Seminary—Atlanta	The first separate school to educate black nurses, who were often denied admission to other schools.

TABLE 4-4	EARLY NORTH AMERICAN TRAINING SCHOOLS FOR NURSES* (*Continued*)	
DATE	**NAME AND PLACE**	**COMMENTS**
1888	Mills School of Nursing at Bellevue Hospital—New York	First school established for male nurses. Prepared them to give general patient care.
1889	Johns Hopkins School of Nursing—Baltimore	Program opened under direction of Isabel Hampton Robb. Mary Adelaide Nutting graduated in 1891.
1890	Montreal General—Montreal, Canada	Although wanting a nursing program as early as 1835, hospital conditions would not allow. Nora Gertrude Livingstone established school in 1890.

*Compiled from Donahue, 1996, and Kalisch & Kalisch, 2004.

Similar movements to establish nursing schools occurred in other countries. In 1868, a school was organized in Sydney Hospital, Australia. In Edinburgh, Scotland, a program was started at the Royal Infirmary. The *Mack Training School* in St. Catherines, Toronto, Canada, was started in 1884.

Characteristics of the Early Schools

The life of the nursing student at the turn of the century was not an easy one. The strong militaristic and religious influences over nursing were embodied in the expectations held for nursing students:

> Monastic and military traditions heavily influenced not only the actual workings of the schools of nursing but also the public's conception of them. The nurse in training was expected to yield to her superiors, obedience characteristic of a good soldier and actions governed by the dedication to duty derived from religious devotion. (Kalisch & Kalisch, 2004, p. 103)

The typical nursing student was about 21 years of age, single, and female. The first weeks or months of their education were spent as probationers, or "probies," and their duties, although helping with the operation of the hospital, did little to educate them as nurses. For example, they spent much of their time washing, scrubbing, polishing, folding, stacking, and the like. Rules of conduct were rigid and unforgiving; early superintendents saw it as their responsibility to discipline pupils, ensuring that they possessed good morals and were honest, conscientious, obedient, respectful, loyal, passive, and devoted to duty. Nursing students were expected to be unselfish, thinking not of themselves but of the happiness and well-being of others (Fig. 4-3).

Initially, nursing education was largely an apprenticeship and resulted in students providing much of the work force of hospitals. The workday was long and arduous, often starting at 5:30 AM and ending with nursing prayers very late at night, and consisted primarily of work on the hospital wards. The superintendent or her assistants provided instruction. There was no standardization of curriculum and no accreditation. The few lectures that were part of the program were usually given by physicians and scheduled at 8 or 9 PM after a long day of work. A 7-day workweek was the standard, and the help needed on the hospital units took precedence over the education of the young women. Lectures were canceled if students were needed to care for patients.

FIGURE 4-3   The duties assigned to probationers may have helped operate the hospital but did little to educate the nurse.

As schools developed, facilities to house nursing students became necessary. Although some of the early programs provided sleeping quarters in the hospital, nursing students usually were housed in a building next to the hospital, often referred to as the "nurses' dormitory." A "housemother" often controlled the nurses' residence. In religious affiliations, a deaconess or Sister served the same purpose. Housemothers ensured that codes of behavior were adhered to and that curfews were enforced. Violations usually resulted in expulsion from the program or the loss of a part of the uniform, such as the bib section of an apron. This signified to all that some infraction had occurred. Young women, who were attracted to nursing because of the imagined glamour of wearing a long, crisp, white apron and ministering to sick (though handsome) young men, often became discouraged with the severe duties and routine. The attrition rate was high in the early schools.

Although there were some changes in the curriculum—work hours were decreased, the length of study was increased, and the theory component was organized into specific areas of care such as medical, surgical, and obstetric nursing—hospital-based programs remained largely unchanged through the 1940s and 1950s. The following is a quote from a special publication developed on the occasion of the closing of a diploma school:

In 1921, a nurse was discharged for "cigarette habit." Skirts of nurses' uniforms were getting shorter but there was periodic measurement to be sure some were not too short.

The year 1924 would see Deaconess' first student protest. Student nurses were required to wear their hair long in those days. A number of them though made arrangements with a barber in the Victoria Hotel to stay open late one evening and they all went down and had their hair bobbed in the latest style. They were deprived of their caps for several weeks and ordered to wear switches and what-nots (separate tresses of hair used by women as part of their coiffure), their punishment comparatively slight, since "banks and other business regularly dismissed employees for social offense" (Deaconess Hospital School of Nursing 1980, p. 10).

Schools proliferated, as even small hospitals established nursing programs, recognizing the valuable commodity available in students who provided the majority of care given. As early as 1905, early pioneers and advocates for nursing, concerned about the proliferation of schools, championed programs that offered a sound educational foundation and reasonable working hours. During the time Isabel Hampton was principal of the Johns Hopkins Training School (a position she accepted in 1889 and continued until her marriage to Dr. Robb in 1894), she arranged for a regular period of 2 hours of free time during a day that was limited to 12 hours. She would have liked to limit the workday to 8 hours, however. Time was allowed for recreation and for meals (Jamieson & Sewall, 1944, p. 432).

Early Textbooks and Journals

There were few textbooks before 1900, a factor that complicated the learning process. Many of the lectures presented by physicians were given from notes they had taken while medical students. The first nursing textbook was reportedly the *Hand-book of Nursing for Family and General Use*, written by a committee composed of physicians and nurses associated with the *Connecticut Training School* at New Haven Hospital and published by Lippincott in 1878. Other books followed over the next 2 years. Table 4-5 describes some of the early textbooks.

Nursing journals also appeared toward the end of the 19th century. Five journals for nurses were published before 1901. The first appeared in 1886 and was entitled *The Nightingale*. In 1889, under the direction of Mary E. P. Davis, a company was formed with 550 cash subscriptions, and a new journal called the *American Journal of Nursing* made its debut in October 1900 (Kalisch & Kalisch, 2004, p. 106). The journal continues to be published today.

Critical Thinking Activity

Imagine that you are an instructor in an early nursing program. There are no textbooks. There are no nursing journals from which you can assign reading. How would you go about teaching the students for whom you are responsible? What would you see as the major concerns? How would the classes differ from those you are in today?

TABLE 4-5	EARLY NURSING TEXTBOOKS*	
YEAR	AUTHOR	TITLE
1878	A committee of physicians and nurses	*Hand-book for Family and General Use*
1885	Clara Weeks Shaw	*A Textbook of Nursing for the Use of Training Schools, Families and Private Students*
1890	Lavinia Dock	*The Textbook on Materia Medica for Nurses*
1893	Diana Kimber	The first anatomy book for nurses, *Anatomy and Physiology*
1889 (about)	Isabel Hampton	*Nursing: Its Principles and Practices for Hospital and Private Use*
1894 (about)	Isabel Hampton Robb	*Nursing Ethics*

*Compiled from Donahue, 1996, and Kalisch & Kalisch, 2004.

DEVELOPING A DEFINITION FOR NURSING

When you entered the nursing program in which you are now enrolled, what was your perception of nursing as a profession? Has that perception of nursing been changed by the experiences you have had as a nursing student? Some might ask, "Why spend so much time and effort trying to define nursing?" Chitty helps answer that question. She states, "They [ie, definitions] are a good place to begin in attempting to understand any complex enterprise such as nursing" (Chitty 1997, p. 143). Over the years, the profession has worked at establishing a definition of nursing.

Defining nursing is difficult. Nurses themselves cannot agree on a single definition, partly because of the history of nursing. Little is known about the work of the nurse in prehistory. A major factor that has made it difficult to define nursing is that it is taught as encompassing both theoretic and practical aspects, but it is pursued (and continues to be defined) primarily through practice, until recently a little-studied area. Benner (1984) states, "Nurses have not been careful record keepers of their own clinical learning. . . . This failure to chart our practices and clinical observations has deprived nursing theory of the uniqueness and richness of the knowledge embedded in expert clinical practice." She further discusses the differences between "knowing that" and "knowing how." When attempting to define nursing, we often stumble over these two concepts and how to combine the distinct and unique aspects of both. Despite the challenges, serious efforts were put into defining nursing in the late 1970s and early 1980s.

Early Definitions of Nursing

A nurse is a person who nourishes, fosters, and protects—a person who is prepared to care for the sick, injured, and aged. In this sense, "nurse" is used as a noun and is derived from the Latin *nutrix,* which means "nursing mother." The word "nurse" also has referred to a woman who suckled a child (usually not her own)—a wet nurse. Dictionary definitions of nurse include such descriptions as "suckles or nourishes," "to take care of a child or children," "to bring up; rear." In this way, "nurse" is used as a verb, deriving from the Latin *nutrire*, which means "to suckle and nourish." References to "the nurse" can be found in both the Talmud and in the Old Testament, and appear more similar to the wet nurse than to someone who cared for the sick.

Over the centuries, the word "nurse" has evolved to refer to a person who tends to the needs of the sick. Florence Nightingale, in her *Notes on Nursing: What It Is and What It Is Not*, described the nurse's role as one that would "put the patient in the best condition for nature to act upon him" (Nightingale, 1954, p. 133), a definition that often is quoted today.

In the past, nurses undoubtedly were more concerned about carrying out their responsibilities than about defining the role of the nurse. Through the years, we have seen the concept of the nurse grow and evolve from the nurse as mother, nourishing and nurturing children, to the nurse without specific reference to gender, with responsibilities encompassing ever-expanding and challenging services to people needing health care.

Not surprising, the development of nursing as a profession, the defining of its role and language for society, and the placing of it among other attractive careers has been inextricably tied to the role of women in society at various times in history, and to the forces that have had an impact on society. If we are frustrated at what appears to be the slow development of nursing as a profession, we need to remember that it was 1916 when Margaret Sanger opened the first birth control clinic in the United States. And not until 1919, after 40 years of campaigning, were women in the United States granted the right to vote, through the 19th Amendment to the Constitution.

Distinguishing Nursing From Medicine

The formulation of clear and concise definitions of nursing also has been hampered by the lack of an obvious distinction between nursing and medicine. For example, it is not unusual to hear a prospective nursing student say, "I've always been interested in the medical field, so I decided to go into nursing." Something of an interdependence exists between medicine and nursing, and they have somewhat paralleled one another in historic development. However, anyone who has been involved in the profession of nursing for any period of time will be quick to assure you that distinct differences exist, and more and more the reference is to health care rather than to medicine.

The primary differences between nursing and medicine are the purpose and goal of each profession, and the education needed to fulfill each role. Although the situation is much changed today, historically medicine was perceived as a profession for men and nursing as a profession for women.

We can dismiss these stereotypes today, but they had an influence on the development of both professions. Finally, the subservient role of the nurse in relationship to the physician in the past—often referred to as the handmaiden of the physician—has been significant in shaping the definition of nursing.

In general, medicine is concerned with the diagnosis and treatment (and cure, when possible) of disease. Nursing is concerned with caring for the person from a holistic perspective in a variety of health-related situations. The caring aspects of nursing are well documented in nursing literature (Benner & Wrubel, 1989; Bevis & Watson, 1989; Carper, 1979; Watson, 1979). We think of medicine as being involved with the cure of a patient and nursing with the care of that patient. The role of the nurse in patient care (today we often refer to this as client care) also involves teaching about health and the prevention of illness, as well as caring for the ill individual. It also may encompass case management and is increasingly being practiced outside the walls of hospitals. Nursing takes place in the community and the home, hospice centers, ambulatory care environments, schools and day care centers, and rehabilitation facilities. In all environments, nurses play a key role in promoting higher standards of health.

With advancing technology in the health care fields, the diverse areas of specialization within those fields, the different routes to educational preparation for nurses, and the distinct practice settings and roles occupied by the nurse, it is critical that nurses provide clear information for themselves and for the public. To state that you are a registered nurse (RN) says little about what you do. It conveys nothing about where you are employed or your educational background. For example, as an RN, you might be employed in a community hospital or in a long-term care facility, have a significant role in a critical care unit, have earned additional credentials and be working in advanced practice, or be a nurse educator.

Thus, you can see that the words "nurse" and "nursing" have been applied to a wide variety of health care activities, in many different settings, performed by people with a variety of education backgrounds. The old adage "A nurse is a nurse is a nurse" is out of place in a highly technical health care delivery system that struggles to keep "high touch" and "high tech" compatible.

Influences on the Definition of Nursing

A number of factors have influenced the definition of nursing. One might first think of technologic advances that have significantly affected the definition of nursing and the role of the nurse. The acute care hospital provides care to patients who are much more acutely ill with conditions from which they would not have survived 25 years ago. Today, recovery is anticipated after careful evaluation and treatment that can require diagnostic imaging, sophisticated laboratory tests, delicate medical procedures, and specialized critical care nursing utilizing a host of variously prepared health care providers. Critical thinking skills are essential to the successful performance of the diverse tasks expected of a nurse. Nurses in many positions have been required to assume ever-greater levels of responsibility. Only recently are nurses beginning to receive the official authority, autonomy, and recognition that should accompany those responsibilities.

Another factor influencing the definition of nursing is the work of nursing theorists. As nursing has grown into a profession, many nursing theorists developed definitions of nursing consistent with their conceptual frameworks. Table 4-6 presents the definitions of some of the theorists.

TABLE 4-6	DEFINITIONS OF NURSING BY MAJOR THEORISTS	
THEORIST	**MAJOR THEME**	**DEFINITION**
Florence Nightingale (1860)	Environment/Sanitation	The goal of nursing is to put the patient in the best condition for nature to act upon him, primarily by altering the environment.
Hildegard Peplau (1952)	Interpersonal process	Nursing is viewed as an interpersonal process involving interaction between two or more individuals, which has as its common goal assisting the individual who is sick or in need of health care.
Faye Abdellah (1960)	Nursing problems	Nursing is a service to individuals, families, and society based on an art and science that molds the attitudes, intellectual competencies, and technical skills of the individual nurse into the desire and ability to help people cope with their health care needs, and is focused around 21 nursing problems.
Ernestine Wiedenbach (1964)	Nursing problems model	Nursing is a helping, nurturing, and caring service rendered with compassion, skill, and understanding, in which sensitivity is key to assisting the nurse in identifying problems.
Virginia Henderson (1966)	Development/Needs	Nursing's role is to assist the individual (sick or well) to carry out those activities . . . he would perform unaided if he had the necessary strength, will, or knowledge.
Myra Levine (1969)	Conservation and adaptation	Nursing means the nurse interposes her/his skill and knowledge into the course of events that affect the patient. When influencing adaptation favorably, the nurse is acting in a therapeutic sense. When the nursing intervention cannot alter the course of adaptation, the nurse is acting in a supportive sense.
Ida Orlando Pelletier (1972)	Interpersonal process	Nursing's unique and independent role concerns itself with an individual's need for help in an immediate situation for the purpose of avoiding, relieving, diminishing, or curing that individual's sense of helplessness.

TABLE 4-6	DEFINITIONS OF NURSING BY MAJOR THEORISTS (*Continued*)	
THEORIST	**MAJOR THEME**	**DEFINITION**
Jean Watson (1979–1988)	Caring	The essence and central unifying focus for nursing practice is caring, a transpersonal value. Nurse behaviors are defined as 10 carative factors. Focuses on the spiritual subjective aspects of both nurse and patient and the "caring moment" relating to the time when nurse and patient first come together (LeMaire, 2002).
Dorothy Orem (1980)	Self-care	Nursing is concerned with the individual's need for self-care action, which is the practice of activities that individuals initiate and perform on their own behalf in maintaining health and well-being.
Dorothy E. Johnson (1980)	Systems approach	Nursing is an external regulatory force that acts to preserve the organization and integration of the patient's behavior at an optimal level, under those conditions in which the behavior constitutes a threat to physical or social health, or in which illness is found.
Imogene M. King (1981)	Open systems approach	The focus of nursing is the care of human beings resulting in the health of individuals and health care for groups, who are viewed as open systems in constant interaction with their environments.
Rosemarie Rizzo Parse (1981)	Man-Living-Health	Nursing is rooted in the human sciences and focuses on man as a living unity and as qualitatively participating in health experiences. Health is viewed as a process.
Betty Neuman (1982)	Systems approach	Nursing responds to individuals, groups, and communities, who are in constant interaction with environmental stressors that create disequilibrium. A critical element is the client's ability to react to stress and factors that assist with reconstituion or adaptation.
Sister Callista Roy (1984)	Adaptation	The goal of nursing is the promotion of adaptive responses (those things that positively influence health) that are affected by the person's ability to respond to stimuli. Nursing involves manipulating stimuli to promote adaptive responses.
Martha E. Rogers (1984)	Science of unitary man	Nursing is an art and science that is humanistic and humanitarian, directed toward the unitary human, and concerned with the nature and direction of human development.
Katharine Y. Kolcaba (1992)	Holistic theory of Comfort	The immediate desirable outcome of nursing care is enhanced comfort. This comfort positively correlates with desirable health-seeking behaviors.

In 1958, Virginia Henderson, a nurse educator, author, and researcher, was asked by the nursing service committee of the International Council of Nurses to describe her concept of basic nursing. Hers is still one of the most widely accepted definitions of nursing:

> The unique function of the nurse is to assist the individual, sick or well, in the performance of those activities contributing to health or its recovery (or to peaceful death) that he would perform unaided if he had the necessary strength, will or knowledge. And to do this in such a way as to help him gain independence as rapidly as possible. (Henderson, 1966, p. 15)

Nursing organizations have also influenced the development of a definition of nursing. Both the American Nurses Association (ANA) and the National Council of State Boards of Nursing (NCSBN) have established definitions of nursing.

In its *Social Policy Statement* published in 1980, ANA stated, "Nursing is the diagnosis and treatment of human responses to actual or potential health problems" (ANA, 1980, p. 9). That definition had a widespread effect, and we see its application in the language used in nursing diagnoses today. The definition presented in the second edition of *Nursing's Social Policy Statement*, published in 2003 is expanded significantly:

> Nursing is the protection, promotion, and optimization of health and abilities, prevention of illness and injury, alleviation of suffering through the diagnosis and treatment of human response, and advocacy in the care of individuals, families, communities, and populations. (ANA, 2003)

Critical Thinking Activity

Compare the two definitions of nursing provided in the first and second editions of ANA's *Social Policy Statement*. Considering especially the nursing activities described and the public served, what differences do you note? Why do you think the content in the second version is so much greater than the first? How has the practice of nursing changed over the intervening 23 years to create the need for an expanded definition?

Through the Model Nurse Practice Act, the NCSBN states,

> The Practice of Nursing means assisting clients to attain or maintain optimal health, implementing a strategy of care to accomplish defined goals within the context of a client-centered health care plan, and evaluating responses to nursing care and treatment. (NCSBN, Article II, Section 1, 2004)

Perhaps nothing so affects the definition of nursing as its legal definition found in each state's nursing practice act (see Chapter 7). This legal definition is critical because it provides the foundation and guidelines for education, licensure, scope of practice, and, when necessary, the corrective actions against people who violate the practice act.

No state adopts the exact wording of any recommended definition, but most states include references to performing services for compensation, the necessity for a specialized knowledge base, the use of the nursing process (although steps may carry different names), and components of nursing practice. Several states include some reference to treating human responses to actual or potential health problems. Most states refer to the execution of the medical regimen, and many include a general statement about additional acts that recognize that nursing practice is evolving and that the nurse's area of responsibility can be expected to broaden.

Defining Nursing for the Future

As the profession grows and responsibilities change, undoubtedly we will continue to refine the definition of nursing. By being responsive to changes, nursing has become more closely aligned with professions such as law, theology, and education, in which changing practices have required greater precision and refinement of definitions of the profession.

Critical Thinking Activity

Analyze the definitions of the major nursing theorists. What concepts found in those definitions are most closely aligned with your perception of nursing? Develop your own definition of nursing and compare it to those of the theorists and to those of your classmates.

CHARACTERISTICS OF A PROFESSION

The meanings of profession and professionalism as applied to nursing have been a subject of debate for many years. From approximately the 1950s through the 1970s or mid-1980s, nursing periodically was reviewed against the **characteristics of a profession** that had been established in the sociologic literature. Some critics believe that nursing falls short of meeting these criteria. Amid these challenges, nurses are working to advance the standing of nursing through the development of a code of ethics, standards of practice, and peer review. Table 4-7 outlines the seven major criteria and briefly discusses how nursing is meeting them or falls short of doing so. This set of characteristics corresponds to those being used by the American Association of Colleges of Nursing (AACN) when they refer to "professional" nursing as requiring a baccalaureate degree in nursing or higher.

Critical Thinking Activity

Select one of the characteristics of a profession that you believe nursing has difficulty meeting. Describe the actions that you believe should occur in the profession that would result in the profession fully meeting that criterion. How would you go about implementing those actions?

Differentiating Between the Terms "Profession" and "Professional"

Nursing involves activities that may be performed by many different caregivers. These people include nursing assistants, practical (vocational) nurses, and RNs prepared for entry into nursing through any of several educational avenues (see Chapter 5). Each of these caregivers contributes to nursing as a profession. To meet the nursing needs of the public, it is essential that caregivers function at various levels of practice. This has led to confusion about the use of the terms **profession** and **professional**. Is there a difference between looking at the practice of nursing in its totality and the "professional" practice of nursing?

TABLE 4-7	HOW NURSING MEETS THE TRADITIONAL CRITERIA FOR A PROFESSION*
CRITERION	**HOW NURSING MEETS THE CRITERION**
• Possession of a Body of Specialized Knowledge	Critics state that nursing borrows from biologic sciences, social sciences, and medical science, and then combines the various skills and concepts. This amalgamation and synthesis may be one of nursing's distinctive qualities. Nursing researchers work to develop an organized body of knowledge unique to nursing along with a specialized language of nursing (discussed later in this chapter). As this body of knowledge expands, this criterion is more nearly met.
• Use of Scientific Method to Enlarge the Body of Knowledge	Much work has been done toward systematically gathering and analyzing data, correctly identifying problems, selecting alternates, and evaluating patient care. Evidence-based practice and evidence-based education are at the forefront of nursing today (see Chapter 6).
• Education Within Institutions of Higher Education	This has been a controversial issue in nursing. Over time, the settings in which nurses are educated have changed, with most programs under the auspices of colleges or universities. Controversy over the length of nursing programs (associate degree versus baccalaureate degree) and the technical aspects of patient care continues.
• Control of Professional Policy, Professional Activity, and Autonomy	Today nurses are responsible for planning, implementing, and evaluating the care patients receive and being accountable for that care. Nursing policies and protocols, standards of practice, and evaluative measures and criteria have been developed by nurses (see Chapter 6). In some settings, nurses are eligible for third-party payment. More collaborative relationships are occurring with other health care team members, including physicians.
• A Code of Ethics	The general standard for the professional behavior of nurses in the United States is the ANA *Code for Nurses,* which is periodically revised. The International Council of Nurses also has developed a code for nurses that sets the standards of ethical practice by nurses throughout the world (see Chapter 9).
• Nursing as Lifetime Commitment	Most nurses view themselves as committed to their profession and continue to identify themselves as nurses long after they retire. However, some do leave the profession due to "burnout" and stress. Better educational and clinical pathways encourage continued growth and retention in the profession.
• Service to the Public	Although discussion occurs with regard to altruism, remuneration for services, and collective bargaining (see Chapter 11), there is no question that nursing provides a service to the public.

*The criteria identified in this table are developed from criteria set forth by Bixler & Bixler, 1945.

A Profession as Defined by Legislation

In at least one instance, federal legislation has helped to establish a list of the characteristics of a professional. Public Law 93-360 (Labor Management Relations Act, 1947 [amended, 1959, 1974]), which governs collective bargaining activities, defines the professional employee as follows:

> (a) any employee engaged in work (i) predominantly intellectual and varied in character as opposed to routine mental, manual, mechanical, or physical work; (ii) involving the consistent exercise of discretion and judgment in its performance; (iii) of such a character that the output produced or the result accomplished cannot be standardized in relation to a given period of time; (iv) requiring knowledge of an advanced type in a field of science or learning customarily acquired by a prolonged course of specialized intellectual instruction and study in an institution of higher learning or a hospital, as distinguished from a general academic education or from an apprenticeship or from training in the performance of routine mental, manual, or physical processes; or
>
> (b) any employee, who (i) has completed the courses of specialized intellectual instruction and study described in clause (iv) of paragraph (a), and (ii) is performing related work under the supervision of a professional person to qualify himself to become a professional employee as defined in paragraph (a).

Based on this definition, all RNs are considered professionals (Figure 4-4).

FIGURE 4-4   Some continue to question whether nursing truly can support the title of "profession."

Popular View of a Professional

A popular view of a professional involves the approach a person has to the role that is required. Most professionals approach their activities earnestly, strive for excellence in performance, and demonstrate a sense of ethics and responsibility in relationship to their careers. Such people consider their work a lifelong endeavor rather than a stepping stone to another field of employment. They place a positive value on being termed professional and perceive being termed nonprofessional or technical as an adverse reflection on their status, position, and motivation. Using this definition, we again find that it would apply to all RNs.

Certain people suggest that professionalism has a great deal to do with attitude, dress, conduct, and deportment. The attributes that are considered professional vary according to the personal values and stereotypes of the person doing the evaluating.

TRADITIONS IN NURSING

Because of its history, nursing has developed many traditions. Some of them are being questioned or eliminated, primarily because they are not practical in today's workplace (eg, the wearing of a nursing cap). It is worthwhile, however, to reflect just a little on the development of these traditions and to discuss their relationship to nursing. Earle P. Scarlett, a Canadian physician, writer, and medical historian, would support such discussion. He wrote:

> The truth of the matter is that any profession worthy of the name must forever be strengthening and re-creating its traditions. A profession is a sensitive organic growing thing, not a static order. And it is particularly important that we should remember this at the present time. (Scarlett, 1991, p. 6)

The Nursing Pin

The nursing pin may date back to the time of the Crusades, when Crusaders marched to Jerusalem to recover the Holy Land. Among the Crusaders were the Knights Hospitallers of St. John of Jerusalem. Their uniform, introduced by a man named Gerard, included a black robe with a white Maltese cross. The Maltese cross became a familiar sight on the battlefields of the Holy Land. Following the capture of Jerusalem in 1099, some of the Crusaders noted the excellent nursing care provided by the Hospital of St. John and decided to join the nursing group. The Maltese cross is an eight-pointed cross formed by four arrowheads joining at their points. The eight points of the cross signified the eight beatitudes that knights were expected to exemplify in their works of charity. When the Knights Templars and the Knights of the Teutonic Order were formed, in 1118 and 1190, respectively, this symbol was carried forward. The Maltese cross later became a symbol of many groups who cared for the sick, including the United States Cadet Nurse Corps.

The actual symbolism of the pin relates to customs established in the 16th century, when the privilege of wearing a coat of arms was limited to noblemen who served their kings with distinction. As centuries passed, the privilege was extended to schools and to craft guilds, and the symbols of wisdom, strength, courage, and faith appeared on buttons, badges, and shields. It was probably this spirit that Florence Nightingale attempted to capture when she chose the Maltese cross as a symbol for the badge worn by the graduates of her first nursing school.

As nursing developed as a profession, each school chose a unique pin, awarded on completion of the program, as a public symbol of work well done. Many of the early schools, particularly those associated with hospitals supported by religious groups, incorporated the cross into their pin. The first Nightingale School of Nursing in the United States was at Bellevue Hospital and is credited with developing the first school badge or pin, which was presented to the class of 1880 (Kalisch & Kalisch, 2004, p. 76). A crane in the center symbolized the nurse's vigilance, an inner circle of blue suggested constancy, and an outer circle of poppy capsules symbolized mercy and the relief of suffering. The nursing journal *RN* has collected nursing pins from across the United States and has occasionally created a cover display of pins from that collection.

The Nursing Cap

The history of the nursing cap is less certain. Several explanations of the origin of the cap have been suggested. It probably evolved during the period of time when nursing was greatly influenced by religion. It may have originated in the habit worn by the Sisters of Charity of St. Vincent de Paul, who established the first modern school of nursing in Paris in 1864. Another opinion suggests that the cap was influenced by the Institute of Protestant Deaconesses, founded by Pastor Theodore Fleidner at Kaiserwerth in Germany, and the institution where Florence Nightingale studied. The white cap of the deaconesses of the early Christian era and the nun's veil of the Middle Ages have been said to be the forerunners of the nursing cap as we know it today (Mangum, 1994). The veil was modified to become a cap and was associated with service to others. We need to remember, also, that in Florence Nightingale's day, every lady wore a cap indoors. If you look at pictures of Queen Victoria, you notice the cap of plain white stiffened muslin framing her face. It was considered proper for women to keep their heads covered; thus, the cap would be viewed as the proper dress for a young woman of the day. The cap worn by students at Kaiserwerth when Florence Nightingale was a student was hood shaped, had a ruffle around the face, and tied under the chin. A final conjecture is that the cap originally was designed to cover and help to control the long hair that was fashionable in the late 19th century, when short haircuts were not acceptable for women (Kalisch & Kalisch, 2004).

In the United States and Canada, the head covering became smaller and lost its scarf or veil as women's hairstyles changed and hair was worn shorter. (The hair-covering aspect remained a part of the cap in many areas of Europe.) As nursing education programs developed in hospitals, they each created their own cap, as with their nursing pin, to symbolize that particular hospital and nursing school. Some of these caps were rather frilly and were fashioned after the cloth cone through which ether was dropped. Again, as hairstyles changed, the size of the cap also changed, until it became one of individual taste or preference. A capping ceremony was part of the ritual of the nursing student and is discussed later.

As the role of nurses changed and as high technology became a significant part of the hospital work environment, nurses found that caps were bothersome as they tried to carry out their duties. They were knocked askew by curtains, equipment, and tubing. By the 1980s, many hospitals no longer required the cap as a part of the uniform. Nursing programs responded by dropping the cap as a required article of dress. If students wished to have a cap, it was purchased from a local uniform store and had no particular identification with the program.

The Nursing Uniform

Like the nursing cap, which is actually a part of the early nursing uniform, the requirement for special dress came from the religious and military history of nursing and has always been significant in nursing. This is due to the fact that dress provides a strong nonverbal message about one's image. The nurse attired in a white uniform, at least in the 1950s and 1960s, communicated an impression of confidence, competence, professionalism, authority, role identity, and accountability. As nurses have adopted more casual dress, some of this identity has been lost, and hospital committees, nursing programs, and nurses have spent considerable time discussing appropriate attire.

Early uniforms were long, usually stiffly starched, and had detachable collars and cuffs. A full uniform often included a long cape that would cover the uniform. Kalisch and Kalisch (2004, pp. 75–78) credit the New York Training School for Nurses at Bellevue Hospital with being the first school to adopt a standard uniform for student nurses in 1876. The uniform consisted of a gingham apron worn in the morning and a white apron worn in the afternoon over a dark woolen dress. A well-bred young woman, Euphemia Van Rensselaer, is credited with updating the basic uniform, which students were opposed to wearing. Given 2 days' leave of absence to have a uniform made for herself, she created a tailored uniform consisting of a long gray dress for winter and a calico version for summer, both worn with a white apron and cap. The attractiveness of her appearance resulted in other students accepting the uniform as standard dress. Later, a more easily laundered dress that could be worn throughout the year replaced both dresses.

A regulation uniform became a distinguishing mark of each nursing school by the end of the 19th century. Typically, the uniform consisted of a bodice and skirt of white material, adjustable white cuffs, a stiff white collar, and a white cap. To maintain the feminine hourglass image popular at the time, a tightly laced corset was worn beneath the uniform and ankles were hidden from view. Some suggest that the adoption of a distinctive and attractive uniform played a significant role in developing a professional image for nursing, giving it status, respect, and authority.

By the 1900s, the uniform became more functional, and the hemline was raised. By the mid-1960s, pantsuits became accepted, and nurses in certain settings, particularly psychiatric and pediatric units, challenged the appropriateness of uniforms, especially white uniforms. By 1970, significant changes occurred in uniforms, with the acceptance of styles that were designed to "make the nurse more approachable." In psychiatric settings, "no uniform" became the standard of the day. Today, athletic shoes are acceptable in many institutions, and scrubs have become so accepted that they are featured in pamphlets advertising uniforms. As dress styles have become increasingly casual, many hospitals have been forced to institute dress codes that restrict dangling jewelry, message T-shirts, and fake fingernails.

In 1987, the Springhouse Corporation conducted a survey of nurses throughout the United States and found that most prefer scrubs or lab coats worn over street clothes. The result of this change has been that nurses today are no longer identifiable by uniform. The stethoscope worn around the neck gives the consumer some clue to a person's position (ie, that the person is a health care worker rather than a maintenance person), and hospital identification badges provide further information, but sometimes do not include the person's full name.

Controversy over the appropriate attire for nurses continues. Some hospitals are instituting dress codes that require a return to white attire in an effort to restore professionalism to the job (Glanton, 2005), while others argue that what nurses wear matters less than what they know and that there are ways to differentiate hospital workers other than returning to a white uniform.

Ceremonies Associated With Nursing Programs

Long-standing traditions embraced by nursing include the ceremonies that mark various points along the educational paths of nursing students. Primary among these are the capping and the pinning ceremonies.

Capping ceremonies are not as common today as pinnings, probably because most nurses and nursing students no longer wear caps. Traditionally, the cap was awarded to students after they completed a certain part of the program. In hospital schools, it may have been awarded on completion of the probationary period, but more often it was given after the completion of the first year. Often held in a nearby church, a special ceremony was planned, to which students invited family and others who were interested in their progress. The director of the school, assisted by other school dignitaries and faculty, solemnly placed the cap on the head of each student. Students proudly wore the cap throughout the remainder of the program. Often a stripe was added to one corner of the cap to signify completion of the second year of study, and a black band was added at the time of graduation. Many colleges included these ceremonies when nursing education moved into institutions of higher education.

The second traditional ceremony in nursing, the pinning, was of even greater significance, and is continued by many schools today. The pinning heralded the completion of the program. Amid much pomp and circumstance, family and friends gathered to watch as the nursing director ceremoniously pinned the school pin on each new graduate. Graduates often recited, in unison, the Nightingale Pledge (Display 4-2) written in 1893 by Lystra E. Gretter, superintendent of Farrand Training School for Nurses at Harper Hospital School in Detroit and a small committee of nurses (Kalisch & Kalisch, 2004). This tradition is often repeated in nursing schools today, although a modified version of the original pledge is often used. Some schools include additional tradition through the "passing of the lamp." A representative of the graduating class hands a lamp (symbolizing the lamp carried by Florence Nightingale) to a representative of the next graduating class, thus reinforcing the concept of the continual caring represented in nursing.

Display 4-2   The Nightingale Pledge

I solemnly pledge myself before God and in the presence of this assembly:

To pass my life in purity and to practice my profession faithfully;

I will abstain from whatever is deleterious and mischievous and will not take or knowingly administer any harmful drug; I will do all in my power to maintain and elevate the standard of the profession, and will hold in confidence all personal matters committed to my keeping and all family affairs coming to my knowledge in the practice of my calling;

With loyalty will I endeavor to aid the physician in his work, and devote myself to the welfare of those committed to my care.

Agnes, G. Deans & Anne L Austin, *The History of the Farrand Training School for Nurses* (Detroit: Alumnae Associate of the Farrand Training School for Nurses, 1936) p. 58, as cited in Kalisch & Kalisch, 2004.

As nursing education moved into institutions of higher education, some of the traditional ceremonies were discontinued. Some argue that the ceremony recognizing program completion in the collegiate environment is the college commencement, and that special celebrations for students of particular areas of study are not appropriate. However, in many large universities, the various disciplines now have separate ceremonies or an additional ceremony for their members. In other cases, the tradition is continued, although there is some tendency for graduates not to purchase a pin.

Critical Thinking Activity

Review the traditions established in nursing. Which is the most meaningful to you, and why? Which is the least meaningful to you, and why? Do you believe traditions should be continued in nursing? Provide a rationale for your answer.

THE IMAGE OF NURSING TODAY

During the late 1970s and early 1980s, much time and energy were invested in studying the image of nursing, with much of this work done by Beatrice and Philip Kalisch, who have written prolifically about the topic. Their writing focuses on segments of an overall study of the image of the nurse in various forms of mass media, including radio, movies, television, newspapers, magazines, and novels. They believe that popular attitudes and assumptions about nurses and what nurses contribute to a patient's welfare can greatly influence the future of nursing. It is their contention that since the 1970s, the popular image of the nurse not only has failed to reflect changing professional conditions, but has been based on derogatory stereotypes that have undermined public confidence in and respect for the professional nurse. Nurses should be concerned about negative or incorrect images because such images can influence the attitudes of patients, policymakers, and politicians. Negative attitudes about nursing also may discourage many capable prospective nurses, who will choose another career that offers greater appeal in stature, status, and salary. This issue is of great concern today, as the shortage of nurses promises to become severe.

Although some might argue that nurses have better things to do than to worry about how the nurse is portrayed in the media, a consistently misrepresented image can negatively affect how the public views nurses. Therefore, nurses have responded to television advertisements or programs that portray nurses and nursing in a negative light with letters and telephone calls. Boycotts on the purchase of products that present nurses poorly in advertisements as well as organized written protests have proved to be an effective way to bring about change. According to the Center for Nursing Advocacy (2003), the adverse responses from nurses resulted in the withdrawal of a commercial for Clairol shampoo that showed a nurse leaving a patient to shampoo her own hair in the patient's bathroom and then dance around his room, waving her hair in ecstasy. In addition, various nursing organizations have waged campaigns to enhance the image of nursing by emphasizing it as a prestigious, desirable, and respected career.

NURSING'S IMAGE AND THE NURSING SHORTAGE

Currently we are experiencing a serious nursing shortage that is affecting the supply of nursing faculty as well as nurses employed in the delivery of care. The shortage is expected to reach serious proportions by 2010, when the gap will widen between the supply of and the requirement for RNs (Geolot, 2000). Authorities believe that the current shortage is not like previous shortages and that extraordinary means will need to be taken to reverse it.

A number of factors are suggested as contributing to the shortfall of RNs. First of all, nurses are getting older. In the United States, the average age of a nurse is 46.8, with many anticipating retirement within the next decade (Preliminary Findings, 2006). Another concern centers on the fact that members of the baby boom generation are beginning to enter their senior years, thus increasing the need for nurses in the health care system. New nurses often enter nursing as a career change in midlife. They will have fewer years in the profession than those who entered as young adults.

However, a factor that demands serious consideration relates to the fact that nursing has always been a female-dominated profession. Women today have more educational and occupational alternatives. Many other careers may seem more attractive than nursing in terms of the salary commanded, the working conditions, and the prestige given to the role. This was realized by an overall dropping enrollment in nursing programs throughout the United States during the 1990s.

The shortage is of such import that various groups that command respect for their work have decided to study the issue or take action to try to encourage more individuals to study nursing. The Robert Wood Johnson Foundation funded a study with findings released in 2002. They recommended that a National Forum to Advance Nursing be created that would draw together a wide range of individuals affected by the shortage. The Forum would focus on helping nursing achieve higher standing as a profession. The Foundation has suggested that the Forum would focus efforts in several strategic areas that include the following:

- Creating new nursing models to address the shortage, study nursing's contribution to health care outcomes and create new models of health care provision.
- Reinventing nursing education and work environments to address the needs and values of and appeal to a younger generation of nurses.
- Establishing a national nursing workforce measurement-and-data collection system.
- Creating a clearinghouse of effective strategies to facilitate cultural change within the profession (Robert Wood Johnson Foundation, 2002).

In February 2002, Johnson & Johnson launched its "Campaign for Nursing's Future," a program that would spend $20 million during a 2-year period to attract more individuals to nursing. The campaign included television advertisements, a Web site (*http://discovernursing.com*), recruitment brochures, and posters and videos directed toward high school-age individuals. The Web site provides a listing of sponsored sites addressing topics such as nursing as a career, schools, scholarships and grants, jobs, salaries, and similar topics. Health care organizations, in collaboration with state nurses associations, have created comparable projects in local television markets. The sponsors of all these efforts hope that this will result in increased enrollment in nursing programs. In Oregon, a major campaign titled "Are you man enough to be a nurse?" was designed to encourage men to enter nursing; the ads contained photos of several different men engaged in challenging nursing roles.

Another factor affecting the nursing supply is the limited number of spaces in nursing programs. As recently as 1993, a Pew report identified an excess of nurses and recommended that some nursing programs be closed (O'Neil, 1993). Fortunately, this recommendation was not acted upon.

Because nursing education is costly, many educational institutions have not been able to increase the size of their programs in the past decade. As applications increase, further efforts will be needed to increase the number of individuals who can be admitted. Some states have instituted major efforts to increase the available spaces for nursing students. The National Council of State Boards of Nursing is maintaining a Web site with information on efforts across the country to increase the nursing supply (*www.ncsbn.org/news/stateupdates_state_shortage.asp#New%20Mexico*).

To provide advice and recommendations to the Secretary of Health and Human Services and Congress on policy matters relating to the nursing work force, the National Advisory Council on Nurse Education and Practice (NACNEP) was established. In 2001, this group focused on the shortage of nurses in practice; at its spring 2002 meeting, NACNEP addressed the shortage of nursing faculty.

As all areas employing nurses feel the effect of the shortage, serious concern has been voiced by educational institutions and organizations supporting educational efforts, such as the National League for Nursing, regarding the supply of educationally prepared nursing faculty. Again, in conjunction with Johnson & Johnson, scholarships have been made available in some geographic areas to nurses who would like to prepare for faculty positions.

Another aspect of the nursing shortage is the retention of current nurses. Some states have identified that there are a large number of RNs not currently working in the profession. Many experts have pointed to working conditions such as mandatory overtime, heavy workloads, and lack of respect in the workplace as reasons for people leaving. The ANA is focusing on actions that will improve the work environment and thus increase retention as means of addressing the nursing shortage.

How this will all play out is yet to be seen. Certainly, at no time in recent history has the need for nurses been more critical and the supply so limited.

Critical Thinking Activity

Interview five of your friends who are not nurses. What is their image of nursing? What do they understand of the role of the nurse? Do they view nursing positively? What recurrent information is mentioned?

COMMUNICATION IN *ACTION*

Affecting Community Images of Nursing

A neighbor consults Susan Williams, an RN, about advising her niece regarding a career choice. The neighbor says, "Julie is a really sweet girl that everyone likes. She isn't very good with academics but is kind, caring, and compassionate with others. I think she would make an excellent nurse, don't you?" Susan replies, "Those are excellent attributes and will be a good foundation for much of life, but registered nursing does require a college level education and is very dependent on sciences, math, and difficult nursing courses. If she finds sciences difficult and is not interested in college-level academics, then nursing is not a good choice for her."

STUDIES FOR AND ABOUT NURSING

Early in the 20th century, the quality of many nursing schools and their graduates was poor; many of Florence Nightingale's admonitions regarding nursing education had been forgotten or ignored. Nurses, doctors, friends, and critics of nursing became concerned that the preparation being offered was inadequate. Before the problem could be corrected, it was necessary to learn more about the programs and how nurses were being used in the employment market. To accomplish this, studies about nursing and nurses were initiated.

We recognize that many students in nursing are not excited by studies, especially those conducted years ago. However, we hope that when you have finished reading this section of the textbook, you will have gained an appreciation of the enduring effort made by nurses and interested colleagues to gain a greater understanding of the profession, with the goal of improving the profession and thus the care provided to the public. As you read you will, no doubt, recognize recurring themes with which we continue to grapple today. Our discussion is limited to those studies that looked at the profession as a whole and does not include any of the myriad studies conducted each year, primarily clinical in focus, that form the basis for evidence-based practice and for the expansion of the body of nursing knowledge.

Although the first nursing studies were not begun until the early 1900s, the number of studies since the 1950s has been voluminous. It is impossible to look at any professional nursing publication and not find mention of some new study in progress. Efforts were made to classify and catalog references to these studies and to report them. One of the first was completed by Virginia Henderson, who prepared *A Nursing Studies Index*. In 1952, a group of nurses, under the sponsorship of the Association of Collegiate Schools of Nursing, launched a new journal called *Nursing Research*, which was designed to disseminate information about nursing research.

A single individual often conducted many of the early studies, typically with a particular purpose in mind. Through the years, studies frequently took the form of a report by a special group of individuals, often appointed by a governmental or professional agency. Although by no means inclusive of all studies and reports, Table 4-8 highlights some of the major significant studies of nursing that have provided benchmarks to the profession, identifies the primary investigator/sponsor, and briefly discusses the focus and recommendation(s) associated with each study.

Critical Thinking Activity

Identify at least three areas in nursing that you believe need further study, and describe how you would begin to conduct those studies. Whom would you involve and why? How and to whom would you like to see the results and recommendations disseminated?

DEFINING A LANGUAGE FOR NURSING

For many, the development of a special language for nursing is a new development. There may be some who feel this is much ado about nothing. However, structured nursing vocabularies allow nurses to use the acquired information to guide evidence-based clinical decisions, manage information in an electronic format, retrieve information for research, and compare clinical outcomes across settings. It also provides a common means of communication (Display 4-3).

TABLE 4-8 MAJOR STUDIES ABOUT NURSING

DATE	NAME OF STUDY	PRIMARY INVESTIGATOR/SPONSOR	FOCUS AND RECOMMENDATION
1912	*The Educational Status of Nursing*	M. Adelaide Nutting/U.S. Bureau of Education	What and how students were being taught and conditions under which they were living. Began to establish nursing as a profession.
1923	*Winslow-Goldmark Report on Nursing and Nursing Education in the United States*	Josephine Goldmark/ Rockefeller Foundation	The educational preparation of students including public health nurses, teachers, and supervisors. It pointed out fundamental faults in hospital training schools and resulted in the establishment of the Yale University School of Nursing.
1923	Committee on the Grading of Nursing Schools—a 3-part study	Francis Payne Bolton and contributions of thousands of nurses	
1928	*(1) Nurses, Patients, and Pocketbooks*	May Ayres Burgess/ statistician	An inquiry into the supply and demand for nurses. Demonstrated that there was an oversupply of nurses.
1934	*(2) An Activity Analysis of Nursing*	Ethel Johns and Blance Pfefferkorn	Looked at the activities that constitute nursing as a basis for improving curricula.
1934	*(3) Nursing Schools Today & Tomorrow*	Ethel Johns	Described the nursing schools of the period and made recommendations about professional schools.
1937	*A Curriculum Guide for Schools of Nursing*— not truly a study of nursing, but often referred to as one because of its far reaching effects	National League for Nursing Education	A revision of a 1917 publication, it outlined the curricula for a 3-year course, emphasizing sound educational teaching procedures. Followed by many schools of the time.
1948	*Nursing for the Future*	Esther Lucille Brown/ Carnegie Foundation, the Russell Sage Foundation, and the National Nursing Council	Done to determine society's need for nursing. Described inadequacies in nursing schools. Resulted in recommendations that nursing education be placed in universities and colleges and encouraged recruitment of large numbers of men and members of minority groups into nursing schools.
1948	The Ginzberg Report or *A Program for the Nursing Profession*— a report of the discussions of the Committee on the Functions of Nursing	Eli Ginzberg/Columbia University	Reviewed problems centering around the shortage of nurses. Recommended that nursing teams consisting of variously educated nurses be developed.
1950	*Nursing Schools at the Mid-Century*	Margaret Bridgman/National Committee for the Improvement of Nursing Services—Russell Sage Foundation	Studied the practices of more than 1000 nursing schools (including organization, costs, curriculum, clinical resources, and student health) and stimulated improvement in baccalaureate schools.
1955	*Patterns of Patient Care*	Francis George and Ruth Perkins Kuehn/University of Pittsburgh	Assessed the amount of nursing service needed by a group of medical/surgical patients and determined how much of that care could be delegated to nursing aides and other nonprofessional people
1958	*Twenty Thousand Nurses Tell Their Story*	Everett C. Hughes/ANA and American Nurses Foundation	Looked at nurses, what they were doing, their attitudes toward their jobs, and job satisfaction. Formed basis for development of nursing functions, standards, and qualifications.

TABLE 4-8   MAJOR STUDIES ABOUT NURSING (*Continued*)

DATE	NAME OF STUDY	PRIMARY INVESTIGATOR/SPONSOR	FOCUS AND RECOMMENDATION
1959	*Community College Education for Nursing*	Mildred Montag/Institute of Research and Service in Nursing Education—Teachers College, Columbia University	Reported the findings of a 5-year study of eight 2-year nursing programs. Led to the establishment of more associate degree programs.
1963	*Toward Quality in Nursing: Needs and Goals*	W. Allen Wallis—Consultant Group on Nursing—a panel of nurses in the health field/U.S. Public Health Service	A report requested by the U.S. Surgeon General to determine funding priorities. Advised on the need for nurses, recruitment concerns, need for nursing research, and improvement of nursing education.
1970	*An Abstract for Action* (a report of the National Commission on Nursing and Nursing Education)	Jerome Lysaught/ANA, ANF, NLN, Mellon and Kellogg Foundations	Looked at current practices and patterns of nursing. Suggested joint practice committees, master planning for nursing education, funding for nursing education and research.
1979	*The Study of Credentialing in Nursing*	Inez Hinsvark/ANA	A review of credentialing—especially of nursing. Resulted in the appointment of a Task Force. Supported a freestanding credentialing center for nursing.
1983	*National Institute of Medicine Study*	Katherine Bauer/DHHS	Required by the Nursing Training Act of 1979, determined the need for continued outlay of federal money for nursing education. Resulted in 21 specific recommendations. Found that the shortage of nurses of the 1960s and 1970s no longer existed, that federal support of nursing education should focus on graduate study, and that the federal government should discontinue efforts to increase "generalist nurses."
1988	*Secretary's Commission on Nursing*	Lillian Gibbons/DHHS	Responded to serious nursing shortage. Validated the shortage. Recommended increased financial support of education and improved status and working conditions for nurses.
1990	*Secretary's Commission on the National Nursing Shortage*	Caroline Burnett/DHHS	Appointed for 1 year to advise on implementation of 1988 report. Had three main foci: recruitment and retention, restructuring of nursing service, and use of nursing personnel and information systems.
1991	*Report of the National Commission of Nursing Implementation Project (NCNIP)*	Vivian De Back/ANA, NLN, AACN, AONE, Kellogg Foundation	Looked at nursing education, practice, management and research, and developed recommendations for the future of nursing.
1993	*Health Professions Education for the Future*	E.H. O'Neill/Pew Health Professions Commission—Pew Charitable Trusts	Reinforced the belief that the education of health professions was not adequate to meet the health needs of America. Identified competencies for 2005 and emphasized the need for nurse-midwives, nurse practitioners, and the role of nurses in health promotion.
1995	*Reforming Health Care Workforce Regulation*	Pew Health Professions Commission	Had as its mission assisting schools preparing health professionals to understand the changing nature of health care, the needs for the future, and how to design and implement the programs preparing these workers. Recommended reform of the licensing process, specifically elimination of exclusive scopes of practice.

The development of nursing languages began as an effort to build a set of terms that would describe the clinical judgments made by nurses that are not in medical language systems. As early as 1909, nurses with a perceptive view of the future recognized that nursing would one day need a language of its own. Ninety years ago, Isabel Hampton Robb wrote the following after attending a meeting of the newly formed International Council of Nurses:

> While attending a special meeting of the ICN in Paris, I was naturally at once struck by the fact that the methods and the ways of regarding nursing problems were . . . as foreign to the various delegations as were the actual languages, and the thought occurred to me that . . . sooner or later we must put ourselves upon a common basis and work out what may be termed a "nursing Esperanto" which would in the course of time give us a universal nursing language. (Hampton-Robb, 1909) (Note: Esperanto was a language developed in 1887 with the goal of being a universal language that could be taught as the second language throughout the world, enabling improved communication among peoples.)

Defining a language for nursing primarily involves the development and refinement of **nursing nomenclatures** and **classification systems** that communicate information and guide data collection about nursing activities. The term "nursing nomenclature" refers to the words by which we name or describe phenomena in nursing. A "classification" is the systematic arrangement or a structural framework of these phenomena. As we move toward an international network of health care, the development of a language unique to nursing is viewed as critical to communication and decision making. Proponents of a specialized language for nursing emphasize the need for objective, science-based information to use in decision making. These data also provide the basis for accountability and the documentation-supporting processes and outcomes of care. The data can be used further to answer research questions about nursing and nursing actions. In the age of information technology, uniform, accurate, and automated patient care data are required to conduct analyses that will result in improving the quality of care and costing out that care. At present, the language of nursing primarily addresses nursing diagnoses, implementation activities, and nursing outcomes. Some would suggest that the existing systems are not adequate to reflect the entire scope of nursing practice and urge further development. Here we discuss the four systems that are currently most popular; others that are approved by the ANA are summarized in Table 4-9.

Display 4-3   Rationale for the Development of a Classification for Nursing

- Permits recognition and communication with others by giving a name to the things nurses do
- Provides a uniform legal record of care
- Supports clinical decision making
- Lays the groundwork for nursing research
- Captures the cost of nursing services for billing and accounting purposes
- Generates a structured retrieval database for quality assurance

NANDA-International

The group originally called the National Group for the Classification of Nursing Diagnosis and then North American Nursing Diagnosis Association (NANDA), and now **NANDA International (NANDA-I)** became a formal organization after its fifth conference in 1982. The Association has two main purposes: to develop a diagnostic classification system (also known as a **taxonomy**) and to identify and approve nursing diagnoses. The list of nursing diagnoses (concepts that are given word labels) continues to grow as nurses encounter diagnoses in clinical practice that have not been included and submit these to NANDA-I for consideration. As a student, you have some familiarity with nursing diagnoses from the nursing care plans you develop for patient care and in the case studies you discuss in your classes. The following is the definition of a nursing diagnosis accepted by NANDA-I:

> Nursing diagnosis is a clinical judgment about individual, family, or community response to actual or potential health problems/life processes. Nursing diagnoses provide the basis for selection of nursing interventions to achieve outcomes for which the nurse is accountable. (NANDA-I, 2005)

Nursing Interventions Classifications

Started in 1996 at the University of Iowa, the **Nursing Interventions Classification (NIC)** is a comprehensive, standardized language that describes actions nurses perform in all settings and in all specialties, and includes both physiologic and psychosocial interventions. The interventions are numbered to facilitate computerization and are organized into classes, and the classes are assigned to domains. The domains are functional health, physiologic health, psychosocial health, health knowledge and behavior, perceived health, family health, and community health. Each intervention has been linked with NANDA nursing diagnoses and with the NOC below and with Omaha system problems. Many institutions have adopted NIC as a standardized terminology for use in computerized documentation systems. An overview of NIC is available on-line (*www.nursing.uiowa.edu/center/cncce*), and a detailed presentation of the entire system is available in print (Dochterman & Bulechek, 2004).

Nursing Outcomes Classification

Also developed at the University of Iowa, the NOC was first published in 1997. An outcome is defined as a variable concept representing a patient or family caregiver state, behavior, or perception that is measurable along a continuum and responsive to nursing interventions. Project developers believed that stating the outcomes as variable concepts rather than goals would allow the identification of positive or negative changes (or no changes at all) in the patient's status. Each outcome has a definition, a list of indicators that assist in evaluation of patient status, a rating scale for evaluation, and a suggested target rating. Listed in alphabetical order, the outcomes are grouped into classes and use the same domains as NIC. Both NIC and NOC are continuing in development. An overview of the NOC is available on-line (*www.nursing.uiowa.edu/centers/cncce*), and the detailed system is available in print (Moorhead, Johnson, & Maas, 2004).

The Omaha System

The **Omaha System**, another example of classification efforts, is based on federally funded research conducted by the Visiting Nurse Association of Omaha from 1975 to 1993. It was

TABLE 4-9	MAJOR CLASSIFICATIONS FOR NURSING CARE RECOGNIZED BY THE AMERICAN NURSES ASSOCIATION

DATA ELEMENT SETS

Title	What It Is	Characteristics
Nursing Minimum Data Set	Identified the four elements of nursing diagnosis, nursing interventions, nursing outcomes, and nursing intensity.	Data must be collected in three arenas: nursing care elements, patient elements, and service elements (Brief Synopsis, 2003)
Nursing Management Minimum Data Set	Provides resources nurse executives need to make informed decisions and manage nursing services delivery and care coordination	Categorizes variables into environment, nurse resources, and financial resources

INTERFACE TERMINOLOGIES

Title	What It Is	Characteristics
NANDA International (formerly North American Nursing Diagnosis Association)	Provides a taxomony of nursing diagnoses. Defines a nursing diagnosis as a clinical judgment about an individual, family, or community response to actual or potential health problems that provides a basis for selecting a nursing intervention	Currently contains 13 domains, 106 classes within those domains, and 183 nursing diagnoses (NANDA-I, 2005)
Nursing Intervention Classification	Provides a comprehensive standardized language, describing treatments that nurses perform in all settings and in all specialties	Includes 514 interventions, each with a definition and a detailed set of activities, organized into 30 classes which are then a part of seven domains (Dochterman & Bulechek, 2004)
Nursing Outcomes Classification	Defines a nursing outcome as a variable concept that represents a patient or family caregiver state, behavior, or perception that is measurable along a continuum and responsive to nursing interventions	Contains 330 outcomes, each of which has a list of indicators in the evaluation of patient status, a measurement scale, and a short list of references grouped in 37 classes and the same seven domains used in NIC (Moorhead, Johnson, & Mass, 2004)
The Omaha System	A system of client problems, interventions,and client outcomes, referred to as the Problem Classification Scheme, the Intervention Scheme, and the Problem Rating Scale for Outcomes	Includes domains, problems, modifiers, and signs/symptoms; intervention categories, targets, and client-specific information; and outcome rating scales for knowledge, behavior, and status (Martin, 2005)
International Classification of Nursing Practice	Collaborative project under the auspices of the International Council of Nursing for classifying nursing phenomena (diagnoses, interventions, and outcomes)	Includes definitions, for nursing phenomena and nursing interventions; provides a unifying framework into which local language, vocabularies, and classifications can be cross-mapped to enable a comparison of data internationally (Coenen, 2003)
Patient Care Data Set (Retired)	Codifies patient problems and actions delivered by all caregivers during a hospital stay	Information gathered from hundreds of terms in patient records

TABLE 4-9	MAJOR CLASSIFICATIONS FOR NURSING CARE RECOGNIZED BY THE AMERICAN NURSES ASSOCIATION (*Continued*)

INTERFACE TERMINOLOGIES (Continued)

Title	What It Is	Characteristics
Clinical Care Classification (previously Home Health Care Classification) Diagnoses and Interventions	Adapted, revised, and expanded NANDA to include additional home health care nursing diagnostic conditions	Consists of two interrelated taxonomies used to track and measure patient/client care holistically over time, across settings, population groups, and geographic locations (Saba, 2003)
Perioperative Nursing Data Set	Standardized language for documenting and evaluating perioperative nursing care	Designed for use in the perioperative nursing area (AORN On-line, 2002)

MULTIDISCIPLINARY TERMINOLOGIES

Alternative Billing Codes	Identifies alternative medicine, nursing, and other integrative health care services and related products	Contains more than 4,400 descriptions of health care services, remedies, and supply items (ABC Coding Solutions, 2006)
Logical Observation Identifiers Names and Codes	A database and universal standard for identifying laboratory observations. Applied to the electronic health record.	Structure includes six factors in its axes: components, kind of property, time aspect, system, type of scale, and type of method
Systematized Nomenclature of Medicine (SNOMED)	Comprehensive system for indexing the entire medical record, including signs and symptoms, diagnoses, and procedures	Allows full integration of all medical information in electronic medical record into a single data source (SNOMED, 2005)

designed as a three-part, comprehensive yet brief approach to documentation and information management for multidisciplinary health care professionals who practice in community settings. It offers terms and codes to classify the client's health-related concerns or problems, the interventions that nurses and other health care professionals use, and the client's outcomes (The Omaha System, 2005). Client problems can be identified for individuals, families, and groups. The interventions describe both plans and interventions for specific client concerns. The outcome scales evaluate a client's health-related changes through the use of problem-specific knowledge, behavior, and status ratings. The Omaha System is recognized by the ANA and has been translated into numerous languages. Automation and technology advances and health care delivery changes have markedly expanded its use nationally and internationally. A survey conducted in 2005 found that with the increased use of electronic health records, 75% of home care and public health organizations reported using Omaha System software (The Omaha System, 2005). An overview of the Omaha System is available on-line (*http://omahasystem.org/index.htm*), and the detailed classification system is in print (Martin, 2005).

Other Classification Systems

Currently, 13 Data Element Sets and Terminologies are recognized by the ANA. All of these are presented in Table 4-9 with a brief description of what each is and its major characteristics.

The Minimum Data Set for Nursing Home Resident Assessment and Care Screening

Although not referred to in terms of nursing language, the **Minimum Data Set for Nursing Home Resident Assessment and Care Screening (MDS)** bears some mention here. When the Omnibus Budget Reconciliation Act was passed in 1991, it required assessment of long-term care facility residents. This assessment, done on admission and every 3 months thereafter, must be standardized, comprehensive, accurate, and reproducible. It must be transmitted electronically to data centers in each state. Whenever problems are identified during the assessment, Resident Assessment Protocols (RAPs) must be instituted. The RAPs lists factors that might be associated with the problem, clarifying information to be considered in making a diagnosis and describing the environment that will help reduce the symptoms. Complete documentation of the situation, including nature of the problem, complications, risk factors, referrals, and rationale for action is required of nurses (Eliopoulos, 1997). The MDS is used as the basis for determining payment to long-term care facilities. The implementation of the MDS nationwide has resulted in a significant collection of data that can be used as a basis for improving the care of the elderly. The MDS 3.0 has been developed and an overview is available on the Centers for Medicare & Medicaid Services (CMS) Web site (CMS, 2005.)

The National Information and Data Set Evaluation Center

The **National Information and Data Set Evaluation Center (NIDSEC)** was established in 1995 by the ANA to review, evaluate against defined criteria, and recognize nursing information systems. Its mission is to "develop and disseminate standards pertaining to information systems that support the documentation of nursing practice, and evaluate voluntarily submitted information systems against these standards" (NIDSEC, 2005, p. 1). Within the framework of the NIDSEC, four dimensions of nursing data sets and systems are evaluated:

- Nomenclature (terms used)
- Clinical content (the linkages among terms)
- Clinical data repository (how the data are stored and made accessible for retrieval)
- General system characteristics (such as performance and attention to security and confidentiality)

Groups or vendors wishing to be recognized by the ANA submit materials to a five-member review panel, who, after examining the application, submit a recommendation to the NIDSEC committee. If accepted by the committee, the recognition extends for 3 years, after which a new application must be submitted. At this writing, 13 groups are recognized by NIDSEC (NIDSEC, 2005).

The International Classification for Nursing Practice Project

The **International Classification for Nursing Practice Project (ICNP)** is an effort of the International Council of Nurses (ICN). The goal of the ICNP is to provide "a unifying framework for existing systems and a system which can be used in countries which have none" (Clark, 1998). It is a classification of nursing phenomena, nursing actions, and nursing outcomes.

Although the United States has been involved in the development of classification and information systems for some time, the need for a unified language is now recognized internationally.

Because cultural and language differences exist, many of the classification systems currently employed in the United States are not useful in other countries. For example, the concept of self-care reflects the cultural values and norms of American society but may be perceived quite differently in other cultures. In 1989, the ICN was asked to encourage member National Nurses Associations to become involved in developing information and classification systems and nursing data sets that could be used by nurses in all countries to identify and describe nursing. The project began a year later. In 1996, an alpha version of the Classification of Nursing Phenomenon and Nursing Interventions was field tested, and a beta version was launched June 1999 at ICN's Centennial Conference. The objectives were reviewed and revised in 2000. The ICNP Programme has established a formal evaluation and review process to advance the project. ICNP® Version 1 is now available on the ICN Web site (ICN, 2005).

Critical Thinking Activity

Analyze the history of the development of a classification and nomenclature specific to nursing. Describe possible future developments, and provide a rationale for your answer. What do you see as major impediments and why? What do you believe will be the long-term benefits and why?

Key Concepts

- In its development as a profession, nursing has struggled with its definition, its image, and its role in the health care delivery system. This is due in part to its history and the fact that it has both theoretic and practical aspects. The role of the nurse in the health care delivery system has probably never been more important than it is today.
- Florence Nightingale dramatically changed the form and direction of nursing. She set down standards for nursing education and made significant recommendations for changes in how hospitals operated and how nursing was practiced.
- The wars in which the United States have been involved have had a significant impact on nursing. Nurses have always played an important role in the care of the wounded and dying.
- Early schools of nursing were established shortly after the Civil War with curricula fashioned much like the Nightingale School in England. Early programs were primarily apprenticeships, with long hours during which students provided much of the workforce of the hospital.
- Nursing is distinct from medicine. Medicine deals with diagnosis and treatment of disease, and nursing is concerned with caring for the person.
- The position nursing occupies as a profession is often judged against sociologically developed characteristics or standards of a profession. Not everyone agrees that nursing meets those standards.
- The standards of a profession typically include seven requirements: (1) possess a well-defined and well-organized body of knowledge, (2) enlarge a systematic body of knowledge and improve education, (3) educate its practitioners in institutions of higher

learning, (4) function autonomously in the formulation of policy, (5) develop a code of ethics, (6) attract professionals who will be committed to the profession for a lifetime, and (7) compensate practitioners by providing autonomy, continuous professional development, and economic security.

- Nursing also has struggled with the terms "profession" and "professional." At times, the characteristics of the professional become confused with the formal concept of a profession.
- Nursing as a profession has many traditions, some of which are challenged today. Among the traditions are the pin, the cap, the uniform, and nursing ceremonies.
- Nursing has struggled with its image. Various groups have waged campaigns to improve the image of nursing and thus make it a more attractive profession. A number of groups have launched campaigns to address this issue. The image of nursing today is viewed as a critical issue because of the nurse shortage. A positive image is needed to attract qualified individuals into the profession.
- Since the beginning of the 20th century, nursing has been a much-studied profession. Early studies dealt with nursing education; later studies dealt with the image of nursing, nurses themselves, and with nursing's role in health care delivery.
- As nursing has developed as a profession, more attention has been directed to establishing a unique classification and nomenclature for nursing. Efforts are being made to do this on an international basis.

Relevant Web Sites

American Association for the History of Medicine: *www.histmed.org*
American Association for the History of Nursing: *www.aahn.org/resource.html*
American Association of Colleges of Nursing (AACN): *www.aacn.nche.edu*
American Nurses Association Centennial Exhibit: Voices from the Past, Visions of the
    Future: *www.ana.org/centenn/index.htm*
American Nurses Association Hall of Fame: *www.ana.org/hof/index.htm*
American Organization of Nurse Executives: *www.aone.org*
Archives of Nursing Leadership:
    www.lib.uconn.edu/online/research/specialib/ASC/dodda2z/Subjectarea.cfm?Area=12
Black Nurses in History: *www4.umdnj.edu/camlbweb/blacknurses.html*
Boston University Nursing Archives: *www.bu.edu/archives/holdings/historical/nursing.html*
British Columbia History of Nursing Group: *www.bcnursinghistory.ca*
Bureau of Labor Statistics: *www.bls.gov*
Canadian Association for the History of Nursing: *www.cahn-achn.ca*
Center for Nursing Historical Inquiry: *www.nursing.virginia.edu/centers/cnhi/index.html*
Center for the Study of the History of Nursing: *www.nursing.upenn.edu/history*
Clendening History of Medicine Library—Florence Nightingale Resources:
    http://clendening.kumc.edu/dc/fn
Florence Nightingale, references regarding: *www.nightingales.com*,
    www.florence-nightingale-avenging-angel.co.uk
Florence Nightingale Museum Web site: *www.florence-nightingale.co.uk;*
    www.countryjoe.com/nightingale

International Council of Nurses: *www.icn.ch*

Johnson & Johnson Nursing Campaign: *www.discovernursing.com*

Margaret M. Allemang Center for the History of Nursing: *www.allemang.on.ca/ index.html*

Men in American Nursing History: *www.geocities.com/Athens/Forum/6011*

National Information Center for Health Services Administration: *www.nichsa.org*

National League for Nursing: *www.nln.org*

Nurses for a Healthier Tomorrow: *www.nursesource.org*

Nursing Classifications: *www.nursingworld.org* (type "Nursing Classifications" into the search box)

Center for Nursing Classification and Clinical Effectiveness: Information about NIC and NOC: *http://nursing.uiowa.edu/centers/cncce*

North American Nursing Diagnosis Association-International (NANDA-I): *www.nanda.org/html/about.html*

National Information and Data Set Evaluation Center (NIDSEC): *http://nursingworld.org/nidsec/index.htm*

Omaha System: *www.omahasystem.org/index.htm*

Nursing Shortage:

National Council of State Boards of Nursing, Inc. (2005). State updates on nursing shortage issues and activities, [On-line]. *www.ncsbn.org/news/stateupdates_state_shortage.asp*

Nursing Theory Page: *www.ualberta.ca/~jrnorris/nt/theory.html*

The Forum on Health Care Leadership: *www.healthcareforum.org*

References

ABC Coding Solutions: Alternative Link. (2006). *About us* [On-line]. *www.alternativelink.com/ali/about_us*. Accessed April 5, 2006.

Abdellah, F. G. (1960). *Patient-centered approaches to nursing*. New York: Macmillan.

American Nurses Association. (1980). *Nursing: A social policy statement*. Kansas City, MO: American Journal of Nursing Co.

American Nurses Association. (2003). *Nursing's social policy statement* (2nd ed.). Silver Spring, MD: Nursebooks.org

Association of Perioperative Registered Nurses. (2002). *Perioperative nursing data set* (2nd ed.) [On-line]. *http://aorn.org/research/pnds.htm*. Accessed September 28, 2005.

Benner, P. (1984). *From novice to expert*. Menlo Park, CA: Addison-Wesley.

Benner, P., & Wrubel, J. (1989). *The primacy of caring*. Menlo Park, CA: Addison-Wesley.

Bevis, E. O., & Watson, J. (1989). *Toward a caring curriculum: A new pedagogy for nursing*. New York: National League for Nursing.

Bixler, G. K., & Bixler, R. W. (1945). The professional status of nursing. *American Journal of Nursing, 45*(9), 730.

Brief Synopsis of the Nursing Minimum Data Set. (2003) [On-line]. *www.nursing.uiowa.edu/NI/collabs_files/Synopsis%20 NMDS%20Nov%202003.pdf*. Accessed September 28, 2005.

Carper, B. A. (1979). The ethics of caring. *Advances in Nursing Science, 3*: 11-19.

Center for Nursing Advocacy. (2003). Procter & Gamble pulls Clairol shampoo commercial and apologizes to nurses [On-line]. *www.nursingadvocacy.org/news/ 2003jun11_clairol.html*. Accessed April 10, 2006.

Centers for Medicare & Medicaid Services. (2005). *SNF Prospective payment system, MDS requirements* [On-line]. *www.cms.hhs.gov/providers/snfpps/snfpps_mds.asp*. Accessed September 28, 2005.

Chitty, K. K. (1997). *Professional nursing concepts and challenges* (2nd ed.). Philadelphia: W. B. Saunders.

Clark, J. (1998). The international classification for nursing practice project. *Online Journal of Issues in Nursing* [On-line]. *http://nursingworld.org/ojin/tpc7tpc7_3.htm*. Accessed October 31, 1999.

Coenen, A. (2003). The international classification for nursing practice (ICNP) programme: Advancing a unifying framework for nursing. *Online Journal of Issues in Nursing* [On-line]. *http://nursingworld.org/ojin/tpc7/tpc7_8.htm.*   Accessed March 29, 2006.

Deaconess Hospital School of Nursing. (1980). *Eighty-one years of nursing: 1899-1980.* Spokane, WA: Deaconess Hospital.

Dochterman, J., & Bulechek G. (Eds.). (2004). *Nursing interventions classification* (4th ed.). St. Louis, MO: Mosby.

Donahue, M. P. (1996). *Nursing: The finest art* (2nd ed.). St. Louis, MO: CV Mosby.

Eliopoulos, C. (1997). *Gerontological nursing* (4th ed.). Philadelphia: Lippincott-Raven.

Geolot, D. (2000). *Resources and funding.* Paper presented at the Nurse Staffing summit (May, 2000) of the American Nurses Association, Washington, DC.

Glanton, D. (2005). White garb returning to hospitals. *Nursing opportunities: Northwest edition, 4,* 1, 6

Hampton-Robb, I. (1909). *Report of the third regular meeting of the International Council of Nurses.* Geneva: ICN.

Henderson, V. (1966). *The nature of a science of nursing.* New York: Macmillan.

International Council of Nurses, (2005). International classification for nursing practice. Version 1 [On-line]. *www.icn.ch/icnp_v1.htm.* Accessed April 10, 2006.

Jamieson, E. M., & Sewall, M. (1944). *Trends in nursing history* (2nd ed.). Philadelphia: W. B. Saunders Co.

Johnson, D. (1980). The behavioral system model for nursing. In J. P. Riehl & C. Roy, *Conceptual models for nursing practice* (2nd ed., pp. 207–216). East Norwalk, CT: Appleton-Century-Crofts.

Kalisch, P. A., & Kalisch, B. J. (2004). *The advance of American nursing* (4th ed.) Philadelphia: Lippincott Williams & Wilkins.

King, I. M. (1981). *A theory for nursing: Systems, concepts, process.* New York: John Wiley & Sons.

Klein, J. A. (1997). Honoring female military nurses. *BRAVO Veterans Outlook,* August-September [On-line]. *www.nursingnetwork.com/veterans.htm.* Accessed January 14, 2000.

Kolcaba, K. Y. (1992). Holistic comfort: Operationalizing the construct as a nurse-sensitive outcome. *Advances in Nursing Science, 1,* 1-10.

Labor Management Relations Act (1947) as amended by Public Laws 86-257 (1959) and 93-360 (1974), Section 2 [On-line]. *www.nlrb.gov/publications/nlrb4.pdf.* Accessed September 28, 2005.

LeMaire, B. (2002). Jean Watson, on her theory of caring. *Nurse Week (Mountain West Edition),* 3(40):7.

Levine, M. E. (1969). *Introduction to clinical nursing.* Philadelphia: F. A. Davis.

Mangum, S. (1994). Uniforms and caps: Do we need them? In O. L. Strickland & D. J. Fishman, *Nursing issues in the 1990s* (pp. 46-66). Albany, NY: Delmar Publishers.

Martin, K.S. (2005). *The Omaha System: A key to practice, documentation, and information management* (2nd. ed.). St. Louis, MO: Elsevier.

Meade, J. (2002). *Health care's human crisis: The American nursing shortage* [On-line]. *www.rwjf.org/newsEvents/nursing.jhtml.* Accessed May 21, 2002.

Moorhead, S., Johnson, M., & Maas M. (Eds.). (2004). *Nursing outcomes classification* (3rd ed.). St. Louis, MO: Mosby.

National Council of State Boards of Nursing, Inc. (2004). *Model Nursing Act and rules* [On-line]. *www.ncsbn.org/regulation/nursingpractice_nursing_practice_model_act_and_rules.asp.* Accessed October 1, 2005.

National Council of State Boards of Nursing, Inc. (2005). *State updates on nursing shortage issues and activities* [On-line]. *www.ncsbn.org/news/stateupdates_state_shortage.asp.* Accessed September 28, 2004.

National Information and Data Set Evaluation Center. (2005). *NIDSEC 3-year recognition* [On-line]. *http://nursingworld.org/nidsec/index.htm.* Accessed September 28, 2005.

Neuman, B. (1982). *The Neuman System model: Application to nursing education and practice.* East Norwalk, CT: Appleton-Century-Crofts.

Nightingale, F. (1954). *Notes on nursing: What it is, and what it is not.* [An unabridged republication of the first American edition, as published by D. Appleton and Company in 1860]. New York: Dover Publications.

Norman, E. M. (1999). *We band of angels.* New York: Random House.

North American Nursing Diagnosis Association-International. (2005). *2005-2006. Nursing diagnoses: Definitions and classification.* Philadelphia: Author.

Nursing Information and Data Set Evaluation Center. (2005). *Standards* [On-line]. *http://nursingworld.org/nidsec.* Accessed September 28, 2005.

O'Neil, E. H. (1993). *Health professions education for the future: Schools in service to the nation.* San Francisco: Pew Health Professions Commission.

Orem, D. (1980). *Nursing: Concepts of practice* (2nd ed.). New York: McGraw-Hill.

Orlando, I. J. (1972). *The discipline and teaching of nursing process.* New York: G. P. Putnam's Sons.

Parse, R. R. (1981). *Man-living-health: A theory of nursing.* New York: Wiley.

Patient Care Data Set. (1998) [On-line]. *www.ncvhs.hhs.gov/990518t3.pdf.* Accessed September 28, 2005.

Peplau, H. E. (1952). *Interpersonal relations in nursing.* New York: G. P. Putnam's Sons.

Public Health Service [PHS]. (n.d.). The Cadet Nurse Corps, 1943–48. [On-line]. *http://lhncbc.nlm.nih.gov/apdb/phshistory/resources/cadetnurse/nurse.html.* Accessed May 19, 2007.

Robert Wood Johnson Foundation. (2002). *The American nursing shortage: Strategies and recommendations for action* [On-line]. *www.rwjf.org/news Events/nursingStrategies.jhtml.* Accessed May 21, 2002.

Rogers, M. E. (May 1984). *Science of unitary human beings: A paradigm for nursing.* Paper presented before the International Nurse Theorist Conference, Edmonton, Alberta.

Roy, C. (1984). *Introduction to nursing: An adaptation model* (2nd ed.). Englewood Cliffs, NJ: Prentice-Hall.

Saba, V. (2003). *Clinical care classification (CCC) system: Background* [On-line]. *www.sabacare.com/background.html.* Accessed April 5, 2006.

Scarlett, E. P. (1991). In M. M. Styles & P. Moccia, *On nursing: A literary celebration* (pp. 6-7). New York: National League for Nursing, Publication No. 14-2513.

SNOMED. (2005). SNOMED International [On-line]. *www.snomed.org/index.html.* Accessed September 28, 2005.

The Omaha System. (2005). Overview [On-line]. *http://omahasystem.org/index.htm.* Accessed April 5, 2006.

The National Archives. (2004). British army: Nurses and nursing services: Military records information 55 [On-line]. *www.catalogue.nationalarchives.gov.uk/RdLeaflet.asp?sLeafletID=169&j=1* Accessed September 28, 2005.

Ulrich, B. (2005). Celebrating nursing's premier trailblazer. *Nurse Week: Mountain West Edition, 6*(9), 3.

U. S. Department of Health and Human Services. (2006). Preliminary findings: 2004 National Sample Survey of Registered Nurses [On-line]. *http://bhpr.hrsa.gov/healthworkforce/reports/rnpopulation/preliminaryfindings.htm.* Accessed March 8, 2006.

Watson, J. (1979). *Nursing the philosophy and science of caring.* Boston: Little, Brown.

Whitman, A. (1985). *American reformers.* New York: H.W. Wilson Co.

Wiedenbach, E. (1964). *Clinical nursing: A helping art.* New York: Springer Publishing Co.

5

Educational Preparation for Nursing

LEARNING OUTCOMES

After completing this chapter, you should be able to:

1. Compare the educational preparation of the nursing assistant, the licensed practical (vocational) nurse, and the graduates of the various types of programs preparing registered nurses (RNs); hospital-based programs; associate degree programs; generic baccalaureate programs; and graduate degree entry programs.

2. Explain the purposes of other forms of nursing education, including external degree programs, RN baccalaureate programs, master's preparation, doctoral studies, non-degree programs, and articulated programs.

3. Discuss some of the innovative approaches to earning a higher degree in nursing.

4. Identify factors that have prompted changes in nursing education, including studies and sociopolitical events, and analyze the effect of each.

5. Analyze the effects the American Nurses Association (ANA) *Position Paper on Nursing Education* would have had on nursing licensure if adopted nationwide.

6. Critique the major points supporting both mandatory and voluntary continuing education, and explain the mechanisms for documenting and recording continuing education.

7. Discuss the concept of differentiated practice and provide a rationale for its development.

8. Discuss the impact of technology on nursing education.

9. Identify factors that have influenced changes in nursing education and analyze the effect of each.

10. Analyze the ways in which nursing theories serve to advance the profession.

KEY TERMS

Accreditation
Advanced nursing practice
Articulation
Associate degree education
Baccalaureate degree education

Career ladder
Community-based practice
Competencies
Continuing education unit (CEU)

Differentiated nursing practice
Diploma programs
Educational mobility
Entry into practice

Evidence-based practice	Mandatory continuing	Scope of practice
External degree	education	Second-degree students
Generic program	Nursing assistants	Theorist/theory
Grandfather clause	Position paper	Titling
Home health aide	Postsecondary education	Unlicensed Assistive Personnel
Hospital-based programs	Practical (vocational) nurse	(UAP)
Internships and residencies	Registered nurse baccalaureate	Virtual university
Interstate endorsement	program	Voluntary continuing education

Most professions provide a single route for the educational preparation of its practitioners. However, the development of nursing as a profession has resulted in three major types of educational programs and additional less common ones that prepare graduates to write the National Council Licensure Examination (NCLEX) for registered nursing. These circumstances have resulted in alternatives and opportunities for prospective students. The benefits of these options for students and the public resulted in the Pew Commission identifying in its 1995 report the multiple-entry points to professional nursing practice as one of nursing's strengths (Pew Health Professions Commission, 1995).

Despite this acknowledged strength, the existence of multiple-entry points has resulted in confusion for both consumers and employers. Health care consumers often find it difficult to understand the various nursing credentials—and probably have little interest in credentials as long as they receive satisfactory care. Employers have difficulty differentiating among the three major types of RN graduates who, at least initially, enter the work environment performing similar activities. This confusion led to another recommendation from the Pew Commission: that nursing distinguish between the practice responsibilities of the graduates educated in each of the different educational environments (Pew Health Professions Commission, 1995). This task has proven difficult at best.

An educator charged with the responsibility of graduating a "safe" practitioner may not have a clear understanding of how the various educational routes to professional preparation differ in purpose, structure, and outcome. Nursing leaders often vigorously debate aspects of the educational preparation of nurses, such as where it should take place, what content should be included in which programs and to what depth, which tests should measure the various competencies, and which credentials should be awarded.

The three traditional educational avenues that prepare men and women for registered nursing are hospital-based diploma programs, 2-year associate degree programs (primarily found at junior and community colleges), and baccalaureate programs (offered at 4-year colleges and universities). It is also possible for students to begin their nursing education in programs that culminate in a master's degree, and several programs now exist in which a student can earn a doctorate before being eligible to write the state licensing examination for registered nursing.

At least two other groups of caregivers are identified with nursing: the nursing assistant, who may be certified, and the practical (vocational) nurse, who is licensed through a separate and different examination from that taken by the RN.

THE NURSING ASSISTANT

For years, individuals called nursing aides or assistants have provided care to patients in hospitals and long-term care facilities. In the past, these caregivers were hired without formal preparation for their responsibilities and were provided on-the-job training. The use of the nursing aides likely started during World War I, and certainly was reinforced during World War II, when approximately 150,000 trained volunteer nursing aides served in wartime hospitals. Nursing aides or assistants have always provided the majority of care in nursing homes. Nursing assistants are within a group that is often referred to as **unlicensed assistive personnel (UAP)**.

In 1987, Congress passed the Omnibus Budget Reconciliation Act, which regulates agencies receiving federal funds and includes an amendment regulating the education and certification of **nursing assistants** who work in nursing homes. The amendment stipulated that by October 1, 1990, all people working as nursing assistants in nursing homes (hospitals and assisted-living units were not included) would be required to complete a minimum of 75 hours of theory and practice and pass both a theory and practice examination to be certified. Certification falls under state jurisdiction, but is guided by federal regulations. In many states, the hours of preparation required exceed the 75 hours established by federal law. Following the federal legislation, the National Council of State Boards of Nursing Inc. developed the Nurse Aide Competency Evaluation Program, which identifies the minimum skills a nursing assistant must attain and can be used to guide programs registering or certifying nursing assistants. The state agency responsible for certifying and maintaining the list of nursing assistants varies from state to state; most commonly, it is the board of nursing or the state department of health services.

The certified nursing assistant (CNA), also referred to as the nursing assistant, certified, functions under the direction of the RN or the licensed practical (vocational) nurse (LPN). Each state determines the skills that may be performed by the nursing assistant. Typically, these include basic nursing skills, such as changing bed linens; measuring temperature, pulse, respirations, and blood pressure; bathing patients and helping with personal care; helping patients with eating, walking, and exercise programs; and supporting patients when they are allowed to get out of bed. The preparation of the CNA emphasizes the importance of a safe environment and includes instruction in patients' rights and the use of side rails and restraints. A number of states also require a designated number of hours per year of continuing education.

There are no national regulations governing the educational preparation and scope of practice of nursing assistants in areas other than long-term care, although some states have legislation to regulate the practice of those in other settings. Typically, training occurs under the sponsorship of the employing facility and without formal certification; student backgrounds may vary from less than a high school diploma to advanced degrees. For example, some physicians licensed in foreign countries but who cannot secure licensure in the United States may work as UAPs in health care settings. A number of states have a category of UAP, known as unlicensed medication administration personnel. Many of these workers are employed within the primary school system and routinely dispense medications to students; in other instances these individuals are employed in assisted living and similar facilities.

The criteria for hospital accreditation established by The Joint Commission (formerly the Joint Commission on Accreditation of Healthcare Organizations) now require that hospitals ensure the competence of all employees, including nursing assistants. This has led many hospitals to the practice of hiring only those who were certified as nursing assistants in long-term care facilities and to the development of courses to prepare individuals as nursing assistants for acute care settings. States vary in their requirements for hospital nursing assistants. Many states expect the hospital to determine what their requirements will be and to then provide their own training.

The **home health aide** is prepared to assist individuals with basic care in their home; thus a program of instruction includes content related to shopping for groceries, cooking, and doing laundry. Some long-term care nursing assistant programs offer an additional period of training and education for roles as home health aides to those who have completed their nursing assistant program. Other states have a shorter program without a certification examination for home health aides. In some states, there is no standardized certification requirement for those who work in homes.

Training for the various types of nursing assistant occurs in many settings, including high schools, long-term care facilities, hospitals, community colleges, regional occupational programs, and privately operated programs. Some consider this preparation the first rung on the ladder of nursing education, and, in some states, the nursing assistant may be exempt from certain classes required in LPN programs. Some registered nursing programs establish certification as a nursing assistant as an admission requirement.

The employment of UAPs has been of concern to nursing. Some state boards have issued a list of tasks that may be performed by UAPs, and both the ANA and the National Council of State Boards of Nursing have issued definitions and guidelines for the use of UAPs. More discussion of UAPs in health care occurs in Chapter 13.

PRACTICAL NURSE EDUCATION

The **practical nurse** (titled **vocational nurse** in Texas and California) is no newcomer to the health care delivery system. In the past, the practical nurse was the family friend or community citizen who was called to the home in emergencies. This person, usually self-taught, learned by experience which procedures were effective and which were not. The practical nurse would perform basic care procedures, such as bathing, and also would cook and perform light housekeeping duties for the family, much like the home health aide does today. Although controls on the licensing of practical nurses and the accreditation of their curricula were slower to evolve than those regulating professional nursing, states gradually enacted licensure laws governing practical nursing. By 1945, 19 states and one territory had licensure laws, but licensure of the practical nurse was mandatory in only one state (Kalisch & Kalisch, 2004). When more states began adopting mandatory licensure laws for practical nurses, many individuals who had been functioning in this capacity were granted a license by waiver and excused from any formal training (see Chapter 7 on credentialing). Most, if not all, of these people are now retired from nursing practice. By 1955, all states had licensure laws for practical nurses.

It is not clear when formal preparation for practical nursing began. Some suggest training programs were started in 1897 (Kalisch & Kalisch, 2004). A more popular belief is that the first programs were initiated through the YWCA in Brooklyn, New York, around 1892. The school established through the YWCA was known as the Ballard School, after Lucinda Ballard, who provided the funding to operate it. The course of study lasted approximately 3 months, and the students, called "attendants," were trained to care for invalids, the elderly, and children in a home setting. By 1930, there were only 11 schools of practical nursing, but between 1948 and 1954, 260 more were opened.

Display 5-1   History of the Development of Practical Nursing

1892   YWCA in Brooklyn, New York, establishes a program in practical nursing named after Lucinda Ballard, who provided the funding for it.

1907   Thompson School is founded in Brattleboro, Vermont.

1908   The American Red Cross founds a practical nursing program.

1918   The Household Nursing Association School of Attendant Nursing begins in Boston.

1938   New York becomes the first state to require licensure for the practical nurse.

1941   The Association of Practical Nurse Schools (APNS) is founded.

1942   Membership in the APNS is opened to practical nurses and the name changed to the National Association of Practical Nurse Education and Service (NAPNES). The first planned curriculum for practical nursing is developed.

1945   NAPNES establishes and accredits service for schools of practical nursing; this program was discontinued in 1984.

1949   The National Federation of Licensed Practical Nurses (NFLPN) is organized.

1957   Working with the American Nurses Association, NFLPN seeks to clarify the role and function of the practical nurse. The National League for Nursing (NLN) establishes the Council on Practical Nursing.

1966   The Chicago Public School Program becomes the first practical nurse program to be accredited by the NLN.

1979   The NLN publishes a list of competencies of graduates of practical/vocational nursing programs.

1996   The National Council of State Boards of Nursing (NCSBN), working with NAPNES, offers a certification examination for licensed practical nurses in long-term care.

A YWCA may seem to many of us to be a strange place for a practical nursing program. But YWCAs were an important source of inexpensive housing for many young women who, in the late 1890s and early 1900s, traveled from their homes to large cities in search of new careers and better lives. Because most of these women were untrained and had no marketable skills, the YWCA was a natural site for a school. Display 5-1 outlines some of the significant history in the development of practical nursing.

The general curriculum for practical nurses, which typically takes 1 year to complete, varies considerably from state to state and even from school to school. In many instances, the education is measured in clock hours instead of credit hours. Most of today's practical nursing education programs stress clinical experience, primarily in structured care settings such as hospitals and long-term care facilities. Basic therapeutic knowledge and introductory content from biologic and behavioral sciences correlate with clinical practice; usually one third of the time is spent in the classroom and two thirds in clinical practice.

The educational preparation of the practical nurse takes place in a variety of settings. High schools, trade or technical schools, hospitals, junior or community colleges, universities, or independent agencies may offer programs. If the rules and regulations of the state board(s) of nursing allow it, practical nursing and associate nursing degree programs can be incorporated in the community college as part of a **career ladder** approach to nursing education. These programs sometimes are referred to as one-on-one programs: 1 year of preparation for practical nursing, followed by 1 more year qualifying the graduate to take the licensure examination for registered nursing. All nursing students in these colleges are grouped together for core courses during the first academic year. At the end of this time, a student has the option of stopping the educational program to seek licensure as a practical nurse, or continuing for an additional year to become an RN. Many students opt to do both. Graduates of these core programs in practical nursing usually have a broader and more in-depth understanding of the biologic sciences, and sometimes the social sciences (often also a part of the core curriculum), especially if these are college-level courses that are transferable to a 4-year institution. Because issues related to educational mobility and articulation between programs have received much attention (discussed later in this chapter), these combined programs have become popular.

Graduates of practical nursing programs take the NCLEX-PN; if they pass the exam, they use the title "licensed practical nurse" (LPN) or, in California and Texas, the title "licensed vocational nurse" (LVN). Their scope of practice focuses on meeting the health care needs of clients in hospitals, long-term care facilities, clinics, and the home. Typically, LPNs or LVNs care for clients whose conditions are considered stable, giving direct patient care; observing, recording, and reporting; administering treatments and medications; and assisting in rehabilitation procedures. They receive direction from an RN or a licensed physician.

As with the associate degree and hospital-based diploma programs for RNs, the educational preparation for practical nurses and the future of practical nursing are topics of much discussion. Some advocate two levels of nurses: the practical nurse prepared with an associate degree and the RN prepared with a baccalaureate degree. Others would eliminate practical nursing altogether. In 1987, North Dakota became the first state (and to date the only state) to require all candidates taking the licensure examination for practical nursing to have completed an associate degree in practical nursing. In 2003, this requirement was rescinded and the state moved back to requiring 1 year for practical nurse licensure and an associate degree for RN licensure.

The nursing shortage has had a major impact on the practice of practical nurses. In many nursing homes, positions that would have been filled with RNs are being filled with LPNs. The effects of this are not all clear, but in many instances LPNs are being asked to practice beyond the scope for which they were originally prepared. With the "graying" of America, and the growing need for nurses in home health care and in long-term care facilities, practical nurses will continue to play a significant role in health care delivery.

TRADITIONAL PROGRAMS THAT PREPARE GRADUATES FOR RN LICENSURE

A number of different avenues of education now prepare individuals for licensure as RNs. The most traditional of these are diploma programs, associate degree programs, and baccalaureate programs. Innovative programs that offer generic masters and doctoral educational routes in nursing are also available.

Diploma Education

The earliest type of nursing education in the United States took place in **diploma programs** administered by hospitals, also referred to as **hospital-based programs**. The first hospital with a nurse training school was the New England Hospital for Women, which accepted five probationers on September 1, 1872 (Kalisch & Kalisch, 2004). The characteristics of these early schools were discussed in detail in Chapter 4.

By the late 1940s and early 1950s, many hospital-based nursing schools had affiliated with nearby colleges and universities; these schools adopted general education requirements, such as anatomy, physiology, sociology, and psychology, as part of the curriculum. During this time, the National League of Nursing Education—later to become two organizations, the National League for Nursing (NLN) and the National League for Nursing Accrediting Commission (NLNAC)—assumed an active role in curriculum guidance and accreditation. Nursing programs gained a stronger educational foundation because they were required to align themselves more closely with other types of **postsecondary education**, that is, education occurring after the completion of high school.

Thus, diploma schools in operation today have sound educational programs that meet the criteria necessary for accreditation. They employ qualified faculty who have developed clinical learning experiences that meet the student's learning needs rather than the hospital's service needs (which often took priority in the past). These programs vary in length from 27 to 36 months. Many diploma schools are affiliated with a college or university so that postsecondary credit can be awarded formally. Graduates are provided with a foundation in the biologic and social sciences, and may have taken some courses in the humanities. There is a strong emphasis in diploma programs on client experiences. The course of study also includes experience in nursing management (for example, being in charge of a nursing unit). Graduates work in acute, long-term, and ambulatory health care facilities, fulfilling the responsibilities established by the scope of practice for RNs as defined by the state in which they are licensed.

During the mid-1960s, there was a significant decline in enrollment in diploma schools, a trend that has continued, so that today diploma programs comprise less than 10 percent of all basic RN education programs (American Association of Colleges of Nursing [AACN], 2004a). As more nursing education programs were moved to institutions of higher education, many hospital-based schools elected to discontinue their programs. Some merged with a local community college or university that assumed administrative responsibility for managing the nursing program and awarded an associate or baccalaureate degree when graduation requirements were satisfied. The elimination of hospital-based programs has occurred most extensively in the western part of the United States, because eastern programs more commonly had strong endowment support.

Finances also played a role in this change. With increasing constraints on funding, many hospitals found that the costs associated with supporting a nursing program were too great. Many diploma programs existing today have strong endowments and private funding support.

Associate Degree Education

The movement toward **associate degree education** began in 1952. Today, associate degree nursing programs prepare more graduates for licensure as RNs than do any of the other programs (Health Resources and Service Administration, Bureau of Health Professions, 2002). Associate degree in nursing (ADN) programs have the distinction of being the first (and, to date, the only) type of nursing education established on the basis of planned research and experimentation.

Four events undoubtedly influenced their beginning. First, these programs followed in the wake of the organization and growth of 2-year community colleges in the United States.

Community colleges were organized specifically to offer the first 2 years of a traditional 4-year college program and bring many vocational and adult education programs to the community. The goal of the community college was to make some form of college education available to everyone. Second, the cadet nurse program, which was created during World War II (see Chapter 4), demonstrated that qualified students could be educated adequately in less than the traditional 3 years of the diploma program. Third, the development of associate degree education was influenced by the studies conducted on nursing education in the United States, as discussed in Chapter 4. The final factor influencing the development of associate degree education was the critical national nursing shortage of the 1950s, which occurred because nurses employed during World War II returned home to raise families. It was anticipated that the 2-year program would put graduates into the work market more quickly, thus helping reduce the shortage of nurses while, at the same time, helping to move nursing education into the overall system of higher education in America.

Associate degree programs have helped to solve the nursing shortages of the 1960s, 1980s, and now. These programs, which focused on preparing graduates skilled in bedside nursing, rapidly increased in number. Associate degree programs particularly appealed to men, minorities, and older students, who had not traditionally pursued educational preparation in nursing. Because most programs were located in community colleges, they tended to be more geographically accessible than the baccalaureate programs in 4-year colleges and universities, typically located in major urban areas.

Characteristics of Associate Degree Education

Associate degree education began with the Cooperative Research Project in Junior and Community College Education for Nursing at Teachers College, Columbia University. The original 5-year research project, which was directed by Mildred Montag, included seven junior and community colleges and one hospital school, located in six regions of the United States. This type of nursing education has expanded from these original programs in 1952 to more than 880 (National Organization for Associate Degree Nursing, 2004).

Accrediting groups ensure that ADN programs are an integral part of the college in which they are housed, that faculty and students have the same rights and privileges as their counterparts, and that the curriculum is sound.

In a typical program, approximately 40% of the credits needed for the associate degree must be fulfilled by general education courses such as English, anatomy, physiology, speech, psychology, and sociology; the rest are to be fulfilled by nursing courses. Clinical learning experiences are carefully selected to correspond with the content delivered in classroom lectures; the pre- and post-conferences help to reinforce the relationship between the two. Some modifications in this structure are occurring, as associate degree educators strive to meet the expectations of employers and the community while remaining true to the concept of associate degree education.

The advent of associate degree education in nursing has brought greater diversity in the students who enroll in nursing programs (Fig. 5-1). Traditionally, nursing students were a homogeneous group—typically single white women, ranging in age from 18 to 35, who graduated in the upper third of their high school classes. Associate degree programs (although they often impose selective admission policies on the "open door" philosophy of the community colleges) attract older people, married women, minorities, men, and students with a wider range of educational

FIGURE 5-1 Associate degree programs attract older people, married women, minorities, men, and students with a wider range of educational experiences and intellectual capabilities.

experiences and intellectual abilities. People who already possess baccalaureate or higher degrees in other fields sometimes seek admission to an associate degree program, often because it can be completed in a shorter period of time than would be needed to earn another baccalaureate degree.

Challenges to Associate Degree Education

Associate degree education, like other educational programs, has experienced change. With these changes have come some challenges.

Pressure to Increase Credits. As programs have developed, there has been a growing tendency to increase the number of nursing credits. Faculty members, who may be struggling to define essential content, often try to comply with requests from advisory committees for graduates who will need shorter orientation programs and possess greater knowledge in certain specialty areas (eg, coronary care). The push to recognize all nurses as managers has led to the addition of management content in most programs. Changes that some colleges have made in the basic requirements for all associate degrees have increased the number of non-nursing credits nursing students must complete; the concept of "core courses" that are taken by all students who graduate from a college has become popular.

The recent shift to **community-based practice** also offers a challenge to associate degree educators. What part of the current curriculum should be cut to provide community experiences? How are community experiences to be supervised? What should be the balance between inpatient care and community experiences? Faculty members who have spent the greater part of their clinical nursing careers in acute care settings are often reluctant to divert even an hour from the time students spend on acute care hospital units.

The Selective Admission Process. Another concern with which educators struggle is the process used in selecting students for a nursing program. This challenge becomes greater when the number of students seeking admission either increases dramatically or drops significantly, a phenomenon many programs have experienced during the past 15 to 20 years. As the demographics of students seeking admission become more diverse, the task of bringing to the program students who can realize success in their endeavors represents additional challenges to nursing faculty. In response to this problem, some programs have developed selective admission processes. Although this is common in 4-year schools and colleges, it is a departure from the open-door policy of most community colleges. Some nursing programs use a waiting list, which honors the concept of first come, first served. Other schools use systems similar to a lottery. Also popular are factoring or point systems that award numeric scores for courses completed, past work experience, cumulative grade-point average, or a combination of all of these, with the students acquiring the greatest number of points being selected for the next class. These factoring systems often require that a student spend at least a year in college to secure a position in the beginning nursing class.

Time Required to Complete the Program. More content and a greater number of credit hours, selective admission criteria (that give preference to students who have completed general education course work), long waiting lists for entry, and students who cannot attend school on a full-time basis are all factors that have contributed to programs that can take as many as 3 to 5 years to complete, rather than the 2 years originally planned.

According to the interpretive guidelines for NLNAC accreditation, the maximum number of credits for an associate degree in nursing is 108 quarter hours or 72 semester hours (NLNAC, 2004). Many schools struggle to meet this criterion.

Misunderstandings About Associate Degree Education

For many years, associate degree education was poorly understood by employers, the public, and, to some extent, nursing educators in baccalaureate and higher degree programs. Although this route to nursing education is now firmly established as credible preparation for a nursing career, it continues to receive some opposition. The controversy regarding "entry into practice" and the preparation needed for "professional" nursing (which will be discussed later in this chapter) is renewed from time to time. Thus, faculty, graduates, and advocates for associate degree education continue to find themselves clarifying facts such as the actual number of nursing credits and the focus on critical thinking and decision-making, not simply technical skills, and emphasizing the contributions made by graduates of the programs.

Baccalaureate Education

Baccalaureate degree education is that which occurs in a 4-year college or university. The first school of nursing to be established in a university setting was started at the University of Minnesota in 1909 as a quasi-autonomous branch of the university's school of medicine. The program was not very different from the 3-year hospital-based program; nothing was required in the way of higher general education, and graduates were prepared for the RN certificate only.

Education took place predominantly through apprenticeship, and students provided service to hospitals in exchange for education. However, nursing education did become a part of an academic organization, with 16 colleges and universities developing programs by 1916.

Many of the early programs offering a baccalaureate degree in nursing extended over a 5-year period. This allowed for 3 years of nursing school curriculum similar to that of the hospital-based programs, and for an additional 2 years of liberal arts. While the increase in the number of schools was not rapid, in 1924, the Yale School of Nursing became the first to be established as a separate department within a university; Annie W. Goodrich was its dean.

Although the development of baccalaureate education for nurses may not seem like a major step to young people today, remember that it was not until 1920 that the 19th Amendment to the Constitution of the United States granted women the right to vote. Many people considered nursing to be a less than desirable occupation: vocational in its orientation; overshadowed by militaristic, religious, and technical characteristics; and confined to women. Liberal education, scholarship, and knowledge were thought to be incompatible with the female personality and capable of interfering with marriage—for many years, nursing students generally were not allowed to marry (Kalisch & Kalisch, 2004). The nursing curriculum, with its emphasis on the performance of skills rather than on the philosophic and theoretic approaches used in the humanities, was not well accepted by universities. Opposition to collegiate education for nurses also came from physicians, who argued that nurses would be over-trained. Physicians were not certain that a sound knowledge base was as important as the technical skills and manual dexterity that could be acquired with brief training at the bedside. Physicians also argued that a baccalaureate education would make nursing services too expensive.

Many nursing leaders advocated for baccalaureate education as the minimum educational preparation for supervisory and administrative nursing roles. Baccalaureate education also provides the background needed for addressing the community as client and incorporating research into practice, and the educational base for entry into graduate education in nursing. In 1965, the ANA recommended baccalaureate preparation in nursing as the minimum educational preparation for entry into professional nursing practice, an issue discussed later in this chapter. The American Nurses' Credentialing Center (ANCC) now requires a baccalaureate degree for what they title "board certification" in a nursing specialty, while the title "certification" is available to associate degree graduates in most of the specialty areas. The ANCC requires a master's degree for initial certification as a clinical specialist or nurse practitioner. Those certified before these new requirements took effect are permitted to maintain their certification. Each specialty organization establishes its own criteria for specialty certification. Some require a baccalaureate degree and some do not. Most advanced practice nursing certifications require the master's degree.

Characteristics of Baccalaureate Education

Baccalaureate nursing programs are located in 4-year colleges and universities. A university nursing program is termed a basic or **generic program** when the program of studies includes an upper division (junior and senior years) nursing major that is built onto 2 years of liberal arts and science courses taken during the freshman and sophomore years.

Five essential components have been identified by the AACN as critical to professional nursing education. They include a liberal education, professional values, core competencies, core knowledge, and role development (AACN, 2005a).

Applicants to such programs must meet the entrance and graduation requirements established by the university, and those of the nursing school. The admission requirements usually specify academic preparation at the high school (or preadmission) level, including courses in foreign language and higher-level mathematics and science, and a high cumulative grade-point average. Relatively high scores on college admission tests also may be required.

During the freshman and sophomore years, students who pursue a nursing education take humanities, social, life, and physical science courses with college students who are preparing for other majors. In some schools, these courses may be completed on a part-time basis; however, this extends the overall course of study beyond 4 years. The number of required liberal arts and science courses may vary from program to program, but usually constitutes about one half the total number of credits specified for graduation—typically 120 semester credits or 180 quarter credits. Students usually begin their study of nursing content during their junior year, thus the term "upper-division major" in nursing. Nursing theory can be taught so that it builds on an understanding of the physical and biologic sciences and liberal arts studied the previous 2 years.

Until the 1980s, most schools offering the baccalaureate degree in nursing required sophomore level nursing courses. Curriculum restructuring and economic pressures gradually led many baccalaureate programs to eliminate sophomore level courses, with all nursing being taught in the last 2 years. More recently, some schools offering a baccalaureate degree in nursing have resumed introducing nursing content during the sophomore year of study. Nursing courses offered at this point often include an overview of the nursing profession and some of the fundamental nursing skills.

Students in baccalaureate nursing programs learn basic nursing skills. They also learn disease prevention and concepts of health maintenance and promotion. Supervisory and leadership techniques and practices are taught, along with an introduction to research. Clinical course work includes experience in community health settings, and leadership responsibility. Emphasis is placed on developing skills in critical decision making, exercising independent nursing judgments that call for broad background knowledge, and working in complex nursing situations in which the outcomes are often not predictable. Acting as a client advocate, the graduate with a baccalaureate degree in nursing collaborates with other members of the health care team in structured and unstructured settings, and supervises those with lesser preparation. Baccalaureate graduates often work with groups as well as with individuals. Baccalaureate programs face some of the same pressures faced by associate degree programs, with a demand for additional content to be added to an already full curriculum.

Changes in Baccalaureate Education

In recent years, the nature of baccalaureate education has changed. Some schools, seeking to add an advanced component, have included courses that permit a degree of specialization at the baccalaureate level (eg, supplemental courses in coronary or critical care nursing). Other schools provide more grounding in research, either as preparation for graduate school or for a more varied role in nursing.

Many baccalaureate nursing programs have taken steps to respond to the need for more RNs prepared at the baccalaureate level. Two innovative methods include the development of accelerated programs and the implementation of articulation agreements with associate degree programs. Both of these will be discussed in detail later in this chapter.

Table 5-1 provides a comparison of these traditional major avenues to RN licensure.

TABLE 5-1	BASIC EDUCATIONAL OPPORTUNITIES FOR REGISTERED NURSING: A COMPARISON		
	DIPLOMA	ASSOCIATE DEGREE	BACCALAUREATE
Location	Is usually conducted by and based in a hospital	Most often conducted in junior or community colleges, occasionally in senior colleges and universities	Located in senior colleges and universities
Length of study	Requires generally 24–30 months, but may require 3 academic years	Requires usually 2 academic or sometimes 2 calendar years	Requires 4 academic years
Requirements for admission	Requires graduation from high school or its equivalent, satisfactory general academic achievement, and successful completion of certain prerequisite courses	Requires that applicants meet entrance requirements of college as well as of program	Requires that applicants meet entrance requirements of the college or university as well as those of program
Program of learning	Includes courses in theory and practice of nursing and in biologic, physical, and behavioral sciences. May require that certain courses in the physical and social sciences be taken at a local college or university	Combines a balance of nursing courses and college courses in the basic natural and social sciences with courses in general education and the humanities	Frequently concentrates on courses in the theory and practice of nursing in the junior and senior years. Provides education in the theory and practice of nursing and courses in the liberal arts as well as the behavioral and physical sciences.
Clinical component	Provides early and substantial clinical learning experiences in the hospital and a variety of community agencies; these focus on an understanding of the hospital environment and the interrelationship of other health disciplines	Requires as a significant part of the program supervised clinical instruction in hospitals and other community health agencies	Provides clinical laboratory courses in a variety of settings where health and nursing care are given
Opportunity for educational advancement	Little or no transferability of courses unless affiliated with a community college or university	Is structured so that some credits may be applied to baccalaureate degree	Provides the basic academic preparation for advancement to higher positions in nursing and to master's degree
Competency on graduation	Graduate is prepared to plan for the care of patients with other members of the health care team, to develop and carry out plans for the care of individuals or groups of patients, and to direct selected members of the nursing team. Has an	Graduate is prepared to plan and give direct patient care in hospitals, nursing homes, or similar health care agencies, and to participate with other members of the health care team, such as licensed practical nurses, nurses aides, physicians, and	Graduate is prepared to plan and give direct care to individuals and families, whether sick or well, to assume responsibility for directing other members of the health care team, and to take on beginning leadership positions. Practices in a

TABLE 5-1	BASIC EDUCATIONAL OPPORTUNITIES FOR REGISTERED NURSING: A COMPARISON (*Continued*)		
	DIPLOMA	**ASSOCIATE DEGREE**	**BACCALAUREATE**
	understanding of the hospital climate and the community health resources necessary for the extended care of patients.	other registered nurses, in rendering care to patients.	variety of settings and emphasizes comprehensive health care, including preventive and rehabilitative services, health counseling and education, and care in acute and long-term illnesses. Has necessary education for graduate study toward a master's degree and may move rapidly to specialized leadership positions in nursing as teacher, administrator, clinical specialist, nurse practitioner, and nurse researcher.
Licensure	Must successfully complete state licensing examination	Must successfully complete state licensing examination	Must successfully complete state licensing examination

Master's and Doctoral Programs That Prepare for Licensure

Our discussion of the various educational programs for registered nursing would be incomplete without mention of the generic master's program. The first generic master's degree in nursing was opened at Yale University in 1974, and several other schools soon followed. Students are admitted with a baccalaureate degree in another area and are granted a master's degree in nursing after completing an established 2-year program of study that prepares them for RN licensure. Case Western Reserve University initiated the first program in which the student earns a doctorate in nursing (ND) before being eligible to take the licensing examination. Most of the graduates of these programs are engaged in teaching and research.

These programs reflect the thinking of some nursing leaders that the minimum preparation for professional nursing should be the master's degree. The programs also provide a higher degree to those people who possess basic baccalaureate preparation in another area of study and are making a career change. With increasing emphasis on the need for a baccalaureate degree for professional practice, this type of program provides a credible opportunity to those with baccalaureate degrees in another area of study. When programs of this type are not available, many students with degrees in other disciplines choose to pursue a 2-year associate degree in nursing.

NONTRADITIONAL PROGRAMS THAT PREPARE FOR LICENSURE

Throughout the years, various adaptations have been made in the traditional ways of educating nurses. These innovative approaches have occurred primarily because of the need to educate more nurses, the need to prepare nurses with higher degrees in nursing, shifts in the economy, and the desire among young people to find work that will make a difference while at the same time making a living.

Accelerated Programs

Accelerated programs are designed to transition adults with baccalaureate and graduate degrees in other fields into nursing and may be completed in 12–18 months, making this the fastest route to licensure as an RN (AACN, 2005d). These fast-track programs have proliferated over the past 15 years and offer nursing education that builds on previous learning experiences resulting in master's and doctoral degrees in nursing. Typical students, referred to as **second-degree students**, are motivated, older, competitive, and have high academic expectations. Programs require a heavy credit load and intense clinical experiences (AACN, 2005d). Accelerated programs resulting in a baccalaureate degree are also available, some in as little as 12 months. More information on this topic can be obtained at *www.aacn.nche.edu?Publications/issues/Aug02.htm*.

The External Degree

The concept of an **external degree** is not new to education in general. Universities in Australia, the Soviet Union, and England have long recognized independent study validated by examination. The University of London has awarded college degrees earned in this fashion since 1836. The major difference between the external degree and the traditional educational experience is that students awarded an external degree are not required to attend classes or follow any prescribed methods of learning (however, they may choose to take some classes).

Learning is assessed through highly standardized and validated examinations. This approach to education was not developed in the United States until about the mid-1950s, and then only in selected areas. New York's Empire State College and the University Without Walls consortium were the first schools in the United States to recognize the value of self-directed learning. Now known as Excelsior University, the New York Regents External Degree Program of the University of the State of New York has become part of this movement.

The nursing program, like other external degree programs in arts, science, and business, uses an assessment approach and is primarily—although not exclusively—designed for those with some experience in nursing. It is philosophically based on principles of adult learning, which advocate flexible and learner-oriented education. Specifically, the responsibility for demonstrating that learning has occurred is placed on the student, and the responsibility for identifying the content to be learned and objectively assessing that this has occurred rests with the faculty. The nursing major is divided into cognitive and performance components. Cognitive learning is documented through nationally standardized and psychometrically valid written examinations. Clinical skills are evaluated through four criteria-referenced performance examinations at regional performance assessment centers throughout the country.

Despite objections, alternative and nontraditional avenues to nursing education appeal to the learner, and these programs continue to evolve. Nursing education, like nursing care, should be tailored to fit the consumer's needs. There are some limitations on the use of external degree programs. Some states do not accept Excelsior degrees for initial licensure because their laws mandate that the educational process include supervised clinical practice. Some states will admit to the licensure examination for RNs only those external associate degree graduates who were LPNs and therefore have had supervised clinical practice in addition to clinical examinations.

COMMUNICATION IN *ACTION*

Dealing With Educational Challenges

Alice Mason, a recent graduate from an associate degree nursing program was working on a unit with a new baccalaureate graduate. On several occasions the baccalaureate graduate made comments such as, "I just don't know how you could learn all you need to know in just two years." Alice invited her colleague to join her for coffee. She initiated the conversation by saying, "From some of your comments, I don't believe you have accurate information about associate degree nursing education, and I'd like to explain a bit about it." Calmly, she explained, "In an associate degree program, we have the same science requirements as in a baccalaureate program in this state. We do have fewer credits in general education, and I would need to obtain those to get a bachelor's degree. We do have 2 full years of nursing, but not as many credits, using the same texts used by programs such as yours. My understanding is that you have spent time studying the community as client, which I did not, and that you have more time devoted to statistics, nursing research, and leadership. While I had a nursing management course, I believe it was fewer credits. In order to complete my bachelor's degree, I will need to take the general education I do not have plus 20 semester credits of nursing." She then said, "Tell me more about your program." Her colleague began to share details of her program, and they both felt they more clearly understood one another's education.

SIMILARITIES AMONG TRADITIONAL ENTRY-LEVEL PRE-LICENSURE PROGRAMS

Currently there are as many similarities in the various avenues to nursing education as there are differences. These similarities may be grouped into several broad classifications, including academic standards, administrative concerns, and areas relating to students.

Academic Similarities

The most obvious similarity is that all programs must academically prepare graduates to pass the NCLEX for registered nursing in their state at the same minimum standardized score used across the nation. All schools must meet criteria established for state board approval in their respective state. There are additional similarities related to administrative problems and students.

Administrative Similarities

Adequate financial support is a major concern for many programs because they are relatively expensive to operate. The economics of the programs are affected by lower student to teacher ratios, expensive laboratories, and limited federal and state funding for nursing education. Another administrative concern focuses on securing appropriate learning experiences. Schools often compete with one another for clinical spaces in hospitals and health care facilities. Certain experiences, such as maternal, child, and psychiatric nursing, may be especially difficult to establish. Developing and maintaining curricula that prepare graduates for current practice often presents a challenge. Demographic changes, with people living longer, technological advances—especially in the area of informatics, changes in venues of care, bioethical concerns, and myriad other changes leave faculty struggling to construct and teach state-of-the-art curricula. Not the least of the administrative similarities is the recruitment and retention of qualified faculty. More lucrative salaries in other positions and the aging and retirement of the present faculty both affect this area, which is already suffering from the current shortage of nurses in most areas.

Similarities Relating to Students

Similarities also exist among students. First of all, recruitment and selection is a major task. Although some schools must turn students away (often because they are unable to find faculty to teach them), at the same time, schools must be responsive to an increasingly diverse population that may not be prepared for college-level studies. This has resulted in the development of selective admission policies that must be scrutinized carefully by school officials and, in some areas, reviewed by the school's attorney for correct legal form and legal ramifications before being accepted by the school's policy-making group.

Programs are caught up in more legal concerns than in the past because applicants and students are seeking their rights as individuals and challenging admission, progression, and dismissal policies. Another legal concern relates to malpractice coverage for students. Some collegiate programs, now removed from the umbrella coverage of the hospital, ask that students purchase malpractice insurance as protection against any lawsuits that might arise as the result of errors committed in the learning process.

There is greater diversity in the student body. Programs are receiving more applications from men, minorities, older adults, and persons who possess degrees in other fields of study. Students with English as a second language present new challenges to nursing faculty in all types of programs. Special courses and other forms of assistance are being developed to enable students with academic challenges to succeed in nursing.

Critical Thinking Activity

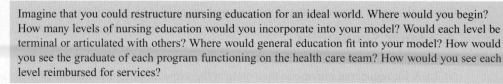

Imagine that you could restructure nursing education for an ideal world. Where would you begin? How many levels of nursing education would you incorporate into your model? Would each level be terminal or articulated with others? Where would general education fit into your model? How would you see the graduate of each program functioning on the health care team? How would you see each level reimbursed for services?

NURSING EDUCATION AT THE GRADUATE LEVEL

The critical need for nurses with additional preparation to work in educational settings, in supervisory roles, as clinical specialists, and to fulfill the expanded role of the nurse has resulted in more programs at the graduate level.

Master's Preparation

As indicated in our earlier discussion of master's education in nursing, there are a variety of models. Some less-traditional approaches include outreach programs, summers-only programs, RN-to-MSN tracks (that provide a direct route to the master's degree for RNs who have graduated from diploma or associate degree programs), programs for students with special needs (such as RNs with non-nursing baccalaureate degrees), and programs that admit non-nurses and foreign graduates. Some schools offer off-campus classes, at times rotating sites, and some deliver core content by way of television or through other distance-learning technology.

Most programs require at least a full year for completion, and many have been expanded to 2 years. Master's programs in nursing typically are found in senior colleges and universities that have baccalaureate programs in nursing. They have the option of seeking voluntary accreditation from the NLNAC or from the Commission on Collegiate Nursing Education (CCNE).

Master's preparation is recommended for leadership positions in nursing, for clinical specialization, and is generally the minimum preparation required to teach nursing. Recently the AACN developed a new role called the clinical nurse leader (CNL) (see Chapter 16). The CNL oversees the care coordination of a distinct group of patients and actively provides direct patient care in complex situations (AACN, 2005b).

Doctoral Studies

The number of requests for admission to doctoral study in nursing has increased greatly since the early 1980s. The impetus for this movement stems from the need for advanced study for academic advancement or tenure in the educational setting and reflects the need in nursing research for the advancement of the profession as a whole.

Before NDs were offered, doctoral study in other fields allowed nurses to benefit from post-master's preparation. A doctorate outside the area of nursing was often the only doctorate available to persons seeking further education; doctorates in nursing are relatively new to the educational milieu, as opposed to such degrees in psychology, sociology, anthropology, or physiology. Certainly nursing can and has benefited from other disciplines.

Doctoral programs in nursing offer various degrees, such as the doctor of nursing science, the doctor of science in nursing, the doctor of nursing education, and the doctor of philosophy in nursing. Other types of doctorates are available to nurses, such as the doctor of education and the doctor of public health.

Recently, the AACN proposed a doctor of nursing practice degree (DNP). The DNP is designed for nurses seeking a terminal degree in nursing practice, as opposed to working in research (AACN, 2004b). Some universities are changing their nurse practitioner programs from master's degree programs to this type of clinical practice doctorates. The AACN has developed a position statement on the DNP that calls for a transformation of nursing education for advanced practice (AACN, 2004c).

The difference in the preparation and function of graduates possessing the various degrees is confusing. Typically, the nurse with a doctorate assumes a leadership role in education, often serving as a faculty member or the dean or director of a nursing program. These nurses also may choose to be involved in the research and development of a body of nursing knowledge.

Critical Thinking Activity

If nurse practitioners are to work collaboratively with physicians, and as primary care providers, what type and level of education do you believe they should complete? How would you ensure that this would occur? What standards regarding continuing education should be mandated for those involved in advance practice? Should it be more stringent than that required at the RN level? Defend your position.

OTHER FORMS OF NURSING EDUCATION

A number of factors have fostered the development of other forms of education for nurses. Most of these are seen in the expansion of higher educational offerings, due in part to the changing role of the nurse in health care delivery, and the need this creates for more adequate education to meet the requirements of that role. Another contributing aspect is the continuing push to make nursing truly professional. To increase nursing's professional component, there is a need for nurses who are interested and competent in research techniques and skills. A third significant reason for advancing nursing education relates to the need for leadership in nursing administration and education. Nurse educators, joining the ranks of other professionals in the academic environment, are required to possess equivalent educational backgrounds. Nurses who assume roles in nursing administration have found the need for a solid understanding of management and finance. Thus, RNs seek baccalaureate, master's, and doctoral degrees to support the complex roles into which they move.

Registered Nurse Baccalaureate Programs

In 2002–2003 increases in the number of nurses enrolling in **registered nurse baccalaureate (RNB) programs** began to be seen (AACN, 2005c). These programs are designed for RNs with either a diploma or an associate degree who wish to return to school to complete a baccalaureate degree in nursing. There are also master's degree programs that admit RNs with associate degrees who, after 3 years, graduate with a master's degree in nursing, receiving a baccalaureate degree partway through the program. Still other master's degree programs in nursing admit RNs with associate degrees in nursing and a baccalaureate degree in another field. Some schools also have added programs designed to admit the LPN, who will emerge with a baccalaureate degree in nursing and be eligible for RN licensure. These programs carry different names in different parts of the country, including baccalaureate registered nurse programs, two-on-two programs, and, in the Midwest, capstone programs.

There are many reasons for the increase in this form of nursing education, several of which have been discussed. In addition, many highly qualified young men and women enter associate degree programs because of cost and time factors and plan for more education several years after completing the original program. The nursing profession is endeavoring to increase the number of nurses prepared with baccalaureate and higher degrees.

The RNB programs vary greatly throughout the United States. In some instances, they exist in universities that already offer the generic baccalaureate program. The students may be completely integrated with generic baccalaureate students, partially separated from them, or in a totally separate program. Another form of RNB preparation is the two-on-two approach, in which RN students transfer into the college or university with junior standing and complete an additional 2 years of upper-division nursing classes. In some instances, this is the only nursing program offered by a college or university; that is, the college may not offer a basic program that prepares a graduate for licensure. Some schools offer nurse practitioner preparation in conjunction with the baccalaureate degree, although the current trend is to place this at the master's level.

Another general trend is to allow the transfer of credits in the natural and biologic sciences, and in basic courses such as psychology and sociology, earned at junior and community colleges. Often, transfer of credit is allowed for nursing courses (eg, 45 quarter credits or 30 semester credits), but the courses may be challenged by examination. Distribution requirements of the particular college or university must be satisfied, and upper-division nursing courses must be completed in such areas as physiologic nursing, community health, understanding nursing research, and supervision. A minimum of 2 years usually is required for completion of the program, although the time may be shorter or longer, depending on the number of requirements satisfied at the time of entry.

Today, RNB education and two-on-two educational programs flourish. Schools with both generic and RNB programs may report more graduates from the RNB program. At least four factors are responsible for the change in attitude toward RNB education. First, the ANA Commission on Nursing Education has provided a push to increase the availability of baccalaureate programs for RNs. Nursing educators are challenged to create and accept more innovative educational strategies.

The second factor comes from pressure within each state. Several states have enacted legislation, sometimes in response to the nursing shortage, which requires the development of a statewide plan for articulation between various types of nursing education programs. In most instances, the legislation establishes a date by which the plan will be implemented.

The third factor influencing the development of RNB programs has been a call for increased educational mobility from organizations in the health care arena. The American Medical Association House of Delegates has suggested career mobility as one way to alleviate the nurse shortage. The Pew Commission recommended strengthening existing career ladder programs to make movement through these levels of nursing as easy as possible (de Tornyay, 1996). Some of the RNB programs currently in operation provide for part-time study or for studies completed through evening courses. The desirability of such approaches for nurses who must work to support their education is obvious. Other innovative RNB programs provide baccalaureate education to people living in areas geographically remote from colleges or universities. These programs use new technologies for distance learning, including the electronic transmission of information.

A final factor influencing the development of RNB programs relates to the allocation of federal dollars to assist students who seek to advance their preparation in nursing. Many of the scholarships and traineeships, once available to all students, have been directed largely to students who wish to continue their education in the area of advanced practice in nursing. Major nursing groups such as the ANA and NLN are lobbying Congress for additional funds directed toward nursing education including the creation of grants to provide scholarships to assist disadvantaged students and individuals entering or seeking advanced education in nursing.

Articulated Programs

Another approach to nursing education is found in programs that are articulated. **Articulation** indicates that the two programs at different levels have well defined links enabling the student to move from one educational level to the next. This can be seen at various levels of nursing education. The major difference between these programs and the ones mentioned earlier is that the curricula are designed so that maximum credit is awarded for work completed earlier.

Today, as increasing numbers of graduates seek education beyond the associate degree or diploma, the career ladder concept in nursing education, mentioned earlier, is growing in popularity. Programs have been developed that provide direct articulation between lower-level and higher-level programs. As mentioned earlier, in some states legislation has been passed strongly encouraging, and in some instances mandating, articulation plans.

The purpose of an articulated program is to facilitate opportunities for students to start nursing education, stop when some goal is reached or degree awarded, or keep moving up the educational ladder. Statewide articulation plans exist in several states. Many of the plans allow most of the work completed at the lower level to meet the requirements of the next degree. Currently 32 states and the District of Columbia have such programs in place. Some have been mandated as part of legislation, some are statewide agreements, and others are school-to-school articulation agreements (AACN, 2005e). Some schools, such as the University of Washington, have formalized RN-to-master's pathways in which the RN graduate of an associate degree program who holds a baccalaureate degree in another field may enter the nursing graduate program without first completing the BSN.

Similar plans exist for articulation between practical (vocational) nurse programs and associate degree programs, and some associate degree programs allow credit for nurse assistant preparation or require it for admission. Again, the articulated program allows students to move up the career ladder from practical nurse to associate degree nurse to the nurse with a baccalaureate degree. Students in an articulated LPN/associate degree program spend a year preparing to be an LPN, and another year completing the associate degree. If they want to continue after this 2-year period, they can earn a baccalaureate degree at another institution after 2 more years of study. Some schools have established LPN-to-baccalaureate degree programs. From that point, a student may continue to work toward a master's degree (Fig. 5-2).

The multiple-entry, multiple-exit programs are not without problems. Initially, they are difficult to develop because of the tremendous amount of joint planning required. Questions arose regarding granting upper-degree credit (course work with 300 and 400 numbers) for studies completed with 100 and 200 numbers in the community college. Understanding what has been taught and determining how to evaluate current knowledge is important. This is particularly relevant to articulation between practical nurse programs and RN programs, where graduates of the practical program may know how to perform many of the nursing skills but may lack the theory base of RNs. Educators need to speak the same language and develop mutual respect.

An Articulated Approach to Nursing Education

Hannah Bledsoe began her nursing education in a practical nursing program. Located in a community college, this program was articulated with an associate degree program. Because of financial concerns, Hannah worked as an LPN for 2 years following completion of the practical nurse program. Eager for more knowledge and the career opportunities it provided, Hannah sought admission to the associate degree program, was admitted, and completed the program. The program she chose had a written articulation agreement with a local 4-year university. On graduation from the associate degree program and successful completion of the RN licensing examination, Hannah was hired at the University Hospital. This employment allowed her to continue to take six credits of study per quarter toward a baccalaureate degree in nursing tuition-free. Working and studying worked well for Hannah, and within a few years she had earned a baccalaureate degree in nursing. She is now considering enrolling in a master's degree program.

The University Without Walls

The University Without Walls approach is being used by a variety of universities and other educational entities to make baccalaureate education more accessible. This approach focuses on making education available through on-line learning, but may also allow academic credit for courses transferred from other colleges and experiences such as past education and work. Part-

FIGURE 5-2   Among innovations occurring in nursing education over the past decade are programs that provide direct articulation between lower-level and higher-level programs.

time study is welcomed. Students benefit because they can continue to work while attending school and experience reduced travel costs. The RN who wishes to obtain a baccalaureate degree from such an institution may take some courses, such as general education requirements, at a local college or community college, attain credit by examination for some nursing courses, and enroll in still other courses on-line, with all accepted as credit by the university granting the BSN degree.

OTHER POST-LICENSURE EDUCATIONAL OPPORTUNITIES

Several opportunities for continued growth and career advancement are available to registered nursing. Most of these do not culminate in an advanced degree, but may be geared to a particular focus or outcome.

Advanced Practice Preparation

Specialized programs have been developed to help individuals prepare for roles of increased breadth and scope. Programs may be incorporated into the preparation leading to a particular degree, exist as part of a school's continuing education program, or result in certification after examination.

Recent health care reform has resulted in an increased emphasis on the role of **advanced nursing practice** in health care delivery, and more demand for educational programs to prepare these practitioners. An advanced practice nurse (APN) is an umbrella term that includes nurse practitioners, clinical nurse specialists, certified nurse-midwives (CNM), and certified registered nurse anesthetists.

The RN anesthesia and midwifery programs both award a certificate after completion of a standardized and rigorous course of study lasting from 18 months to 2 years. At one time, admission requirements stipulated RN licensure only; however, a baccalaureate degree in nursing is now required for admission to schools of anesthesia, with a master's degree awarded on completion. The American College of Nurse Midwives hopes to establish a master's degree on completion of a CNM program by 2010. Some states require a master's degree for the nurse anesthetist or nurse-midwife.

More recent programs offer nurse practitioner and nursing specialist preparation in areas of nursing practice such as pediatrics, gerontology, family health, genetics, and women's health care. In the 1990s, the Pew Commission encouraged growth in the number of master's level nurse practitioner training programs and many more were developed (de Tornyay, 1996). Programs that prepare nurse practitioners concentrate study in specific areas during a period lasting from several months to a year or more. Requirements for admission vary tremendously. Most programs require a bachelor's degree in some field and a current RN license to enter and award the master's degree on completion. Still others require that the education occur at the post-master's degree level or be part of the new ND. The ANCC requires the master's degree for all those seeking initial nurse practitioner certification, and some states now require the master's degree for those seeking initial licensure as a nurse practitioner.

The development of new APN programs has been so great that a complete listing is impossible. A student interested in pursuing such preparation is encouraged to write to the college or university of choice for information about available programs.

Residencies and Structured Orientation for the New Graduate

When nursing education moved from hospital-based diploma programs into higher education, a new problem arose. Employers of the new graduates expected these graduates to function as experienced and qualified professionals on the day after graduation and complained that the graduates were not prepared to assume staff nurse positions within their institutions.

As nursing education moved into institutions of higher education, all clinical time was recognized in credit hours. If students worked on hospital units on weekends, they did so as hospital employees, not as a requirement of their education. As a result, students spent less time in the clinical area. Many graduates of diploma schools in the 1950s would have had as much as 4,000 clock hours of clinical experience, albeit more as apprenticeship and service to the hospital than as a learning experience. Graduates of associate and baccalaureate degree programs, with integrated curricula and objective-based learning experiences, joined the work world with clinical learning time of 800 or fewer clock hours. Hospital-based programs also decreased their clinical hours as curricula were reorganized. Students in all programs now receive their clinical experience in a variety of settings as opposed to one primary health care facility where they become very familiar with policies, procedures, and the physical plant.

All of this resulted in individuals graduating today needing orientation to the work facility and their new role, and time to become efficient in using their newly learned skills. Although few would question the need for internships and residencies for new physicians, the need for similar experiences for new nursing graduates has not been readily accepted. The new graduates, unable to live up to expectations placed on them, often became frustrated and discouraged; some opted for less stressful situations, sometimes even outside nursing. Nursing educators, in defending the education provided, cited other professions, such as law and engineering, in which graduates needed time to adapt to the world of work.

As a result of efforts to address this concern, orientation programs, **internships**, and **residencies** for new graduates were instituted by hospitals. The programs were intended to ease the transition from the role of student to that of staff by providing the opportunity to increase clinical skills and knowledge, as well as self-confidence. These programs can last from several weeks to a year, and are designed for graduates of all nursing programs—associate degree, diploma, and baccalaureate. They often include rotations to various units in the hospital, including specialty areas, and they accommodate different shifts. Usually, some formal class work is associated with the experience, but the majority of the time is spent in direct patient care, often under the supervision of a preceptor.

Institutions receive some direct benefits from such programs in addition to securing a better-prepared employee who remains employed. Inadequacies in policies and procedures have been uncovered and, as a result, rewritten. Performance evaluation tools that are more objective in format have emerged. Nursing practice throughout some agencies has become more standardized. Job satisfaction has increased. It is no longer unusual for hospitals to advertise planned orientation and internships as benefits offered to the new graduate seeking employment, a strong recruitment tool in times of nurse shortages.

The major disadvantage voiced by hospitals is the cost of operating such programs. When cost containment is crucial, hospitals may not be anxious to deal with these additional costs. Another problem is that some employees who benefit from such programs may resign from their positions soon after completing an internship. This has resulted in hospitals stipulating a period of required employment following the orientation or internship.

Continuing Education

Continuing education in nursing is defined as

> planned learning experiences beyond a basic nursing educational program. The learning experiences are designed to promote the development of knowledge, skills, and attitudes for the enhancement of nursing practice, thus improving health care to the public. (ANA, 1974)

Continuing education programs are widely publicized in today's nursing literature. They often are presented just before and during major nursing conventions. Some professional meetings carry continuing education credit. Other continuing education programs exist as extensions of nursing programs at colleges and universities.

Like so many other areas of nursing, continuing education is not new. In an article entitled "Nursing the Sick," written around 1882, Florence Nightingale wrote:

> Nursing is, above all, a progressive calling. Year by year nurses have to learn new and improved methods, as medicine and surgery and hygiene improve. Year by year nurses are called upon to do more and better than they have done. It is felt to be impossible to have a public register of nurses that is not a delusion. (Nightingale, as cited in Seymer, 1954, p. 349)

The first continuing education courses for nurses probably would be considered postgraduate instruction today. In 1899, Teachers College at Columbia University instituted a course for qualified graduate nurses in hospital economics. Nursing institutes and conferences were first offered to nurses in the 1920s; often these were given to make up for deficiencies in basic nursing curricula. The first hospital inservices or staff development programs were discussed in nursing literature around this time. Today most hospitals employ someone who is responsible for the staff education program. By 1959, federal funds became available for short-term courses, giving much thrust to continuing education. In 1967, the ANA published Avenues for Continued Learning, its first definitive statement on continuing education; and in 1973, the ANA Council on Continuing Education was established. The Council, which is responsible to the ANA Commission on Education, is concerned about standards of continuing education, accreditation of the programs, the transferability of credit from state to state, and development of guidelines for recognition systems within states. In 1974, the first edition of *Standards for Continuing Education in Nursing* was published by the ANA, and the federal government altered the Nurse Traineeship Act of 1972 to include an option that would provide continuing education as an alternative to placing more students into programs receiving federal capitation dollars.

By the 1970s, most nursing publications had something to say about continuing education for nurses. Practically all states were organizing or planning to organize some method by which the nurse could receive recognition for continued education. These systems were called continuing education approval and recognition programs, or continuing education recognition programs, and most state systems followed the guidelines and criteria prepared by the ANA.

The **continuing education unit (CEU)** became a rather uniform system of measuring, recording, reporting, accumulating, transferring, and recognizing participation in nonacademic credit offerings. The National Task Force on the Continuing Education Unit, which represented 34 educational groups, developed the definition of a CEU. Although nursing was not one of the groups, the profession has accepted the definition. Ten hours of participation in an organized continuing education experience under responsible sponsorship, with capable direction and qualified instruction, is equal to one CEU. Many states and organizations, however, simply report clock hours of instruction. Following a system for accreditation and approval of continuing education in nursing that was developed and implemented by the ANA in 1975, programs or individuals offering courses for continuing education now receive authority to do so from a recognized body, thereby ensuring quality programs and standardization in their approach.

Today, colleges, universities, hospitals, voluntary agencies, and private proprietary groups all offer continuing education courses to RNs (Fig. 5-3). The cost of this education varies tremendously.

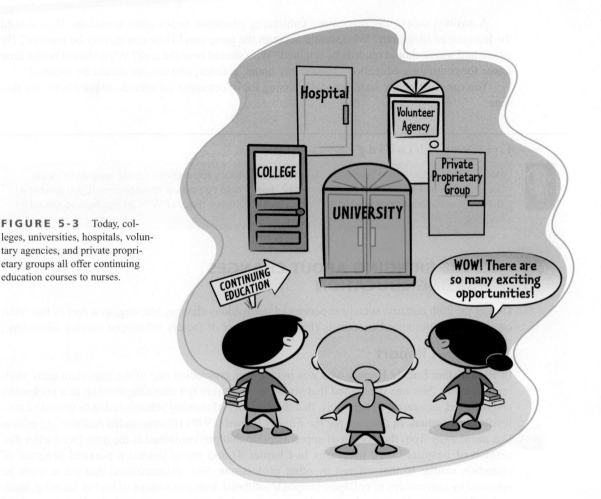

FIGURE 5-3   Today, colleges, universities, hospitals, voluntary agencies, and private proprietary groups all offer continuing education courses to nurses.

Nurses can earn continuing education credits for merely attending meetings and conferences. Attempts to assess whether learning has occurred vary tremendously. Professional journals include sections of programmed instruction that can be completed in the comfort of one's living room. These have an evaluation mechanism. Telecourses are offered by television. Workshops, institutes, conferences, short courses, and evening courses abound. Additionally, courses are available on the Internet.

However, some nurses do not feel the need to keep up with these offerings. An issue today is whether continuing education should be mandatory or voluntary. **Mandatory continuing education** affects licensure, meaning that any nurse renewing a license in a state requiring (mandating) continuing education will have to satisfy that requirement. **Voluntary continuing education** is not related to relicensure. Government agencies and state legislatures are exerting pressure on nurses, as they have on physicians, attorneys, dietitians, dentists, pharmacists, and other professionals, to provide evidence of updated knowledge before license renewal.

A position supporting mandatory continuing education raises some questions. How should the learning be measured? Who should accredit the programs? How can quality be ensured? By whom and where should records be retained? Who should bear the cost? What should be the time frame for continuing education? How many hours, courses, and credits should be required?

You can contact any state board of nursing for information on specific requirements for that state.

Critical Thinking Activity

Do you believe continuing education should be a mandatory requirement for the renewal of one's license? Why or why not? If your answer is no, how would you ensure competence? If you believe it should be mandatory, what kind of record keeping would you require? Who do you believe should keep the records?

FACTORS BRINGING ABOUT CHANGES IN NURSING EDUCATION

During the 20th century, society experienced tremendous change. Nursing, as a part of that society, has also experienced enormous change. A number of factors influenced nursing education.

The Brown Report

In 1948, Esther Lucille Brown, who was not a nurse, conducted one of the important early studies of nursing. She was concerned that young women were not choosing nursing as a profession and believed, as a result of her study, that the majority of nursing schools failed to provide a professional education. In *Nursing for the Future*, Brown (1948) recommended that nursing education move away from the system of apprenticeship that predominated at the time (see earlier discussion of hospital-based programs in Chapter 4) and move toward a planned program of education similar to that offered by other professions. She recommended that the schools be operated by universities or colleges, hospitals affiliated with institutions of higher learning, medical colleges, or independently. She also recommended that programs periodically be examined or reviewed, and that a list of accredited schools be published and distributed.

The Brown report attracted the attention of many nursing leaders, who shared her concerns about recruiting qualified women into nursing. The study took place shortly after World War II, and nurses who had been involved in the military had a new sense of autonomy and independence that they were not willing to leave behind. Committees formed to respond to the suggestions put forth in the Brown study, particularly those related to the accreditation of programs. At the same time, the National League for Nursing Education (NLNE), later to become the NLN, recommended that hospital schools of nursing consider transferring control and administration of their programs to educational institutions. The NLNE also urged that federal grants be provided to nursing schools to allow for their improvement.

Development of a National Examination Standard

Along with the push for the improvement of nursing education, licensing authorities were pressured to establish a uniform licensing examination. The development of the State Board Test Pool

Examination, which gradually expanded until all states required that same examination, helped all schools to focus on common goals and laid the foundation for interstate endorsement of licenses. The tests required to obtain licensure is now known as the NCLEX for Registered Nursing (or Practical Nursing for practical nursing program graduates) (see Chapter 7).

National Accreditation of Nursing Programs

By 1952, the NLN had a temporary accreditation program in place and was helping schools to find ways to improve their programs of instruction. Accreditation of all kinds requires that the institution study its own practices in relationship to standards. Peers then examine the institution and a determination is made as to whether it meets the standards. The **accreditation** of programs had a noticeable effect on standards of nursing education. As a result of accreditation activities, schools were forced to look at the educational preparation of faculty, the workload of faculty and students, the structure of clinical teaching, withdrawal rates, and the state board examination scores. This system of program assessment enhanced the quality of education; graduation from a nationally accredited school meant added opportunities for advanced education or certain types of employment. Today accreditation of nursing programs is carried out by the NLNAC for practical, associate degree, baccalaureate, and master's programs in nursing. For baccalaureate and master's programs, accreditation is also available through the CCNE.

Changes in Nursing Service

While changes were occurring in the education of nurses, nurses in the workplace also experienced significant changes. With the advent of antibiotics and other major advances in medical protocols and medical technology during the mid-1900s, the public received care in hospitals rather than treatment in the home. Births that previously took place at home now occurred in hospitals. Federal funds were allocated for the construction of hospitals. Increased hospitalization drove the need for qualified nurses to a new high. Hospitals were desperate to find nurses to fill needed positions, and nurses represented half of all hospital personnel. Today RNs constitute the largest health care occupation, with 2.3 million jobs (Bureau of Labor Statistics, 2004–2005).

The role of the nurse changed in response to changes in the workplace. Nursing staff began assuming responsibilities formerly associated with physicians. Unfortunately, they also assumed responsibilities that could have been assumed by housekeeping, dietary, laboratory, and pharmacy departments. Nurses began spending more time managing personnel, delegating responsibilities, and carrying out other administrative duties. Nurses at higher levels in the organization needed higher levels of education (ie, baccalaureate and master's degrees).

The Report of the Surgeon General's Consultant Group

In 1961, the Surgeon General of the U.S. Public Health Service appointed a group to advise him of the federal government's role in providing adequate nursing services to the country. This group was known as the Surgeon General's Consultant Group on Nursing, and they published their report in 1963.

The report emphasized the need for more nurses, and identified the lack of adequate financial resources for nursing education as a major problem. Several other major concerns also were reported. Of critical importance were the reports that too few schools were providing adequate nursing education, that too few college-bound young people were being recruited into the profession, and that more nursing schools were needed in colleges and universities. (By now you are recognizing this as a recurrent theme regarding nursing.) Educational preparation at the baccalaureate degree level was recommended as the minimum preparation for nurses assuming leadership roles (U.S. Public Health Service, 1963).

The Surgeon General's Consultant Group on Nursing also recommended that federally funded low-cost loans and scholarships be made available to students in both professional and practical nursing programs. It advocated the use of federal funds to construct additional nursing school facilities and to expand educational programs. The Nurse Training Act of 1964 was an outgrowth of these recommendations.

The American Nurses Association Position Paper

In the early 1960s, the educational preparation of nurses became a major concern of the ANA. The ANA believed that the improvement of nursing practice and the profession as a whole depended on the advancement of nursing education. After studying the issue for 3 years, *A Position Paper on Educational Preparation for Nurse Practitioners and Assistants to Nurses* was published in December 1965. In 2000, the ANA reaffirmed this position (ANA, 2000). The positions of the paper are listed in Display 5-2. It resulted in the **entry into practice** controversy.

No other single action or position has affected nursing more or has there been any issue that has been more divisive than the ANA position paper. Gosnell (2002) states, "Overall, entry into practice has been one of the most contentious issues in all of nursing." For almost 40 years, the profession has been plagued with the issues it brought forth. A basic concern related to the fact that the roles, functions, and responsibilities (competencies) of programs offering three different routes to preparation for registered nursing were not clearly differentiated for graduates. All graduates took the same examination and performed similar activities when hired as new graduates in acute care facilities.

Associate degree nursing programs in community colleges and hospital-based diploma programs took serious exception to the paper. To this group, not being considered professional was unacceptable, and they were unwilling to compromise title or licensure. Because of the dissension the position paper created among nursing groups, little immediate action followed.

Display 5-2   Four Major Positions of the ANA Position Paper on Educational Preparation

1. The education of all those who are licensed to practice nursing should take place in institutions of higher education.
2. Minimum preparation for beginning professional nursing practice at the present time should be baccalaureate degree education in nursing.
3. Minimum preparation for beginning technical nursing practice at the present time should be associate degree education in nursing.
4. Education for assistants in the health service occupations should be short, intensive pre-service programs in vocational education institutions, rather than on-the-job training programs.

(ANA, 1965, p. 107).

However, groups slowly began to take action regarding the paper, with many nursing organizations supporting the position, and others adamantly opposed to it. The controversy continues today.

Problems Associated with Changing Educational Requirements for Licensure

Several problems are associated with making any changes in educational requirements for licensure. Four major problems are related to titling, scope of practice, grandfathering, and interstate endorsement.

Titling. One of the most controversial problems associated with changing requirements for licensure involves **titling**, or the use of titles. The RN title has a long history and is clearly recognizable to the public and to the health care community. Currently graduates of all nursing programs use this title. If a differentiation were to be made between those with a baccalaureate degree, those with associate degrees, and those prepared in hospital-based programs, which graduates would use the title Registered Nurse? What alternate titles would be available for graduates from the other programs currently preparing individuals for licensure?

Scope of Practice. Of equal concern is the description and delineation of the **scope of practice** for the two levels of caregivers. The scope of practice (discussed in Chapter 7) is that section of the Nurse Practice Act that outlines the activities a person with a particular license may legally perform. This would mean the separate testing of each level as it currently exists between the RN and the practical nurse licensure examination. This problem might be of less concern if the nursing profession could agree on an approach to differentiated practice. In some suggestions for two levels of practice, the process of making nursing diagnoses and developing nursing care plans was at times included in the scope of practice of the baccalaureate-prepared nurse only, a position totally unacceptable to associate degree advocates. Again, the diploma graduate was left out of the discussion.

The Grandfather Clause. The application of a **grandfather clause** presents another challenge to nurses. Traditionally, when a state licensure law is enacted, or if a current law is repealed and a new law enacted, a grandfather clause has been a standard feature that allows persons to continue to practice their profession or occupation after new qualifications have been enacted into law. The legal basis for the process is found in the 14th Amendment to the U.S. Constitution, which declares that no state may deprive any person of life, liberty, or property without due process of law. The Supreme Court has ruled that the license to practice is a property right. A grandfather clause has been used in nursing at various times in the past. For example, when psychiatric nursing became a requirement of all programs, nurses who graduated and were licensed without psychiatric nursing experiences were grandfathered into the new role. In other words, they continued to practice as RNs without taking a formal course in psychiatric nursing, and without being required to write a psychiatric examination to maintain their licenses. If nursing began to require a baccalaureate degree for individuals using the RN title, under the provisions of a grandfather clause, all associate graduates licensed before the implementation date for the change would continue to use the title "registered nurse." Those licensed after the change would use whatever new title was established. Although this serves to protect the title of currently licensed nurses, it does not prevent employers from writing job descriptions stipulating a baccalaureate degree as the minimum educational preparation acceptable for a particular position.

Complicating this matter is the fact that some nurses believe a grandfather clause should be conditional. If it were conditional, nurses licensed before the changes in the licensure law would continue to use their current title for a stipulated period of time—for example, 10 years. At the end of that period, if they had not completed the education mandated in the changes (or any other conditions that might have been added), they would have to use the title stipulated in the new law for nurses with their educational preparation. Because of the complexity and the difficulties associated with implementation, it is unlikely that conditional grandfathering will ever become a reality.

Interstate Endorsement. A fourth concern is that of **interstate endorsement**. Nursing is one of the few professions to have developed a process whereby national examinations with standardized scores are administered in each state or jurisdiction, thus allowing a nurse who has passed the licensing examination in one state to move to another state and seek licensure without the need to retake and pass another examination. (However, with the exception of those states participating in the licensure compact [see Chapter 7], they do need to secure licensure in each state in which they practice.) Because nurses can be highly mobile, this has been a great advantage. As the profession examines multistate licensure, this issue takes on new dimensions.

The Position Paper and Nursing Today

Because the initial thinking and work on the **position paper** occurred 40 years ago, nursing leaders are raising questions about its relevancy today. Gosnell (2002) points to differences in practice demographics, stating that in the early 1960s, 75% of all nurses were educated in diploma schools of nursing, that 16% came from baccalaureate programs, and that associate degree nursing was in its infancy. By the year 2000, diploma programs had dramatically declined to just 6%, baccalaureate programs had doubled to 30%, and associate degree programs had risen to produce nearly 60% of all new graduates. Certainly the goal to place nursing in institutions of higher education was being realized, but two thirds of the graduates possess less than a baccalaureate education, resulting in nurses being the least educated of all health professionals.

The AACN (an organization of baccalaureate and higher degree nursing programs) has taken a position on licensing of associate degree graduates. Its Web site (*www.aacn.nche.edu*) clearly states that it does not advocate changing licensure for associate degree nurses. It recognizes the valuable role of associate degree nurses in health care and encourages articulation and continued education. It does support the baccalaureate degree as entry into "what the organization holds to be professional-level nursing practice."

At the spring 2000 meeting, the ANA board of directors reaffirmed the long-standing position that baccalaureate education should be the standard for entry into professional nursing practice. Just prior to that decision, the ANCC decided to offer a new certification examination for nurses who hold a bachelor's of science in nursing with the credential of Board Certified and to offer the current exams, with the credential of Certified to nurses with diplomas or associate degrees (ANA, 2000).

As some nursing groups set 2010 as the target year for requiring the baccalaureate in nursing as the educational preparation for entry into practice as an RN (Barter & McFarland, 2001), it becomes clear that this contentious issue is not one of the past but, rather, is one with which the nurses of tomorrow will continue to grapple.

Critical Thinking Activity

Take a stand on the ANA position on nursing education. Provide a rationale for the position you have taken. What do you see as the outcome of the position paper? How would your position be implemented in the future? What implications might it have for nursing practice? Do you believe the salaries of nurses educated at different levels and practicing at differentiated levels should differ? Why or why not? If so, how?

DIFFERENTIATED PRACTICE

In the 1990s, some nursing leaders began to reassess the entry-into-practice issue. Although the nursing shortage of the late 1980s and the push toward cost cutting in the 1990s may have encouraged its reevaluation, the review also may reflect a new thinking regarding the role of nurses and nursing and the role of all education in the United States. Many nursing leaders encouraged recognition of the need for different types of practitioners, prepared with different types of education, or differentiated practice. **Differentiated nursing practice** can be defined as "the practice of structuring nursing roles on the basis of education, experience, and competence" (Boston, 1990, p. 2).

Today, many groups support the concept of differentiated practice. The report of the Pew Commission (1995) advised that nursing distinguish between the different levels of nursing. The Commission recommended associate degree preparation for the entry-level hospital setting and nursing home practice, baccalaureate degree preparation for hospital-based care management and community-based practice, and master's degree preparation for specialty practice in the hospital and independent practice as a primary provider. The National Commission Nursing Implementation Project also strongly supported differentiated practice.

The AACN and the American Organization of Nurse Executives established a Task Force on Differentiated Competencies for Nursing Practice funded by the Robert Wood Johnson Foundation. This group was later expanded to include representatives from The National Organization for Associate Degree Nursing. A joint publication of these three organizations, titled *A Model for Differentiated Nursing Practice*, is available at *www.aacn.nche.edu* (click on "Publications"). It recognizes that nurses with differing educational preparation bring different capabilities to the patient care system.

Competency Expectations and Differentiated Practice

The task of describing and differentiating the **competencies** and the scope of practice of nurses graduating from various types of programs is one of the major challenges facing nursing today. As stated earlier, graduates of baccalaureate nursing programs, associate degree programs, and hospital-based programs all write the same licensing examination, designed to ensure minimum safe practice. This approach fails to recognize the broad range of functions in nursing, and the potential for improving the quality of care given, if different roles and responsibilities were identified. In the work environment of acute and long-term care facilities, little differentiation exists in beginning staff nurse positions.

If developed and implemented, realistic statements about competencies of each level or category of nursing education will facilitate the effective and efficient use of each category of graduate within the health care delivery system. Validated competencies also will provide a basis for the development of curriculum patterns to ensure adequate preparation of each category of care-giver, without running the risk of over- or undereducating at any one level. The competencies also can serve as a foundation for educational mobility patterns in the profession, job descriptions in the health care system, and responsive reimbursement packages.

The Work of Organizations in Defining Competencies

Some work has been done toward describing the competencies of graduates of different programs in nursing. In 1978, the Council of Associate Degree Programs (CADP) of the NLN developed a document, *Educational Outcomes of Associate Degree Nursing Programs: Roles and Competencies*. In 1990, the CADP revised this document and identified three roles that are still in use by many associate degree nursing programs: provider of care, manager of care, and member within the discipline of nursing (NLN, 1990). Later in 1999, another document was published by the NLN that restructured the roles and competencies into five roles. This document never achieved the widespread acceptance and use of the 1990 document.

The *Characteristics of Baccalaureate Education in Nursing*, revised by the Council of Baccalaureate and Higher Degrees of NLN in 1994, was an initial approach to describing a standard for baccalaureate education. In 1998, the AACN revised an earlier publication and published *Essentials of Baccalaureate Education for Professional Nursing Practice*. This document includes the role of the baccalaureate-prepared nurse, professional values for baccalaureate nursing education, an outline of essential curriculum content, baccalaureate core competencies and knowledge, as well as suggested teaching strategies (AACN, 1998).

Similarly, the Council of Diploma Programs and the Council of Practical Programs of NLN developed competencies for graduates. Since 1999, all the educational councils of NLN have been merged into one group, and there has been no further activity in the area of role definition.

In 1986, and every 3 years following that, the National Council of State Boards of Nursing has conducted several studies aimed at role delineation and job analysis of entry-level RNs. The purpose of these studies is to validate the NCLEX-RN. During 1997, the National Council developed a protocol for conducting a study to identify similarities and differences in the practice of all levels of licensed nurses within and across employment settings; it conducted the study in 1998 (National Council of State Boards of Nursing, 1998). In 1999 it published the *Role Delineation Study*, which describes the similarities and differences in the roles of nurse aides, LPNs, RNs, and APNs.

Some of the most recent work related to defining competencies has come from the Pew Health Professions Commission's final report. The fourth report, which continued the theme of reforming health professions, addressed skills needed to function in health care in the 21st century. Twenty-one competencies were identified as critical to practice (Display 5-3) (Bellack & O'Neil, 2000).

Special Projects to Differentiate Practice

Several projects have been conducted throughout the United States in an effort to achieve a regional consensus among nursing service persons and educators on differentiated statements of scope of practice for each level of graduate. Some of the early projects included the Midwest Alliance in Nursing Projects, the first project funded by the W. K. Kellogg Foundation and the second project by a grant from the Division of Nursing of the Department of Health and Human Services (Primm, 1987); the Healing Web Project, composed of representatives of nursing education and practice from six midwestern and western states; and the Sioux Falls Experience, a detailed project implemented to differentiate educational design.

Display 5-3   Competencies Defined by the Pew Health Professions Commission

1. Embrace a personal ethic of social responsibility and service.
2. Exhibit ethical behavior in all professional activities.
3. Provide evidence-based clinically competent care.
4. Incorporate the multiple determinants of health in clinical care.
5. Apply knowledge of the new sciences.
6. Demonstrate critical thinking, reflection, and problem-solving skills.
7. Understand the role of primary care.
8. Rigorously practice preventive health care.
9. Integrate population-based care and services into practice.
10. Improve access to health care for those with unmet health needs.
11. Contribute to continuous improvement of the health care system.
12. Advocate for public policy that promotes and protects the health of the public.
13. Continue to learn and help others learn.
14. Practice relationship-centered care with individuals and families.
15. Provide culturally sensitive care to a diverse society.
16. Partner with communities in health care decisions.
17. Use communication and information technology effectively and appropriately.
18. Work in interdisciplinary teams.
19. Ensure care that balances individual, professional, system, and societal needs.
20. Practice leadership.
21. Take responsibility for quality of care and health outcomes at all levels.

Bellack & O'Neil, 2000

Other states have developed sets of recommendations to enable differentiated practice. For example, the 1988 Colorado Experiment recommendations first asked for a statewide plan to facilitate articulation of nursing education programs, allowing nurses to move from one educational credential to another without unnecessary replication of learning or curricular experience. The second recommendation called for a differentiated model for nursing practice that would facilitate appropriate use of nurses with varying educational credentials and degrees of experience. This would be accompanied by a differentiated pay scale, to allow appropriate compensation of nursing personnel as career advancement or growth occurred. Movement from one role to another required completion of the appropriate additional degrees, although growth within each role was possible without acquiring formal education. Wide-scale implementation of this model has not yet occurred.

In 1995, the AACN, working with the AONE and the National Organization for Associate Degree Nursing, published *A Model for Differentiated Nursing Practice.* This document outlined a model for differentiated learning and practice identifying separate and distinct roles that could be delineated for associate degree nursing, BSN, and master's of science in nursing levels, with each needed and valued for comprehensive health care delivery (AACN, 1995). Another approach focused on the development of competency models. These models were frequently the outgrowth of the work of one of the 20 Colleagues in Caring project throughout the United States that were funded by the Robert Wood Johnson Foundation. Frequently incorporated into the models were ANA's standards of care or the levels of practice identified by Benner (1984) of novice, advanced beginner, competent, proficient, and expert. One such model, originating in New Jersey, was developed for two levels of practice and licensure. Other states, including California, Mississippi, New Mexico, Alaska, South Dakota, Arizona, and South Carolina, initiated pilot projects for differentiated practice (Ellis & Hartley, 2005).

All the above points to the fact that, despite interest and desire, the implementation of differentiated practice is slow in coming. If it is to be realized it will continue to take high levels of commitment and perseverance.

Critical Thinking Activity

Given the situation we have today, with three routes to preparation for registered nursing, how would you suggest that the skills of the graduate of each program be differentiated? How should that influence nursing practice? How would you implement differentiated practice on a unit on which you were working? If it is to be realized, it will continue to take high levels of commitment and perseverance.practice on the unit on which you currently are working? Do you believe that there should be a difference in salary? What is the rationale for your answer?

FORCES FOR CHANGE IN NURSING EDUCATION

As the nursing profession advances and education remains responsive to the changes that occur, it is imperative that nursing education undergo modifications. A discussion of some of the most significant challenges follows.

Incorporating Computer Technology in Nursing Education

It is safe to say that in the past 10 years nursing education has experienced no transformation more dramatic than the incorporation of computer technology into all aspects of teaching, learning, and health care. These changes encompass activities covering everything from entire degrees that can be earned via on-line courses to separate courses that are taught on-line to the incorporation of computer technology in the classroom and learning laboratory. In the health care setting, computers are used for patient records, business functions, and increasingly as a support to effective decision making.

Computer Technology in the Classroom

The computer plays a major role in nursing education and is as essential to the operation of colleges and universities as it is to the operation of hospitals. Additionally, it is an important instructional tool. The computer offers a variety of approaches to instruction that are appealing and helpful to a diverse student population. Classroom lectures and presentations are augmented by computer-assisted instruction in the form of interactive and linear video programs, patient simulations, drill and practice routines, problem-solving programs, and tutorials, to name a few examples. Faculty also use computers for word processing, literature review, and the development and scoring of tests. Some faculty use computers in the classroom to augment their lectures and discussions through Power Point presentations and other computer technology. E-mail and the Internet are also a part of most teaching environments. Some instructional programs are delivered to sites far from the main campus through distance learning modalities using computer technology. At the end of their program of study, all students demonstrate their ability to practice safely on computerized licensing examinations in the form of computerized adaptive testing. In the nursing skills laboratory, mannequins that can blink their eyes, have dilating pupils, breathe, and have a heartbeat and a pulse assist students in the process of learning about heart attacks, diabetic shock, and other emergencies.

Computer literacy among students and faculty is no longer an issue—they possess computer skills. Nursing educators express concern about the initial cost of the equipment and programs needed for this instruction, as well as the increasing cost of keeping both equipment and programs current. For example, the mannequin mentioned above carries a price tag of $215,000. At a time when the budgets of educational institutions are experiencing severe cuts, people responsible for purchasing supplies and equipment increasingly must find creative ways to acquire needed items. Another challenge to faculty is finding time to evaluate the existing software and integrate it into the approved curriculum.

Computers in the Hospital Environment

Today's health care settings could not operate without computers and computerized equipment. Computers are used for business operations, medical records, and collection of clinical data, such as vital signs and hemodynamic values. Computers may be voice activated for charting at the bedside, for use with nursing care plans, for communication from the physicians' office to nursing stations, for regulating the administration of medications, and for many other facets of operation and patient care. Most of the equipment used in today's modern hospital is computerized. New graduates move into a highly technical world when they seek their first nursing positions. The education they receive to prepare them for these positions also must include the skills necessary to work in this highly computerized environment.

Distance Learning Options

Many students who are geographically bound and unable to relocate to a community offering a baccalaureate or master's education in nursing have found distance learning convenient and flexible. It also appeals to the nurse who cannot quit work to attend school. Essentially, distance learning refers to a teaching/learning situation in which the student and the teacher are not present in a classroom. Distance education may be accomplished through on-line courses, through courses broadcast to distant sites and courses taught in areas distant from the campus. A wide variety of approaches and methods are used, including courses that are Internet-enabled, Web-based, computer-mediated, on-line, synchronous, and asynchronous.

For on-line courses, sometimes referred to as a **virtual university**, students register for a class and are given passwords and access to the system. They work with an instructor and other class members, discussing issues, sharing ideas, and testing theories without the need to gather physically. Often individuals in the group share a mailbox, which serves as an electronic classroom, facilitating a group forum among students. Research material is available through an electronic library. Students usually concentrate on one subject at a time, with courses being sequenced but offered outside the constraints of established times. Students may sign on at any hour, day or night. The instructor may have posted a short lecture and provided discussion questions. Students complete reading and written assignments as in traditional learning situations, except that the written assignments are sent to the instructor, graded, and returned on-line. Computer conferencing allows the students to participate in class discussion, ask questions, and receive feedback. After completing one course, the students move to the next until degree requirements are met.

Although these programs offer much flexibility to students, they also demand a great deal of discipline on their part. A single course may require as much as 15 to 20 hours of study time per week. A student attempting such a program needs to be an independent learner. Sufficient faculty time also must be provided for students to receive effective feedback regarding their efforts. Library resources are always a concern for distant learners, and colleges need to provide access to appropriate learning resources for distance learners. Mechanisms for evaluating the learning must be developed thoughtfully to ensure the integrity of resulting credentials.

Establishing Programs That Provide for Educational Mobility

The concept of **educational mobility** in nursing has been discussed earlier in this chapter in the section dealing with articulation. In current times, it certainly must be included as one of the forces for change in nursing education.

Increasing Community-Based Practice Experiences

Another significant change in nursing practice is the trend toward community-based practice. Most nursing programs, especially hospital-based and associate degree programs, have a history of being strongly oriented toward the hospital as the primary clinical teaching environment. "Community," as the term was used in nursing education, was associated with public health nursing and was to be found in baccalaureate education only.

Earlier hospital discharge to the home and an increasing emphasis on prevention has created new demands on nursing. Nurses are expected to provide care in clients' homes, the workplace, schools, nursing homes, community health agencies, clinics, shelters, and community gathering places. As the arena in which nursing is practiced begins to shift, nursing educators are challenged to define what part of the nursing curriculum should be taught in a community setting. Often this requires different clinical teaching strategies and approaches. Some faculty are reticent to shorten any time in acute care facilities; many are uncertain how a community experience should be provided and evaluated. Others worry about the legal ramifications associated with having students in many different environments and in less-controlled situations. Tremendous strides have been taken in developing innovative approaches to community-based nursing; more will follow.

Increasing Emphasis on Nursing Theories and Research

As the nursing profession continues to grow, one of the areas receiving more emphasis is nursing theory and research. As nursing education keeps pace with the advancement of nursing knowledge, there has been a push to develop curricular patterns that respond to the work of nursing theorists. Most approval bodies, state and national, now stipulate that a nursing program must have a coherent organizing or conceptual framework around which the program of learning is developed. Some programs have chosen to select the approach of a particular nursing **theorist**, and structure the program of learning around that theorist's work. The program in which you are enrolled may reflect this trend. Perhaps one of the hospitals to which you are assigned for clinical experience also uses the principles of a nursing theory to structure the delivery of care, although this is less common than using a theory in curriculum development.

A **theory** is a "scientifically acceptable general principle which governs practice or is proposed to explain observed facts" (Riehl & Roy, 1974, p. 3). Because nursing as a developing profession is seriously involved in research, theories are valuable to use in building a sound body of nursing knowledge. They provide the bases for hypotheses about nursing practice. They make it possible for us to derive a sound rationale for the actions we take. If the theories are testable, they allow us to build our knowledge base and to guide and improve nursing practice.

Today, there are many published nursing theories. In an attempt to structure and organize those theories, various authors have categorized or classified them. Not all are classified similarly. Included are general classifications such as the art and science of humanistic nursing, interpersonal relationships, systems, and energy fields. Other categories include growth and development theories, systems theories, stress adaptation theories, and rhythm theories.

Examples of growth and development theories with which you are probably familiar are those of Maslow, Erikson, Kohlberg, Piaget, and Freud. Most basic nursing texts incorporate a discussion of the concepts developed by these theorists. The theories are so named because they focus on the developing person. They have the common characteristic of arranging this development in stages through which a person must pass to reach a particular level of development. They allow nurses to monitor progress through the stages and evaluate the appropriateness of that progress. You will recognize Maslow for his approach to self-actualization, Erikson for his psychosocial development, Kohlberg for his theories of moral reasoning, Piaget for his approach to cognitive development, and Freud for psychosexual theories on which medicine later based the school of psychoanalysis. These theories are not truly theories of nursing, however, because they were not developed for the purpose of explaining, testing, and changing the practice of nursing. They represent some of the borrowed knowledge around which we build our profession.

Most nursing theories are developed around a combination of concepts. Among these concepts, four approaches usually include those directed to the human person, health and illness, the environment (or society), and nursing.

Nursing theories usually are classified according to the structure or approach around which they are developed. Theories that speak to the art and science of humanistic nursing were among the earliest pure nursing theories developed. Some authors have looked back at the contributions of Florence Nightingale and have included her work in that grouping. Among others are Virginia Henderson and her *Definition of Nursing*, Faye Abdellah and the *Twenty-one Nursing Problems* (which is often cited as one of the early attempts at classification of nursing behaviors), Lydia Hall and her *Core, Care, and Cure* model, and Madeleine Leininger's *Transcultural Care Theory*.

Interpersonal process theories deal with interactions between and among people. Many of these theories were developed during the 1960s. Included in this grouping could be Hildegard Peplau's *Psychodynamic Nursing*, Joyce Travelbee's *Human to Human Relationship*, Ernestine Wiedenbach's *The Helping Art of Clinical Nursing*, and Imogene King's *Dynamic Interacting Systems* model, although the last also could be classified as a systems theory.

Systems theories are so named because they are concerned with the interactions between and among all the factors in a situation. A system usually is viewed as complex and in a state of constant change. It is defined as a whole with interrelated parts and may be a subsystem of a larger system as well as a suprasystem. For example, a person may be viewed as a system composed of cells, tissue, and organs. The person is a subsystem of a family, which in turn is a subsystem of a community. In a systems approach, the person usually is considered as a "total" being, or from a "whole" being viewpoint. Systems theories also provide for input into the system and feedback within the system. The systems approach became popular during the 1970s. Included in this group of theorists are Dorothy Johnson, Sister Calista Roy, and Betty Neuman.

TABLE 5-2	NURSING THEORIES AND THEORISTS
THEORIST	**THEORY OR MODEL**
Lydia Hall	Viewed illness and rehabilitation as learning experiences in which the nurse's role was to guide and teach the patient through personal caregiving. Role involves therapeutic use of self (core), the treatment regimen of the health care team (cure), and nurturing and intimate bodily care (care).
Dorothy Johnson	A behavioral systems approach that focuses on health viewed as a state of equilibrium that the nurse assists in maintaining or balancing.
Imogene King	A model in which three open systems interact with the environment: personal, individual, and social. Nurse's role is to assist individual to perform daily activities and includes health promotion and maintenance. Involves goal attainment.
Madeleine Leininger	Focused on a caring model that must be practiced interpersonally. Emphasized a transcultural approach.
Myra Levine	Developed around the four concepts of conservation of energy, structural integrity, personal integrity, and social integrity. Supports a holistic approach to nursing based on recognition of the total response of the person to the interaction between the internal and external environment.
Betty Neuman	A systems model influenced by Gestalt theory, stress, and level of prevention. Employs lines of resistance and lines of defense in creating a healthy being. Nurses are to identify the stressors and assist the individual to respond. Involves primary, secondary, and tertiary prevention.
Dorothea Orem	Recognized as a self-care theory of nursing, supports the concept that each person has a need for the provision and management of self-care actions to achieve "constancy." When the individual is unable to provide these, a self-care deficit exists. The role of the nursing system is to help eliminate the self-care deficit through wholly compensatory, partially compensatory, or supportive-educative actions.
Martha Rogers	Includes complicated approaches to health that involve helicy, resonancy, and complementarity. The holistic individual moves through time and space as part of an expanding universe with potential states of maximum well-being. Nurses act to promote symphonic interaction between man and environment by repatterning the human and environmental fields.
Sister Calista Roy	Identified as an adaptation model that conceives of the individual as being in constant interaction with a changing environment, thus requiring adaptation. Four adaptive modes, or ways in which a person adapts, are identified through: (1) physiologic needs, (2) self-concept, (3) role function, and (4) interdependence relations. The nurse's role is to assess a patient's adaptive behaviors and the stimuli that may be affecting the person to manipulate the stimuli in such a way as to allow the patient to cope or adapt.

Stress adaptation models are based on concepts that view the person as adjusting or changing (adapting) to avoid situations (stressors) that would result in the disturbance of balance or equilibrium. The adaptation theory helps to explain how balance is maintained and therefore directs nursing actions. One often finds Sister Calista Roy's adaptation model and Betty Neuman's work included in this group, but both also may be considered systems models, as mentioned above.

One of the most recent classifications of theories is by energy fields. These theories, although developed earlier, received growing recognition during the 1980s. Included in this group are the works of Myra Levine, Joyce Fitzpatrick, Margaret Newman, and Martha Rogers.

Humanistic models are also fairly recent. These focus on man's humanness and needs for love, caring, personal meaning, and living in concert with the environment. Theorists noted for developing these theories include Jean Watson, Rosemarie Rizzo Parse, and Margaret Newman.

It is not our purpose to discuss and critique the many approaches to nursing theory. The student who wants to pursue nursing theorists further is encouraged to consult the section on further reading at the end of the chapter or follow links provided on the Web available at *www.enursescribe.com/nurse_theorists.htm*. Table 5-2 outlines the approaches of several recognized nursing theorists.

Critical Thinking Activity

Select one nursing theorist. Describe what you find interesting and attractive about her nursing theory. Give a rationale for your decision, and describe how using her theory might affect your practice of nursing.

Education Supporting Evidence-Based Practice

The term **evidence-based practice** has a variety of definitions and interpretations. Evolving from evidence-based medicine, it generally refers to the integration of the best evidence available into expert nursing care. It requires that nurses and other health care providers have access to the latest research, expert opinion, and understandings of cultural and personal values as a basis for planning and delivering nursing care. Evidence-based practice is discussed in detail in Chapter 6.

Key Concepts

- Three major avenues to preparation for licensure as a registered nurse exist in the United States: the hospital-based diploma, the university-based baccalaureate degree, and the associate degree (usually offered in community colleges). Many similarities exist among these programs. In addition, various nontraditional approaches to nursing education have evolved.
- Educational programs prepare nursing assistants and licensed practical (vocational) nurses for roles in the health care delivery system. As these programs have grown, greater oversight of the programs by approval bodies has occurred. The education of unlicensed assistive personnel can vary tremendously.
- The nursing shortage of the 1990s, coupled with recommendations or mandates from important groups, has resulted in greater creativity and collaboration in educational approaches.
- Master's and doctoral programs that prepare nurses for leadership positions in the profession continue to grow, with more emphasis on the master's degree for advanced practice. The actual degree awarded at the end of doctoral studies varies. A variety of new educational approaches to higher degrees in nursing has evolved.
- One of the most rapidly growing areas is that of advanced practice; this growth was accelerated by health care reform. Recommendations from major commissions have urged continued expansion of advanced practice programs and the educational qualifications for such positions.
- Continuing education, whether further education that results in a higher degree or rather in the form of classes, seminars, or workshops that update and increase expertise,

is being encouraged by more and more organizations. Staying current in practice is critical to safe client care.

- Many changes are occurring in nursing education. These include more emphasis on articulation and career ladder programs and a shift in educational settings from acute care facilities to community-based experiences.
- No change has affected nursing education as greatly as has the computer age. Entire programs can be completed on-line. Computer technology has changed the structure of the typical nursing classroom, and instructors prepare graduates who will be able to function in a health care environment that makes heavy use of computerized services.
- Nursing education has been influenced by the ANA position on nursing education that advocated the baccalaureate degree as the minimum educational preparation for professional practice. Many nursing educators, particularly those in diploma and associate degree programs, disagreed with this position. This issue may take on new life in the 21st century.
- Models for differentiated practice are being encouraged; these models recognize and use graduates according to the competencies inherent in the program from which they graduated.
- Nursing theories continue to influence nursing and nursing education. Nursing theories assist us in building a body of nursing knowledge and describing and defining nursing practice.
- The advent of evidence-based practice is impacting the curricula of nursing education programs.

Relevant Web Sites

American Association of Colleges of Nursing (AACN): *www.aacn.nche.edu*
American Association of Nurse Anesthetists (AANA): *www.aana.com*
American College of Nurse Midwives (ACNM): *www.acnm.org*
Commission on Collegiate Nursing Education (CCNE): *www.aacn.nche.edu/Accreditation*
National Council of State Boards of Nursing (NCSBN): *www.ncsbn.org*
National League for Nursing (NLN): *www.nln.org*
National League for Nursing Accreditation Commission (NLNAC): *www.nlnac.org*
National Organization for Associate Degree Nursing (NOADN): *www.noadn.org*
Nursing theorists: *www.enursescribe.com/nurse_theorists.htm*

References

American Association of Colleges of Nursing. (1995). *A model for differentiated nursing practice.* Washington, DC: Author.

American Association of Colleges of Nursing. (1998). *The essentials of baccalaureate nursing education for professional nursing practice.* Washington, DC: Author.

American Association of Colleges of Nursing. (2002). *Associate degree in nursing programs and AACN's support for articula-* tion. [On-line]. *www.aacn.nche.edu/Media/Backgrounders/ADNFacts.htm.* Accessed September 22, 2005.

American Association of Colleges of Nursing. (2004a). *Nursing fact sheet.* [On-line]. *www.aacn.nche.edu/Media/FactSheets/nursfact.htm.* Accessed March 30, 2006.

American Association of Colleges of Nursing (2004b). *AACN adopts a new vision for the future of nursing education and* practice. [On-line]. *www.aacn.nche.edu/Media/NewsReleases/DNPRelease.htm*. Accessed September 22, 2005.

American Association of Colleges of Nursing. (2004c). *AACN position statement on the practice doctorate in nursing*. [On-line]. *www.accn.nche.edu?DNP/DNPPositionStatement.htm*. Accessed September 22, 2005.

American Association of Colleges of Nursing. (2005a). *The essentials of baccalaureate education for professional nursing practice*. [On-line]. *www.aacn.nche.edu/Education/bacessn.htm*. Accessed September 22, 2005.

American Association of Colleges of Nursing. (2005b). *The clinical nurse leader*. [On-line]. *www.aacn.nche.edu/Media?FactSheets?CNLFactSheet.htm*. Accessed September 22, 2005.

American Association of Colleges of Nursing. (2005c). *Annual state of the schools: July 2003-June 2004*. [On-line]. *www.aacn.nche.edu/Media/pdf/annualreport04.pdf*. Accessed March 30, 2006.

American Association of Colleges of Nursing. (2005d). *Accelerated programs: the fast-track to careers in nursing*. [On-line]. *www.aacn.nche.edu/Publications/issues/Aug02.htm*. Accessed September 22, 2005.

American Association of Colleges of Nursing. (2005e). *Articulation agreements among nursing education programs*. [On-line]. *www.aacn.nche.edu/Media/FactSheets/AA.htm*. Accessed March 30, 2006.

American Nurses Association. (1965). American Nurses Association's first position on education for nursing. *American Journal of Nursing, 65*(12*)*, 106–107.

American Nurses Association. (1974). *Standards for continuing education for nursing*. Kansas City, MO: American Nurses Association.

American Nurses Association. (2000). *ANA reaffirms commitment to BSN for entry into practice-supports new certification program to be offered by ANCC*. [On-line]. *http://nursingworld. org/pressrel/2000/pr0225b.htm*. Accessed March 30, 2006.

Barter, M., & McFarland, P. L. (2001). BSN by 2010: A California initiative. *Journal of Nursing Administration, 31*(3), 141–144.

Bellack, J. P., & O'Neil, E. H. (2000). Recreating nursing practice for a new century. *Nursing and Health Care Perspectives 21*(1), 14-21.

Benner, P. (1984). From novice to expert. Menlo Park, CA: Addison-Wesley.

Boston, C. (1990). Differentiated practice: An introduction. In C. Boston, *Current issues and perspectives on differentiated practice* (pp. 1-3). Chicago: American Organization of Nurse Executives.

Brown, E. L. (1948). *Nursing for the future*. New York: Russell Sage Foundation.

Bureau of Labor Statistics, U.S. Department of Labor, *Occupational handbook, 2004-2005 edition, registered nurses*. [On-line]. *www.bls.gov/oco/ocos083.htm*. Accessed September 14, 2005.

de Tornyay, R. (1996). Critical challenges for nurse educators. *Journal of Nursing Education, 35*(4), 146-147.

Ellis, J. R., & Hartley, C. L. (2005). *Managing and Coordinating Nursing Care* (4th ed.). Philadelphia: Lippincott Williams & Wilkins.

Gosnell, D. J. (2002). Overview and summary: The 1965 entry into practice proposal-is it relevant today? *Online Journal of Issues in Nursing*. [Online]. *http://nursingworld.org/ojin/topic18/tpc18ntr.htm*. Accessed March 30, 2006.

Health Resources and Service Administration, Bureau of Health Professions. (2002). *The registered nurse population*: Findings from the 2000 national sample survey. Washington, DC: U.S. Department of Health and Human Services.

Kalisch, P. A., & Kalisch, B. J. (2004). *American nursing: A history* (4th ed.). Philadelphia: Lippincott Williams & Wilkins.

National Council of State Boards of Nursing. (1998). National council update. *Issues, 19*(4), 10-11, Chicago: Author.

National League for Nursing. (1990). Educational outcomes of associate degree nursing programs: Roles and competencies. (Publication No. 23-2348), Council of Associate Degree Programs, New York: Author.

National League for Nursing Accreditation Commission. (2004). *Interpretive guidelines for standards and criteria 2004: Associate degree programs in nursing*. New York: Author.

National Organization for Associate Degree Nursing. (2004). Associate degree nursing (ADN) facts. [On-line]. *www.noadn.org/and-facts.htm*. Accessed March 30, 2006.

Pew Health Professions Commission. (1995). *Critical challenges: Revitalizing the health professions for the twenty-first century*. San Francisco, CA: UCSF Center for the Health Professions.

Primm, P. L. (1987). Differentiated practice for ADN- and BSN-prepared nurses. *Journal of Professional Nursing, 3*(4), 218-225.

Riehl, J. P., & Roy S. C. (1974). *Conceptual models for nursing practice*. New York: Appleton-Century-Crofts.

Seymer, L. R. (1954). *Selected writings of Florence Nightingale*. New York: Macmillan.

U. S. Public Health Service. (1963). *Toward quality in nursing: Needs and goals. Report of the Surgeon Generals' Consultant Group on Nursing*. Washington, DC: U.S. Government Printing Office.

6

Nursing for the Future

LEARNING OUTCOMES

After completing this chapter, you should be able to:

1. Describe an effective strategy for evaluating information resources.
2. Discuss the value of the research in nursing.
3. Explain the role of the staff nurse in nursing research.
4. Explain the term "evidence-based practice" (EBP) and its application to nursing.
5. List the types of evidence that may be used for EBP, moving from the most reliable to the least reliable.
6. Outline a process for establishing an evidence-based nursing practice in an institutional setting or in your own personal practice.
7. Discuss the role of technology in nursing.
8. Assess your own competence in the realm of nursing technology.
9. Identify factors contributing to the shortage of nurses.
10. Assess the effect of the current nursing shortage on your own career path and your ability to practice effectively.

KEY TERMS

Computerized order entry
Computerized physician order entry
Control group
Convenience sample
Dependent variable
e-ICU
Evidence-based practice (EBP)
Experimental group
Hypothesis
Independent variable

Informatics
Information technology
Informed consent
Institutional review board (IRB)
Level of significance
Nursing supply
Nursing demand
Participant
Population
Probability

Qualitative research
Quantitative research
Random sample
Randomized controlled trial (RCT)
Reliability
Sample
Subject
Telehealth
Validity
Variable

As you look toward the future, it is hard to imagine what nursing will be like. What new insights will nursing research bring? What expectations for practice responsibilities will rest with each nurse? How will evidence-based practice (EBP) change nursing? What technology will be a part of nursing practice? What is happening in regard to the shortage of nurses? How will the nursing shortage affect your practice? While we do not have the ability to predict the future, looking at trends and some of the concerns that are surfacing may help you consider how you can be prepared to move into future practice.

VALUING NURSING RESEARCH

In this brief section of text, it is not possible to present all the information you would need in order to effectively read and understand nursing research. If you are in a baccalaureate nursing program, a course in statistics and one in understanding nursing research are usually requirements. While a course in nursing research is usually not an essential part of associate degree (AD) education, more AD programs are presenting a brief introduction to research as the emphasis on EBP increases in all settings. Many students come to AD nursing having taken courses related to statistics research in other fields. Here we will provide an overview of the development of research for nursing practice along with some basic concepts and information to guide your reading.

The Development of Nursing Research

Nursing research essentially began after World War II, when academic nursing programs expanded rapidly. Nurses began obtaining graduate degrees and learning how to conduct research. *Nursing Research*, which began in 1951, was the first nursing publication to focus on research. Gradually more journals, both in the United States and in the United Kingdom and Canada, began to focus on nursing research. Table 6-1 provides an overview of the nursing research journals available and the dates they were first published to help you see how nursing research has grown. In addition to the journals, whose total content is research, many other nursing journals devote a significant number of their pages to research along with articles related to policy and current practice descriptions. This increase in nursing research publications has been a reflection of the increasing emphasis of the profession on scholarly work and the growing number of nurses academically prepared to conduct effective research.

For many individuals, a key landmark along the path toward a research-based profession was the authorization of the National Center for Nursing Research (NCNR) in 1986 (National Institute of Nursing Research [NINR], n.d.). Prior to this, nursing research was found in a variety of federal endeavors, such as the Division of Nursing within the Office of the Surgeon General and the various sections with the National Institutes of Health (NIH). While the NCNR was an important milestone for nursing research, it did not have the prestige or funding that was provided for the NIH. Based on an increasing recognition of the importance of nursing research, the NCNR was changed into a full-fledged NINR within the NIH in 1993 (NINR, n.d.). In October 2005, the NINR celebrated its 20th anniversary at a national nursing research conference.

Each October, a conference titled the National Congress on the State of the Science in Nursing is held in Washington DC. Close to 800 individuals attend this conference. This is a reflection of the number of nurse researchers and the status of nursing research. In 2004, the

TABLE 6-1	INITIAL PUBLICATION DATES FOR NURSING RESEARCH JOURNALS
YEAR OF FIRST PUBLICATION	**RESEARCH JOURNAL**
1951	*Nursing Research*
1968	*Journal of Nursing Scholarship: International* (Sigma Theta Tau)
1969	*Canadian Journal of Nursing Research*
1976	*Journal of Advanced Nursing* (UK)
1979	*Western Journal of Nursing Research*
1988	*Applied Nursing Research*
1991	*Clinical Nursing Research* (Canadian editors)
1992	*Nurse Researcher: The International Journal of Research Methodology in Nursing and Health Care* (UK)
1993	*Online Journal of Knowledge Synthesis for Nursing*
1995	*International Journal of Psychiatric Nursing Research*
1995	*Journal of Nursing Research* (UK)
1998	*Evidence Based Nursing Online Journal* (UK)
2000	*BMC Nursing Online* (UK)
2000	*Southern Online Journal Of Nursing Research: Electronic Publication Of Research (http://snrs.org/publications/journal.html)*
2004	*World Views on Evidence Based Nursing (www.blackwell-synergy.com/links/toc/wvn/1/1)*

opening address of this conference emphasized the role of nurses in leading interdisciplinary research teams and recognized the fact that 50% of NINR-funded research is published in non-nursing journals. Nursing research truly is patient-oriented research and supports goals of improved health outcomes for the nation (Kennedy, 2004). In 2006 the conference's focus was "Nursing Research–Improving Life: Development and Dissemination of Nursing Innovation."

An Overview of the Nursing Research Process

A research study begins with one unanswered question. Literature is reviewed thoroughly to determine what is already known about the question. The question is then refined based on the knowledge available and identified **variables** (things in the setting that vary or change) and questions about how they are inter–related. In a traditional research study, a **hypothesis** (statement of the expected relationships) is established. A research study is designed to gather information that will help to answer the question. The study is carried out carefully, and afterward the information collected is analyzed. Any concerns with the study are presented. Then the researcher reaches a conclusion about what has been learned from the study, discusses the application of the study to nursing, and identifies further research needed. See Display 6-1.

A group of individuals within the institution who have research expertise is appointed to review research proposals and assure that they conform to standardized guidelines. This group

---

Display 6-1   Steps of the Traditional Nursing Research Process

- Developing the research question
- Reviewing the literature
- Developing the hypothesis
- Designing the study
- Carrying out the study

- Analyzing the data
- Identifying concerns about the study
- Drawing conclusions and applications
- Identifying future research needed

---

is usually titled the **institutional review board (IRB)**, and it oversees the entire research process in any organization. The IRB determines whether the question is appropriate, the means of study fit the question, the study is ethical, and most especially, the rights of any subjects or participants are protected (see discussion of participants below). No research is allowed in an institution that has not been approved by the institution's review board. For research that occurs outside of institutions, private organizations serve as review boards to ensure the protection of the public.

While this greatly oversimplifies the research process, it provides a foundation to help you understand some of the important concepts and terms in nursing research we are about to discuss.

Basic Research Terminology

The **independent variable** in a research study can be controlled by the researcher and is applied, or manipulated, to determine its effect on the **dependent variable**. The dependent variable is the phenomenon being studied. In health care, the dependent variable is usually a health problem of some kind.

Validity refers to the ability of the research to actually measure or accurately describe the variables in the study. A physical measure, such as blood pressure, may easily be shown to be valid. However, the device used for measuring, such as the particular blood pressure cuff, must be checked for accuracy. Questionnaires must also be examined for validity. For example, a questionnaire that purports to measure depression (such as by numbering severity using a scale of 1–10 or by using words indicating severity: none, mild, moderate, and severe) must have evidence that it really is measuring depression. The concern also arises that a questionnaire may be valid in one group (such as college-educated students on whom it was tested) and not valid in another group (such as clients with limited education who may not understand the terminology used in the questionnaire). There are many different processes for establishing validity in the setting in which the research is conducted. An important role of the researcher is determining the appropriate method for demonstrating validity of the research.

Reliability refers to the ability of the research instrument or tool to yield consistently the same results over repeated testing periods. Again there are multiple methods for establishing the reliability of any instrument, and the researcher must establish the reliability of any instrument used. Reliability and validity are closely related and often are discussed together.

In a study, the **population** is the entire group of people affected by the problem under scrutiny. The **sample** is that small group of people who will actually be studied. How representative the sample is of the entire population is one factor affecting whether the study will be useful. Selecting a **random sample** involves some type of nonbiased approach to selecting the individuals from the population that ensures that all persons in the population have an equal and independent chance of being chosen to be sampled. The use of a random sample increases the likelihood that the sample adequately represents the population. This often is not possible, and a **convenience sample** (a group that may be conveniently accessed) is used. The **subject** or **participant** is the individual person in the sample. Although the term "subject" has been traditionally used, many people now encourage the use of the term "participant" to emphasize the choice that is made to be in the study and the important partnership that occurs.

At least two groups of participants are usually formed. One group is considered the **control group**, sometimes also referred to as the comparison group. The control group will not receive any special treatment or procedure being studied. The **experimental group**, however, will receive the new treatment or procedure. Sometimes there are multiple experimental groups to test different treatments, but one group continues to be the control group that demonstrates the outcome if no treatment is given. In some instances, having no treatment is not possible. In such cases, two or more treatments might be compared. For example, if the focus of the study was the effectiveness of treatments of pressure ulcers, it would be unethical to not treat a pressure ulcer at all. Therefore, the study might compare different methods of treatment to determine the most successful one. Assigning individuals to the groups using a random method may be done even if the sample selected is not random.

An essential part of any research study is the provision for **informed consent** of the participants. Informed consent for research has the same attributes as informed consent for medical treatment. The individual must be informed of both potential risks and potential benefits of participating. The researcher must disclose that the participant may or may not receive the treatment under consideration. As part of the consent process, any restrictions on other types of health care that may occur while in the study must also be disclosed. Participation must be voluntary, with no adverse consequences occurring if subjects choose not to participate. Further, participants must be informed of their right to withdraw from the study at any time without needing a reason for doing so.

Quantitative Research

Quantitative research refers to a study in which items can be counted or measured and statistics can be used to analyze the results. There are many types of quantitative studies, but in experimental research, in which a new or different treatment is given to a sample group, it is important to demonstrate in an objective way the effectiveness of the treatment being studied.

The Randomized Controlled Trial. The type of experimental research emphasized most often in medicine is the double-blind, randomized controlled trial, often referred to more simply as the **randomized controlled trial (RCT)**. Double-blind means that neither the participant receiving the treatment nor the person administering the treatment knows whether the participant is receiving the real or active treatment or a placebo. Randomized indicates that the participants are assigned to either the treatment group or the control group by some type of random process. Controlled, as we have discussed, means that there is both a treatment group and a group that does not receive the treatment (Fig 6-1).

FIGURE 6-1   Double-blind random controlled trials are often not possible when researching nursing care.

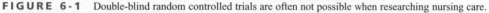

EXAMPLE

A Double-Blind Randomized Controlled Trial

Pharmaceutical Company X is testing a new medication for joint pain. People are asked to participate in the research study. They are informed about the study in detail, and they are told that there will be a random control group which will not receive any actual medication. Those agreeing to participate are asked to not take any other medication for joint pain during the study. The researcher uses a random number table to assign the individuals to the two groups: one that receives the new medication and one that will not. Those not receiving the medication will receive an identical tablet that is an inert substance (a placebo). The knowledge of which persons are receiving the active medication is not shared with either the participants themselves or with those who distribute the medications to the patients. All participants are evaluated for joint pain on a regular schedule using the same pain assessment tools. Those assessing the participants do not know who has received the active medication. At the end of the trial, the pain scores over time will be analyzed statistically to determine whether the new medication had a significant effect on joint pain.

RCT research is valued for determining appropriate medical care. Although this might be the best evidence for choosing a medical therapy or drug, even within medicine this emphasis is narrow. RCTs are often impossible for testing the nature of nursing. One cannot hide from a patient that he or she is receiving extra or different nursing care. Nursing activities such as special education, spending time on psychosocial interactions, or even monitoring more frequently are all highly visible to patients and providers. Further, an RCT would not be able to accurately capture individual settings for care, the skills of the practitioners, or the attributes of the individual patient, which include cultural background, expectations, preferences, and abilities.

Other Types of Quantitative Research. There are a variety of other types of quantitative research that may be more useful for nursing. It is sometimes possible to have a treatment group and a control group to be studied that occur naturally (ie, existing by nature and without artificial aid), rather than assigned as randomized groups. Research may be done by studying the same sample of people across time; this is called a longitudinal study. Other types of quantitative research studies include descriptive studies that collect naturally occurring data such as infection rates or complication rates. Methodological research is another type of quantitative research that is used to develop research instruments.

Analysis of Quantitative Research. Quantitative studies are analyzed using statistical techniques. In a statistical test, the aim is to determine whether any difference between the control group and the experimental group may be due to chance rather than to the effect of the treatment. There are many statistical tests, but most result in the determination of the **probability** of the result occurring by chance. The probability is expressed as a decimal fraction. For example, a probability of <0.10 means that there is less than a 0.10 or 10% possibility that the result was due to chance. A probability of <0.01 means that there is less than 0.01 or 1% possibility that the result was due to chance.

Often a researcher sets a **level of significance** ahead of time. The level of significance is the level at which the researcher believes that the study results most likely represent a non-chance event. A level of significance of <0.01 (less than a 1% probability that the result is due to chance) is commonly used. A result that meets the appropriate level of significance is often referred to as a "significant" result.

Statistical significance is not the same as clinical significance. While the effect of the treatment might have made a change, this change may not make a difference in the outcome for the patient. Clinical significance relates to the effect on actual patient outcomes.

Qualitative Research

Qualitative research involves studying phenomena as they naturally occur. By doing this, the researcher achieves a "more comprehensive, contextual understanding of the topic in question" (Ellis & Hartley, 2005, p. 403). Qualitative research in nursing is frequently used to gain greater understanding of the experience of the patient and family and may help the nurse to identify areas to explore with the client and family. This type of research may include interviews, lengthy observations, and detailed case histories. Analysis of qualitative research attempts to find themes within the data.

Types of Qualitative Research. Specific types of qualitative research include phenomenology, ethnography, case studies, and life histories.

In phenomenology, extensive and unstructured interviews are conducted with a limited number of participants. The goal is identify the themes and patterns within their discussions. Phenomenology frequently results in extensive descriptive discussions of the "lived experience" of persons with a certain health concern.

Case studies and life histories provide detailed information about a single individual. These may serve as an example that will present the various concerns and potential health professional responses. Case studies help the reader to see the specific and particular circumstances of the individual more clearly and then apply that same comprehensive inquiry to their patients. A life history helps the nurse to understand how a health problem might fit into an entire life.

Analysis of Qualitative Research. Analysis of qualitative research differs from analysis of quantitative research. No statistical tests are used, and there is no effort made to try to determine probability in regard to the information.

The analysis of the data gathered in a qualitative study involves an extensive immersion of the researcher into the data to begin to detect themes and patterns. The report is usually a lengthy narrative discussion with the liberal use of quotations from the data to illustrate the topic being presented. Some qualitative research results in the development of conceptual models of relationships. The results of a qualitative research study enable the reader to gain increased depth of understanding about the research topic.

A Staff Nurse's Role in the Research Process

For the results of nursing research to be successful, it must be carried out by an individual who has the educational background to thoroughly understand and direct the process. This may be a nurse with a master's degree; but for large studies, for funded research, and in large institutions, the principal researcher is usually a nurse with a doctorate. The research itself is most often conducted by a team that includes individuals who provide the treatment (if this is a part of the research design), those who collect the data, and specialists in statistics who assist with data analysis. The staff nurse may fulfill a treatment role or a data collection role in this process.

A major role for staff nurses is to identify questions or problems. Within an institution, there may be a specific method for a staff nurse to communicate questions to an individual or a committee that might plan research. If you believe a topic should be studied, do not be concerned if your question is not clearly formulated. Any question will need refinement and reconsideration as it goes through the process. Your question may just be the beginning of gathering important information.

Another role of the staff nurse is to guard the welfare of the patients for whom he or she cares. This means asking questions to be sure the research proposed has gone through the appropriate institutional processes before agreeing to participate as a data gatherer or the nurse providing the research intervention. There should be a formal consent process that is clear to the participants. Just as the staff nurse is not responsible for medical consent, the staff nurse is not responsible for research consent. If patients who have agreed to participate exhibit ambivalence or uncertainty about participating, do not try to convince them to participate. Ask the person from the research team who is managing consents to speak with concerned patients about the study. Patients do have the freedom to withdraw from a research study at any time. Additionally, nurses need to be sure that effective care can be provided to the patient. For example, they need to be able to assess for possible side effects or adverse reactions. Protocols for managing such side effects must be in place for patient protection.

■■■ **COMMUNICATION IN** *ACTION*
■■

A Staff Nurse's Concern About Consent

Isabel Andretti was a staff nurse on the oncology unit at a large hospital where a double-blind controlled trial of a new medication was being researched. The researcher had talked with the potential participants and obtained consent. When Isabel went in to administer the first dose of the study medication to Mrs. Wilson, Mrs. Wilson asked, "Can you explain what this research thing is all about? I didn't understand half of what that woman said when she was here." Isabel said, "Tell me what you do know." Mrs. Wilson explained, "Well, I am going to get this new medicine, but I wonder if it is dangerous. Do you think it is?" Isabel then said, "That is a good question, and you should have an answer before we start this. The best person to explain this is the researcher in charge of this project. We will wait to give you this medication until she has talked with you again and you have made your decision about participating. We don't want you to agree to something you don't understand." Isabel immediately left the room and called the researcher. She explained to the researcher, "Mrs. Wilson, who signed the consent forms for the research project, just said that she did not understand what this was all about. She did not seem to understand that she might not be receiving the new medication, and she was concerned about whether it was dangerous. I know that you talked with her before, but she seems not to have been able to process the information you gave. I am holding the first dose that was due to be given to her until you are able to talk with her again. When do you think you might be able to discuss her concerns with her?"

Using research in practice is perhaps the most important role of the staff nurse. The process of using research in practice is discussed below as part of evidence-based nursing.

EVIDENCE-BASED PRACTICE IN NURSING

One major thrust for the future of nursing revolves around the development of **evidence-based practice (EBP)**. EBP first began in medicine and is expanding to all of health care. EBP in nursing is being instituted in many health care organizations.

Establishing a Definition of Evidence-Based Nursing

DiCenso, Cullum, and Ciliska (1998, p. 38) provide a comprehensive definition for evidence-based nursing: "Evidence based nursing practice is clinical decision making based on the best available scientific evidence, combined with clinical nursing expertise, and considering patient preferences and available resources." This definition provides an excellent foundation both for the individual nurse and for the institution to establish evidence-based nursing practice (Display 6-2).

Let us examine this definition carefully. The major focus is on clinical decision making. Nurses are accountable for decisions, and they need to base those decisions on supporting evidence, not custom or habit. Another significant part of this definition is the emphasis on clinical nursing expertise. The expertise of nurses in applying information to the care of specific patients is essential. Nurses have an obligation to continually work to improve their own knowledge base and ability to identify appropriate applications of information to specific patient situations.

An important aspect found in the DiCenso definition is the autonomy of the client. This supports views set forth by Melnyk (2004), who suggests that patient values and preferences should always be added to any discussion of the use of EBP. Although the definition states "patient," this can be expanded to consider the client, whether that is the individual, family, or community.

An issue included in this definition is the consideration of the available resources. This would include both human and material resources and is strongly related to the cost effectiveness

Display 6-2   Evidence-Based Nursing Practice

"Clinical decision making based on the best available scientific evidence, combined with clinical nursing expertise, and considering patient preferences and available resources."

From DiCenso, A., Cullum, N., & Ciliska, D. (1998). Implementing evidence based nursing: Some misconceptions [Editorial]. *Evidence Based Nursing, 1*, 38.

of an intervention. Rodwin (2001) points out that cost effectiveness constrains decisions that individual patients make, as well as the decisions made by health care providers. The individual patient may decide that the marginal difference between a new brand-name wound therapy and the older therapy is not worth several hundreds of dollars a month in costs. A system itself may reject providing certain high-cost options that demonstrate marginal improvement in outcomes. The human resources needed for implementation of some therapies may critically change the cost-effectiveness data. For example, some expensive wound management products may so significantly reduce nursing time and shorten the days of hospitalization that they are, in fact, still cost effective. Thus considering cost effectiveness is critical for nursing.

Determining Adequate Evidence

This brings us to the question of what constitutes adequate evidence upon which to base practice. Melnyk and Fineout-Overholt (2005) provide a rating system for examining the hierarchy of evidence that might be used as a basis for evidence-based nursing practice (see Display 6-3). RCTs stand at the top of this list, with types of research studies encompassing the first four levels

Display 6-3   Commonly Used Rating System for the Hierarchy of Evidence

Level I: Evidence from a systematic review or meta-analysis of all relevant randomized controlled trails (RCTs), or evidence-based clinical practice guidelines based on systematic reviews of RCTs.
Level II: Evidence obtained from at least one well-designed RCT.
Level III: Evidence obtained from well-designed controlled trials without randomization.
Level IV: Evidence from well-designed case-control and cohort studies.
Level V: Evidence from systematic reviews of descriptive and qualitative studies.
Level VI: Evidence from a single descriptive or qualitative study.
Level VII: Evidence from the opinion of authorities and/or reports of expert committees.

From Melnyk, B. M., & Fineout-Overholt, E. (2005). *Evidence based practice in nursing & healthcare. A guide to best practices*. Philadelphia: Lippincott Williams & Wilkins.

Display 6-4   Sources Used for Evidence-Based Nursing Practice

1. Research reports of all types
2. Retrospective or concurrent chart reviews
3. Quality improvement, risk management, and benchmarking data
4. International, national, and local standards or guidelines developed by expert panels evaluating a variety of information resources
5. Infection control data
6. Pathophysiology information
7. Cost-effectiveness analysis
8. Patient preferences
9. Clinical expertise of individuals

of evidence. Qualitative studies and single descriptive studies, as well as reports of expert committees, are included at the end of the list. Qualitative studies are often used in nursing because they are more likely to reveal the patient's perception of the problem or of the intervention. This attention to patient preferences is impossible in the RCT.

While the Melnyk & Fineout-Overholt list (2005) provides a good starting point, nursing generally relies on a broader array of evidence for determining the best practice for a nursing situation. Display 6-4 provides a list of the types of evidence commonly used to support nursing practice. Although they are in an approximate order of reliability, there is not a clear-cut hierarchy. Research reports (the first on the list) include all the types of research that are listed in Display 6-3 as Levels I to VI. Retrospective or concurrent chart reviews, quality improvement, risk management, and benchmarking data are all site specific and useful to nurses.

Guidelines for practice developed by groups of experts based upon the best available evidence are a useful tool for EBP. These panels of experts—whether international, national, or local—use a variety of evidence and information resources as they seek to determine best practices. Their guidelines may be an excellent source for nursing decision making. The Agency for Healthcare Research and Quality (AHRQ) convenes expert panels to develop guidelines for some situations of common concern. It also maintains a clearinghouse of guidelines that have been developed by other authoritative groups. These guidelines may be accessed on AHRQ's Web site at *www.ahrq.gov* and are an excellent resource for staff nurses seeking to use EBP.

Infection control data provides an important foundation for nursing decision making as well. For example, the infection control data of an individual setting may be stronger evidence for the effectiveness of a certain practice than a research study conducted in a very different setting. The infection control data reflects this individual setting with its providers, patient population, and physical set-up. In the same way, quality improvement data may help an institution to target its own processes in a way that an RCT might not.

Shine (2001, in the second paragraph of the Web page section titled "The Meaning Of Evidence And The Practice Of Evidence Based Medicine") points out that "evidence of an effect under ideal conditions, such as double-blind, randomized controlled trials, and 'effectiveness,' evidence of what actually works in practice, is a subtle and important one for all users of evidence." Real life situations lack the controls of research studies. Both patients and health care settings are more varied than typical research subjects and settings. Patients often have multiple health problems and confounding interactions that make their situations unique. Issues such as patients' view of quality of life profoundly affect decisions about appropriate health care. Health care settings have differing resources, both material and human.

Nurses must also face the reality that there is **no** evidence regarding some aspects of nursing practice. One cannot just delay making decisions and withhold care until data are forthcoming. That is why the list in Display 6-4 also contains the use of basic scientific information in regard to pathophysiology.

Patient values and preferences are unique to each patient situation, although there may be trends across patient populations treated in some settings. An understanding of these values and preferences may guide decisions about what interventions to investigate. In some situations, patient preferences may rise to the top of the list of appropriate evidence when a decision must be made and may outweigh all other evidence.

EXAMPLE

Ensuring the Inclusion of Patient Preference In Evidence-Based Practice

Mildred Ogilvie was a 78-year-old woman diagnosed with multiple myeloma. A meeting between Mildred, her oncologist, her husband of 54 years, her family physician, and her primary nurse was scheduled after Mildred had failed to respond to the chemotherapy initially prescribed. During this meeting, the oncologist presented the option of a stem cell transplant. He explained that the statistics for successful treatment were not excellent, but that this was the only option left. He then presented the risks, side effects, and benefits of the proposed treatment, along with a detailed analysis of the information. He emphasized that she had good health before this diagnosis and no co-existing health problems, which would help the situation. Her insurance company had been contacted and it would fund this care. To everyone's surprise, Mrs. Ogilvie said, "No, I really don't want to go through anymore treatment. I have had enough." She was then given more reasons why this was a good treatment option and the evidence for possible success was presented more strongly. The oncologist asked her husband to help convince her that she should have this treatment. Mrs. Ogilvie turned to her husband and said, "Dan, help me. I cannot do this." Her husband turned to the oncologist and said, "I don't want to lose her, but I can't ask her to do what she doesn't want to do." The oncologist began again to discuss the treatment. When he paused, the primary nurse spoke up. "I think that Mrs. Ogilvie has clearly told us what she wants. I think they both understand the consequences that you have so clearly explained. Perhaps now is the time to give them privacy so they can talk about the situation together." This nurse recognized that the patient's decision and values were going to be the determining factor and was supporting their autonomy in decision making.

The expertise of the staff is also a factor in determining the most appropriate practice. Expert staff members may attend conferences, read widely, and access resources that they then may use when problem solving in regard to appropriate nursing interventions. Additionally, the expertise of the staff is a factor in deciding whether certain types of actions can be implemented.

When looking for evidence, many believe this to be an entirely scientific inquiry. There is an element of politics in examining evidence for practice. That means that there are competing interests involved as well as simply the evidence. Rodwin (2001) points out that evidence is rarely so clear that there is no room for differences of opinion in regard to the meaning of the evidence. When decisions involve competing values such as safety, quality of life, length of life, or cost, the process of determining the appropriate path becomes complex. Managed care organizations, insurance providers, and hospitals may make some decisions based on their own best interests more than those of the client. Nurses need to be aware of these political factors and recognize that adopting a new EBP may require astute attention to the politics of the setting.

The Evidence-Based Practice Process

Many different models for evidence-based nursing practice have been developed. One of the first was the Conduct and Utilization of Research in Nursing Project in the late 1970s, which was designed to encourage the translation of nursing research into practice (Twin Cities Evidence-Based Health Care Project, 2001). Later in the 1980s, the Stetler Model of Research Utilization was developed as a process for the individual to incorporate research into practice (Twin Cities Evidence-Based Health Care Project, 2001). The Iowa Model of Research in Practice, developed in the 1990s, grew out of the quality improvement process and was designed for institutions moving toward EBP. That model has been broadened into the Iowa Model of Evidence Based Practice to Promote Quality Care (Titler et al., 2001), The Iowa Model has been the basis for the project in evidence-based care at the University of Iowa Hospitals and Clinics from which many publications on specific evidence-based projects have arisen. Many institutions and specialty nursing organizations are developing or adopting their own model of instituting EBP. All of these models have features in common in regard to the process of identifying and using evidence to support practice.

At the University of North Carolina (UNC), a simple rubric of "5 As" has been established to stimulate individuals to adopt EBP. The steps in this rubric are "Ask, Acquire, Analyze (or Appraise), Apply, and Assess" (UNC, n.d.). See Display 6-5. These words relate to a process first described by Flemming (1998.)

For the beginner, the University of North Carolina model is easy to understand and follow. You may use this process to improve your own practice, but, more important, a group of nurses may use it to establish an EBP protocol or procedure. The use of the UNC model is described below.

Display 6-5   The Five A's Of The Evidence-Based Practice Process

Ask   Convert information needs from practice into focused, structured questions.

Acquire   Use the focused questions as a basis for literature searching in order to identify relevant external evidence from research and to identify relevant internal data from quality improvement, risk management, or infection control data.

Analyze   Critically analyze the evidence found for validity and the ability to generalize it.

Apply   Use the best available evidence alongside clinical expertise, the patient's perspective, and knowledge of available resources to plan care.

Assess   Evaluate performance through a process of self reflection, audit, or peer assessment.

Adapted from University of North Carolina. (n.d.). *Evidence Based Nursing*. [On-line]. *http://www.hsl.unc.edu/services/tutorials/ebn/practice.htm*. Retrieved February 16, 2006. And from Flemming, K. (1998) Asking answerable questions. *Evidence Based Nursing*, 1 (2), 36–37.

Asking Appropriate Questions

The first step, "Ask," involves developing a clear, focused question. This is essential to obtaining the information needed for decision making. Vague questions about "best care for [any given health problem]" are seldom helpful. Flemming (1998) suggested that a good question has three parts: the situation, the intervention under consideration, and the desired outcome. It should be framed to address a specific clinical problem in order to facilitate the literature search but at the same time remain focused on the patient or the patient population. The situation might be for an individual patient or for a group of patients.

> **EXAMPLE**
>
> **Developing a Question Regarding Nursing Practice**
> A staff nurse frequently cared for patients with long-term central intravenous (IV) catheters. All the patients with long-term IV catheters became her "population" of interest. The nurse had read about several approaches to caring for these catheters. One of the complications she had observed was catheter-related septicemia. The results of these serious infections were often life threatening. The interventions of interest were the various ones that had been presented in the literature for catheter care. The outcome of concern was the incidence of catheter-related infection. The question might be stated as, "What is the most effective central venous catheter care for preventing infection in individuals with a long-term central venous catheter in place?"

Thompson, Cullum, McCaughan, Sheldon, and Raynor (2004) identified a variety of decision-making questions that often face nurses. The effectiveness of the intervention may be the one that is thought of most often. Other questions relate to the timing of the intervention. Still others relate to referral patterns. Questions regarding assessment strategies are important. Which assessments provide clinically relevant data and which are merely custom? How frequently should assessments be done? Another category of questions are those that relate to communication and teaching strategies. Nurses must continually strive to find the most effective ways to communicate with and teach clients in order to achieve the desired outcomes.

Acquiring Information for Decision Making

The next step is to "Acquire" information related to the concern. This requires a systematic review of the literature in your search for scientific evidence to answer the question. You need to be able to access and effectively use information resources in order to gather the needed data. The information might include research studies, practice guidelines produced by authoritative bodies, infection control data from one's own institution, benchmarking data regarding infection of central venous catheters from other institutions, information on processes used in other settings along with their infection control data, and costs (both human and material) of processes that are suggested. Haynes (2005) states that original studies; syntheses of studies, such as those available from agencies such as the Cochrane Review; evidence-based journal articles; and computerized data support systems may all be appropriate sources of information. Gathering all this information may require the collaboration from many people and consultation with a reference librarian and those responsible for budgeting for supplies. A team approach often is set up to include relevant contributors to the data-gathering process. Accessing information for practice is discussed later in this chapter.

Analyzing Information for Application

After the information is acquired, it's time for "Analysis." Analysis of a whole group of research studies is challenging. Often a clinical nurse specialist or other advanced practice nurse takes the lead in analyzing the research data. You will want to determine that the research studied is valid, relevant, and can appropriately be applied to the given situation. Analysis does not end with traditional analysis of the research studies. There must be an integrative approach in which all the data are examined in relationship to other data. You must consider resources, your own patient population, and how this might fit with patient preferences. The analysis results in a decision about a course of action. Again, a group discussion to analyze the data may be most productive. One result of analysis may be that no change is warranted. If that is the case, then the analysis and report need to be written so that it can be accessed by others at a later time if a change is again contemplated.

Applying New Information

When the analysis has been completed and it has identified a need for a change in practice, then preparations are made to "Apply" the new information. A protocol or procedure must be developed or adopted and a plan for implementation is needed. Will this plan be implemented for the entire facility, for a particular unit or units, or as a pilot project in one area with a decision about the entire facility made after results of the pilot are completed? How will this change in practice be introduced? When will it be introduced? What steps will be taken to ensure that the patient's values and desires are considered? Are resources available? The application of a new intervention needs the thoughtful use of information related to change and how change can be implemented.

Assessing Outcomes of New Practices

Introducing the change by itself is not enough, however. The next step is to "Assess" the change using the quality improvement process in place in the institution. It may involve assessing the response of a single patient or of a group of patients. Is the desired outcome being achieved? What are the strengths as well as the drawbacks of the change in practice? Are nurses committed to the change in practice?

Individual Accountability for Evidence-Based Practice

While this discussion has focused on the EBP process for an institution as a whole, individual nurses also have accountability for EBP. Nurses increasingly find the expectation that they must be critical decision makers in their own practice. This requires an ongoing commitment to asking questions and choosing paths.

The nurse as an employee, not an independent practitioner, has an obligation to identify how a change in personal practice will affect others and the system. Part of applying a new nursing intervention or assessment process may involve consulting with others, especially with the nurse manager. What may be needed is for the individual nurse to become the change agent to affect the practice within the system (see Chapter 14 on leading change).

Example of the Use of Infection Control Data for Evidence-Based Nursing

The manager of an intensive care unit (ICU) was contacted by the infection control nurse of the hospital about the series of urinary tract infections that had been identified in patients in that unit. All had had the same strain of serratia as the infective agent, and one patient in the unit was currently infected. A committee was appointed to review data and make recommendations. The committee identified that all patients had had indwelling urinary catheters and all had been in the same "pod" in the ICU. In addition, there were no infections among the patients who had been having hourly urine measurements. The staff members were interviewed in regard to care practices for patients with catheters. One interviewer talked with a nursing assistant who worked nights. This nursing assistant explained that he was responsible for emptying the urinary drainage bags when intake and output were measured at the end of the shift. When asked carefully about his technique, he revealed that he would commonly obtain one measuring container and use it as he moved from patient to patient. All measuring containers were immediately removed for cultures and replaced with clean ones. Education in using a measuring container for only one patient was provided along with the rationale for that action. Subsequent results revealed that the container for the infected patient cultured positive for the serratia. Using this container could easily have transmitted the organism to another patient's catheter, and the infectious agent could be spread from patient to patient in this manner.

Barriers to Evidence-Based Nursing Practice

Although the production of nursing research has grown, the use of nursing research as well as other types of evidence to inform practice has not moved forward as quickly as some nursing leaders would like This has its roots in many different issues.

Access to Information Resources

Factors affecting nurses are the availability of information resources and the access to search capabilities. Many people mistakenly believe that all needed information is available without charge on-line. While many government sources of information, such as guidelines through the AHRQ and the Medline database, are available at no charge, the majority of databases that provide full text articles require subscriptions for on-line access. Subscribing to one or more journals in your field provides some information for practice, but most nurses will find that they need the resources of a good library to find and retrieve all the information they need.

Academic medical centers may have a wide array of resources; however, there are many hospitals and other employment settings with little or no access. The libraries in smaller hospitals have historically focused on supporting medical practice rather than nursing practice. Some hospitals and nursing homes have blocked any Internet access in order to deter inappropriate use and create a stronger firewall against unauthorized entry into their own computer system. The side effect of this action is decreased access to on-line resources for staff.

Lack of Time for Seeking Information Resources

Within most employment settings for nurses, there is no time in the workday to seek new information for practice. While general reading in one's field may be appropriately expected to occur on one's own time, seeking specific information regarding a patient currently receiving care would seem appropriate to the workplace. Integrating this need into a very busy workplace is a challenge.

Lack of Background in Understanding and Valuing Research

Another issue that may affect the utilization of all types of evidence is the fact that the largest number of currently practicing nurses received their nursing education in an AD or diploma program in which the research process was not emphasized. Without an academic background in research understanding and utilization, these nurses may find it challenging to effectively interpret research results and weigh that research against other evidence. This suggests that having nurses work in teams to evaluate evidence for practice might alleviate this concern as those with greater knowledge and expertise in research evaluation take a leadership role. Baccalaureate- and master's-prepared nurses who have a more in-depth background can be effective leaders for this process.

An ongoing concern is whether nurses are committed to supporting the use of research and other evidence to improve their practice. If nurses do not value and support the development of nursing research in their own settings, nursing as a profession will be hampered in its growth (Fig. 6-2).

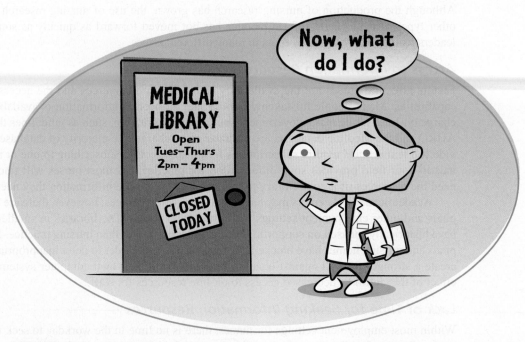

FIGURE 6-2   The lack of resources may be a barrier to evidence-based nursing practice.

Critical Thinking Activity

In the facility in which you have clinical experience, research the resources available for EBP. Is there a library? What resources for nursing in terms of databases, references, journals, and so forth are available? Can a nurse access the Internet? If so, what are the rules or restrictions? Does the institution have a committee or committees that have responsibilities in terms of evidence-based nursing practice? Are there nurse specialists who provide support and guidance for EBP? Analyze the resources and try to determine whether the resources are sufficient to meet the needs of the nursing staff for evidence-based nursing practice.

ACCESSING INFORMATION RESOURCES FOR EVIDENCE-BASED PRACTICE

With the rapid changes occurring in health care, all providers find themselves needing to access the most current information about specific illnesses, medications, and other treatments. Providers need strategies for finding information. Additionally they need to be able to evaluate the information retrieved.

Strategies for Finding Information

When all bibliographic databases were in print form, the information lagged behind publication by many months. Additionally, searching databases was cumbersome and missing important information was not uncommon. With the computerization of databases, the search function provides flexibility in the language used and the combination of terms that can be entered. This sets the framework for specifically targeted searches of the health care literature. Many nursing programs require that students learn to use bibliographic references to support their education. This is a skill that will continue to be of importance throughout your career.

The most comprehensive database is Medline, a resource of the National Library of Medicine (NLM), which may be searched through the PubMed search site. PubMed provides a thesaurus of specific terms that are used by the NLM librarians to index articles into relevant categories within the Medline database. Additionally, the Medline database can be searched in terms of key words that might appear in the title or in the abstract or even within the article itself. PubMed searches are free and available on-line. After the search has enabled the identification of appropriate references, a source for those references is needed. The NLM operates a document retrieval service in which specific articles may be photocopied (for a charge) and mailed to a library that subscribes to the service. PubMed may also be used to identify resources and then the specific documents may be sought in a hospital, college, or medical center library.

The Cumulative Index of Nursing and Allied Health Literature (CINAHL) is a bibliographic resource organized around nursing-related terms as well as broader health-related terms. The thesaurus for CINAHL includes nursing diagnoses and steps of the nursing process as well as terms related to common nursing interventions. CINAHL is available by subscription only and may be included in a library's subscription base.

There are several databases that include health-related publications to which libraries may subscribe. These include Ebsco Host and Proquest. Many of these databases provide abstracts and some full-text articles. Access to these databases is restricted to those belonging to the agencies that purchase them, such as students and faculty of college and university libraries and employees of institutional subscribers. Cochrane Library is a database of systematic reviews available on-line (see discussion of systematic reviews below). It includes four databases: the Cochrane Database of Systematic Reviews, the Database of Abstracts of Reviews of Effectiveness, the Cochrane Controlled Trials Register, and the Cochrane Review Methodology Database.

On-line journals are indexed in databases along side print journals, but many online journals are also accessible through Internet search engines such as Google and Yahoo Search. On-line journals may require a paid subscription to access full-text articles. These Internet search engines may also reveal government and organization recommendations or standards, papers, conference proceedings, reports, and other resources that are available on-line.

Critical Thinking Activity

Identify a medical diagnosis with which you are not familiar. Using PubMed, seek information on the nursing care needs of individuals with that particular medical diagnosis. Once you have identified specific articles using PubMed, use whatever databases are available in your school library to seek articles. After that, use an Internet search engine such as Google, MSN Search, or Yahoo Search to look up the same medical diagnosis. Compare the resources you found from each of the different search techniques.

Evaluating Information Retrieved

Regardless of the resource used for accessing data, critical judgment regarding the reliability and validity of information retrieved is essential. You will need to ask a series of questions about the source and content of the material you have accessed. These same questions may be taught to patients who are often researching information about their health conditions using on-line references (Display 6-6).

The first question to ask is about the source of the information. If this is a journal, who publishes it? It may be a nursing or medical organization, an independent party, or a pharmaceutical company. Look at the editorial board. What are the credentials of those individuals? Do you know of any of them? If this is a Web site, who controls the content on this site? Is it identified by a date? By an author? Examine the policies regarding publication. There is often a page or section of a Web site designed to give information to potential authors or contributors. This may provide you with information about how content is reviewed. Is there a process in which appropriate professionals peer-review any manuscript before publication? Individuals are eligible to be peer reviewers when they have both subject matter expertise and an understanding of research. The journal selects appropriate peer reviewers, who read and critique the article and make recommendations as to whether it should be published. Peer review strengthens the reliability of the content. Consider the potential accuracy of the material and whether the source might be biased.

Look at the biographical material on the authors. What are their credentials for writing? If this is a report of a clinical practice in a particular institution, what is the author's role in that institution? If it is a research report, what are the author's credentials for research? Who funded the research?

Display 6-6   Key Strategies for Evaluating Information Resources

1. Source of Information:
   - Who controls the journal or Web site?
   - Is it peer reviewed?
2. The author or authors:
   - Are the authors or editors apparent in the resource?
   - What are the credentials of the authors or editors?
   - What are the affiliations of the authors or editors?
   - Who funded their research?
3. Content of the resource
   - How closely does the resource speak to your situation or need?
   - Where was the provided information obtained? Consider the various sources for evidence-based care.
4. Consensus of multiple resources
   - Are there other resources that agree with this one?
   - Is this resource suggesting actions that are outside the generally accepted standard?
5. Comparison of new information with previous information
   - What are the differences from what you previously understood?
   - Are differences explained so that you can understand them?

As you read the material, consider the content from different perspectives. Consider how closely the basis of the report matches your situation or need. For example, a protocol used in a major medical center may be unrealistic for a small community hospital with fewer resources. Interventions that work well with a college-educated population may not work well for a low-income, low-educational-level group. An intervention that has limited study may be useful for an individual patient for whom the standard interventions are not being successful. However, this same intervention might be inappropriate as a standard of care. Is the information anecdotal only or was there a planned method of measuring outcomes and results that are being reported?

When using references for practice, you will find it useful to look for multiple references. What worked in one small study may have been unsuccessful when a similar study was done. What might have contributed to this disparity in outcomes? If multiple sources all achieved the same outcome or made the same recommendation, this strengthens the recommendation. Consider how the recommendations fit in with prior standards of practice. While new standards will emerge, changing dramatically from known standards requires a higher level of proof than would be required when making a minor change.

For some problems, a systematic review may be available from a source such as the Cochrane Review or in an article. A systematic review examines a broad spectrum of research regarding a specific problem. The review presents the strengths and weaknesses of the various research studies and then provides an analysis of the meaning of all them combined. Often this review is done by an expert panel. Such a review provides excellent information on which to base decisions.

Always compare new information with old. Make sure that you clearly understand the similarities and differences. Sometimes the long-established practice is not based on research, but rather is simply customary. If you do not understand the current practice, you will have difficulties making judgments about changing practices.

Critical Thinking Activity

Working with a small group of students, identify a nursing care concern that is of interest to you. Using the EBP process discussed, seek evidence for the best nursing practices in relationship to this concern. Be sure to document all references you used in your process. Based on the evidence you found, formulate a policy and/or protocol to address the nursing care concern and present it to your class.

TECHNOLOGY IN HEALTH CARE

Technology in health care is found in many places. It is found as an approach to managing general knowledge related to health care, as well as computerized patient care data. Computerized management of patient care is available through many devices that gather data and manage the health care environment. The use of computerized systems in health care has increased steadily, and all information will eventually be managed by computer. This poses challenges to nursing to maintain a "high touch" relationship with the patient in the midst of the high tech environment of health care.

Increasingly, the vast amount of information that is used to inform practice in general as well as the care of a specific patient is managed through computerized technology. **Information technology** is being used to store research data, disseminate research and practice information, and retrieve information for use. The study and management of information technology is often referred to as the field of **informatics**. There is a national specialty group in nursing that focuses on nursing informatics.

Computerized Patient Records

Computerization of patient data began in most facilities with the computerization of payment and billing data. While forward-looking health care institutions began computerizing patient care records beginning in the early 1980s, the beginning of the 21st century was characterized by directives from Medicare and Medicaid to computerize patient records and communication. The Health Information Privacy and Portability Act (HIPAA) mandated that all billing to the federal government be done electronically. In order to facilitate this, all providers submitting bills were required to use standardized documentation.

Computerization of Financial and Reporting Data

The International Classification of Diseases, which is now in its 9th edition and the Current Procedural Terminology both use a numbering system to enable the coding of diseases, treatment modalities, and procedures performed. Health information specialists became essential to manage these complex systems for data entry and retrieval. Billing of third-party payers is dependent on exact use of the correct codes. Deliberately using incorrect codes in order to generate increased income has been prosecuted as fraud. All statistical management became computerized with birth and death records, cancer registries, and other data-gathering requirements met by skilled coders taking each patient's handwritten chart and extracting and coding the data into computer systems.

As health information specialists became responsible for reviewing patient charts for billing purposes, they were given responsibility for monitoring charts for complete documentation. Their sphere of responsibility in most facilities also includes management of the patient privacy mandates such as HIPAA and may involve quality monitoring processes.

Computerized Pharmacy and Laboratory Data

Pharmacy and laboratory records usually followed billing data in the process of computerization. Computerized records could then be accessed more quickly by those who needed them. Pharmacy and laboratory records are, by their nature, specific, concrete, and objective, thus making them adaptable to and suitable for computerization.

Nurses are able to access laboratory data more quickly and respond by providing the appropriate intervention that is based on data. Many hospitals have made laboratory data available to providers who are not in the hospital to enable them to respond more effectively to information as it becomes available. The availability of data on the computer has freed the nursing department from a major collection, filing, and notification role. Although this was often delegated to a unit secretary, the nursing staff was responsible for ensuring that this was accomplished.

Computerized pharmacy records have decreased the nurses' need to process large volumes of paperwork related to medication administration. Information regarding allergies, drug interactions, and other concerns are often immediately available.

Computerized Nursing Care Records

Computerizing the nursing patient care record has been a complex task in computerization. Many different people need to enter data into the record, and many need to extract it. Data that are nonstandardized and more qualitative in nature are more difficult to computerize. The increase in checklists and charting by exception paved the way for an easier entry into computerized data for some aspects of nursing care. The need for detailed narrative was lessened by these various tables, checklists, and charts. Many institutions are turning to the various nursing terminology systems such as the North American Nursing Diagnosis Association, Nursing Intervention Classification, Nursing Outcomes Classification, the Omaha system, and others to systematize the language used in documentation. By systematizing the language, uniform data can be extracted for quality assurance purposes as well as for research.

For nurses, there are still problems with computerized data systems. Some have been designed without the input of direct caregivers and are time-consuming and cumbersome to use. The need for large numbers of computer entry stations for nursing units has been a problem in other settings. The move toward computerization of the nursing record will continue until all records are computerized. Learning a new computer system is becoming a standard part of any orientation to a new facility.

Computerized Order Entry

Computerized order entry (COE) systems, sometimes referred to as computerized physician order entry or physician order entry systems, are gaining in use. To institute COE, prescribers, whether physicians, dentists, nurse practitioners, or physician assistants, must be willing to change their practice patterns. One major advantage of COE is that errors based on handwriting difficulties are eliminated. Nurses do not have to decipher handwritten orders or spend time trying to contact the provider to clarify the order. In addition, Evans, Pestotnic, Classen, et al. (1998) pointed out that computer prompts may be used to indicate such items as default doses and a range of potential doses for each medication, and to indicate a requirement to enter dosage, route, and frequency for each order. This has helped to eliminate the time-consuming process for nurses of contacting providers to obtain complete information when it was overlooked at the time of writing the order. There may also be prompts to suggest the need for laboratory monitoring, and the computer may be programmed to display values already in the patient record. Most systems provide for a cross-check with patient drug allergy data and drug–drug interactions for the medications already prescribed. The system may be set to reject the use of abbreviations that appear on a "do not use" list. All of these provide greater safety for the patient and have the potential to decrease nursing workload in a time of nursing shortage.

Reese (2005) points out that COE can be used to facilitate the use of standard protocols for care. When the standard protocol with options for individualization is offered on the screen, it becomes easy for a physician to use the standard protocol. Institutions seeking to systematize best practices find this a valuable asset.

However, COE may contribute to different kinds of errors. A study of one hospital COE system found attributes of the systems itself that were problematic (Koppel et al., 2005). In this system, the researchers identified fragmented displays that prevented a "coherent view of patients' medications" (Koppel et al., 2005, p. 1197). In addition, it was possible to mistake which display was being viewed. The pharmacy inventory display of dosages currently available could be mistaken for the dosage guidelines display. There was a separation of functions that made double dosing and incompatible orders possible. Not all screens showed the patient's name, so mixed identities were possible. These and other problems with the system prompted the researchers to recommend that institutions considering COE investigate the problems as well as the benefits of any system being considered. Nurses need to be aware of these problems and not become complacent that COE will decrease the need for nursing knowledge and critical thinking in regard to the administration of medications.

Patient Privacy and Computerized Records

Concerns about privacy become magnified when information is available to many people in many sites far removed from where the patient is located. All systems require passwords for entry and contain tracking capabilities to determine who has accessed which record from which location. This is essential to enforce the restrictions that govern not accessing a record when one does not have a genuine professional need to know that information. Of even greater concern than the individual who violates confidentiality is the wholesale access to large databases for illegal purposes. As ambulatory care data are merged into overall systems with hospital data, the potential for misuse of information is expanded. HIPAA legislation has mandated that institutions using computerized records have safeguards for patient privacy in place. Agencies that fail to implement appropriate privacy policies are subject to substantial fines.

▪▪ COMMUNICATION IN *ACTION*
▪▪

Maintaining Integrity With Computerized Records
Jose Martinez was a new RN working on the evening shift. One of the nursing assistants approached him and said, "My sister was admitted to the Birth Room just before I came on the shift. Would you check the computer and see if she has had the baby yet? I think it will appear on the new admissions." Jose replied, "I wish I could help you. I know how anxious you have been about your sister. But I really can't access the computer for that information; it wouldn't be appropriate because I am not involved in her care. But I can watch your patients for you so that you can go to the maternity area and see if you can talk with her or her husband."

Advantages of Computerized Patient Records

Computerized records have many advantages for patients and health care providers. Some of those were discussed in relationship to specific aspects of the record.

A major advantage of the computerized record is that it can be available at the point-of-care without the need to obtain a copy of the written record. Continuity of care is also facilitated when the information follows the patient from setting to setting. Many health systems are integrating ambulatory care data with hospital data so that wherever the patient is, the provider has access to the needed care information. Even when the records are not integrated, it may be possible to send electronic forms of the record to the setting where it is required.

Computerizing Management of Patient Care

The use of technology for direct care has increased gradually throughout the past 30 years. Within nursing, computerized devices initially became available in ICUs as monitors for cardiac rhythms. Computerized pumps and controllers were introduced to monitor IV infusions. Automatic blood pressure–measuring devices provide for frequent measurements accompanied by alarms for readings outside preset parameters. Small blood glucose monitors that allow for more precise control of blood sugar for the patient with diabetes have become common. After beginning slowly in many places, the introduction of new technology for direct care has increased at a rapid pace.

Following the Institute of Medicine report that identified a high incidence of errors that compromised health and even caused death within the hospital, hospitals were encouraged to begin using technology to provide safeguards against human error. Computerized drug cabinets (such as Pyxis and Omnicell) make it more difficult (although not impossible) to access and give a medication at the incorrect time. Computerized drug inventories provide increased protection against drug diversion. Computerized checks in the pharmacy will identify drug incompatibilities and alert the pharmacist to allergies, but only if that information is first entered into the system. The use of bar codes on medication administration records, the medications themselves, and patient identification bands have all created greater protection against errors in medication administration. Many additional computerized safety systems are being introduced to decrease the incidence of error in health care.

Distance Monitoring Using Technology

The ability for someone to monitor a critically ill patient from another site has created the opportunity to develop what is being called the **electronic ICU (eICU)**. The eICU includes both monitoring equipment and video cameras connected to a separate monitoring center. In the monitoring center, an expert ICU nurse assumes the role of overseeing the electronic monitoring of patients, analyzing data, and recognizing patterns. The eICU nurse uses the video monitor to view a patient as well as review monitor information. The bedside nurse manages the direct care of two or three patients. The eICU nurse communicates with the bedside nurse to alert that individual to problems that occur and may initiate calling a physician if necessary. Working together, the bedside nurse and the eICU nurse form a strong team to ensure that the patient receives optimum care (Federwishch, 2006).

Expert ICU nurses typically rotate through the eICU role as one of their assignments, but work as bedside nurses on other days. This ensures that the eICU nurse remains skilled in bedside care. A critical role of the eICU nurse is in mentoring beginning ICU nurses. The eICU nurse assists the new nurse in developing toward an expert role.

While in its infancy, the concept of the distance monitoring is expanding. Long-distance monitoring is one suggested expansion. An expert ICU nurse at a distant site also could assist by monitoring patients in a smaller hospital where there are fewer ICU experts.

Personal Digital Assistants for Nurses

Personal digital assistants (PDAs), which are small, handheld computers, provide the technology for nurses and physicians to have information resources immediately available. A PDA may be loaded with a drug reference book, a laboratory reference book, a resource on diseases and their management, a medical dictionary, a calculator, and nursing references. The technologically proficient nurse can access information immediately when it is needed. Some nursing education programs have developed projects in which all students must have a handheld computer and, rather than purchasing print versions of reference books, purchase versions to be loaded on the handheld.

Another use for PDAs is to manage assessment data as they are collected and to track nursing actions taken. For nursing students, this might include using the PDA to develop all of the paper work required for clinical experiences. The instructor may use a PDA to manage student data. There are Web sites that offer programs for organizing and managing assessment data.

When used in these ways, concerns arise about privacy and the protection of information for both patients (in accord with HIPAA) and students (who are protected under federal Family Educational Rights and Privacy Act). A health care agency may have specific rules regarding entering patient data into a PDA. However, in settings where these are still uncommon, the institution may not have developed policies and procedures around their use. The nurse who uses a PDA has an obligation to use the available security provisions to protect the patient. This includes setting up effective passwords to access the information and deleting information as soon as it is not needed for care. PDA loss prevention is another important responsibility.

Telehealth

Telehealth is "the use of electronic information and telecommunications technologies to support long-distance clinical health care, patient and professional health-related education, public health and health administration" (Office for the Advancement of Telehealth, n.d.).

Telehealth has the potential for supporting effective care of rural populations that have difficulty accessing certain types of health care. Through on-line technology, nurses and physicians may be available to patients who reside far from the provider. Cameras can be used to facilitate long-distance assessment, and specific laboratory and physical assessment information can be communicated to the provider through the Internet.

One area of practice for nurses in telehealth is in telephone triage. Patients and families call the telephone help line, and the nurse uses evidence-based protocols to assess and direct patients in self care or in accessing medical care as needed. Telephone help lines are often supported by health plans to decrease the use of expensive emergency room care for less serious problems that could be managed in other ways. For patients, the consultation with the nurse provides expert advice and relieves anxiety over which steps appropriately may be taken.

Licensure and practice laws affect the practice of those in telehealth. One concern relates to the control of practice vs. the control for patient safety. If the patient is in one legal jurisdiction and the provider is in another (which often occurs), to whom is the provider accountable for care? Many states are addressing this specifically within their licensure laws. The *Telemedicine Licensure Report* identifies aspects of licensure laws across all states that affect both nurses and physicians engaged in telehealth (Center for Telemedicine Law, 2003). These may be accessed on-line at *http://telehealth.hrsa.gov/lincensure.htm#2*.

The value of technology for the education of health professionals has become more apparent as opportunities arise. There are on-line degree programs, on-line continuing education for providers, and on-line conferences in which individuals may participate. Technology is overcoming the barriers to staying up to date that occur because of distance and funding for health care professionals living in smaller communities or rural areas.

Telehealth may also be used to facilitate improved screening and detection of illness, to improve patient self-management of chronic conditions, for short- and long-term symptom monitoring, and the delivery of appropriate health interventions. To address all of these areas, the OAT is supporting research and projects that can be used to implement effective telehealth programs.

Clinical Decision Support Systems

Clinical decision support systems are computer programs designed to integrate a medical knowledge base and patient data and provide specific advice on how to manage the individual patient case. The goal of clinical decision support systems is to provide the best of evidence-based practice to patients in an efficient and cost-effective manner that maintains patient safety. A wide variety of different computer systems have been developed for this purpose. A meta-analysis (integrative review of multiple resources) concluded that while computerized clinical decision support systems hold great promise, their benefits are yet to be realized (OpenClinical, 2006).

THE EFFECT OF THE NURSING SHORTAGE

Prominent among current concerns about nursing is the worldwide shortage of the nursing supply relative to the demand for nurses. A survey of chief executive officers of hospitals identified an 8.5% vacancy rate for registered nurses (RNs) in 2005. This compares with a 2004 vacancy rate of 8.1% (Evans, 2006). The **nursing supply** is the number of nurses available based on new individuals entering the nursing profession and those leaving the profession. The **nursing demand** represents the number of jobs or potential jobs that require an RN. Many new nursing positions, such as telephone triage, quality assurance, risk management, nurse informatics specialist, RN first assist in surgery, and advanced practice, did not previously exist. Television advertisements, help wanted ads, and the newspapers are filled with stories of the shortage of RNs. The nursing shortage has many implications for your future practice.

Exploring Origins of the Shortage

As we entered a new century, the nursing shortage became the subject of considerable concern throughout health care. The demand for nurses rose. The client of the downsized hospital was more acutely ill and older than before. To maintain short stays and early discharge, patient teaching and planning for discharge assumed more importance than before. Hospitals that downsized too abruptly found that they needed to replace RNs. As the population ages, with an expected increase of 54% in those 65 and older, the demand for RNs is expected to increase in all settings, with an overall increase in demand of 40% between 2000 and 2020 (National Center for Health Workforce Analysis, 2002).

Concerns that the nursing shortage will continue and even grow more acute are based on the convergence of several factors. The RN workforce is aging, with a majority of nurses over 45 years of age. This trend is expected to continue until 2020 (National Center for Health Workforce Analysis, 2002). The workload is high, and the pace is demanding. As a consequence, older RNs often choose to work less than full time or retire early, further depleting the supply. Positions for those with baccalaureate and higher degrees and for those with specialty training, such as intensive care or operating room nursing, are growing faster than the job market in general. There also are regional differences in the nursing supply (Spratley, Johnson, Sochalski, Fritz, & Spencer, 2000).

Meanwhile, the number of new graduates entering the employment market decreased during the second half of the 1990s. Some programs failed to meet targets for admissions, and, subsequently, graduations from nursing schools declined. Although this trend is now reversing, the supply of new RNs is expected to increase by only 6% by 2020 if no actions are taken to increase the number of spaces in nursing schools (National Center, 2002).

Some have asked, "How did we get to this place?" Looking back at the changes occurring during the 1980s and the early 1990s gives us some perspective on the issue. In the late 1980s, health care faced major challenges financially as reimbursement systems changed. Technology changed the approach to medical care; with minimally invasive surgery leading to short stays, early discharge, and more care being provided on an ambulatory or home care basis. There were predictions that the need for nurses would drop. Hospitals and health care systems began consolidating, and there was a move to more private for-profit institutions and away from non-profit institutions.

In the 1990s, the pressures of a changing health care system and cost containment created many changes for nursing. Hospital stays shortened so dramatically that hospital censuses decreased across the country.

As these changes occurred, many hospitals identified that their largest single employee cost was nursing. They began looking for ways to decrease their nursing staffs. A focus on "right sizing" meant that the hospital did not want to staff for more than the actual patient census at any given time. Units were closed or consolidated, and hospitals stopped hiring RNs. Care patterns were changed, and primary nursing or total patient care was abandoned and replaced with a variety of patterns that included a mix of nurses and unlicensed assistive personnel. Hospitals adopted the strategy of notifying people not to come to work or even to go home if the census dipped, thus creating "no-pay" days. For the majority of nurses, a dependable income was essential, and this created a great deal of stress. The prior nursing shortage of the 1980s appeared to end abruptly, as hospitals began reassessing their needs. These factors contributed to layoffs of nurses from hospitals. Long-term care and home care increased, although funding of home care remained a problem.

Hiring was often at a standstill, and the current nursing workforce continued to age. If there were layoffs, newer nurses went first. Those currently in the system had the most to lose in terms of wages and benefits (especially retirement) and chose to stay. As the nursing workforce average age crept upward, those observing the system began to recognize that a time was coming when retirements would occur at a rapid rate, further decreasing the number of working RNs. This was going to be especially true for the staff nurse arena, where the physical demands are very heavy.

All the changes in the workplace occurred on the assumption that there would be fewer patients needing care. This did not really happen. The population continued to age; shorter stays meant that the hospitalized patient population was sicker and had more needs. Nurses felt that they were working harder than ever with decreased satisfaction because of the fragmentation of their relationships with patients, the demands of constantly changing technology, and the use of assistive personnel. Satisfaction with the work role decreased; there was increased burn-out, and nurses began to leave nursing for other careers. As one nursing colleague put it, "If nursing employment were a bucket, the bucket has holes in it. You cannot fill it up if it keeps leaking out the bottom." So instead, nurses found that the critical thinking skills, communication abilities, and work ethic they had learned for nursing were transferable to other occupational fields.

As employment opportunities in nursing narrowed and other fields broadened their appeal to the women traditionally attracted by nursing, the number of applicants to many nursing programs decreased. Some colleges were unable to fill all their student positions. While the population continued to grow, the number of nursing graduates remained static in some areas but dropped in other areas of the country. Those who did graduate were increasingly people changing careers later in life rather than the traditional young adult. Although these individuals brought much strength to nursing, their total years of career practice were clearly going to be fewer.

The Current Situation

According to studies conducted in 2002 and 2004, nurses themselves perceived that the supply of nurses was decreasing the gap relative to the nursing demand. In 2004, salary and benefits were not perceived as the major cause of the shortage, but most did not see that the recruitment and retention strategies recommended were being implemented (Buerhaus, Donelman & Ulrich, 2005a). More than 80% of the nurses in the 2004 survey reported that they were satisfied with their jobs, with 46% reporting that they were "very satisfied" (Donelman et al., 2005). This holds promise for stopping the loss of currently working nurses (Fig. 6-3).

An aspect of the current nursing shortage of great concern is the shortage of nursing faculty that are needed to expand and even continue current levels of nursing education. The average age of nursing faculty members is 51.6 years, and many are nearing retirement (AACN, 2004). A report from Oregon released in 2001 predicted that 41% of nursing faculty in place at that time would retire by 2005, and an additional 33% by 2010 (Northwest Health Foundation, 2001). A similar situation existed across the country, and it stimulated national efforts to increase the numbers of individuals preparing to teach nursing. Another factor in the shortage of nursing faculty is that faculty roles have not paid as well as clinical roles for nurses with advanced education.

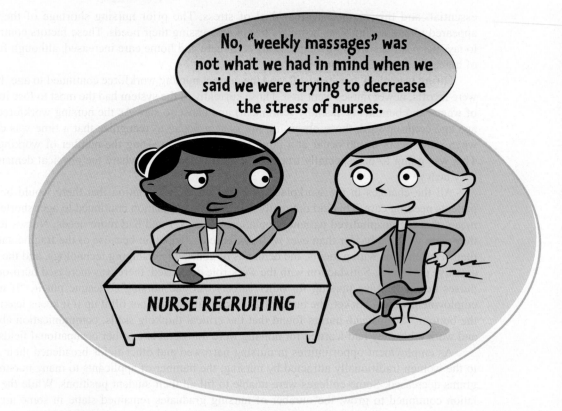

No, "weekly massages" was not what we had in mind when we said we were trying to decrease the stress of nurses.

NURSE RECRUITING

FIGURE 6-3 Improving the work environment for nurses has been identified as a key component in addressing the nursing shortage.

Multiple efforts have been instituted across the country in an effort to address the concern about the nursing faculty shortage. They are identified on the AACN Web site (AACN, 2004).

Future Directions for the Nursing Workforce

Meanwhile, nurses express concerns that emphasis on patient safety and quality improvement will not be successful until the shortage is alleviated (Buerhaus et al., 2005b). In 2003, the AHQR asked the Institute of Medicine (IOM) to explore key aspects of the work environment for nurses that likely would have an impact on patient safety and potential improvements in health care working conditions that likely would increase patient safety (IOM, 2004). This report recommended actions to be taken by individual health care organizations, regulatory agencies, professional associations and philanthropic agencies, and labor partners that would address the work environment and support a culture of safety. These recommendations identify the importance to patient safety of a work environment in which nurses are not overburdened with too many patients and are not overly fatigued from working too many hours. The report emphasizes that nurses individually cannot create the work environment that will lead to the goals of improved patient outcomes.

Nurses must unite in their efforts to speak up for the importance of workplace initiatives that improve the work climate and thus support improved patient safety and outcomes. While leaving the setting when it threatens to become overwhelming is understandable, working together to change the system has long-term benefits for nurses and patients. Technology must be harnessed in a manner that supports nursing practice and does not simply demand more nursing time. An environment must be created that supports and sustains efforts by nurses to move to EBP.

Key Concepts

- Nursing research has grown and developed since the middle of the twentieth century and now is supported through the NINR, which is part of the NIH.
- Nursing research involves the development of a research question, a literature review, a plan for seeking answers, implementation of the plan, analysis of the data gathered, a discussion and evaluation of the results of the study, and recommendations for further research.
- Understanding research terminology and the types of research that can be conducted are essential to reading and using any nursing research.
- The staff nurse's role in relationship to conducting nursing research includes identifying research questions, safeguarding patients who participate in a study and collecting data and performing treatments.
- "Evidence based nursing practice is clinical decision making based on the best available scientific evidence, combined with clinical nursing expertise, and considering patient preferences and available resources." (Dicenso et al, 1998, p. 38). This definition provides an excellent foundation both for the individual nurse and for the institution to establish evidence-based nursing practice.
- A wide variety of evidence, including research reports, chart reviews, quality improvement, benchmarking, and data regarding risk management, infection control, pathophysiology information, cost effectiveness, and patient preferences, may be used to support nursing practice.
- While many models for EBP exist, a simplified process is incorporated in the terms Ask, Acquire, Analyze, Apply, and Assess.
- Barriers to EBP include the availability of resources, time availability, educational preparation, and nursing commitment.
- Accessing information resources requires knowledge of information resources and the use of databases, as well as an understanding of data such as quality improvement and infection control data from the institution.
- Information must be evaluated in relationship to its source, the authors, its relevance to your own practice setting, support from multiple resources, and how this relates to current practice.
- Information technology is dramatically changing how individual patient care information and provider planning for care are entered into the record, stored, and retrieved. PDAs are allowing individual health care providers to manage large volumes of information more easily. Security and privacy of patient information remain both an ethical and legal challenge.

- Computerized devices increasingly are used to manage the direct care of patients, from automatic blood pressure measuring devices to IV controllers to monitoring equipment both locally and from a distance. They are changing the way nursing is practiced.
- The nursing shortage affects the safety and outcomes for patients and also affects nurses' job satisfaction. A key concern is the shortage of nursing faculty, which restricts the ability to expand the nursing work force because schools cannot take more students due to inadequate numbers of faculty.
- The improvement of the nursing work environment to support quality, safe care is essential to overcoming the nursing shortage.

Relevant Web Sites

Evidence-Based Practice

Agency for Health Care Research and Quality (AHRQ): *www.ahrq.gov*
Cochrane Collaboration: *www.cochrane.org*
Cumulative Index of Nursing and Allied Health Literature (CINAHL): *www.cinahl.com*
Joanna Briggs Institute: *www.joannabriggs.edu.au/about/home.php*
Medline Plus: *www.nlm.nih.gov/medlineplus/aboutmedlineplus.html*
National Institute for Nursing Research: *http://ninr.nih.gov/ninr*
National Library of Medicine: *www.nlm.nih.gov*
PubMed Online: *www.pubmed.gov*

Computers in Nursing and Personal Digital Assistants—PDA (Handheld Computers)

Online Journal of Nursing Informatics: www.eaa-knowledge.com/ojni
PDA Listserv for Nurses: www.rnpalm.com/nursing_pdas_listserv.htm

Patient Safety

Veteran's Administration Center for Patient Safety: *www.patientsafety.gov/rca.html*

References

American Association of Colleges of Nursing. (2004). *Nursing faculty shortage fact sheet*. [On-line]. www.aacn.nche. edu/Media/Backgrounders/facultyshortage.htm. Accessed April 20, 2006.

Buerhaus, P., Donelman, K., Ulrich, B. T., & Norman, L. (2005a). Is the shortage of hospital registered nurses getting better or worse? Findings from two recent national surveys of RNs. *Nursing Economic$*. [On-line]. *www.nursingeconomics.net*. Accessed January 31, 2006.

Buerhaus, P., Donelman, K., Ulrich, B. T., Norman, L., William, M., & Dittus, R. (2005b). Hospital RNs' and CNOs' perceptions of the impact of the nursing shortage on the quality of care. *Nursing Economic$*. [On-line]. *www.nursingeconomics.net*. Accessed January 31, 2006.

Bureau of Labor Statistics, U.S. Department of Labor. *Occupational outlook handbook, 2006–07 edition, registered nurses*. [On-line]. *www.bls.gov/oco/ocos083.htm* . Accessed January 17, 2006.

Center for Telemedicine Law. (2003). *Telemedicine licensure report*. [On-line]. *http://telehealth.hrsa.gov/lincensure.htm#2*. Accessed April 20, 2006.

DiCenso, A., Cullum, N., & Ciliska, D. (1998). Implementing evidence based nursing: Some misconceptions [Editorial]. *Evidence Based Nursing, 1*, 38–40.

Donelman, K., Buerhaus, P., Ulrich, B. T., Norman, L., & Dittus, R. (2005). Awareness and perceptions of the Johnson & Johnson Campaign for Nursing's Future; Views from nursing students, RNs, and CNOs. *Nursing Economic$*. [On-line]. *www.nursingeconomics.net*. Accessed January 31, 2006.

Ellis, J. R., & Hartley, C. L. (2005). *Managing and coordinating nursing care* (4th ed.) Philadelphia: Lippincott Williams & Wilkins.

Evans, M. (2006). Hospitals say RN vacancies high, recruiting harder. *Modern Heathcare Online*. [On-line]. *www.modernhealth care.com*. Accessed May 8, 2006.

Evans, R. S., Pestotnik, S. L., Classen, D. C., Clemmer, T. P., Weaver, L. K., Orme, J. F., Jr., et al. (1998). A computer-assisted management program for antibiotic and other anti-infective agents. *New England Journal of Medicine, 338*(4), 232–238.

Federwishch, A. (2006). From a distance. *Nurseweek: Mountain Edition, 7*(1), 10–11.

Flemming, K. (1998). Asking answerable questions. *Evidence Based Nursing, 1*(2), 36–37.

Haynes, R. B. (2005). Of studies, summaries, synopses, and systems: The "4s" evolution of services for finding current best evidence. *Evidence Based Nursing, 8*(1), 4–6.

Institute of Medicine. (2004). *Keeping patients safe: Transforming the work environment of nurses.* Committee on the Work Environment for Nurses and Patient Safety, Page, A. (ed.), Washington, DC: National Academies Press. [On-line]. *http://newton.nap.edu/books/0309090679/html.* Accessed February 17, 2006.

Kennedy, M. S. (2004). The state of the science on nursing research. *American Journal of Nursing, 104*(12), 28–29, 31.

Koppel, R., Metlay, J. P., Cohen, A., Abaluck, B., Localio, A. R., Kimmel, S. E., et al. (2005). Role of computerized physician order entry systems in facilitating medication errors. *Journal of the American Medical Association, 293*, 1197–1203.

Melnyk, B. M. (2004). Integrating levels of evidence into clinical decision-making. *Pediatric Nursing, 30*(4), 323–326.

Melnyk, B. M., & Fineout-Overholt, E. (2005). *Evidence based practice in nursing & healthcare. A guide to best practice.* Philadelphia: Lippincott Williams & Wilkins.

National Center for Health Workforce Analysis, Bureau of Health Professions. (2002, July). *Projected supply, demand, and shortages of registered nurses: 2000–2020.* Rockville, MD: Health Resources and Services Administration.

National Institute of Nursing Research. (n.d.). *A brief history of the NINR.* [On-line]. *http://ninr.nih.gov/ninr/about/history.html.* Accessed February 22, 2006.

Northwest Health Foundation. (2001). *Oregon's nursing shortage: A public health crisis in the making.* [On-line]. *www.nwhf.org/assets/nursing_shortage_health_crisis.pdf.* Accessed April 20, 2006.

Office for the Advancement of Telehealth. (n.d.). *What is telehealth?* [On-line]. *http://telehealth.hrsa.gov.* Accessed April 20, 2006.

OpenClinical. (2006). *Potential benefits and drawbacks of the use of CDSSs; Factors which may help determine the success-ful use of CDSSs in clinical practice, Summary.* [On-line]. *www.openclinical.org/dssSuccessFactors.html#preamble.* Accessed April 20, 2006.

Pravikoff, D. S., Tanner, A. B., & Pierce, S. T. (2005). Readiness of U.S. nurses for evidence based practice. *American Journal of Nursing, 105*(9), 40–51.

Reese, S. (2005, April 1). Computerized order entry brings practice protocol off the shelf. *Managed Healthcare Executive.* [On-line]. *www.managedhealthcareexecutive.com/mhe/article/articleDetail.jsp?id=155758&&pageID=2.* Accessed February 11, 2006.

Rodwin, M. A. (2001, April 2). The politics of evidence based medicine. *Journal of Health Politics, Policy and Law, 26,* 2. [On-line]. *www.ahrq.gov/clinic/jhppl/rodwin.htm.* Accessed February 16, 2006.

Seymour, R. (1999, August). Cooking ham and the masters nursing thesis. *Graduate Research in Nursing, 1*(1). [On-line]. *www.graduateresearch.com/seymour.htm.* Accessed February 12, 2006.

Shine, K. I. (2001). The meaning of evidence and the practice of evidence based medicine. *Journal of Health Politics, Policy and Law, 26,* 2. [On-line]. *www.ahrq.gov/clinic/jhppl/havighurst1.htm#meaning.* Accessed February 14, 2006.

Spratley, E., Johnson, A., Sochalski, J., Fritz, M., & Spencer, W. (2000). *The registered nurse population: Findings from the National Sample Survey of Registered Nurses.* U.S. Department of Health and Human Services, Health Resources and Services Administration. [On-line]. *http://bhpr.hrsa.gov/healthworkforce/rnsurvey/rnss1.htm.* Accessed April 15, 2006.

Thompson, C., Cullum, N., McCaughan, D., Sheldon, T., & Raynor, P. (2004). Nurses, information use, and clinical decision making: The real world potential for evidence based decisions in nursing, *Evidence Based Nursing, 7*(3), 68–72.

Titler, M. G., Kleiber, C., Rakel, B., Budreau, G., Everett, L. Q., Steelman, V., et al. (2001). The Iowa Model of evidence based practice to promote quality care. *Critical Care Nursing Clinics of North America, 13*(4), 497–509.

Twin Cities Evidence-Based Health Care Project. (2001). *Evidence based nursing.* Minneapolis University, University of Minnesota. [On-line]. *http://evidence.ahc.umn.edu/ebn.htm.* Accessed February 22, 2006.

University of North Carolina. (n.d.). *Evidence based nursing.* [On-line]. *www.hsl.unc.edu/services/tutorials/ebn/practice.htm.* Accessed February 16, 2006.

U N I T   I I I

Legal and Ethical Responsibility and Accountability for Practice

This unit begins by exploring the credentialing of health care providers. It discusses the basic concerns related to credentialing, provides a rationale for credentials, and emphasizes the responsibility of health care providers (especially nurses) to the public.

A well-grounded understanding of the legal and ethical dimensions of practice provides the foundation for professional nursing. The first chapter of this unit continues with a discussion of the legal ramifications of practice. Concrete examples provide help in understanding specific legal issues of importance to consumers and health care providers. The chapter concludes with the role of the nurse as a witness.

Ethical and bioethical issues associated with health care constantly challenge us as professionals and as members of society. Each technologic advance brings additional questions and concerns to our attention. The second and third chapters of the unit explore these issues and their ramifications on nursing practice. The unit concludes with a discussion of major questions posed by ethical and bioethical issues, provides an understanding of the basis of ethical decision making and the factors that significantly affect it, and outlines a framework for ethical decision making. Some of the specific problems you will encounter as you move into a professional role are explored in the hope that considering them before you become directly involved will help you to address them more comfortably.

7

Credentials for Health Care Providers

LEARNING OUTCOMES

After completing this chapter, you should be able to:

1. Define and discuss the concept of credentialing in the health professions.
2. Describe how each of the following types of credentials differ: diploma, certificate, and license.
3. Outline the purposes of accreditation and the general process for seeking accreditation.
4. Identify and analyze the major elements addressed by nursing practice acts.
5. Outline the role of the state boards of nursing or other state regulatory authority.
6. Differentiate between licensure by examination, licensure by endorse-

ment, and mutual recognition of licensure.
7. Discuss personal strategies to avoid violating the provisions of the nursing practice acts and encountering the disciplinary process.
8. Discuss issues in licensure, including ensuring continued competence, multistate licensure, and licensure for graduates of foreign nursing schools.
9. Explain the various uses of certification in nursing.
10. Discuss current trends in credentialing within the health care workforce.

KEY TERMS

Accreditation
Administrative law
Advanced practice registered nurse (APRN)
Certificate of completion
Certificate/Certification
Computerized adaptive testing (CAT)
Credentials
Criticality
Degree
Diploma
Disciplinary action

Enacted (statutory) law
Frequency
Grandfathering
Home state
Injunctive relief
License
Licensure by endorsement
Licensure by examination
Mandatory licensure
Mutual recognition of licensure
NCLEX-PN

NCLEX-RN
Nurse practice act
Party state
Permissive licensure
Reciprocity
Remote state
Revocation
Rules and regulations
Site-based certification
Site-based examination
State Board of Nursing
Sunset laws
Telenursing

Credentials are written documents that communicate to others the nature of one's competence and provide evidence of one's preparation to perform in a specific occupation. Credentials include certificates, degrees, and diploma awarded by educational institutions; legal licenses awarded by a government body; and recognition by a professional organization (usually termed "certification") that focuses on a specialty area. Members of health professions have supported the need for credentials of all kinds to protect the public; those who are engaged in careers in health occupations want to be assured that the standards of practice in their discipline remain high. They do not want to be replaced by people with less educational preparation and skill who are willing to work for lower wages. Credentials also are used by organizations or institutions to demonstrate the quality of the care provided to the public. These institutional credentials are usually referred to as approval or accreditation by a specific body. All these types of credentials are discussed below.

APPROVAL AND ACCREDITATION OF INSTITUTIONS AND PROGRAMS

Institutions are approved by government bodies to operate within their state borders. States have varying standards and processes for approval of educational institutions such as technical institutes, colleges, and universities. The approval of most educational institutions is carried out by a state board of education or similar educational authority. States also have approval processes for programs that provide education for licensed health professions. These are most commonly carried out by professional boards.

Educational institutions and programs also may have voluntary accreditation for both their general educational programs and for specialized programs. Most **accreditation** represents "a voluntary process by private agencies which is an external quality review by peers to assure that an educational program meets established standards for structure, function, and performance" (Sheets, 2002, p. 4). Organizations that have the authority to offer national or regional accreditation of educational institutions must be approved by the United States Department of Education. Some accreditation recognizes the entire educational institution, such as the accreditation offered by regional bodies for colleges and universities. If an institution's programs meet standards developed and published by that regional body, it is awarded accreditation. The standards include agreed-upon criteria designed to measure quality and value. An associate, baccalaureate, or master's degree awarded by this accredited institution would reflect a standard of postsecondary education approved by the accrediting organization. In many instances, educational credentials are acknowledged only if offered by an accredited educational institution. Although a nonaccredited institution might award a degree, there is no guarantee that the school meets educational standards; therefore, the degree might not be accepted as adequate evidence of qualifications. Similarly, only course work completed at an accredited institution may be accepted for transfer. You may have experienced the need for this type of accreditation if you transferred academic credits from one college to another. A regionally accredited college or university usually limits direct transfer of coursework into its programs.

Some academic accreditation is specialized, meaning that it applies only to a particular program in an institution, or to a particular type of professional–technical education. Specialized accreditation requires that the specific program meet professional standards for excellence established by a specialized accrediting agency. An educational institution might have general accreditation for its degrees but still not have specialized accreditation. Sometimes this is because of the cost of the accreditation process, or because of a philosophic stance that additional accreditation is not needed if the institution has general accreditation. Certain educational organizations are not degree-granting institutions, and therefore are not eligible for general accreditation, but they are still eligible for specialized accreditation. This is true of hospital-based diploma schools of nursing.

Government Approval of Nursing Programs

For its graduates to be eligible to take the National Council Licensure Examination (NCLEX) in any state, it is a legal requirement that a nursing program be approved by a state board of nursing or another designated state government department. In most states this is called approval, but in a few states it is called accreditation (a term most commonly associated with a voluntary process described above).

In most states, the approval/accrediting activities for nursing programs are carried out through the state board of nursing. After registration laws were passed, state boards of nursing began to emerge for the purpose of licensing nurses and protecting the public. Inspectors from the boards began making program visits for approval. Through the ANA, the Council of State Boards of Nursing was created to have a common forum for those who had the responsibility to regulate the practice of nursing in each state. In 1978, the National Council of State Boards of Nursing, Inc. (NCSBN) was formed to replace the ANA Council. NCSBN provided greater independence of the regulatory authorities from the professional organization.

When a new nursing program is to be initiated, it must provide preliminary information to the appropriate state government department while in the planning phase, often in the form of a feasibility study or a self study or both. The nursing program must be approved prior to admitting students to assure prospective students that the program will provide the preparation they seek. Each state also has a designated time frame to renew its approval of existing nursing programs. This often involves a comprehensive evaluation study, done by the program/school, that is submitted to the state. Representatives of the state approval authority then visit the program. In some jurisdictions, a school that has received national accreditation from the National League for Nursing Accreditation Commission (NLNAC) or the Commission on Collegiate Nursing Education (CCNE) is not required to be further reviewed for state approval (see below).

Accreditation of Nursing Education Programs

Nursing programs may seek national accreditation from an approved organization. The origin of specialized accreditation of nursing education programs arose from concerns about the quality of nursing education among nurses. Accreditation helps to strengthen uniform national standards for nursing education. The national accreditation of nursing programs is voluntary and specialized.

In 1893, the American Society of Superintendents of Training Schools for Nurses was established to develop and maintain a universal standard for nursing education. It was renamed the National League for Nursing Education in 1912, and in 1917 it released the first Standard Curriculum for Schools of Nursing. Throughout the first half of the twentieth century, the National League for Nursing Education continued to provide guidance for quality in nursing education. In 1952, seven organizations combined into one and became the National League for Nursing (NLN), which assumed responsibility for accrediting nursing education programs. In 1997, in response to the Department of Education's expectations for greater separation of the membership organization and the accrediting process, the NLN formed the NLNAC as an independent subsidiary to provide accreditation of nursing programs. The NLNAC accredits nursing programs at all levels: practical nursing, hospital diploma nursing education, associate degree nursing education, and baccalaureate and higher-degree education programs.

In 1999, another organization entered into the nursing program accreditation process: The CCNE, a subsidiary of the American Association of Colleges of Nursing, also offers accreditation to baccalaureate and higher-degree nursing programs only. Advanced practice nursing organizations such as the American Association of Nurse Anesthetists provide specialized accreditation for institutions offering advanced practice/nurse practitioner programs.

Voluntary accreditation by any organization has a similar process. Accreditation is based on a systematic self-study and evaluation by the nursing program itself that focuses on the standards and criteria for accreditation. Peer evaluators from the accrediting organization visit the nursing program, review the self-study, and provide an independent evaluation. Their visit includes meetings with officials throughout the institution, faculty, and students, as well as a review of records and documents. The report and recommendations of the visiting evaluators, along with the self-study document, is submitted to a panel in the organization composed of peer educators. A nursing program may be granted accreditation, granted accreditation with conditions that must be remedied, placed on a warning status for being deficient, or denied accreditation. A program that is accredited has met the national standards of the organization for quality in nursing education.

■■ COMMUNICATION IN *ACTION*
■■

Jerry Wilson was a student in an associate degree nursing program. His program was being evaluated for reaccreditation, and an evaluator visited his clinical site. As part of the process, the evaluator interviewed Jerry. She said, "Please tell me about your objectives for today's clinical experience." Jerry was nervous but pleased to be able to be prepared to respond. "I am working on my neurological assessment skills today," he said. "Although I have performed them in the lab, this is my first opportunity to use those skills with a patient and to interpret their meaning in a real-life situation. This assignment is also giving me an opportunity to increase my abilities to relate to the family as well as the patient, because a family member is always with the patient." The evaluator then asked, "Would you give me some feedback on the adequacy of this clinical site in providing opportunities for the learning that you need?" Jerry responded, "This unit has been an exceptionally good learning environment. The nurses are very helpful and supportive. They go out of their way to help us find good learning experiences. I am always able to find patients that will help me meet the course objectives." Jerry's communication was clear, was direct, and provided important information to the evaluators.

Accreditation of Continuing Education Programs

The American Nurses Credentialing Center, which is best known for providing certification for individual nursing specialties (discussed later in this chapter), also provides an accreditation mechanism for institutions or organizations that want to be approvers or providers of nursing continuing education programs. State nurses associations and specialty organizations often seek accreditation as *approvers of programs*. These organizations then approve specific continuing education offerings as meeting appropriate standards for content and process. Accreditation as a *provider of a program* assures the nurse consumer that the specific continuing education offering meets appropriate standards.

Many of the states that require continuing education for renewing a nursing license require that the offering be approved or accredited by some official group. This ensures that the continuing education is of high quality and will be meaningful for a nurse. Some states operate their own approval systems. When evaluating continuing nursing education offerings, it is important to know whether that class, workshop, or course has been approved and by whom.

CREDENTIALS FOR INDIVIDUALS

Individuals may hold multiple types of credentials. As people progress in their careers they are likely to attain additional credentials.

Diplomas, Degrees, and Certificates of Completion

A school or business offering instruction awards a **diploma** or **certificate** to those who complete a designated program of study. A business that provides instruction in using computer programs might present certificates to those who complete the course. Licensed practical nursing (LPN) programs offer a **certificate of completion**. Hospital-based programs preparing registered nurses (RNs) offer a diploma. College-based nursing programs offer academic **degrees**, such as the associate, baccalaureate, or master's degree, which require the fulfillment of certain general education courses and course work specific to a particular career, such as nursing. The value of a diploma or educational certificate or degree is related to the quality of the educational institution or program as well as to the actual title of the certificate or degree. So, when deciding which institution to attend, check on both the approval of the institution and the specific accreditation of the program.

Licensure

A **license** is a legal credential awarded by an individual state that grants permission to that individual to practice a given profession. The individual seeking licensure must have demonstrated an essential amount of competency necessary to perform a unique scope of practice prior to receiving the license (NCSBN, 2002b). Most states require licensing only of those who have more direct contact with clients. Physicians, dentists, pharmacists, and nurses are licensed in all states. The licensing of other health care workers varies. An individual state or province determines eligibility for licensure and the type of testing required for that profession within that state. Each state develops and enforces its own practice act, which includes the scope of practice for the profession the license represents. We will discuss practice acts later in this chapter.

Certification

For some groups, a standard credential is available in the form of **certification** provided by a nongovernmental authority, usually a professional organization. Workers with this credential are referred to as "certified" or "registered." This type of credential should not be confused with a legal license or a simple certificate of completion (nursing is an anomaly in that the term "registered nurse" was adopted early in this century and refers to legal licensure.) Certification usually is granted on completion of an education program and the passing of a standardized examination.

The program usually has been approved by the professional organization and the organization that administers the examination. Certification does not include a legal scope of practice. Scope of practice will be discussed later in this chapter.

While some professional organizations conduct their own certification, in most instances they have established an independent national affiliated organization whose sole purpose is credentialing. By having an independent organization that focuses all of its efforts on accreditation, they better ensure objectivity and enhance the confidence of others in the process.

Some organizations provide certification for several related occupational groups. One such organization is the National Accrediting Association for Clinical Laboratory Sciences. Members of the various professional groups involved in laboratory science cooperated in setting up this association. The purpose of this organization is to make the laboratory science credentialing system more independent and as objective as possible. This organization awards the title medical laboratory technician and medical technologist (MT) to those who have met the educational standards and passed the certification examination for each of those credentials. All groups in the field of laboratory science recognize these as professional credentials. Some states have made certification by this body the required criterion for practice in clinical laboratory sciences.

One of the concerns regarding certification is the potential for confusion that exists because regulatory agencies (such as state boards of nursing) and professional associations may use the term "certification" differently and in different contexts. In nursing, certification is used for identifying licensed RNs who have specialized or advanced competence in a specific area of nursing. Certification in nursing will be discussed in more detail later in this chapter, after the discussion of basic licensure.

Critical Thinking Activity

Choose an allied health occupation found in a health care facility in which you have clinical practice. Investigate the credentials needed for that occupation and how they would be obtained in your state. Analyze a way in which you could work collaboratively with an individual in this health occupation.

NURSING LICENSURE IN THE UNITED STATES

Nursing leaders historically have maintained an ethical position that accountability to the public for quality nursing care is essential. The public, however, often has no method for evaluating the competence of an individual nurse. Therefore, the nursing profession has tried to ensure that nurses have credentials that can be recognized by everyone. The basic rationale for legal credentials in health care occupations is that legal licensure provides a standard mechanism for judging competence and therefore protects the safety of the public (Fig. 7-1).

Through the efforts of nurses working collectively, a licensure process was developed and state agencies were established to regulate the practice of nursing. Through a regulatory process set up in each state, only individuals who meet predetermined qualifications are permitted to practice nursing. The government agency that has the legal authority to regulate nursing is usually named the board of nursing (although some states use different titles). This body enforces the licensure law enacted by the legislature of each state and the administrative rules and regulations regarding practice.

FIGURE 7-1 Various forms of credentialing ensure the public of qualified caregivers.

The History of Licensure in Nursing

Recognizable credentials were not always available for nurses. Before the Nightingale schools became prevalent in England and nursing schools were established in the United States, little training was available to those who wanted to provide nursing care. Nurses with some training and those without typically worked side by side. After schools of nursing became common, a rudimentary means of identifying the qualifications of a caregiver was the certificate of completion issued by the nursing school. This was the first true nursing credential.

However, because the quality of education offered in the nursing schools varied greatly—programs varied in length from 6 weeks to 3 years—it became apparent that a completion certificate was not an adequate guarantee of competence. Nursing leaders were concerned about this situation; they believed that clients had no way to judge a particular nurse's competence, or whether they might suffer from the care administered by a poorly prepared nurse.

England first debated the issue of self-regulation versus legal regulation. Florence Nightingale did not support individual licensure for nurses because she believed the focus should be on the societal/moral standards of the professional nurse. She believed that only continuing education and practice could ensure competence and that a license approved at one time could not. While England debated whether to initiate some form of licensure, New Zealand became the first country to enact an independent licensing law in 1901. Similarly, Canada began to regulate nurses in the early 1900s. England followed in 1919 (NCSBN, 2004a).

Meanwhile in the United States, the Nurses' Associated Alumnae of the United States and Canada was created in 1896. This organization later evolved into the ANA. One of the major concerns of the Association was the establishment of legal licensure for nurses. The ANA campaigned vigorously for the adoption of state licensing laws. Nurses, legislators, and the public had to be educated about the value of licensure for the profession and encouraged to support it. The set of laws regulating the practice of nursing is termed the **Nurse Practice Act**.

The early laws provided for permissive licensure. **Permissive licensure** is a voluntary system whereby an individual may choose to become licensed to provide evidence of competence, but a license is not required to practice. The requirements for permissive licensure included graduating from a school that satisfied certain standards established in the practice act for that state and passing a comprehensive examination. Only those who had met these standards could use the title RN; others used the title "nurse." Under this system, no one was required to have a license to practice nursing and there was much variability in standards from one state to another.

North Carolina passed the first permissive licensure law in 1903, followed by New York, New Jersey, and Virginia. However, the early laws did not define the scope of practice; New York first did this in 1938 (NCSBN, 2004c). By 1923, all the existing 48 states had permissive licensure laws. Alaska and Hawaii passed licensure laws while they were still territories, and continued to recognize these laws when they became states.

After permissive licensure laws came into being, nurses' activity regarding licensure became less intense because most individuals graduating from nursing schools sought and received licenses to practice. However, there was still concern that some individuals were practicing nursing without having demonstrated skill and knowledge. The majority of those functioning without licenses were nursing school graduates who had failed the licensing examinations; they were referred to as "graduate nurses," rather than RNs. Other nurses who practiced without licenses included individuals who had been educated as nurses in foreign countries.

To end this situation and provide greater protection to the public, many nurses began to call for **mandatory licensure**. Mandatory nursing licensure requires that all persons who wish to practice nursing meet established standards for education, pass standardized examinations, and secure a license to practice in the state, province, or territory in which they wish to work.

The first mandatory licensure law took effect in New York in 1947. Today, mandatory licensure is the standard in the United States, Canada, and most other countries. Therefore, if you wish to work as a nurse in any state, territory, province, or other country, you must obtain a license that is valid in that jurisdiction before you begin working. Even though you are licensed to practice in one place that does not allow you to practice elsewhere without meeting the requirements of the new jurisdiction (see Display 7-1 for the chronology of nursing licensure).

Although the terms "RN" and "LPN" (or licensed vocational nurse [LVN], as used in Texas and California) were protected in law, the more general term "nurse" has not been protected traditionally. Many individuals describe themselves as nurses, when their roles in health care are

Display 7-1   The History of Nursing Licensure

1867	Dr. Henry Wentworth Acland first suggested licensure for nurses in England.
1892	American Society of Superintendents of Training Schools for Nurses organized and supported licensure in the United States.
1901	First nursing licensure in the world: New Zealand
1903	First nursing licensure in the United States: North Carolina, New Jersey, New York, and Virginia (in that order)
1915	ANA drafted its first model nurse practice act.
1919	First nursing licensure in England
1923	All 48 states had enacted nursing licensure laws.
1935	First mandatory licensure act in the United States: New York (effective 1947)
1946	Ten states had definitions of nursing in the licensing act.
1950	First year the same examination used in all jurisdictions of the United States and its territories: State Board Test Pool Examination
1965	Twenty-one states had definitions of nursing in the licensing act.
1971	First state to recognize expanded practice in the nursing practice act: Idaho
1976	First mandatory continuing education for relicensure: California
1982	Change to nursing process format examination: National Council Licensure Examination for Registered Nurses (NCLEX-RN)
1986	Only state to require baccalaureate degree for initial RN licensure and associate degree for licensed practical nurse licensure: North Dakota (effective 1987 and rescinded in 2003)
1994	Computer-adapted testing initiated nationwide
1998	Mutual Recognition Nurse Licensure Compact finalized. Utah is the first state to become part of the Compact.

assistive. Their employers also may refer to them as nurses to support those individuals' status. Some states (for example, Washington) have made "nurse" a protected term. In these states, only RNs or LPNs may use the title nurse. Others, such as certified nurses' aides/assistants and medical assistants, may use only their specific title.

Current Nursing Licensure Laws

The authority for establishing a licensure law lies with the legislature of each jurisdiction. A proposed change in the law enters the legislative process through an elected member of the legislature who has been persuaded that the change is in the best interest of the public. That individual introduces a bill (see Chapter 3 for an overview of how a bill becomes a law). A group, such as the nurses association, wishing to instigate this action may spend months preparing and planning the content for a bill and gaining the support of legislators who might introduce the legislation.

During the legislative process, individuals and organizations may affect the content of the proposed legislation by influencing the legislators to amend the bill. Amendments to a bill may change the content dramatically and cause the original supporters of the bill to reconsider their support. Once the appropriate legislative body passes a bill, it becomes the **enacted** or **statutory law**. This law cannot be changed without another vote of the legislative body.

Rules and Regulations

Each state has its own set of administrative **rules and regulations** to carry out the provisions of laws regulating nursing. These rules are termed the **administrative law**. They are established by an administrative body, usually the **state board of nursing** that is given responsibility for administering the Nurse Practice Act. This responsibility is authorized in the Nurse Practice Act itself (see the section later in this chapter on the role of the board of nursing). Most states require that public hearings be held regarding proposed rules and regulations, but the board has the authority to make the final decision. The rules and regulations must be within the scope outlined by the legislation that was passed. Those that are accepted by the appropriate board have the force of law unless they are challenged in court and are found not to be in accord with the legislature's intent.

In some states, the Nurse Practice Act is detailed and specifies most of the critical provisions regarding licensure and practice. In other states, the practice act is broad, and the administrative body is given a great deal of power to make decisions through rules and regulations. Both the Nurse Practice Act and state rules and regulations govern nursing in every state.

Nursing Licensure Law Content

In the early 1900s, the ANA, assuming its leadership role in nursing licensure, formulated a model nurse practice act to be used by state associations when planning legislation. The last ANA revision of this model was in 1990 by the ANA Congress for Nursing Practice (ANA, 1990). When the responsibility for overseeing the licensure process shifted to the NCSBN, that group also developed a model nurse practice act. In addition, it wrote the Model Nursing Administrative Rules. The NCSBN continues to update its model act and model rules and regulations as part of its role in supporting the state boards of nursing, with the most recent update in 2004 (NCSBN, 2004a). This latest update includes both model law provisions and model regulations in a side-by-side format to facilitate understanding of their reciprocal nature.

Carefully read the Nurse Practice Act for the state in which you will practice. A copy of the Act may be obtained from the state board of nursing (check the NCSBN Web site, *www.ncsbn.org*). Many states make these documents available on-line. In some states, one act includes both practical nursing and registered nursing; other states have separate, but similar, acts. Historically, the role of the nursing assistant was not outlined in nursing laws. As federal legislation mandating classes and certification for nursing assistants in long-term care took effect, some states modified laws and rules and regulations to address the role of the nursing assistant. In other states, regulations governing nursing assistants rest within a different department of the state government.

The following general topics usually are covered in state licensure laws for nursing.

Purpose

The purpose of regulating the practice of nursing is twofold: Regulations protect the public and make individual practitioners accountable for their actions. Note that the protection of the status of the licensed individual is not the reason for licensure. With this in mind, you can better understand the inclusion of some other topics in the act.

Definitions and Scope of Practice

All of the significant terms in the act are defined for the purpose of carrying out the law. This is where the legal definition of nursing and the scope of practice are spelled out. The NCSBN has given the following definition:

> Nursing is a scientific process founded on a professional body of knowledge; it is a learned profession based on an understanding of the human condition across the lifespan and the relationship of a client with others and within the environment; and it is an art dedicated to caring for others. The practice of nursing means assisting clients to attain or maintain optimal health, implementing a strategy of care to accomplish defined goals within the context of a client-centered health care plan, and evaluating responses to nursing care and treatment. Nursing is a dynamic discipline that is continually evolving to include more sophisticated knowledge, technologies and client care activities. (NCSBN, 2004a)

The document then proceeds to distinguish between RN and LPN practice.

No state adopts the exact wording of any recommended definition, but many states include references to performing services for compensation (which has been deleted from the NCSBN definition), the necessity for a specialized knowledge base, the use of the nursing process or its parts (although steps may be named differently), and components of nursing practice. Several states include some reference to treating human responses to actual or potential health problems; this was first addressed in New York State's license law and was later incorporated in the ANA's *Nursing: A Social Policy Statement* (ANA, 1980). Most states refer to the execution of the medical regimen, and many include a general statement about additional acts that recognize that nursing practice is evolving and that the nurse's area of responsibility can be expected to broaden.

Definitions of practical nursing are more restrictive, and usually state that the individual must function under the direction of an RN or physician, in areas demanding less judgment and knowledge than is required of the RN. In the NCSBN model act, this is referred to as "a directed scope of nursing practice" (NCSBN, 2004a). Practical nurse standards usually focus on data collection rather than comprehensive assessment, and they specify that the practical nurse contributes to the plan and evaluation of care rather than being accountable for them.

The scope of practice for any profession includes those activities, processes, and skills that are part of that profession and is directly tied to the legal definition. The education of the professional provides the basis for scope of practice and therefore differs for RNs, advanced practice nurses, and LPNs. The scope of practice also differentiates those activities that are nursing from those that are a part of other professions.

Because the definition of nursing in the law is written in broad terms, it is sometimes difficult to determine whether a specific action is permitted as part of the scope of practice. Figure 7-2 provides a decision-making process to help you examine whether any action is within your scope of practice as an RN. In some instances, when the issue is very complex, an advisory opinion regarding whether a specific action is within a nursing scope of practice may be sought from the state board of nursing.

Health care facilities employ a variety of nursing assistants, in the way of mental health technicians, nursing assistants, or medication technicians. The preparation and scope of practice for these individuals are a matter of serious concern to the public. Laws regarding educational requirements and legal definitions of scope of practice have been adopted for nursing assistant practice. Through the Omnibus Budget Reconciliation Act of 1987 regulations for long-term care

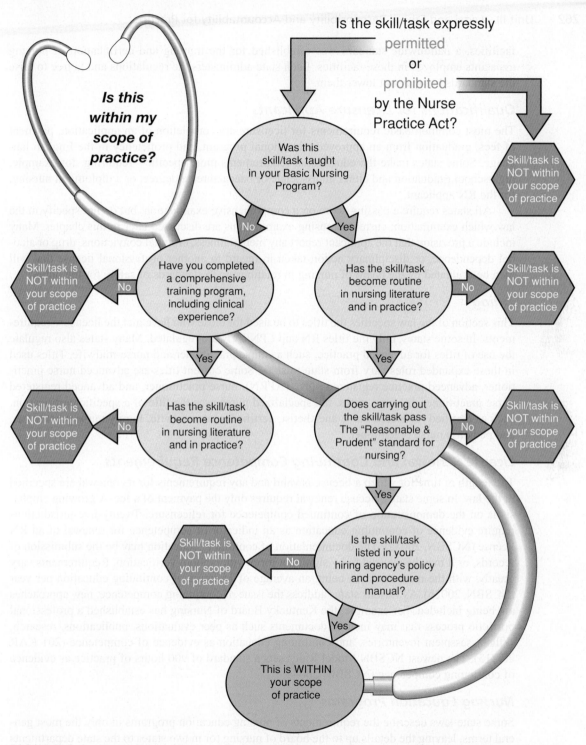

FIGURE 7-2 Nursing Scope of Practice: A Decision-Making Model (with permission of South Dakota Board of Nursing).

facilities, a nationwide standard was established for the training and certification of nursing assistants employed in these facilities. Each state administers the regulations and is free to raise the standards but may not lower them.

Qualifications for Licensure Applicants

The most common basic requirements for licensure are completion of an application, payment of fees, graduation from an approved educational program, and proficiency in the English language. Some states make the educational requirements more specific—requiring, for example, high school graduation and either an associate or baccalaureate degree, or a diploma in nursing, for the RN applicant.

All states require a passing score on a comprehensive examination, but do not specify in the law which examination; current licensing examinations are discussed later in this chapter. Many include a provision that the applicant report any mental illness, criminal convictions, drug or alcohol dependence, or disciplinary action taken in regard to another professional license that will then be evaluated by the board of nursing in relationship to standards of safety for the public.

Titling

This section of the law specifies the titles to be used for those who have met the licensure requirements. In some states, only the titles RN and LPN/LVN are regulated. Many states also regulate the use of titles for advanced practice, such as nurse practitioner and nurse-midwife. Titles used in these expanded roles vary from state to state. Some current titles are advanced nurse practitioner, advanced practice registered nurse (APRN), nurse practitioner, and advanced registered nurse practitioner. In some states, the specialized nurse uses the title of a specific certification, such as certified registered nurse anesthetist, certified nurse-midwife, family nurse practitioner, and pediatric nurse practitioner.

License Renewal and Continuing Competence Requirements

The length of time for which a license is valid and any requirements for its renewal are specified in the law. In some states, license renewal requires only the payment of a fee. A growing emphasis is on the demonstration of continued competence for relicensure. Twenty-five jurisdictions require evidence of continuing education as an indicator of competence for renewal of an RN license (NCSBN, 2005a). The documentation of continuing education may be the submission of records, or it may be attested to by signing a form with random verification. Requirements vary greatly, with the most common being an average of 15 hours of continuing education per year (NCSBN, 2002b). As various states address the issue of continuing competence, new approaches are being included. For example, the Kentucky Board of Nursing has established a professional portfolio process that may include documents such as peer evaluations, publications, research, skills assessment inventories, and continuing education as evidence of competence (201 KAR 20:215). The newest NCSBN Model Rules sets a standard of 900 hours of practice as evidence of continuing competence (NCSBN, 2004a).

Nursing Education Programs

Some state laws describe the requirements of nursing education programs in only the most general terms, leaving the details up to the board of nursing (or in two states to the state departments of education); in other states, the laws are specific. The law may specify the number of years of education required, which courses or what content must be included, and the approval process for particular programs. If the law is general, then the board sets more specific standards. Some jurisdictions are establishing outcomes that must be met by the nursing education program. A nursing education program in those states must fulfill the requirements of the state law for graduates to be eligible for licensure.

Grounds for Disciplinary Action

Disciplinary action refers to all penalties that may be imposed against an individual who has violated provisions of a licensing law. The Nurse Practice Act for a state identifies the basis for disciplinary action, and the board is empowered to prosecute those who violate the law. Disciplinary actions may include fines, reprimands, restrictions on practice (such as working only under supervision), suspension of a license for a specified period, or **revocation** (removal) of a license. The board may be authorized to ask a court to halt a specific practice that it believes is contrary to the law until a full hearing can be held. This is called **injunctive relief**. This term refers to the court order called an injunction that requires an individual or organization to stop a particular activity. The board also may immediately suspend a license, pending investigation, if the situation holds a serious threat to the public.

Disciplinary action can only be taken based on criteria stated in the law (Fig. 7-3). Most courts have supported revocation of a license only when the offense was related in some way to practice issues that affected the public safety. Thus, most modern nurse practice or disciplinary acts contain specific concerns such as the following:

- Fraud or deceit in obtaining a license
- Criminal conviction
- Unethical conduct

FIGURE 7-3 A nursing license may be revoked by the State Board of Nursing.

- Drug diversion
- Unsafe or unprofessional practice (including practicing while chemically impaired)
- Practicing outside the scope of practice

Some states also have clauses that call for license revocation for individuals who default on government-sponsored education loans or on agreements regarding service in return for scholarship aid.

Exceptions

Certain provisions may allow those who are not licensed to act as nurses in specific situations. Performing as a student while in an education program is usually the primary exception. Those who care for family members or friends without pay are also exempted from license regulations. Those who practice nursing in a federal agency, such as a military hospital, are exempted from seeking a license in the state where they are stationed as long as they maintain a current license in another state. Some states are adopting exceptions for self-directed care by the disabled. In these situations, a paid care provider may perform certain care that is usually considered nursing when directed to do so by the mentally competent, physically disabled client. This includes administering medications in the home and carrying out specific care procedures, such as catheterization.

Administrative Provisions

Each law requires administrative specifications detailing when the law will become effective and when a previous act will no longer be in force. Such provisions are of particular interest to nurses when a law is first passed, because nurses want to know when changes affecting them will take place.

Although the Nurse Practice Act itself usually does not specify the fees to be charged for obtaining or renewing a license, general restrictions on the method of calculating fees and on how the fees may be used are often included in the act. The act may specify how the expenses of the board of nursing are to be met and who has legal authority to make decisions regarding the use of funds.

All states charge a fee for processing an application for licensure. At initial licensure, there is also a fee for taking a licensing examination (approximately $200), which is paid to the company that prepares and scores an examination. In addition, there is a fee each time a license is renewed. There may be fees associated with providing documentation to another state regarding credentials when the nurse is seeking licensure from another jurisdiction. For specific information about current fees, contact your state board of nursing or visit its Web site.

Grandfathering

When a new law is written, it usually contains a statement specifying that anyone currently holding a license may continue to hold that license if and when requirements for the license change. This is termed **grandfathering**. Without this provision, the enactment of a new law would require individuals who are currently licensed to reapply and to show that they meet the new standards.

However, not all changes in the law are grandfathered. When new requirements are instituted that the legislature believes are important for the safety of the public, all currently licensed individuals may be required to meet the new standards within a given time period. A good example is the requirement for continuing education for relicensure. When this requirement was added, all applicants had to meet the requirement by a specific date.

Sunset Laws and Nurse Practice Acts

Most laws remain in effect until the legislature votes to rescind or replace them. Because this has resulted in archaic laws remaining in effect for many years, some states have passed what are known as "sunset laws." **Sunset laws** provide that any regulatory act, such as the Nurse Practice Act, will automatically be rescinded after a predetermined length of time if not reauthorized. In states with sunset laws, nurses cannot wait for an opportune time to support changes in the Nurse Practice Act. Instead, they must identify when "sun-setting" will occur and work in advance to sustain the current law or make changes. The advantage of sunset laws is that they guarantee that the legislature will review and evaluate agencies and programs.

Advanced Practice Registered Nurses

Advance practice registered nurses (APRN) include nurse practitioners, nurse anesthetists, nurse–midwives, and, in some states, clinical nurse specialists. Licensure requirements for advanced practice vary from state to state, although work is being done to develop uniform APRN licensure. Many, but not all, require the master's degree in nursing. Gradually, states are moving toward the master's degree as the standard. None of the states administers a state licensing examination for advanced practice nursing.

Often the law requires that a person be certified for advanced practice by the American Nurse Credentialing Center (ANCC) or a nursing specialty organization (see section on certification later in the chapter) to receive a license as an APRN. This certification includes testing. The requirements and methods for obtaining certification remain with the organization granting the certification, but the nurse receives a license from the state to practice in the expanded role. This is true of certified nurse anesthetists, who are all certified through the Council on Certification of Nurse Anesthetists, but who receive legal status to practice in anesthesia by the appropriate authority in their state. Some states do not specifically mention APRNs, but the board of nursing approves specialty practice based on the provisions in the basic act. In still other states, APRNs are governed under the Medical Practice Act. Contact the board of nursing in the state in which you are interested for information about advanced practice.

Some of the laws regulating advanced practice have provided for physician review of nursing's scope of practice. The ANA is concerned that these laws will take autonomy away from nursing and allow medicine to control some aspects of the nursing profession. The ANA also is concerned about the rigidity of these laws, which may not allow for evolving nursing roles. The ANA holds the position that the licensure law should regulate minimum safe practice, and that the profession should regulate advanced practice. A parallel process is used in medicine, in which there is only basic licensure and specialty practice is regulated by specialty boards in the profession.

The NCSBN has adopted the position that the licensing of nurses in advanced practice is an appropriate responsibility of the legal jurisdiction governing nursing practice. Therefore, the NCSBN has entered into discussions with the various organizations providing advanced practice certification regarding the validity and reliability of their testing and whether that testing is legally defensible if the state board chooses to use it in the process of APRN licensure. The NCSBN has developed a set of uniform requirements for advanced practice licensure that would facilitate interstate endorsement (NCSBN, 2002b) and a position paper on advanced practice in nursing (NCSBN, 2002a).

The Role of the State Board of Nursing

The state boards of nursing (or their equivalent) are the administrative department of the government legally empowered to carry out the provisions of the Nurse Practice Act. Board membership, the procedures for appointment and removal, and the qualifications of board members are determined by the Nurse Practice Act. Boards have the power to write the rules and regulations used in daily operations.

The governor of the state usually appoints the members of the board. The law specifies the occupational background of the candidates; nominations may be made by nurses' organizations and other interested parties. North Carolina is the only state in which the RN members of the state board are elected by the RNs in the state.

Boards of nursing range in size from 7 to 17 members. Prerequisites for educational background of nurses who serve as board members vary across states. Some states require that the board include nurses from different occupational areas, such as education and nursing service. Most states have at least one public member of the board. And a few have at least one physician on the nursing board.

Most states have a single board for RNs and LPNs. In some states, separate boards exist. Each state board has a paid staff that usually is headed by an RN with advanced education who is employed as the executive director of the state board of nursing. The executive director is responsible for administering the work of the board and seeing that rules and regulations are followed. This individual also represents the state board on the NCSBN.

Duties related to professional licensure may be performed by a centralized state agency acting in that capacity for all licensed occupations. The responsibilities of these centralized agencies may range from administrative matters (such as collecting fees, managing routine license renewals, and providing secretarial services) to decision making, relegating individual boards, like the board of nursing, to an advisory status.

Each state board must operate within the framework of its own state law regarding the practice of nursing, but all cooperate through the NCSBN. For example, state boards acting together through the NCSBN contract with the company that prepares the licensing examinations for RNs and practical nurses that are used throughout the United States. They also cooperate with other organizations, such as the ANA, the NLN, and the NLNAC, in some matters, but maintain the separation that is required of a group whose focus is protection of the public through effective licensure of nurses.

The board of nursing typically performs the following functions:

1. Establishes standards for licensure
2. Examines and licenses applicants
3. Provides for interstate endorsement
4. Renews licenses, grants temporary licenses, and provides for inactive status for those already licensed who request it
5. Enforces disciplinary codes
6. Provides rules for revocation of license
7. Regulates specialty practice

8. Establishes standards and curricula for nursing programs
9. Approves nursing education programs

OBTAINING A NURSING LICENSE

There are two procedures for obtaining a nursing license; one is used for obtaining an initial license and the other for obtaining a license when the nurse is already licensed in another jurisdiction. The initial licensure process is called **licensure by examination**. Obtaining a license in a second jurisdiction is called **licensure by endorsement**. In both instances, the applicant for licensure must meet all provisions of the law (such as educational preparation, language proficiency, and legal residency status) in the state where he or she seeks licensure. In the initial licensure process, the applicant must take and pass the NCLEX. When seeking licensure by endorsement, the applicant is not required to take another examination—the licensing examination results from the initial state are accepted as proof of minimum safe practice—but other requirements must be met. This process is discussed later in the chapter.

Licensure by Examination

The establishment of a licensing examination was an important part of early efforts to achieve a professional standard for the RN. When each state adopted a licensing law, it also established a mechanism for examining license applicants. A major achievement in the history of nursing licensure was the formation of the Bureau of State Boards of Nurse Examiners, which eventually led to the use of an identical examination in all states in 1950. The original examination, called the State Board Test Pool Examination, was prepared by the testing department of the NLN, under a contract with the state boards. Although each state initially determined its own passing score, eventually all states adopted a common passing score. The current examination, called the **NCLEX-RN** for registered nursing and the **NCLEX-PN** for practical nursing, is used in all states and territories of the United States. Beginning in October 2002, a new testing company, Pearson Professional Testing of Minnesota, was granted the contract for preparing and administering all NCLEX examinations.

Content of the Examination

Historically the State Board Test Pool examination content was divided into the categories of medical, surgical, obstetric, pediatric, and psychiatric nursing. Because nursing had changed in nature and these categories no longer adequately reflected nursing practice, the NCSBN adopted a different examination plan, which was implemented in July 1982. For this examination, the National Council supported a research study, called the RN Job Analysis, which identified nursing behaviors critical to maintaining a safe and effective standard of care. This research is repeated periodically to ensure that the test plan remains relevant to current nursing practice.

In all of these studies, newly licensed, practicing RNs are studied to determine both the frequency and the criticality of various behaviors. **Frequency** refers to how often the behaviors are required of the newly practicing RN. **Criticality** refers to those actions that, if performed incorrectly or omitted, could cause serious harm to the client. These studies are reflected in the *Test Plan for the NCLEX for Registered Nurses* (NCSBN, 2004b). The NCLEX-RN examination questions are organized into categories based on the interaction of client needs and the steps of the nursing process. The four client needs (safe effective care environment, health promotion and

TABLE 7-1	2004 TEST PLAN FOR NCLEX-RN
CLIENT NEEDS CATEGORIES/SUBCATEGORIES	PERCENTAGE OF ITEMS
Safe Effective Care Environment	
Management of care	13%–19%
Safety and infection control	8%–14%
Health Promotion and Maintenance	6%–12%
Psychosocial Integrity	6%–12%
Physiological Integrity	
Basic care and comfort	6%–12%
Pharmacological and parenteral therapies	13%–19%
Reduction of risk potential	13%–19%
Physiological adaptation	11%–17%

maintenance, psychosocial integrity, and physiologic integrity), and their subcategories, form the basis of the exam (see Table 7-1). The nursing process is divided into five steps: assessment, analysis, planning, implementation, and evaluation. These two sets of concepts form a matrix in which each question tests a step of the nursing process and one subcategory of client need. Another set of broad concepts (caring, communication and documentation, cultural awareness, and self-care) is integrated into the test. The multiple-choice questions in the examination typically are based on situations that require a nursing response. They are designed to test judgment and decision making, not simply knowledge of facts. Setting priorities, delegating, and communicating with the health team are aspects of that judgment. The entire test plan is explained in the test plan booklet distributed to those who apply to take the examination. The test plan is also available for downloading without charge from the NCSBN Web site (NCSBN, 2004b).

The NCLEX-PN has a similar construction pattern. A "PN Job Analysis" study is conducted, and then the test plan is developed. The most recent PN Job Analysis was completed in 2003; the newest test plan for the PN was approved in 2004 and implemented in April 2005. The practical nurse is expected to assume a more dependent role in assessment; therefore, that step is titled data collection. Analysis is not part of the test plan. Whereas the RN examination includes management of care, the PN examination focuses on coordination of care. Even when topics are the same, the level of judgment expected of the PN differs from that expected of the RN. The newest test recognizes that many LPNs are employed in long-term care settings, with clients older than 65 years of age; therefore, it focuses on the older population (NCSBN, 2005b).

Preparing and Administering the Examination

Preparing questions for the examination is a complex process. Nursing educators and RNs who work with new graduates are brought together to write exam questions based on the test plan. Content experts who are also nurses currently working with new graduates review all questions. Another panel of individuals reviews the questions for bias. Each question then is verified for accuracy by using current nursing references; test-construction experts also review the structure of all of the questions. The final versions of all questions are tested by inclusion in a nongraded part of the license examinations being given to new graduates; the questions are evaluated for their level of difficulty and appropriate use as part of a future scored examination.

In addition to assuming responsibility for test preparation, the testing service administers the computerized tests through contracted testing centers, scores the examinations, and reports scores to the state boards. The testing service is authorized to sell statistical information related to the examinations to the states and to individual schools.

Computerized Adaptive Testing

All NCLEX examinations (both RN and PN) are now administered through **computerized adaptive testing (CAT)**. CAT consists of a bank of examination questions administered through a computerized system. It was first field tested in 1990, then across the country in 1993, and finally adopted for all testing beginning in April 1994.

In this computerized test, the multiple-choice questions are delivered on a computer screen. The computer contains a large bank of questions, and different individuals may be presented with different questions. The computer program evaluates each response, and then selects an appropriate question to present next, choosing a slightly harder question if the previous question was answered correctly, or an easier question if the response was incorrect. The computer program ensures that all essential aspects of the test matrix plan are part of every examination. The development of questions and the design of the computer program ensure that all tests are equivalent, even when they're not identical. On the NCLEX-RN, the minimum number of questions that might be administered is 75 and the maximum is 265. The maximum length of time for the examination is 5 hours, but a candidate performing either especially well or very poorly might complete the exam in just 1 hour. One break is required after 2 hours of testing, and others may be taken at the discretion of the applicant. Testing ends when the scoring analysis clearly indicates a pass or fail, the maximum number of questions has been answered, or the maximum time has been completed.

Each candidate for licensure makes an individual appointment at a testing site. Security at the center is tightly monitored using photo identification and thumb prints. The computers are located in a quiet room without distractions. No test study materials are allowed at the testing center and no food or drink is allowed in the test environment. An erasable note board is provided for notes or calculations. An optional on-screen calculator is provided.

Only one question, along with its possible answers, is presented on the screen at a time; if there is a brief situation, however, the question may appear on the same screen. The space bar moves between the alternative answers, and the "enter" key must be pressed twice to make a selection. A mouse is also available for movement and selection. A selection must be made to move to the next question. It is not possible to go back to a question previously answered. In April 2003, two new types of questions in addition to the one correct answer were introduced. One involves keyboard entry of short answers, and the other allows the person to select several answers from the multiple options. A tutorial on how to use the computer, including the on-screen calculator, along with some practice questions are provided to ensure that the individual understands the process. When the individual has completed enough questions for the computer program to determine whether the student has passed or failed, the testing session is ended.

Scoring the Examination

The computer calculates the score as the applicant answers questions. Based on the computation made as the applicant progresses, additional questions are presented to clearly determine whether the applicant meets the standards for safe, effective practice in all areas of the test plan.

The score used to determine whether a student passed or failed is not a raw score (ie, the number correct), but is derived from a complex statistical process that takes into consideration both the difficulty of a question and whether the response was correct. As soon as the statistical computation provides a clear prediction of pass or fail, the test is terminated. If the computerized score has not provided a clear prediction of pass or fail by the end of the examination (because either time is up or the maximum number of questions are answered), the performance on the last 60 questions becomes the basis for determining pass or fail. The test was not designed for the purpose of differentiating levels of excellence, only for demonstrating basic safe practice, and this is what the pass or fail communicates.

Although the computer immediately determines a score (upon the completion of the examination), the individual is not notified of the result at that time. The scoring information is communicated to the testing service, which then notifies the appropriate board. The board of nursing then notifies the individual whether he or she passed or failed.

Every 3 years, the NCSBN considers the appropriateness of the passing standards for both the PN and RN examinations and may modify them. Additionally, every 3 years a study of essential functions is repeated and the test plan itself may be modified based on this research.

Preparing for the NCLEX

Individuals must determine how best to prepare for the licensure examination based on their background and preferred study style. A review of the knowledge basic to nursing is important for most individuals. This may be done using course notes and texts. Those who become anxious in testing situations may want to focus on exercises to decrease anxiety during the examination. Those who find the process of test taking difficult can gain greater self-confidence by practicing test-taking techniques. This can be done through printed tests in books or computerized test preparation programs.

For both the NCLEX-RN and the NCLEX-PN, many commercial study aids are available. To prepare applicants to take the examination, the NCSBN has authorized the preparation of a study book that explains the examination, how it was written, and the scoring system, and that provides sample questions to familiarize applicants with the way the test is written. The NCSBN also provides an on-line NCLEX-RN study program available by subscription. Many companies also prepare NCLEX-RN and NCLEX-PN review books, sample examination questions, audiotapes, and computerized practice examinations that are used to prepare for the licensing examinations. Manuals that outline standard nursing practice relative to many different health care problems may be useful for reviewing nursing content. Live and videotaped review courses, produced both by individual schools of nursing and by commercial publishers, are available to those who want assistance with preparation. During your preparation, remember that the goal is to solidify your knowledge and skills and to develop your critical-thinking and problem-solving skills. Memorizing answers to test questions presented in study books will not help you with the problem solving in regard to the unique questions presented in the actual examination.

Critical Thinking Activity

A student about to graduate from an RN program in New York wishes to practice nursing in New Jersey. What options are available to her? Investigate the steps she should take to ensure that she may legally practice nursing in New Jersey as soon after graduation as possible.

Licensure by Endorsement

The process of obtaining a nursing license in a new state (while already licensed in another state) is called licensure by endorsement. Sometimes people incorrectly assume reciprocity exists among all states for nursing licenses. Technically, **reciprocity** is the type of recognition provided for such items as a driver's license; you can drive in any state as long as your license from your state of residence is valid. A similar type of recognition for nursing licensure has been developed between some states, but is not the universal pattern.

In licensure by endorsement, each case is considered independently, based on the rules and regulations of the state. However, due to the uniformity of licensing laws throughout most of the United States and its territories, nurses have enjoyed easy mobility between geographic areas.

Because the same licensure examination and passing standards are used nationwide, no state requires that the examination be retaken. Basic educational and legal requirements of the individual state where a license is sought must be met. Sometimes a nurse moving to a new state must meet the current criteria for new licensure. In other states, a nurse must fulfill only the requirements that were in effect at the time of the original licensure. A state may require a nurse to meet other criteria, such as those for continuing education, before granting licensure by endorsement. In all cases, appropriate paperwork must be completed, necessary fees paid, and a license obtained before a nurse may begin employment.

A temporary license, which allows the applicant for licensure by endorsement to be employed while credentials are being verified and processed, is available in some states. Other states require that a permanent license be obtained before any employment is legal in those jurisdictions.

If a nurse wishes to maintain licensure in more than one state, this may be done by paying the renewal fees and meeting other requirements for continued licensure, such as continuing education, in each state. Some nurses hold licenses in several states to be able to work as a traveling nurse or to choose work in different locations. Nurses working close to state lines may need more than one license to be employed by an agency that operates in more than one state. This might also be true of a nursing education program that has clinical sites in two adjacent states or a home care agency with clients in two states.

Critical Thinking Activity

An RN who has been working in San Jose, California, for 10 years decides to relocate to Orlando, Florida. What are the steps that the nurse must take to ensure that she is able to work as an RN in Florida? Where should she seek information about the needed steps?

Mutual Recognition of Licensure

Mutual recognition of licensure is based on a multistate agreement called the Nurse Licensure Compact. Mutual recognition of licensure involves an individual receiving an RN license in the state where he or she resides and being legally permitted to practice in additional states without obtaining additional licenses for those states. This is sometimes referred to as "multistate licensure." The Nurse Licensure Compact is the agreed-upon standard for mutual recognition of registered nursing licensure that was adopted by the NCSBN. Those states that have entered into the NCSBN Nurse Licensure Compact have all passed legislation adopting the terms of the Compact into their licensure laws (NCSBN, 1998). At this writing, 18 states have entered the compact agreement, and three other states have passed legislation and are planning implementation. For the most current information on states participating, go to the NCSBN Web site and link to Nursing Licensure Compact.

Processes Involved in Mutual Recognition

All of the states that have signed the compact are referred to as **party states**. A person's **home state** is the state in which he or she resides and has a registered nursing license. An individual maintains only one license, the license granted in the home state, but is legally permitted to practice in any party state. When renewing a license, the individual renews in the home state. The individual nurse cannot hold a license in two party states at the same time. When an individual changes residence to a new party state, he or she applies for a new home state license based on residency. Individuals who wish to practice in a nonparty state still need to apply for a license in the nonparty state before practicing nursing.

A **remote state** is a party state other than the nurse's home state where the patient or recipient of nursing practice is located. For purposes of this law, nursing care location is based on where the patient is, not where the nurse is. The individual nurse must comply with the state laws regulating nursing practice in the state in which the client is located. Any party state where nursing care occurs (whether the home state or the remote state) may institute disciplinary action based on appropriate procedures. The home state is notified of the action being taken in the remote state through a coordinated information data bank system called NURSYS. When a remote state institutes disciplinary action, it may revoke a nurse's privilege to practice in that state only. Only the home state may revoke the license itself. If an individual has been assigned to some type of alternative program (such as drug treatment and monitoring) as part of the disciplinary process by any party state, the conditions of the disciplinary process must prohibit the individual from practicing in other states in the compact until the problem is resolved.

NURSYS was completed in 2000. This data bank contains licensure and disciplinary information from approximately 33 states that have chosen to use the system. NURSYS can be used by any state to track disciplinary concerns (NCSBN, 2006). Noncompact states may also submit disciplinary information through the Health Care Integrity and Protection Data Bank maintained by the NCSBN.

As you can see, the RN who is licensed in a Nurse Licensure Compact state who chooses to work outside the home state must follow the directives contained in the compact and become familiar with the nursing practice act in any state in which clients are located. The state board of any state participating in the compact will provide complete information on the specific requirements to be met. A separate APRN compact has also been developed. That compact has not yet been implemented.

Reasons Nurses Seek Mutual Recognition of Licenses

Under standard licensing laws, the nurse who practices in more than one state must hold multiple nursing licenses. This is both costly and complex. As the health care system grows more diverse, it is not uncommon for a health care–providing organization to operate across state boundaries.

Telenursing includes the use of telecommunications technology (eg, telephone, fax, computers, teleconferencing, interactive television, and video phone) to provide nursing services to individuals and groups. A telenurse in one state may care for a client in a distant state, thus raising questions regarding licensure requirements for a nurse who serves clients in more than one state. Does the nurse who provides telephone monitoring and advice for the client in another state need to be licensed in that client's state? Another area of concern is the nurse who works for an agency that serves clients across state borders. This nurse needs to visit clients in more than one state. The nursing case manager may follow clients in several states. All of these situations create a demand for a simpler licensing system for working in multiple states.

Concerns Regarding Mutual Recognition of Licenses

Not all nurses have supported mutual recognition of licenses. The ANA has identified that nurses who have differing requirements for relicensure could be practicing side-by-side; for example, one home state requires continuing education and another does not. Some state attorneys general have given opinions that it would be unconstitutional in their state to allow another state to control the requirements for practice. Issues of privacy regarding the data stored in the NURSYS system are another area of concern. The mutual recognition of licenses system may save money for the nurse who practices in multiple states because only one license would be purchased. However, if fewer nurses are licensed in the state, but the same number practice in the state, one would expect that disciplinary costs would remain even. The cost of licenses for all nurses, therefore, would have to rise to ensure adequate funds to support disciplinary costs (ANA, 2006).

A major concern is the disciplinary process. Although the board of nursing can investigate nursing practices and enforce its own standards in the state, it cannot change the licensure status of the person whose licensure originates in a different state; this fact is troubling to some boards of nursing. They are concerned that this doesn't allow them to protect the public adequately. A person disciplined in a remote state will still possess what would appear to be a valid home state license, but perhaps would not legally be able to practice in the remote state. For the individual nurse, the differences in licensure regulations could result in the same behavior being the cause of disciplinary action in one state but not in others; however, if the license were removed by the home state, then it would be invalid in all states.

Simpson (1999) suggests that technology can solve most of these concerns if it is applied effectively. The ANA has expressed concern that mutual recognition of licenses would facilitate bringing in out-of-state nurses for strike breaking and thus interfere with valid collective bargaining (see Chapter 12 for a further discussion of collective bargaining).

The future holds many exciting possibilities for nursing, but also poses many potential pitfalls. This is a complex issue, because state licensing agencies are charged with protecting the public and have legitimate concerns regarding such areas as disciplinary action.

REVOCATION OR LIMITATION OF A LICENSE

A license to practice any occupation becomes a property right of the individual once the state has awarded it. As long as the individual renews a license by paying the appropriate fees and meeting any requirements, such as continuing education, the license cannot be revoked without cause. The possible reasons for revoking or limiting a license are spelled out in the law.

The procedure for revoking a license includes a fact-finding process and a hearing, which functions in many ways like a court proceeding. The state board or a specially designated hearing board is responsible for conducting the hearing and making a decision. The board may provide a license with conditions, suspend a license until certain conditions are met, or revoke a license completely. For example, a nurse faced with charges of chemical dependency might be directed to enter a treatment program, to refuse employment involving direct responsibility for clients who need controlled substances or access to drugs, and to be monitored for compliance. If these conditions are met, the individual may be allowed to work in a restricted environment and then be reinstated to full rights and privileges of licensure when treatment is completed. The board's decision may be appealed in a court of law in most states. If a board of nursing finds that the individual's actions constitute a felony, the board is obligated to report that to the criminal authorities for prosecution.

The individual being investigated for any violation of the Nurse Practice Act, or who is in the hearing process, should have an attorney who is knowledgeable about professional disciplinary issues from the time of notification of the complaint. According to Malugani (2000), the majority of nurses facing disciplinary action fail to take this important step to protect themselves. The state nurses association or the local chapter of the National Association of Nurse Attorneys can often provide referrals of attorneys who are familiar with the disciplinary process. Although attorney costs are substantial, a license to practice nursing is extremely valuable to the individual nurse. Some malpractice insurance policies include payment for attorney fees in the case of disciplinary action (see Chapter 8).

As a licensed professional, be aware that you are responsible to your clients and to the state in which you practice. You can act to protect your license through maintaining current knowledge and appropriate standards of practice. Also understand and abide by the scope of practice as described in your individual nursing practice act. If you take a position in a new state, be sure to become informed about that state's Nurse Practice Act.

Critical Thinking Activity

A nurse in your state receives a notification from the board of nursing that a complaint has been lodged with the board regarding his practice. Find out what the process would be in your state for this nurse to respond to the complaint. What resources will this nurse need? What are the possible consequences if the complaint is sustained?

 ## LICENSURE OF GRADUATES OF FOREIGN NURSING SCHOOLS

Many nurses from other countries have immigrated to the United States and sought licensure to be able to work in their new home. Some nurses have come to the United States for additional education and need a license to engage in clinical practice associated with that education. Still others are attracted by the higher salaries and better living conditions for nurses in the United States. During the nursing shortage of the early 1980s, and again in the current nursing shortage, employers in the United States actively recruited foreign nurses, sometimes providing support for travel and relocation expenses.

Several concerns have been expressed regarding the recruitment of foreign-educated nurses to the United States. In many of the countries from which nurses emigrate to the United States, there are also nursing shortages. Thus, the United States depletes other countries of an important health resource. And some U.S. nurses believed that overseas recruitment took the place of addressing the workplace problems that contribute to the shortage.

For the foreign-educated nurse, there are two requirements that must be met in order to work in the United States. The first of these is a visa that permits employment. This might be a visa granted to a permanent immigrant or it might be a visa granted to a temporary worker. The employer is required to verify the individual's eligibility for employment in the United States.

The second requirement that the foreign-educated nurse must meet is to obtain a state license to practice nursing. To obtain a license, all graduates of foreign nursing schools who want to practice nursing in the United States must provide verification to the state licensing authority that their nursing education meets state requirements and they must take the appropriate NCLEX examination. In the past, institutions would sometimes hire foreign nurses into lower-paying positions until they obtained a license. When many did not pass the examination, the nurses felt exploited by the system.

Committee on Graduates of Foreign Nursing Schools

The U.S. Department of Labor, the Department of Health and Human Services (HHS), the Immigration and Naturalization Service (INS), the ANA, and the NLN are all concerned about the safety of the public and about the well-being of the foreign-educated nurse. To address these problems, these organizations and government agencies collaborated in the development of an independent organization called the Commission on Graduates of Foreign Nursing Schools (CGFNS).

CGFNS provides a variety of services to graduates of foreign nursing schools to enable them to meet the requirements both for licensure and for eligibility for employment. One service is the evaluation of education credentials, including course-by-course evaluations that can be submitted to licensing boards. Another service is the English language proficiency examination. A third service is the CGFNS examination, which is a predictor of potential success on the NCLEX. This exam is offered around the world for individuals to take before emigrating. Because many foreign-educated nurses still come to the United States without having taken the CGFNS examination, it also is offered in selected cities in the United States. Some states require only verification of credentials, and others require that the examinations also be completed prior to admission to the NCLEX. Up to 88.7% of foreign-educated nurses who have obtained CGFNS certification pass the licensing examination. Those who failed the CGFNS exam had an NCLEX pass rate of only 49.3%. This contrasts to the 5% to 10% who passed the licensing examination without CGFNS screening (Yocum & Davis, 2002).

While some nurses who come to the United States possess regular immigrant visas, the majority come on special-preference visas. Special immigration regulations allow a foreign nurse to obtain a special-preference visa from the INS, or a work permit from the U.S. Labor Department because of the nursing shortage. To obtain this special-preference visa, an individual nurse must obtain a visa certificate from an HHS-approved agency, such as CGFNS. Under the North Atlantic Free Trade Agreement (NAFTA), nurses from Mexico and Canada were originally exempt from the requirement of obtaining the visa certification; they could directly seek licensure. However, a ruling of the Department of Homeland Security changed that, requiring a visa certificate for Mexican and Canadian nurses after July 2005.

The CGFNS service called *VisaScreen*^{TM} provides this visa certification. The certification does the following:

> satisfies the U.S. Citizenship and Immigration Services (USCIS) requirement for healthcare professionals seeking a temporary or permanent occupational visa in order to work in the U.S., or who are working in the U.S. under Trade NAFTA status. (CGFNS, 2005).

This program includes (1) a review of the foreign nurse's education, (2) evaluation of all current and previous licenses to practice, (3) assessment of English language proficiency (Canadian nurses are exempt from the language assessment except those from Quebec province), and (4) completion of either the CGFNS Qualifying Examination or the NCLEX-RN. The same documentation used for obtaining the visa certification can then be used to apply for licensure in one of the states.

The Trilateral Initiative for Nursing

In 1994, representatives from nursing organizations from Canada, Mexico, and the United States met together as the Trilateral Initiative for North American Nursing to discuss the nursing needs of the three countries and identify opportunities presented by NAFTA. Three goals were established to guide future study and activities:

1. To encourage the development of mutually acceptable standards for education, education program approval and accreditation, licensure/registration, and specialty certification among Canada, Mexico, and the United States in order to advance the nursing profession across North America.
2. To establish a viable, lasting network of key nursing organizations and professionals across North America.
3. To create a methodology that would demonstrate how other professional groups in the three countries could consult, develop goals and programs, and institute policies to increase cross-border cooperation. (Trilateral Initiative, 1996)

The outcomes of the Trilateral Initiative for North American Nursing were published as *An Assessment of North American Nursing* (Trilateral Initiative, 1996). This collaborative effort has served as the foundation for continuing relationships and dialogue among nursing organizations from the three countries.

International Centre on Nurse Migration

The International Centre on Nurse Migration is a project of the CGFNS and the International Council of Nurses (ICN). The goals of the Centre relate to both effective patient care and the well being of nurse migrants. To achieve its goals, the Centre works on policies worldwide that affect nurse migration, collects and reports data on nurse migration, and serves as a resource for those working with regulations regarding nurse migration. (International Centre on Nurse Migration, 2006). Because there is a worldwide shortage of nurses and a wide disparity of wages and recognition between developing and developed countries, nurse migration will continue to be an important international issue.

INTERNATIONAL NURSING LICENSURE

Nursing education and nursing licensure differ greatly throughout the world. Additionally, practice patterns and expectations of nursing behaviors may differ between countries. In Australia, nursing education has been moved into university settings, and future applicants for licensure in that country are required to have a university education. In Italy, nursing education is now consolidated under broad, multisite programs administered by university nursing departments. The European Union is moving toward a system that allows freer movement of professionals between its nations. The nations of Eastern Europe face many drastic changes in their health care systems as they change internally and form different relationships with the West. Nursing education was restricted during Soviet domination, and many nurses had limited nursing educational opportunities, with basic nursing education sometimes occurring at the high school level. This pattern is changing rapidly, as nursing in those countries moves into modern expectations.

Because of educational and practice differences as well as language barriers, nursing credentials are not easily transferred internationally. The ICN has supported the development of effective licensure legislation worldwide. In 1988, it launched a project called "Nursing Regulation: Moving Ahead," which was funded by the W. K. Kellogg Foundation. This ongoing project involved nurses and officials from 77 countries in seminars and studies. To date, nursing licensure laws in the United States have not been affected by this study, but it has supported the development of licensure laws in some parts of the world.

In 1995, the ICN was asked to prepare a guide for an approval system for schools of nursing. This was difficult because many countries lacked approval systems or the ones that existed functioned poorly. In May 2005, the ICN supported an international conference on issues relating to professional nursing regulation worldwide. Information from the presentations at that conference is available on-line at *www.icn.ch*. Presentations focused on standards and competencies, education, and trends and models.

Individuals who are interested in international nursing need to consider both their language proficiency and their educational backgrounds. Organizations actively working in the international health field, such as the World Health Organization and medical relief organizations, usually will provide information on opportunities and licensure requirements in various countries. The ICN in Geneva can provide addresses of appropriate government authorities to contact regarding licensure in other countries. During times of emergency, such as the tsunami in the Indian Ocean, countries may welcome nurses as part of relief groups without requiring licensure in that country. And there are opportunities for short-term health care work in developing countries through charitable agencies and international missions.

CERTIFICATION IN NURSING

As mentioned earlier, certification in nursing is primarily a professional, not legal, credential, and it focuses on knowledge and skills related to a particular area of practice. The definition of certification adopted by the Interdivisional Council on Certification of the ANA (1978) states, "Certification is the documented validation of specific qualifications demonstrated by the individual registered nurse in the provision of professional nursing care in a defined area of practice." Certification is available from many professional nursing and health care organizations (Fig. 7-4).

American Nurses' Credentialing Center Certification

In 1988, the ANA established the ANCC, which assumed all of the ANA credentialing activities. The ANA invited all other organizations providing credentialing for nurses to join; some joined, but many retained their individual programs.

ANCC certification is a method of recognizing nurses who have special expertise. Applicants must demonstrate current practice and knowledge beyond that required for licensure as an RN. After submitting evidence of completing all requirements, a nurse may take the national examination for a specific certification. Certification is granted for a period of 5 years, after

FIGURE 7-4   Certified nurses provide an expert level of practice and may serve as a resource to others.

which a nurse may renew the certification by submitting new evidence of current practice and ability. Table 7-2 lists the various certification credentials available from the ANCC.

Effective in 1998, as approved by the House of Delegates in 1991, individuals seeking certification as generalists in all specialties were required to have a baccalaureate in nursing; those seeking certification as specialists or advanced practice nurses needed a master's degree in nursing. In 2000, responding to the voices of RNs, the ANCC revised its certification program. There are now two basic types of certification. Registered Nurse, Certified (RN, C) is awarded to those with diplomas or associate degrees in nursing who meet the certification requirements for the areas in which this level of certification is offered. Registered Nurse, Board Certified (RN, BC) is awarded to nurses with a baccalaureate or higher degree who meet differing certification requirements for some of the same areas and for additional areas of practice. The master's degree remains the requirement for certification as a clinical nurse specialist, a nurse practitioner, or other advanced practice roles. See Table 7-2 for a list of ANCC certifications available.

Other Nursing Certifications Available

In 1991, eight national nursing certification programs joined to establish the American Board of Nursing Specialties. These organizations included the ANCC of the ANA, the American Board for Occupational Health Nursing, the American Board of Neuroscience Nursing, the Association of Rehabilitation Nurses, the Council on Certification of Nurse Anesthetists, the National Board of Nutritional Support Certification, the Nephrology Nursing Certification Board, and the Orthopaedic Nurses Certification Board. Since that time, a number of other nursing organizations that provide certification have joined this organization. The goals of this board are to ensure quality in specialty nursing, improve the public's perception of specialty nurses, and provide specialty nurses who bring a consistent standard of education and experience to their practice. This

TABLE 7-2	NURSING CERTIFICATION AVAILABLE THROUGH THE AMERICAN NURSES' CREDENTIALING CENTER
CERTIFICATION TITLE	**CREDENTIAL AWARDED**
Advanced Practice Exams *Acute Care Nurse Practitioner* *Adult Nurse Practitioner* *Family Nurse Practitioner* *Gerontological Nurse Practitioner* *Pediatric Nurse Practitioner* *Adult Psychiatric and Mental Health Nurse Practitioner* *Family Psychiatric and Mental Health Nurse Practitioner* *Clinical Specialist in Gerontological Nursing* *Clinical Specialist in Medical-Surgical Nursing* *Clinical Specialist in Pediatric Nursing* *Clinical Specialist in Adult Psychiatric and Mental Health Nursing* *Clinical Specialist in Child and Adolescent Psychiatric and Mental Health Nursing*	Advanced Practice Registered Nurse, Board Certified (APRN,BC)
Advanced Diabetes Management—Clinical Specialist Advanced Diabetes Management—Nurse Practitioner	Advanced Practice Registered Nurse, Board Certified—Advanced Diabetes Management (APRN,BC-ADM)
Nursing Administration, Advanced	Registered Nurse, Certified in, Nursing Administration, Board Certified (RN,CNA,BC)
Baccalaureate-level Exams *Informatics Nurse: Baccalaureate degree in nursing* *Informatics Nurse: Baccalaureate degree in other relevant field of study* *Nursing Professional Development*	Registered Nurse, Board Certified (RN,BC)
Nursing Administration	Registered Nurse, Certified in Nursing Administation, Board Certified (RN,CNA,BC)
Exams for RNs With Any Pre-licensure Preparation *Cardiac/Vascular Nurse* *Gerontological Nurse* *Medical-Surgical Nurse* *Pediatric Nurse* *Perinatal Nurse* *Psychiatric and Mental Health Nurse*	Registered Nurse, Board Certified (RN,BC)
Associate Degree/Diploma-Level Exams Perinatal Nurse	Registered Nurse, Certified (RN,C)
Other Specialty Exams for Associate, Baccalaureate, or Other Preparation *Ambulatory Care Nursing* *Nursing Case Management* *Pain Management*	Registered Nurse, Certified (RN,C)

is a major breakthrough in the entire certification process for nursing. This board has established a peer review process for certification organizations that provides evaluation and recognition of the certification granted (Table 7-3).

There are additional organizations providing certification that are not part of the American Board of Nursing specialties. The American College of Nurse Midwives certifies for practice as

TABLE 7-3	NURSING CERTIFICATIONS AVAILABLE FROM OTHER ORGANIZATIONS
ORGANIZATION	**CREDENTIAL(S)**
American Association of Critical Care Nurses Certification Corporation	Critical care registered nurse (CCRN) Critical care nurse specialist (CCNS)
American Academy of Nurse Practitioners Certification Program	Nurse Practitioner-Certified (NP-C)
American Association of Nurse Life Care Planners Certification Board	Certified Nurse Life Care Planner (CNLCP)
American Board of Neuroscience Nursing	Certified Neuroscience Registered Nurse (CNRN)
American Board for Occupational Health Nurses	Certified Occupational Health Nurse (COHN) Certified Occupational Health Nurse- Specialist (COHN-S) Certified Occupational Health Nurse/Case Management (COHN/CM) Certified Occupational Health Nurse Specialist/Care Manager (COHN-S/CM)
American Board of Perianesthesia Nursing Certification, Inc	Certified Post Anesthesia Nurse (CPAN) Certified Ambulatory Perianesthesia Nurse (CAPA)
American Legal Nurse Consultant Certification Board	Legal Nurse Consultant Certified (LNCC)
Board of Certification for Emergency Nursing	Certified Emergency Nurse (CEN) Certified Flight Registered Nurse (CFRN)
Competency & Credentialing Institute (formerly Certification Board for Perioperative Nursing)	Certified Nurse Operating Room (CNOR) Certified Registered Nurse First Assistant (CRNFA)
Certifying Board of Gastroenterology Nurses and Associates	Certified Gastroenterology Registered Nurse (CGRN) Certified Gastroenterology Licensed Practical/Vocational Nurse (CGN)
Council on Certification of Nurse Anesthetists	Certified Registered Nurse Anesthetist (CRNA)
Dermatology Nursing Certification Board	Dermatology Nurse, Certified (DNC)
Infusion Nurses Certification Corporation	Certified Registered Nurse Infusion (CRNI)
Medical-Surgical Nursing Certification Board	Certified Medical Surgical Registered Nurse (CMSRN)
National Alliance of Wound Care	Wound Care Certified (WCC)
National Board for Certification of Hospice and Palliative Nurses	Advanced Practice Registered Nurse, Board Certified-Palliative Care Management (APRN, BC-PCM) Certified Hospice and Palliative Nurse (CHPN) Certified Hospice and Palliative Licensed Nurse (CHPLN) Certified Hospice and Palliative Nursing Assistant (CHPNA)
National Board for Certification of School Nurses	National Certified School Nurse (NCSN)
National Certification Board for Diabetes Education	Certified Diabetes Educator (CDE)
National Certification Corporation for the Obstetric, Gynecological and Neonatal Specialties	Registered Nurse Certified (RNC); add one of the following designators: • Inpatient Obstetric Nursing (INPT) • Maternal Newborn Nursing (MN) • Low Risk Neonatal Nursing (LRN) • Neonatal Intensive Care Nursing (NIC) • Telephone Nursing Practice (TNP)
Nephrology Nursing Certification Commission	Certified Nephrology Nurse (CNN) Certified Dialysis Nurse (CDN)

TABLE 7-3	NURSING CERTIFICATIONS AVAILABLE FROM OTHER ORGANIZATIONS (*Continued*)
ORGANIZATION	**CREDENTIAL(S)**
Oncology Nursing Certification Corporation	Oncology Certified Nurse (OCN) Certified Pediatric Oncology Nurse (CPON) Advanced Oncology Certified Nurse (AOCN) Advanced Oncology Clinical Nurse Specialist (AOCNS) Advanced Oncology Certified Nurse Practitioner (AOCNP)
Orthopaedic Nurses Certification Board	Orthopedic Nursing Certified (ONC)
Pediatric Nursing Certification Board	Certified Pediatric Nurse Practitioner (CPNP) Certified Pediatric Nurse (CPN)
Rehabilitation Nursing Certification Board	Certified Rehabilitation Registered Nurse (CRRN) Certified Rehabilitation Registered Nurse-Advanced (CRRN-A)
Wound, Ostomy and Continence Nursing Certification Board	Certified Wound, Ostomy, Continence Nurse (CWOCN) Certified Wound Care Nurse (CWCN) Certified Ostomy Care Nurse (COCN) Certified Continence Care Nurse (CCCN) Certified Foot Care Nurse (CFCN) Certified Wound Ostomy Continence Nurse- Advanced Practice (CWOCN-AP)

a nurse-midwife. Other nurses seek certification from non-nursing organizations, such as lactation consultants, which are certified by LaLeche League.

Critical Thinking Activity

An RN with 5 years of general medical-surgical acute care experience is interested in working in the critical care unit of a hospital in your community. Seek information regarding how this nurse could obtain a critical care position in your community. Compare that process with what would be required of you as a new graduate to move into such a position.

Certification for Licensed Practical Nurses

Certification for LPNs/LVNs is available for those practicing in long-term care. The National Association of Practical Nurse Education and Service determined that many LPNs have responsible positions in long-term care and that recognition of their abilities through certification would be appropriate. They contracted with the NCSBN to develop and administer a certification examination. Those taking this examination use the title CLTC (Certified in Long-Term Care). Other certifications available to LPNs are listed in Table 7-3.

THE FUTURE OF CREDENTIALING IN HEALTH CARE

Because credentialing in nursing involves so many aspects of education, licensure, and certification, it has confused the public, nurses, and other health care professionals. The ideal credential clearly communicates qualifications and competence; therefore, it is important for nursing to have a credentialing system that can be understood by others. Current changes are moving nursing closer to an effective credentialing system.

Institutional Control of Credentials

Many new health care occupations related to new procedures and processes in medical care are being developed as new technology develops. Those who believe the state should take positive action to protect the public continue to exert pressure to license additional health care providers. Those who oppose credentialing of additional individual groups of health care workers believe that modern-day employers are able to assess workers and to differentiate among them on the basis of competence. Some who oppose credentialing of individual health occupations believe that licensing the institution that hires the employees would be an adequate safeguard for the public.

Another approach to credentialing in health care is certifying specific competencies rather than an entire field of practice. Those advocating this approach believe that it would facilitate the development of individuals with a broad range of competencies suited to a particular setting. For example, in a rural area one individual might be certified as competent to perform certain basic x-ray examinations (such as for simple fractures), basic laboratory studies (such as complete blood count and urinalysis), and some basic client care procedures (such as bathing, toileting, feeding, and positioning). Because more complex procedures are sent to a larger center and there is no need for a full-time person in any of these positions, basic care would be made available in a convenient and low-cost manner. Certification of specific competencies by the employing agency is sometimes referred to as **site-based examination** and **site-based certification**. One concern about this method of certifying competencies is its focus on technical skills, without adequately recognizing the knowledge base needed for decision making and judgment. Other concerns are the complexity of keeping track of the many specific competencies and the difficulty with job mobility when competencies are not standardized.

Pew Report

A comprehensive reform of all health care workforce regulation was first proposed by the Center for the Health Professions (Finocchio, Dower, McMahon, Gragnola, & the Taskforce of Health Care Workforce Regulation, 1995). Based on a study supported by the Pew Charitable Trust, the report, titled, *Reforming Health Care Workforce Regulation* (commonly referred to as one of the "Pew Reports on Health Care Workforce Regulation"), made 10 recommendations for changes in regulations. These are found in Display 7-2. These recommendations are based on what is termed a SAFE focus: Standardized where appropriate, Accountable to the public, Flexible to support optimal access, and Effective and Efficient in protecting and promoting the public's health, safety, and welfare. Many of the recommendations, such as educating the public about health professional regulations and collecting data on the health professions, are supported by almost everyone. Others, such as developing, implementing, and evaluating continuing competency requirements, raise many questions in the minds of both health professionals and regulatory boards.

The NCSBN provided leadership in a national meeting in December 1995 to discuss the Center for Health Professions' recommendations and their implications for nursing regulation. The response of those in attendance was that nursing has supported the broad goals of the recommendations and has achieved goals in many areas. However, there was concern that the stated

---

Display 7-2   Recommendations for Reforming Health Care Workforce Regulation

1. Standardize regulatory terms.
2. Standardize entry-to-practice requirements.
3. Remove barriers to the full use of competent health professionals.
4. Redesign health professional board structures and functions.
5. Educate the public.
6. Collect data on the health professions.
7. Develop, implement, and evaluate continuing competency requirements.
8. Reform the professional disciplinary process.
9. Develop tools to evaluate regulatory effectiveness.
10. Understand the organizational context of health professions regulation; develop partnerships to streamline regulatory structures and processes.

The Center for the Health Professions. *What's the fuss?* Front & Center, San Francisco: University of California, Summer, 1996.

---

goals are unfocused and go beyond what can be accomplished through regulation alone. Although some of the policy suggestions in the report were controversial, constructive dialogue has built on that framework and encouraged the participation of legislators, consumers, and health professionals in decision making about health professional regulations.

Institute of Medicine Recommendations

In the Institute of Medicine (IOM) report *Health Profession Education: A Bridge to Quality* (2003), the study committee came to some conclusions around the issues confronting health professions education. One concern is the fact that each profession tends to educate, practice, and dialogue within a "silo." These narrowly constructed walls make it difficult for interdisciplinary collaboration to occur. The languages used by the differing groups are a major barrier.

One of the recommendations of the report was that there should be an interdisciplinary focus on building a common language of health care with the ultimate aim of creating a set of core competencies for all health professionals.

Another recommendation was that those with responsibility for oversight of the various health professions (approval and accreditation bodies) meet to develop specific core competencies that relate to the following:

- Delivering patient-centered care
- Working as part of interdisciplinary teams
- Practicing evidence-based health care
- Focus on quality improvement
- Using information technology

A third recommendation is that accreditation bodies should revise their processes to require outcomes related to these core competencies. Two other recommendations related to the oversight of continued competence by health professionals. The IOM report recommended that both licensing bodies and specialty certification bodies require health professionals to demonstrate in some way their continued competence in the previously determined core competencies.

There is concern for how educational institutions could implement the core competencies once they are developed. The report acknowledged the many barriers to implementation of these recommendations and identified that the current health care delivery system will need to change in order for changes to occur in education. It also identified that changes in health professional education will require interdisciplinary education of faculty into new roles and ways of teaching. To this end, the report recommended that major foundations in education and practice should take the lead in funding demonstration centers that focus on teaching and assessing the core competencies.

The Future of Approval/Accreditation of Nursing Education Programs

As nursing grows and moves forward, the dual expectations of state approval and national accreditation create a substantial workload and cost for the individual nursing program. The NCSBN developed a *White Paper on the State of the Art of Approval/Accreditation Processes in Boards of Nursing* (NCSBN, 2004c). The group preparing this paper investigated the current processes in place for approval and accreditation and identified the models being used. The report notes both benefits and costs of the current system and discusses the value of using interdisciplinary faculty in order to enhance disciplinary practice. The report also recommends that future approval processes include the five areas of competence identified by the IOM (IOM, 2003).

Key Concepts

- Credentials are written proof of qualifications and may include diplomas awarded by educational programs, certification, or registration by professional groups, and legal licenses awarded by governmental agencies.
- Permissive licensure allows for those meeting certain standards voluntarily to be licensed, whereas mandatory licensure requires that all individuals who wish to practice in the field be licensed to practice.
- Nursing leaders began efforts to obtain legal licensure in 1896. The first permissive licensure law was passed in 1903 by North Carolina, and the first mandatory licensure law was passed in New York in 1947.
- Legal rules governing nursing practice are found in the licensure law passed by a legislative body. Further provisions governing nursing are found in the rules and regulations established by the administrative agency in which the legislation vests authority.
- The state nursing practice acts usually contain a definition of nursing and address qualifications for licensure applicants, use of titles, renewal and continuing competence requirements, grandfathering, financial concerns, nursing education programs, disciplinary action, violations and penalties, administrative provisions, and expanded nursing roles.
- The state boards of nursing (or their equivalent) are the administrative agencies that have the authority to carry out the provisions of the Nurse Practice Act.

- A license to practice nursing must be obtained from the state or province in which you wish to work, except in the case of states that belong to the Multistate Compact. An initial license is termed licensure by examination, and subsequent licenses may be obtained in other jurisdictions through licensure by endorsement.
- Advanced practice nurses are regulated by each state. Most require professional certification in an advanced practice nursing specialty to be licensed in that role.
- Mutual recognition of licensure involves a compact between certain states that allows nurses who are licensed in one of those states to work freely among all the compact states without the need for obtaining additional licenses.
- The NCLEX-RN examination is administered through a computerized plan that covers the five steps of the nursing process and four areas of client needs, and that identifies competence for entry-level safe nursing care.
- Graduates of foreign nursing schools must have their credentials reviewed and may be required to take the CGFNS examination, which reviews both nursing content and English language ability, before being admitted to take the NCLEX examination.
- A license may be revoked by the state board of nursing, a designated disciplinary board, or a court of law based on specific reasons stated in the Nurse Practice Act.
- Certification provides evidence of specialized clinical knowledge and ability beyond the basic level. Certification as a nurse practitioner may be used as a basis for legal approval to practice in an expanded role.
- Concerns about the future of health care worker credentialing include issues of public accountability and continued competence.
- The IOM report on health professions education made a series of recommendations, several of which focus on developing a set of core competencies that could be used for both education and ongoing professional regulation.
- The NCSBN has endorsed the core competencies identified by the IOM and encourages movement toward outcomes assessment as part of approval and accreditation decisions.

Relevant Web Sites

Certification information:

American Nurses Association (ANA): *http://nursingworld.org*

Lippincott/AJN: *www.nursingcenter.com/prodev/ce_certification.asp*

Licensure information:

Commission on Graduates of Foreign Nursing Schools (CGFNS): *www.cgfns.org*

National Council of State Boards of Nursing (NCSBN): *www.ncsbn.org*

References

201 KAR 20:215, Kentucky Board of Nursing, Administrative Rules. [On-line]. *www.kbn.ky.gov/education/ce*. Accessed October 20, 2005.

American Nurses Association. (1978). A study of credentialing in nursing: A new approach, vol. 1, The Report of the Committee. Kansas City: MO, Author.

American Nurses Association. (1980). Nursing: A social policy statement. Kansas City, MO: American Journal of Nursing Co.

American Nurses Association, Congress for Nursing Practice. (1990). Suggested state legislation: Nursing Practice Act, Disciplinary Diversion Act; Prescriptive Authority Act. Kansas City, MO: Author

American Nurses Association. (2006). *Multistate licensure compact: areas of concern.* [On-line]. *http://nursingworld.org/gova/concerns.htm.* Accessed September 1, 2006.

Committee on Graduates of Foreign Nursing Schools. (2005). Overview. [On-line]. *www.cgfns.org/sections/prog/overview.shtml.* Accessed October 19, 2005.

Finocchio, L. J., Dower, C. M., McMahon, T., Gragnola, C. M., & the Taskforce of Health Care Workforce Regulation. (1995). *Reforming health care workforce regulation: Policy considerations for the 21st century.* San Francisco: Pew Health Professions Commission.

International Centre on Nurse Migration. (2006). Mission, vision, and goals. [On-line]. *www.intlnursemigration.org.* Accessed September 1, 2006.

Institute of Medicine. (2003). *Health Professions Education: A Bridge to Quality.* Washington, DC, National Academies Press.

Malugani, M. (2000). Nurse, interrupted: A disciplinary action can put a wrinkle in your career and tie you up in knots. *Nurseweek.* [On-line]. *www.nurseweek.com/news/features/00-08/discip.html.* Accessed August 10, 2002.

National Council of State Boards of Nursing. (1998, November 6). *Nurse licensure compact: Final version* Chicago: Author. [On-line]. *www.ncsbn.org.* Accessed October 15, 2005.

National Council of State Boards of Nursing. (2002a). *Regulation of advanced practice nursing: NCSBN position paper.* Chicago: Author. [On-line]. *www.ncsbn.org/pdfs/APRN_Position_Paper2002.pdf.* Accessed November 15, 2005.

National Council of State Boards of Nursing. (2002b). Uniform advanced practice registered nurse licensure/authority to practice requirements. Chicago: Author. [On-line]. *www.ncsbn.org/pdfs/uniformaprn.pdf.* Accessed October 20, 2005.

National Council of State Boards of Nursing. (2004a). *Model nursing practice act and rules.* Chicago: Author. [On-line]. *www.ncsbn.org/regulation.* Accessed October 15, 2005.

National Council of State Boards of Nursing. (2004b). *Test plan for the NCLEX for registered nurses.* Chicago: Author. [On-line]. *www.ncsbn.org/pdfs/RNTestPlan_Apr04.pdf.* Accessed October 18, 2005.

National Council of State Boards of Nursing. (2004c). *White paper on the state of the art of approval/accreditation processes in boards of nursing.* Chicago: Author. Retrieved on-line, November, 7, 2005, from *www.ncsbn.org/pdfs/Approval_White_Paper_Final_09_05.pdf*

National Council of State Boards of Nursing. (2005a). *Meeting the ongoing challenge of continued competence.* Chicago: Author. [On-line]. *www.ncsbn.org/pdfs/Continued_Comp_Paper_TestingServices.pdf.* Accessed October 18, 2005.

National Council of State Boards of Nursing. (2005b). *Test plan for the NCLEX for practical nurses.* Chicago: Author. [On-line]. *www.ncsbn.org.* Accessed October 18, 2005.

National Council of State Boards of Nursing. (2006). *Nurses Licensure Verification.* Chicago: Author. [On-line]. *www.nursys.com/Common.asp?pt=LICENSEVERIFICATION.* Accessed September 1, 2006.

Sheets, V. (2002). *An overview of the accreditation of healthcare education and the regulation of healthcare practitioners* (Unpublished manuscript). In National Council of State Boards of Nursing, *White paper on the state of the art of approval/accreditation processes in boards of nursing.* [On-line]. *www.ncsbn.org/pdfs/Approval_White_Paper_Final_09_05.pdf.* Accessed November 3, 2005.

Simpson, R. L. (1999). Tech talk on multistate licensure. *Nursing Management, 30*(1), 12–13.

Trilateral Initiative for North American Nursing. (1996). *An assessment of North American nursing.* Philadelphia: Commission on Graduates of Foreign Nursing Schools.

Yocum, C. J., & Davis, C. R. (2002). *The CGFNS validity study: commission on graduates of foreign nursing schools qualifying examinations as predictors of success on the United States registered nurse licensing examination — April 2001 through March 2002.* [On-line]. *www.cgfns.org/sections/research/validity.shtml.* Accessed October 18, 2005.

8

Legal Responsibilities for Practice

After completing this chapter, you should be able to:

1. Differentiate the two general sources of law and explain how they apply to nursing.
2. Explain the role of institutional policies and protocols in legal decision making.
3. Describe situations in which inappropriate nursing actions may violate criminal law.
4. Discuss liability in relationship to nursing practice, including situations in which liability is shared by employers or supervisors.
5. Analyze how you could benefit as an individual nurse from purchasing professional liability insurance.
6. Explain the nurse's role in supporting patient rights through informed consent and advance directives.
7. Identify specific issues that can constitute malpractice and discuss the nurse's responsibility in relationship to them.
8. Describe the most commonly recurring legal issues in nursing.
9. Identify factors that contribute to a suit being instituted against a health care professional, and explain how an individual nurse might prevent legal suits.
10. Explain the various aspects of a legal action.
11. Outline the role of the nurse when testifying for a legal proceeding.

Administrative ruling	Discovery	Health Insurance Portability
Advance directive	Durable power of attorney for	and Accountability
Assault	health care	Act (HIPAA)
Battery	Emancipated minors	Informed consent
Civil law	Enacted law	Intentional tort
Common law	Ethics	Judicial law (decisional or
Constitutional law	Expert witness	case law)
Criminal law	False imprisonment	Lawsuit
Criminal negligence	Felony	Liability
Defendant	Fraud	Living will
Deposition	Futile	Malpractice
Directive to physicians	Health care proxy	Mature minor

Misdemeanor	Procedure	Standard of practice
Negligence	Protected health	Statutory law
Patient Self-Determination	information	Substitutionary decision-
Act (PSDA)	Protocol	maker
Perjury	Prudent professional	Testimony
Plaintiff	Reckless endangerment	Tort
Policy	Regulatory law (administrative)	Unintentional tort
Privileged communication	Standard of care	Witness to fact

Every newspaper contains reports of sensational cases being considered in our courts and legal arenas. Concerns about lawsuits and liability are voiced in every business. Health care remains at the forefront of professions where legal issues constitute a major area of concern. The prudent nurse considers legal issues before a crisis arises and uses sound information to help guide action in situations where questions arise. This chapter provides basic information you will need in that process.

UNDERSTANDING THE SCOPE OF THE LAW

Legal issues are those that are decided by law. Law may be defined as "a rule of conduct or action prescribed or formally recognized as binding or enforced by a controlling authority" (Judson & Hicks, 1999, p. 4). They are put in place to ensure that behavior that would threaten public safety is controlled. **Ethics** are the principles of conduct governing one's relationships with others— basic beliefs about right and wrong. Legal and ethical issues are often discussed together because they go hand in hand, with one supporting the other. Ethics also may address questions that are entirely different from those addressed by the law. Hall (1996, p. 49) stated, "Law is the minimum ethic, written down and enforced; behavior that is not merely desired but mandated." In this chapter, we focus on how the law affects nursing practice. Ethics are introduced here and are discussed in more detail in Chapter 9.

Examples and situations relating to legal issues discussed throughout this chapter are given to help you understand the application of the specific concepts. Many more factors would be considered in arriving at an actual legal decision than can be presented in a paragraph or two. It is the interaction of multiple factors that makes it impossible to provide absolute predictions regarding legal outcomes in specific situations; that is, data may be interpreted differently by judges and juries, resulting in different outcomes, even though cases may appear similar.

If you have a question about a specific personal situation, you would be well advised to consult an attorney who is experienced in medicolegal matters. The facility where you are employed may have a legal counselor who is available to you. Another source of legal aid is your nurses association attorney. If you desire private counsel, suitable names may be recommended by the nurses association in your state or the local bar association. And, of course, you may always identify and seek the services of an attorney in your community who works in the area of law about which you are concerned.

SOURCES OF LAW

If nurses know the source of law, then they know how it can be challenged and changed, and how powerful it can be. There are three general sources of law: *statutory law*, *regulatory* (also known as administrative) *law*, and *common law*. All are relevant to nursing practice (Fig. 8-1).

Statutory Law

A statute is a rule or formal regulation established by government legislative authority, such as the Congress, the state legislature, or the city council, that appears in writing. A violation of a statute is legally punishable. Statutory law is published in codes. A key aspect of all statutory law is that it is broken down into specific rules. In the United States, **statutory law** includes constitutional law and enacted law. All laws fall in a hierarchy of authority, with constitutional law having the greatest authority and enacted law the next. Regulatory law, to be discussed later, has less authority than statutory law.

Constitutional Law

Constitutional law is established by the federal government and based on the U. S. Constitution. The Constitution was developed and passed by the Continental Congress and then ratified by all the states. It establishes the general organization of the federal government, and specifies the federal

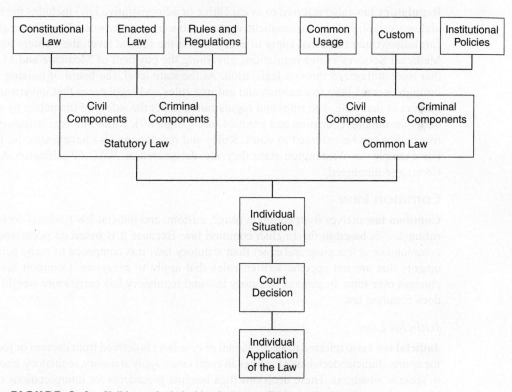

FIGURE 8-1 Civil law and criminal law both may affect a nursing situation.

power and limitations to that power. The powers not specifically given to the federal government in the Constitution are retained by the states. The Constitution can be amended (ie, changed), with the amendments having the same status as the original provisions. Amendments to the U.S. Constitution require similar passage and ratification by the states. The first 10 amendments are called the Bill of Rights and were passed between 1789 and 1791. The last amendment in 1992 was number 27, which limited pay raises for members of Congress. In addition, each state has its own constitution that acts as the highest law for that state. Many other nations, such as Great Britain, do not have a constitution or equivalent document. In those countries, the enacted law is the highest level of law.

Enacted Law

Enacted law includes all bills passed by legislative bodies, whether at the local, state or province, or national level. Enacted laws of the U.S. federal government all carry the designation USC (United States Code) in their official title. The federal Social Security Act (42 USC 401) is an example of federally enacted law. Enacted laws of states or other governing bodies carry a similar designation, specified by the individual state. For example, in Washington state the enacted laws are designated RCW (Revised Code of Washington) and numbered. Nurse practice acts in the various states are examples of enacted law at the state level.

Regulatory Law

Regulatory law (also referred to as executive or administrative law) includes the rules and regulations established by government agencies to carry out enacted law. These also appear as carefully written rules that apply to everyone. At the federal level, the Centers for Medicare & Medicaid Services writes regulations governing the payment of Medicare and Medicaid funds that were authorized through legislation. At the state level, the board of nursing is authorized through enacted laws to establish and enforce rules and regulations that govern the practice of nursing in that state. The rules and regulations protect the safety of the public by defining standards for nursing education and practice (see Chapter 7). Rules and regulations of administrative bodies can be enforced in court. Rules and regulations also have a specific identification. For example, in Washington state they are designated as WAC (Washington Administrative Code) and numbered.

Common Law

Common law derives from common usage, custom, and judicial law (judicial decisions or court rulings). It is based in the English common law. Because it is based on occurrences of events, common law is less clear and exact than statutory law; it is composed of many actions and documents that are not specific written rules that apply to everyone. Common law is fluid and changes over time. In general, statutory law and regulatory law carry more weight in court than does common law.

Judicial Law

Judicial law (also referred to as decisional or case law) is derived from decrees or judgments from the courts. Judicial decisions or rulings in court cases apply statutory, regulatory, and common law to specific situations. These decisions then become precedents for interpretations of all types of law in other cases. Court rulings are binding within the jurisdiction of the particular court that determines them, but are used in a more general way (as guidelines) in other jurisdictions. In any specific situation, the final determination of the application of all types of law is the decision of the court in that case, although in most instances a decision may be appealed to higher courts.

Common Usage and Custom

As the term seems to imply, courts are empowered through the concept of common law to examine the common usage and custom in a community for patterns that reflect the community's standards for behavior. Common usage and custom are not usually written down and specific. However, written documents can be used to support common usage and custom in specific cases. For example, when examining standards of professional practice in a court case, the court may examine documents that specify standards of professional practice as reflecting common usage. These documents may be changed by the organization writing the standard and thus are not fixed.

The issue of abandonment of a patient illustrates how common usage applies to nursing. An individual state may not have a written law that dictates that a nurse cannot leave a seriously ill patient without ensuring that someone else will provide care, but common practice and custom (which could be supported through the testimony of nurses and other health care workers) require that nurses do not abandon their patients. Failure to meet this standard might be deemed a violation of common law even when no statute exists.

OTHER FACTORS AFFECTING LEGAL DECISIONS

In addition to the sources of law discussed above, several other factors can affect how laws are interpreted and enforced. These factors also play an important role in our legal system.

Administrative Rulings

An **administrative ruling**, also referred to as an advisory opinion, made by a state board or by an attorney general provides a guideline based on an interpretation of the enacted and regulatory law relative to a specific situation. It is not considered a final legal decision, and different boards and attorneys general might vary in their opinions. The validity of an opinion stands until the issue is brought before a court and the court rules on the situation and provides a final decision. The court decision may or may not support the advisory ruling.

Rights and Responsibilities in Health Care

Rights and responsibilities have both legal and ethical aspects. In the United States, basic rights are specified in the first 10 amendments to the Constitution and are part of statutory law. This section of the Constitution is called the Bill of Rights and is an example of one of the limitations placed on the federal government. These rights protect the individual from government interference in basic areas of life. From these primary rights, other rights are deduced. For example, although the right to privacy of medical records is not specifically discussed in the Bill of Rights, the right to be secure in one's own home against unreasonable search and seizure is guaranteed. This basic right has led to court decisions supporting the right to privacy regarding one's own affairs, including medical records.

In some countries, rights may be part of the statutory law and thus carry less weight than a constitution does. Some countries have no counterpart to the rights found in the United States that are guaranteed through the constitution.

Some of the rights of which we commonly speak are not legally supported, but are based on ethical beliefs. For example, we often speak of a "right to health care." There is no legal basis for this right in the United States, but many people believe an ethical basis exists. In some countries, such as Canada and Great Britain, health care is a right supported by the law. In these countries, health care for all has been established through legislation and administrative rules and regulations.

In the United States, patient rights within the health care system have received considerable attention by both government and consumer bodies. The federal **Health Insurance Portability and Accountability Act (HIPAA)** enacted in 1996, with rules and regulations implemented in 2003, contains a significant section regarding the privacy of **protected health information**. Protected health information refers to individually identifiable data about a person's health or health care. This act made privacy in regard to health care a legally supported right at the federal level. All health care agencies and health plans are required to provide training for all employees in regard to the privacy rules and the procedures in place to ensure compliance. There are significant monetary penalties for breaches of privacy. Many facilities have adopted employment policies that include dismissal for certain types of breaches of patient confidentiality.

Recent attention has been directed to the patient's right to pain management. While managing pain has always been a health care goal, most providers did not think of it in terms of the patient's right to pain relief. The Joint Commission has added requirements to accreditation standards requiring that agencies have comprehensive plans for effectively managing pain and demonstrating that those plans are used. In at least one instance, a family successfully brought suit against a nursing home for the failure to manage terminal pain in their loved one (Furrow, 2001). Therefore, all health care providers need to recognize this as a newly developing legal right.

Responsibilities often accompany rights. If a right is guaranteed, the government and designated others have legally mandated responsibilities to ensure that the right is upheld. In the matter of the right to privacy of medical records, for example, all health care workers have legally mandated responsibilities to ensure that privacy is upheld.

Institutional Policies, Protocols, and Procedures

Institutional **policies** provide guidance in the proper actions to be taken in specific situations and identify the individuals responsible for taking action. Established agency policies may be considered the **standard of practice** for that agency and, therefore, common usage (common law) by the court, and may become important as a basis for legal decisions. Policies may protect the institution and its employees from legal difficulties if they are based on current practice and sound legal advice.

Members of the hospital staff who have expertise in the practice area under consideration usually develop the specific policy. An attorney also may be consulted to ensure that policies conform to legal requirements. Many larger institutions have a hired risk manager who often is a nurse attorney. Final approval of policies often rests with the board of trustees, directors, or commissioners, who have ultimate responsibility for the financial and legal management of the organization.

Institutional policies are changed in response to new situations and new expectations in society. Usually there is an established institutional route for the change or expansion of a hospital policy. Nurses may be in a position to recognize the need for such a change as they use a policy and compare it with the latest professional information.

Protocols, as the term is used in the health care environment, provide a list of actions for managing a specific problem that may involve the use of more than one procedure. For example, a protocol on the care of a central venous catheter might include frequency of tubing change, the type of fluid used for flushing, the frequency of dressing change, the type of dressing materials to be used, and other aspects of care. Protocols for nursing often include aspects of care that might be part of the medical orders for patient care. Therefore, they are usually developed with consultation between nursing and physician representatives and may be approved by the medical practice committee as well as by a nursing committee before implementation.

Specific institutional **procedures** outline the steps in a particular task. In the example of the central venous catheter, a procedure would be the list of steps to be taken when flushing the catheter to maintain patency. A procedure for nursing would be developed by the relevant nursing committee or sometimes by a clinical nurse specialist.

The purpose of protocols and procedures is to ensure that there is consistent, sound practice in an institution. Just as policies must be updated, so should protocols and procedures (see Chapter 11).

COMMUNICATION IN *ACTION*

Making Changes in a Procedure

Stan Wilson, a registered nurse (RN) was reading a nursing journal. He was surprised to learn that, according to an article, the procedure they were using at his hospital for intravenous (IV) site care was specifically not recommended. In fact, that practice was identified as increasing the incidence of site inflammation and infection. The next day he took the journal with him to work. He said to his coworkers, "Look at this article during your break if you can. It has some information that has made me concerned about our current IV site care. I am going to show this to our manager Nancy and ask if we can start a study process to figure what really is best to do." He contacted the manager and asked for a time to sit down and talk with her about a concern. When they sat down to talk later in the day he introduced the subject: "Nancy, I just read this article about IV site care. This is a peer-reviewed journal, and the article quotes some impressive research. According to the information here, our IV site care procedure does not meet current standards. Some specific concerns are our cleaning procedure and the ointment we are using at the site. Would you read this article and then meet with me again so we can talk about the possibility of updating our procedure?"

CLASSIFICATION OF LAWS

Law is divided into civil and criminal components. Both statutory law and common law may be subdivided in this way.

Criminal Law

Criminal law addresses the general welfare of the public. A violation of criminal law is called a crime, and it is prosecuted by the government. On conviction, a crime may be punishable by imprisonment, parole conditions, a loss of privilege (such as a license), a fine, or any combination of these. The punishment is intended to discipline the violator and deter further such actions by this person as well as discourage others from committing the crime. A crime may be classified as either a **misdemeanor** or as a **felony**. A misdemeanor is a lesser infraction of the law and is punishable by a fine or an imprisonment of less than a year. A felony represents a more serious violation of the law and carries heavier fines and longer periods of imprisonment, and in the most serious of cases, perhaps even death (Guido, 2001).

Civil Law

Civil law regulates conduct between private individuals or businesses and is enforced through the courts as damages or money compensation. A **tort** is a violation of a civil law in which another person is wronged. Private individuals or groups may bring a legal action (a **lawsuit**) to court for breach (or breaking) of civil law. The judgment of the court results in a plan to correct the wrong and may award a monetary payment to the wronged party. Nurses may find themselves involved with both civil and criminal laws, either separately or within the same situation.

CRIMINAL LAW AND NURSING

Because a violation of any law governing the practice of any licensed profession may be a crime, you must be aware of the extent of the Nurse Practice Act of the state in which you are practicing. Where the Nurse Practice Act requires that actions (such as administering drugs) be performed only under the direction of a physician, that explicit authorization must exist. Standing orders or protocols that refer to specific situations, as well as the usual orders written for an individual patient, may both be adequate authorization. However, custom or usual practice will not substitute for the specific authorization required by law. A violation of a professional practice act may be prosecuted as a crime even if no actual harm occurred to the patient.

It is costly to the state to undertake criminal prosecution; therefore, even when they are discovered, some violations of criminal law are not prosecuted in court. Knowing this, some nurses make the error of believing that "minor" violations are acceptable. Even when not prosecuted in court, criminal action could result in the loss of a job and a license to practice nursing.

For example, the Nurse Practice Act does not give the nurse the authority to diagnose disease and prescribe medication, regardless of the situation. The Medical Practice Act and the Nurse Practice Act on Advanced Nursing Practice contain this authorization. To give a medication without an order is a violation of the law and is a crime, even if doing so does not harm the client.

Violation of laws related to the care and distribution of controlled substances is also a crime. Altering or changing narcotic records is a crime even if no diversion of drugs occurred. While finding where the error in a narcotic record occurred may be a tedious and time-consuming process, as a nurse, you need to look beyond temporary inconvenience to the potential consequences of your action.

Nurses also have been charged by states with committing crimes while in the role of caregiver. These legal actions may be based on such charges as **reckless endangerment** or **criminal negligence**. For example, if a nurse left a long-term care facility at midnight knowing that the nurse for the next shift had not yet arrived, this might be considered reckless endangerment. To leave incapacitated residents without a nurse is abandoning them and is considered reckless because it shows a lack of appropriate regard for the well-being of the patients. These are situations in which the actions of the professional fall outside the bounds of simple error and reflect a serious lack of concern or attention to the safety of the patient.

Errors that result in the serious injury or death of a patient are investigated and may be prosecuted and tried by the criminal courts. A license to practice nursing may be temporarily withdrawn while such charges are investigated and tried. If the individual is found innocent, the license then may be restored. If the individual is convicted of the crime, however, the nursing license may be revoked, in addition to sentencing and other penalties.

In Colorado, criminal charges were brought against three nurses for negligent actions that resulted in the death of an infant. Through a series of actions carried out by the nurses, the infant was given a 10-fold overdose of IV penicillin. This case clearly shows that the state has the power to prosecute as a crime professional conduct that results in serious harm or death (Fiesta, 1999). Commenting at the time of the incident, Curtin (1997) noted that many nurses are distressed by the actions of the prosecutor in the Colorado case because the facts as presented did not seem to indicate a criminal level of negligence.

Nurses who commit felonies such as theft, abuse, or deliberate harm in which a patient is a victim are usually charged under both criminal laws and the laws regulating nursing practice. Nurses who commit felonies outside of the care setting can be prosecuted under criminal law and under the law regulating nursing practice if the felony reflects on their fitness to practice nursing. For example, an individual prosecuted for selling narcotics usually will have action taken under the Nurse Practice Act as well.

CIVIL LAW AND NURSING

Civil law relates to legal disputes between private parties. Malpractice actions brought in health care situations involve civil law.

Torts

Torts are civil wrongs committed by one person against another person or a person's property (Guido, 2001). The wrong may be physical harm, psychological harm, harm to livelihood, or some other less tangible value, such as harm to reputation. The action that causes a civil wrong may be either intentional or unintentional. An **intentional tort** is one in which the outcome was planned, although the person involved may not have believed that the intended outcome would be harmful to the other person. For example, preventing a patient from leaving against medical advice may be based on concern for the patient, but it is illegal and to do so is an intentional tort.

An **unintentional tort** is a wrong committed against another person or property that was not intended to happen. The most common cause of an unintentional tort is negligence.

Negligence

Negligence is a general term that refers to conduct that does not show due care (Guido, 2001). If harm is caused by negligence, it is termed an unintentional tort and damages may be recovered. All negligence has the following four essential characteristics (Fiesta, 1994):

1. Harm must have occurred to an individual.
2. The negligent person must have been in a situation where he or she had a duty toward the person harmed.
3. The person must be found to have failed to fulfill his or her duty. This is called "breach of duty." This might include either doing what should not have been done (commission of an inappropriate action) or failing to do what should have been done (omission of a necessary or appropriate action). This is also referred to as failing to act as a reasonably prudent person. A reasonably prudent person in this context means someone who demonstrates careful and thoughtful action. Some authorities emphasize that this

FIGURE 8-2   A reasonably prudent nurse uses common sense as well as nursing theory.

includes the responsibility to foresee possible results of a situation and act appropriately (Guido, 2001).

4. The harm must be shown to have been caused by the breach of duty.

Malpractice

Malpractice is a term used to identify a specific type of negligence. It refers to the negligence of a specially trained or educated person in the performance of his or her job. Therefore, malpractice is the term used to describe negligence by nurses in the performance of their duties.

Malpractice is professional negligence—liability resulting from improper practice based on standards of care required by that profession (Shinn & Curtin, 2001). The professional person must have had a professional duty toward the person receiving the care. For example, the nurse was performing the professional activities of a nurse for the person needing the care (in either a paid or volunteer capacity). Additionally, the harm that occurred to this person or to the property must be based on a failure to act as a **prudent professional** and in accordance with professional standards in the situation (Fig. 8-2). This is a higher standard than is required of the general public; it demands appropriate professional judgment and action (Guido, 2001) (Display 8-1).

Display 8-1   Essential Elements of Malpractice

- Harm to an individual
- Duty of a professional toward an individual
- Breach of duty by the professional
- Breach of duty as the cause of harm

Just as all parts of the situation are clear in some general negligence situations and not in others, the same can be said of professional duty. The nurse who is assigned to care for a patient in a hospital clearly has a duty to that patient. In some situations, duties overlap and more than one nurse might have a duty toward the same patient; whether a supervisor, another nurse on the unit, or a nurse visitor has a professional duty to a patient might be in dispute. In general, all nurses within a facility are considered to have a duty toward all patients and even toward visitors, in case of emergency, and are expected to act on behalf of the institution in that regard. For example, if a visitor falls, any nurse present is expected to respond, institute action, and summon help. Again, the court would decide whether a duty was present if any legal action occurred.

Critical Thinking Activity

You have taken a new position as a home health nurse. One of your patients is an elderly woman who has a leg ulcer and a long history of diabetes. Your role is to assess the patient in relationship to her diabetic management and wound care and teach as needed. While you are in the home, her husband tells you that he has been having pain in his knee and asks if you would examine it and tell him whether it is all right to use a heating pad on it, and whether he should take ibuprofen or some Tylenol. Do you have a duty to help him? Why or why not? What will your response be? What legal issues are involved in this situation? If you advise him and your advice turns out to be incorrect, what legal action could he take?

A breach of duty, as mentioned earlier, is a failure to act as a prudent professional, that is, according to the **standard of care** for the profession in a particular situation (Killion & Dempski, 2000). Standards of nursing care are determined in variety of ways. State boards of nursing set some standards; accrediting agencies such as The Joint Commission and professional nursing organizations set others. Federal administration codes may set standards, such as nurse–patient ratio in federally funded institutions. Standards of care also appear in policies, protocols, and procedures of the institution. Current nursing references, educational material, and articles may contribute to an understanding of an appropriate and current standard of care. Still other standards of care are determined by seeking the input of an expert professional. To determine that a breach of duty was present in a particular case, a court will officially determine what constitutes a professional standard of care for that situation. This includes the application of both statutory law and common law, as previously discussed.

The final question becomes one of identifying the cause of the harm that occurred. Malpractice is present only if a breach of duty was the cause of the harm. The presence of harm is often clear. For example, if the outcome of a situation is a fractured hip, no one will dispute that this is harm. However, the cause of a fractured hip might be the person's own responsibility, not the responsibility of someone else. When the harm is so clear and the responsibility for the harm so straightforward that it does not need to be proved in court, the legal term *res ipsa loquitur* is used. This is Latin for "the thing speaks for itself." In this case, the harm and responsibility do not need to be proved, because all would agree that harm occurred and who was responsible. This may be invoked in a case where a surgical instrument is left in an abdomen and causes harm. There is no way that the instrument could be in the abdomen if the surgical team had not placed it there and overlooked its removal. Everyone would agree that a surgical instrument in the abdomen that caused pain and failure to heal was harm to the person. Expert witnesses would not be needed to make this determination. Remember that, as discussed earlier in the chapter, a breach of duty may be either the omission of a correct action or the commission of an incorrect action.

LIABILITY

A **liability** is an obligation or debt that can be enforced by law. In the case of malpractice, a person found guilty of any tort (whether intentional or unintentional) is considered legally liable, or legally responsible, for the outcome. The person legally liable usually is required to pay for damages to the other person. These may include actual costs of care, legal services, loss of earnings (present and future), and compensation for emotional and physical stress suffered. Although liability is legally determined by a court, an individual who believes that he or she would be held legally liable if a court were consulted, may agree to pay damages (or that individual's insurance company may agree to pay) without actually going to court. This may be done even when the person denies true negligence or malpractice, but chooses to settle the issue because a court case would be more costly than the damages to be paid.

Personal Liability

As an educated professional, you are always legally responsible or liable for your actions (Bernzweig, 1996). Thus, if a physician or supervisor asks you to do something that is contrary to your best professional judgment and says, "I'll take responsibility," that person is acting unwisely. The physician or supervisor giving the directions may be liable also if harm results, but that would not remove your personal liability.

EXAMPLE

Personal Liability

The RN who gives medications on a large medical unit at night notes that an order for dopamine is considerably larger than the usual dose. She looks up the medication in a reference book and finds that she is correct about the dosage: The ordered dose is several times the usual dose. The nurse then calls the supervisor and explains the situation and suggests that the physician be called (in this facility, night calls to physicians must be approved by the supervisor).

The supervisor double-checks the order with the RN and then states, "Dr. Jones is an outstanding physician. I am sure he has a good reason for ordering this dose. Go ahead and give the medication as ordered. I'll take responsibility. I don't believe it is worth bothering him at night." The RN then gives the medication, and the patient suffers a toxic reaction.

The RN could be held liable for giving the incorrect amount of medication. She had the knowledge and judgment to recognize that the dose was much larger than usual, and she failed to check with the physician. A statement by the supervisor does not remove the nurse's personal responsibility for her own actions. Because even a competent physician might make an error, the nurse had a responsibility to clarify the order. The supervisor and the physician could be held liable in addition to the nurse, but not instead of her.

Although each person is legally responsible for his or her own actions, the example above illustrates that there are also situations in which a person or organization may be held liable for actions taken by others.

▰▰ COMMUNICATION IN *ACTION*
▰▰

Clarifying Your Actions

In the above situation, the RN might have responded differently and protected both herself and her supervisor. After being reassured that the supervisor would take responsibility for administering what appeared to be an excessive dose of the medication, the prudent nurse might reply, "I know you mean to be reassuring, but if the dosage is wrong I will be liable because I am the nurse administering the drug. I think it is best to call Dr. Jones and clarify the order. He has the same goal that we do: the safety and well-being of the patient. I will be glad to make the call now."

Employer Liability

The most common situation in which a person or organization is held responsible for the actions of another is in the employer–employee relationship. In many instances, an employer can be held responsible for torts committed by an employee. This is called the doctrine of *respondeat superior* (Latin for "let the master respond"). The law holds the employer responsible for hiring qualified persons, establishing an appropriate environment for correct functioning, maintaining correct policies and procedures, and providing supervision or direction as needed to avoid errors or harm. Therefore, if a nurse, as an employee of a hospital, is guilty of malpractice, the hospital also may be named in the suit. The employer's liability may exist even if the employer appears to have taken precautions to prevent error.

It is important to understand that this doctrine does not remove any responsibility from the individual nurse, but it extends responsibility to the employer in addition to the nurse. If, for example, a hospital has a procedure that does not conform to good nursing practice as you know it, and you follow that procedure, you will still be liable for any resulting harm. You are expected to use your education and experience to make sound judgments regarding your work.

●●● Employer Responsibility for a Staff Nurse

EXAMPLE

A nurse working in a long-term care facility is responsible for planning and coordinating the care of a severely debilitated resident. This elderly man is totally dependent for all activities of daily living due to a recent stroke. He is not eating and drinking adequately. He faints and is discovered to have very low blood pressure and a rapid weak pulse. He is sent to the local hospital, where he is admitted for dehydration secondary to inadequate fluid intake. An investigation reveals that no assessment of his fluid or nutritional status had been recorded, nor was there any written plan to ensure that nutritional and fluid needs were met.

Both the nurse and the long-term care facility in this situation might be found liable for harm that resulted. The nurse had a personal, professional responsibility to accurately assess the resident and to institute care to meet his basic needs. And the facility had a responsibility to guarantee that policies, procedures, and protocols were in place to ensure appropriate assessment and care, and that employees followed through on them.

Supervisory Liability

In the role of clinical leader, charge nurse, unit manager, supervisor, or any other role that involves delegation, supervision, or direction of other people, the nurse is potentially liable for the actions of others. The supervising nurse is responsible for exercising good judgment in a supervisory role, including making appropriate decisions about assignments and delegation of tasks. If an error occurs and the supervising nurse is shown to have exercised sound judgment in all decisions made in that capacity, the supervising nurse may not be held liable for the error of a subordinate. If poor judgment was used in assigning an inadequately prepared person to an important task or oversight was inadequate, the supervisory nurse might be liable for resulting harm. The extent of the subordinate's responsibility would depend on his or her level of education and training. People with limited education or training might not be liable for some errors; the more education subordinates have, the more likely they will be liable also (see Chapter 13 for more discussion of delegation).

EXAMPLE

Supervisory Responsibility for an Educated Staff Member

Two sudden admissions to the coronary care unit (CCU) create a situation in which additional help is needed to care for the patients in the unit. A "float" nurse is sent to the CCU to assist. The charge nurse does not ask the temporary float nurse whether she has education or experience in coronary care, nor does the temporary float nurse volunteer this information. In fact, the temporary float nurse has no background or experience in coronary care.

The temporary nurse is assigned by the charge nurse to the complete care of two patients. Because of the float nurse's inability to accurately interpret the monitors, a potentially life-threatening problem is not identified until the patient "arrests." Resuscitation efforts are successful, but the patient suffers some brain damage.

In this scenario, both the charge nurse, who assigned the inadequately prepared nurse to total care, and the temporary nurse could be found liable: the charge nurse for incorrectly assigning the nurse, and the temporary nurse for not recognizing her own limitations. The educational preparation of the temporary nurse gave her the background to understand that she did not possess the expertise needed in this situation. If the situation were changed so that the temporary nurse was reviewed for expertise in coronary care and found to have that expertise, then the charge nurse might not be liable for the error of the temporary nurse. The supervisory function of ascertaining level of preparation and ability to meet the standards of the job would have been carried out.

EXAMPLE

Supervisory Responsibility for a Staff Member With Limited Education

An RN is working on a unit that assigns a nursing assistant to work with each RN. One evening, the regular nursing assistant is absent due to illness. A new nursing assistant is assigned to work with the RN. During the evening, the RN asks the nursing assistant to monitor the new postoperative patient. The RN lists for the nursing assistant the items that are to be checked: vital signs, hourly urine output, pain, and condition of the dressing. Each hour, the RN stops the nursing assistant, asks if the patient is doing okay, and receives an affirmative reply. When the RN stops to chart, he reviews the past 4 hours of flow sheet information listed by the nursing assistant. He sees that the urine output has been only 15 mL/hr for the past 4 hours. When he questions the nursing assistant, he learns that the nursing assistant had no idea what information needed to be reported immediately. The RN completes an assessment and calls the physician. The patient is found to have developed renal failure.

The RN might be found negligent in this case for assigning the nursing assistant to monitor a critical postoperative patient without proper direction or supervision. The nursing assistant might not be found negligent because she had no basis for recognizing the seriousness of the situation or for recognizing her own lack of ability to meet the responsibilities involved in this assessment. She could carry out the tasks assigned and had done those correctly.

Limits on Patient's Claim to Negligence

Several situations may be viewed by the court as a valid defense to a patient's claim that negligence has occurred. Contributory negligence is based on the concept that the patient contributed to the injury by not acting prudently in that circumstance. For example, the patient may not have followed instructions, may have provided false information that led to improper treatment, or may not have followed warnings about the side effects of medications (Killion & Dempski, 2000).

Courts also may incorporate the use of comparative negligence. If this is used, the court would determine what percentage of the injury resulted from the patient's negligence and what part rested with the nurse, and reduce the damage award accordingly (Killion & Dempski, 2000).

Charitable Immunity

Charitable immunity refers to a situation in which an individual or an organization is held to a lesser standard of care because of the provision of charitable care. This lesser standard is that the person must be guilty of gross negligence, often referred to as "willful, wanton, or reckless conduct" instead of the usual standard of simple negligence in order to be liable (Hattis, Staton, & Walton, 2004). Thus, they are protected from liability.

Institutional Charitable Immunity

Historically, charitable immunity covered all the work of some hospitals and churches. Charitable immunity was granted if all the income for the institution was derived from charitable giving. Some laws even provided specific dollar amounts of liability limitation for charitable organizations. This type of liability for institutions is rapidly disappearing because there are few major hospitals that do not provide both compensated care and uncompensated care. There is also a strong public interest in holding all organizations accountable for the actions of those who work under their auspices.

Charitable Immunity for Volunteers in Health Settings

Forty-three states and the District of Columbia have some type of charitable immunity laws covering health professionals who volunteer (Hattis, Staton, & Walton, 2004). Many of these provide charitable immunity laws for physicians or other medical providers who work in "free" clinics or other settings in which they are not paid for services. This does not mean that a person cannot sue a volunteer care provider; however, it makes it much less likely that they could win and therefore, less likely that an attorney would help them to pursue such a case. Legislation in some states requires that the clinic inform clients in writing that by accepting free care they are agreeing to the limited liability of the care providers. This has been done to encourage health professionals to volunteer their services where they are greatly needed.

A few states have sought to protect volunteer health care providers with laws that limit their liability as if they were state employees and by providing a fund to compensate anyone who is injured through the actions of a volunteer health professional. In these states, there are generally very specific rules as to who qualifies for this protection. The legislation focuses on individuals working in clinics or other such settings where neither the clinic nor the individual received compensation for the care provided. The organization often must meet strict criteria, and the health care provider must be working within that organization.

In 1997, the federal government passed the Volunteer Protection Act to encourage the development of free clinics to serve the uninsured and poor. The Volunteer Protection Act "provides immunity from lawsuits filed against a nonprofit's volunteer where the claim is that he carelessly injured another in the course of helping the nonprofit" (Non-Profit Coordinating Committee of New York, 1998). This act protects the volunteer in health care against claims of simple negligence, but does not protect against gross negligence. Anyone rendering aid in an emergency is expected to behave as a reasonably prudent person would in such a situation; however, simple negligence refers to causing harm in any way, and gross negligence is defined as "failure to use even the slightest amount of care in a way that shows recklessness or willful disregard for the safety of others" ('Lectric Law Library, 2006). This is a very difficult standard for a plaintiff to meet. This is an especially important protection for health professionals who volunteer in free clinics, screening programs, and other settings.

Good Samaritan Laws

Another type of charitable immunity is found in laws that relate to people responding to emergencies. These are often referred to as Good Samaritan laws. These laws are meant to encourage anyone to render assistance in an emergency situation without fear of liability for simple negligence. Liability is only for gross negligence. The nurse rendering aid in an emergency must behave as a reasonably prudent nurse in that situation. Thus, the standard is higher than for the nonprofessional person. For example, a person on the street might bend an injured person's neck in an effort to help the person, but a nurse might be found to be reckless for doing that because the nurse has more formal education regarding proper actions in accidents. However, in this scenario, the nurse is not expected to perform as if he or she were operating in a health care setting. The physical situation and the psychological situation are both considered when determining what is a reasonably prudent nursing action, but the courts have supported those rendering aid. An additional aspect of the professional responsibility is to not abandon the person until care can be turned over to another competent person. So the professional may relinquish responsibility to emergency services personnel who arrive on the scene, but not to a simple bystander. To date, there has been no instance of a nurse being sued for coming to the aid of someone in an emergency situation (Bernzweig, 1996).

The automatic external defibrillator (AED) is now being placed in public settings throughout the nation for the treatment of cardiac arrest victims. In 2002, the federal government passed the Community Access to Emergency Devices Act (Community AED Act), which provided grants for the purpose of placing AEDs in public locations and training individuals in their use, thus further expanding the presence of AEDs. The liability of those who use the devices became an immediate concern after their use was implemented. All 50 states have now enacted laws relative to the liability of those who use these devices. These laws again protect individuals from charges of simple negligence (National Conference of State Legislatures, 2006).

Each nurse must make an individual decision about rendering emergency aid in a specific situation unless the law mandates that people respond to emergencies. Vermont is the only state to mandate that anyone encountering an emergency render assistance (Guido, 2001). Check to see whether such a statute has been enacted in your state. In Canada, the province of Ontario requires a person to render assistance in an emergency. In other provinces, no specific duty to render assistance exists (Search and Rescue Society of British Columbia, 1995).

The decision to render aid involves ethical as well as legal considerations. If the profession of nursing is a public trust and nurses are truly involved in the business of caring, then failure to aid an individual who is in serious danger is an ethical violation of that trust. Professional liability insurance does provide coverage when the nurse assists in this way, which may make a nurse feel more comfortable about rendering emergency aid in the first place.

LIABILITY INSURANCE

Liability insurance transfers the legal and any settlement costs related to a suit from the individual to an insurance company, which spreads the risks to a large group of policy holders. The expectation is that most individuals will not be sued, and that the pool of premiums collected from policy holders therefore will adequately cover the costs of those who are sued, the administrative costs of managing the policies, and the profit for the insurance company. Individuals benefit by transferring risk from themselves to the insurance company for the cost of the insurance policy.

A liability insurance crisis exists in the United States. The cost of liability insurance for primary health care providers (such as physicians and nurse practitioners) has escalated at an extraordinary rate. Some of the factors that have caused this are the large judgments that have been made, the number of suits that have been brought, the large fees that attorneys receive, and the high profits of insurance companies. Nurses in independent advanced practice have been especially affected by the increase in premiums, because their incomes have traditionally been moderate and they cannot charge fees sufficient to cover insurance costs that may equal those of physicians. Nurses who are employed in more traditional roles are able to obtain malpractice insurance for a modest cost.

Some states have initiated legislation that allows for awards to cover actual losses and costs of care, while limiting awards for pain and suffering and other nontangible factors. Sometimes this legislation has been accompanied by restrictions on insurance company rates. Laws in some states are being amended to restrict the monetary liability of any party according to the percentage of responsibility. Liability laws continue to be a major concern for nurses, because nurses are being named in an increasing number of suits, although the total number is still low.

Institutional and Individual Insurance

Many hospitals and other institutional employers carry liability insurance that covers both the institution and its employees. Some hospitals may limit the coverage that their policies provide for individual employees in an effort to hold down costs. Kihm (1999) pointed out that when health care institutions merge, are bought out, or go bankrupt, liability insurance coverage might be called into question. Some institutions have chosen to self-insure part of their liability requirements. If such an institution goes bankrupt, there are no funds left to pay liability claims and pending claims may revert to individuals named in the suits.

Even if an employer carries liability insurance, it is usually advisable for the individual professional to carry an independent policy. An independent policy provides coverage in voluntary activities as well as on the job. It is also transferable from one employer to another. Some policies may provide for personal liability (for such things as a person tripping on a rug and being injured) as well as professional liability. If a legal action is instituted against you, the individual liability insurance policy provides independent legal counsel. If the institution has charitable immunity and nurses are paid employees, the policy supports the individual nurse who may be sued when the institution is protected from a lawsuit. Many nursing liability policies also provide coverage for legal expenses incurred in defending your license in a disciplinary proceeding.

Keep in mind that insurance is not the only source of payment for a judgment. Judgments may be levied against most tangible assets, including houses, cars, and savings; judgments also may be levied against future earnings. Married nurses who reside in community property states should realize that one half of the assets of a family may be vulnerable to a judgment. Community property states at this time include Arizona, California, Idaho, Louisiana, Nevada, New Mexico, Texas, Washington, and Wisconsin. These factors combine to support the need for the individual professional to carry liability insurance that will provide legal counsel and protection in the case of any judgment.

Analyzing Liability Insurance Coverage

Individual liability insurance for RNs is available from a variety of insurance companies (directly through their agents) and through professional organizations that offer coverage as a service to members. When investigating individual liability insurance, ask the agent or company the questions in Display 8-2. Of particular importance is the difference between a "claims occurred" and a "claims made" policy. A claims occurred policy is safer because if you subsequently drop the

---

 Display 8-2   Questions to Ask Regarding Individual Liability Insurance

1. In what situations would I, as an individual, be covered?
2. In what situations would I not be covered?
3. How is my coverage affected by my actions? For example, if I failed to follow hospital policy, would I still be covered?
4. What are the monetary limits of the policy?
5. Does the policy provide me with an attorney?
6. Is the policy renewable at my option? What factors affect renewability?
7. Does the insurance cover incidents that occurred while the policy was in force, regardless of when the claim is brought (claims-occurred insurance coverage), or does it cover incidents only if I am currently insured (claims-brought insurance coverage)?
8. What is the cost compared with other policies?

Display 8-3   Additional Questions Regarding an Institutional Liability Policy

1. Does the policy provide me with a personal attorney, or will the same attorney be working for the hospital?
2. At what point would the hospital no longer be responsible and would I become personally responsible?
3. How would my job be affected if a lawsuit were filed or payment awarded based on an action against me? (Check institutional policy as well as the insurance company policy.)
4. Does the insurance company have the right to seek restitution from me if it pays a claim based on my actions?

(It is important that you have accurate answers to these questions so that you can make an informed decision regarding your need for an individual policy.)

policy, it will still be in effect for any incident that occurred while you were covered. If a claims made policy was chosen, then the coverage for any claim ends when the policy premium is no longer being paid. Because the time limit on liability claims is substantial, you would have to continue to hold the policy and pay the premiums even if you were no longer employed in health care (Brooke, 2006b).

The questions in Display 8-2 can help you to compare policies from different insurance carriers. When coverage appears equal, you might ask how long a company has been in business and how long it has been providing nursing liability insurance. You want to be insured with a reliable, stable company.

The nurse employee should investigate just as carefully liability insurance coverage that is carried by the hospital. Questions 1 through 4 in Display 8-2 apply to institutional insurance policies as well as to individual insurance policies. In addition, ask the questions in Display 8-3 about any institutional policy.

Critical Thinking Activity

You are accepting a position in a clinic. When might you ask about professional liability insurance coverage? Formulate specific questions. Identify the person who would be the best source of this information. How will you proceed if this person does not have the information you seek? If the interviewer tells you that the clinic is well covered by liability insurance, will you purchase personal malpractice insurance? Why or why not?

NATIONAL DATA BANK

In the United States, the federal government maintains a national data bank on all licensed health care providers. This is separate from and has a purpose different from the data collected by the National Council of State Boards of Nursing. By law, the court or relevant board must report to this data bank all judgments, settlements paid, or convictions for malpractice, and all situations in which a health care provider's privileges to practice are curtailed or withdrawn. All institutions must consult this data bank for information before giving any health care provider privilege to practice in the institution. This reflects the privileges given to physicians, physician assistants, nurse practitioners, dentists, and any other independent practitioner that the institution allows to practice in that setting while not being employees. Institutions have always been required to check the credentials of those that they employ. The purpose of the national data bank is to protect the public from incompetent professionals who could continue to practice by moving from one place to another.

LEGAL ISSUES COMMON IN NURSING

Some legal issues recur frequently in nursing practice. It is wise for the nurse to understand these particular issues as they relate to individual practice.

Duty to Report or Seek Medical Care for a Patient

A nurse who cares for a patient has a legal duty to ensure that the patient receives safe and competent care. This duty requires that the nurse maintain an appropriate standard of care and take action to obtain an appropriate standard of care from other professionals when necessary. For example, if a nurse identifies that a patient needs the attention of a physician and fails to make every effort to obtain that attention, the nurse has breached a duty to the patient. In a recent study, the "failure to rescue" individuals experiencing life-threatening complications was linked to the shortage of RNs on duty in the facility (Needleman, Buerhaus, Mattke, Stewart, & Zelevinsky, 2002). This is a critical RN function.

EXAMPLE

Failure to Seek Medical Care for a Patient

The RN is caring for a postoperative patient during the night. The patient's blood pressure begins to drop, and the pulse begins to rise. The nurse's assessment indicates that the patient may be bleeding internally. The nurse institutes a plan for close nursing monitoring and calls the surgeon to describe the situation. The surgeon gives a telephone order to increase the IV fluid rate and states that she will see the patient in the morning. The patient's condition continues to deteriorate, but the nurse does nothing further to ensure that a physician examines the patient.

If the outcome is unfavorable, the nurse can be found to have breached a duty to the patient. The patient relies on the nurse to provide appropriate care and to identify when a physician is needed. The nurse could have made more telephone calls to the surgeon and, failing the success of that, could have followed the facility's procedure for asking another physician (such as the emergency department physician) to see the patient.

The nurse has a duty to continue all efforts to obtain appropriate medical care for the patient. If the nurse had followed all procedures, sought another physician, and continued efforts when initial attempts were unsuccessful, the nurse would not have breached a duty. The nurse cannot guarantee a physician's care, but can guarantee that the patient will not be left without an advocate.

Nursing Responsibility for Medical Orders

The nurse has a responsibility to critically examine medical orders that are written for a patient. Although the nurse is not responsible for the medical order itself, the nurse's education provides a background to identify obvious discrepancies or problems. In one reported case (Anonymous, 1997), two doctors left conflicting orders, which the charge nurse then transcribed. The court ruled that the nurse had a duty to understand the patient's plan of care and to communicate with the doctors who had written the conflicting orders.

Another area of important nursing responsibility is in relationship to telephone orders. The Joint Commission discourages these whenever possible, encouraging instead written orders that are faxed or communicated in writing in some way. However, there are situations when telephone orders are essential to timely care. In these instances, there should be clear guidelines as to how orders are documented and verified. The preferred method is for the nurse to speak directly to the prescriber, write down the order as received, and then read it back to the prescriber for verification. The prescriber must then review and sign the order as soon as practical.

In some states it is legal for the nurse to take a verbal order from the agent of the prescriber. This agent may be the nurse or medical assistant in the office. When receiving an order through an agent, the nurse should verify and document the identity and position of the agent, verify that the order did come from the prescriber (not at the discretion of the agent), and then follow the same procedure for verifying and documenting the order (Brooke, 2006a).

■ ■ **COMMUNICATION IN *ACTION***
■ ■

Obtaining a Telephone Order

Evan Wilson was an RN on a medical unit. He called Dr. Marie Stevens regarding the needs of a patient Esther Moran. The nurse in Dr. Stevens's office answered the phone. Evan stated, "Hello, this is Evan Wilson, the RN on 4W at Mercy Hospital. I am caring for Dr. Stevens's patient Esther Moran, who was admitted this morning for management of her heart failure. She is complaining of indigestion and has asked for an antacid, which Dr. Stevens has directed her to use while at home. I would like to speak with Dr. Stevens about this." The nurse replied, "Dr. Stevens is with a patient now, but I am familiar with Mrs. Moran and I am sure that Dr. Stevens would order the antacid. Go ahead and give it to her. I will talk with Dr. Stevens and get her O.K. as soon as she is available." Evan replied, "I appreciate your interest in facilitating care for Mrs. Moran, but I can only accept an order that the physician has initiated after assessing the situation. It will be fine if you contact me after talking with Dr. Stevens. Thanks for your help. Dr. Stevens can call me on my cell phone for additional information." While in his state it was legal for an RN to accept an order through an agent of the physician, Evan knew that the order must originate with the prescriber, not with the agent.

Confidentiality and Right to Privacy

Confidentiality and the right to privacy with respect to one's personal life are basic concerns in our society. All information regarding a patient belongs to that patient. This right has been inferred from interpretation of the federal constitution, but is explicitly stated in some state laws. HIPAA demands major efforts of all health care providers in regard to protecting patient privacy. In theory, the rights identified in HIPAA should protect a patient's privacy. Only information that the patient specifically releases may be shared with others. However, third-party payers (such as insurance companies and health maintenance organizations) will not reimburse for care if they do not receive the records they request. The result is that patients often must sign statements giving blanket approval for all information to be sent to the third-party payer. They may be unaware of exactly what information is sent or who may see it.

When computerized records are transmitted to insurance companies, they no longer contain only a brief statement of diagnosis and treatment; they may also contain detailed accounts of interactions between a patient and a mental health professional, health information of a sensitive nature, and genetic information that could be used inappropriately. Because increased use of computerized records can result in easier retrieval and cross-referencing of records from many sources, the general public, health care providers, and government officials are becoming more concerned about potential invasions of privacy. Safeguards must be built into all computerized medical record systems that prevent unauthorized access and the tracking of those who do access the system.

A nurse who gives out information without authorization from the patient or from the legally responsible guardian can be held liable for any harm that results. If you have question about who the legally responsible guardian of a patient is, be sure to consult with your administrative authority. If there is not a court-appointed legal guardian, then specific state laws identify who becomes the responsible guardian when the person is unable to give personal consent. The hospital administration should be able to ascertain the correct guardian.

Only those professional persons involved in the patient's care who have a need to know about the patient are allowed routine access to the record. A physician who is not involved in the patient's care or who does not have an administrative responsibility relative to that care is not allowed routine access. Persons not involved in care may be allowed access to the record only by specific written authorization of the patient or by court order. Be cautious about what information you share verbally and with whom.

Medical records professionals state that it is not uncommon for attorneys, family members, media representatives, or law enforcement officials to request access to patient records or specific patient information without having express consent from the patient or a legal court order to view the records or be given information. Those unfamiliar with laws regarding privacy sometimes reveal information inappropriately. If you are ever approached for patient information by someone who purports to have authority, your best course of action is to refer that individual to appropriate administrative personnel, who can determine the validity of the request.

EXAMPLE

Breach of Confidentiality

A nurse in a small community hospital discusses with a friend the admission of a female member of the community for treatment of cancer. The nurse's friend then talks to others, who talk to still others, until there is widespread knowledge of the patient's cancer in the community. The woman's daughter hears about her mother's cancer diagnosis at school and is very upset.

In a suit charging breach of privacy and confidentiality, the nurse in this example could be held liable for revealing this information. The harm is the emotional distress to the woman and her family. If the breach of confidentiality could be traced to the nurse's conversation, the nurse's action would be considered the direct cause of harm.

A newer concern is that more health care agencies are using fax machines to send patient information to one another and even between departments within an institution. Faxes have a legitimate purpose in that continuity of care is enhanced when information is shared. When you send a document via fax machine, it is difficult to ensure that confidentiality is maintained. Facilities are being mandated by HIPAA to keep fax machines in areas not accessible to the public. Some facilities have a policy requiring that you call ahead and designate a specific person to be present to receive the fax. The cover page often states that this is confidential material and should not be read by anyone other than the designated recipient. If your facility or agency has no policy regarding the safeguarding of faxed information, you would be wise to raise the concern.

Other new areas of concern are the Internet and e-mail. Through these avenues, a health care provider may consult with other professionals to provide the best diagnostic and treatment services to the patient. However, on-line computer communications are not private. Those with the necessary skill may intercept and read any e-mail or Internet message. Therefore, the identity of patients must be protected in any such communication.

Defamation of Character

Any time that shared information is detrimental to a person's reputation, the person sharing the information may be liable for defamation of character. Written defamation is called libel. Oral defamation is called slander. Defamation of character involves communication that is malicious and false. Sometimes such comments are made in the heat of anger. Occasionally, statements written in a patient's chart are libelous. Severely critical opinions may be stated as fact. An example of such a statement might be, "The patient is lying," or "The patient is rude and domineering." Patients may charge that comments in the chart adversely affected their care by prejudicing other staff against them. Libel and slander may also be charged when written comments or verbal statements are made regarding another health care provider. Thoughtless or angry comments that impugn the abilities of a physician or that might cause a patient to lose trust in a physician can be slander. The astute nurse will chart only objective information regarding patients and give opinion in professional terms, well documented with fact. In conversations, the prudent nurse avoids discussing patients and carefully considers any comments about other health care providers before making them.

■■ COMMUNICATION IN *ACTION*
■■

Accurate and Responsible Documentation

William Whittier was caring for a patient who was brought in by an ambulance after being found unconscious on the sidewalk. There was considerable side discussion among the staff about whether the patient was drunk. In his documentation, William notes, "Skin red, flushed, and warm. Strong breath odor that resembles alcohol. Patient responds only to shaking and loud verbal stimulation." Later, when the patient has become more responsive and awake, he documents, "Patient states, 'I really tied one on last night. What happened?'" This provided factual information for the reader without making potentially libelous accusations.

Defamation of character also may be charged by a health care provider who believes that statements made by another professional are false, malicious, and have caused harm. There are accepted mechanisms for confidentially reporting inappropriate care or errors; be sure to use them and do not make critical statements to uninvolved third parties. In many states, licensed professionals are required to report poor practice or illegal acts on the part of other professionals. Criticism reported without malice and in good faith, through the appropriate channels, is protected from legal action for defamation.

Privileged Communication

Privileged communication refers to information that is shared by an individual client with certain professionals but that does not need to be revealed, even in a court of law. This professional is said to possess "privilege"—that is, has the privilege of not revealing information. All states consider certain types of communication (between client and attorney, between patient and doctor, or between an individual and a member of the clergy) privileged. Not all states recognize the nurse–patient relationship as one in which privileged communication takes place; even those states that recognize nurse–patient communication as potentially privileged do not consider *all* communication between patients and nurses to be privileged. Privilege is a limited concept. Only a court can determine whether privilege exists in any specific case. If a court does not determine information is privileged, then you are legally obligated to testify about the communication.

Informed Consent

Every person has the right to either consent (agree) to or to refuse health care treatment. The law requires that a person give voluntary and **informed consent**. Voluntary means that no coercion exists. Informed means that a person clearly understands the choices being offered.

Consent for Medical Treatment

Consent for medical treatment is the responsibility of the medical provider (eg, physician, dentist, nurse practitioner). Information to be shared with the client includes a description of the procedure, any alternatives for treatment, the risks involved in the procedure, the probable results, including problems of recuperation, and anything else generally disclosed to patients (Shinn & Curtin, 2001). This consent may be either verbal or written and indicates a patient has decided to go ahead with the procedure based on a clear understanding of the options. Written consent usually is preferred in health care to ensure that a record of consent exists, although a signature alone does not prove that the consent was informed. A blanket consent for "any procedures deemed necessary" usually is not considered adequate consent for specific procedures. The form should state the specific proposed medical procedure or test.

The courts do not accept the patient's medical condition alone as a valid reason for withholding complete and accurate information when seeking consent. Currently, there are no clear guidelines as to what constitutes complete information. What constitutes adequate information about various alternative approaches to treatment is often unclear. Is it always necessary to discuss a treatment the physician does not believe is a good choice? Must all risks be discussed? Courts have generally supported the idea that commonly accepted alternatives and usual risks need to be disclosed, but that marginal or unusual treatments and rare or unexpected risks do not have to be discussed.

The law places the responsibility for obtaining consent for medical treatment on the provider who will perform the procedure. It is that person's responsibility to provide appropriate information, and he or she is liable if the patient charges that appropriate information was not given. A nurse may present a form for a patient to sign, and the nurse may sign the form as a witness to the signature. This does not transfer the legal responsibility for informed consent for medical care to the nurse. If the patient does not seem well informed, the nurse should notify the provider so that further information can be provided to the patient. Although the nurse would not be liable legally for the lack of informed consent, the nurse has ethical obligations to assist the patient in exercising his or her rights and to assist the provider in providing appropriate care.

Consent for Nursing Measures

Nurses must obtain a patient's consent for nursing measures undertaken. This does not mean that exhaustive explanations need to be given in each situation, because courts have held that patients can be expected to have some understanding of usual care. Consent for nursing measures may be verbal or implied. The nurse may ask, "Are you ready to ambulate now?" The patient answers, "Certainly," providing verbal consent. Alternatively, the nurse may state, "I have the injection the doctor ordered for you. Will you please turn over?" If the patient turns over, this is implied consent.

Similarly, consent for care should be requested in emergency situations, such as those mentioned earlier in the discussion of Good Samaritan policies, if the injured is able to give that consent. A simple statement such as, "I am a registered nurse. Do you want my help?" is sufficient.

The nurse should remember that the patient is free to refuse any aspect of care offered. Like the physician, the nurse is responsible for making sure that the patient is informed before making a decision. Good nursing care requires that you use all means at your disposal to help the patient comprehend the value of proposed care. For example, the postoperative patient needs to understand that getting into a chair is part of the plan of care, not a convenience for the nurse or simply a change to prevent boredom. Thus, a patient's refusal of care is accepted only after the patient has been given complete information. The nurse would then carefully document this situation.

Competence to Give Consent

A person's ability to make judgments based on rational understanding is termed competence. Dementia, developmental disabilities, head injuries, strokes, and illnesses creating loss of consciousness are common causes of an inability to make judgments. Determining competence is a complex issue. The patient's illness, age, or condition alone does not determine competence. Legal competence is ultimately determined by the court. The general tendency of the courts has been to encourage whatever decision-making ability an individual has and to restrict personal decision making as little as possible.

When a person is determined legally to be incompetent, a legal guardian is appointed and consent is obtained from the legal guardian. A legal guardian is constrained from making some types of decisions. For example, if the health care action could be identified as injurious to the individual involved, a court may need to be consulted regarding consent for that specific action. An example would be the decision about discontinuation of dialysis for an incompetent individual. When such an individual leaves no clear indication regarding personal wishes, the health care providers might insist on getting a court decision before accepting the consent of the guardian to terminate the dialysis.

Health care providers often encounter clients for whom no legal determination of competence has been made, but who do not seem able to make an informed decision; examples include the very confused elderly person, the inebriated person, and the unconscious person. There are usually institutional guidelines to follow in determining that a person cannot give his or her own consent. The guidelines may require examination by a physician and documentation of the patient's condition. More than one physician may be required to examine the patient.

This patient may not have a legally designated guardian or substitute decision maker. The law in each state specifies who is allowed to give consent in such situations. Frequently, this is the spouse, parent, children, or siblings. Your facility policy should contain directions to guide you in obtaining legal consent; if it does not, consult a supervisor for a decision. In situations where there are several persons in the category, such as children of an elderly person, agreement regarding decisions is needed before proceeding. Determining who is able to give legal consent in such a situation is not a nurse's responsibility.

Competence may change from day to day, as a person's physical illness changes. The person who has had major surgery and is receiving large doses of narcotics for pain may not be able to reason clearly. Forty-eight hours later, this same individual may be perfectly alert and capable of considering complex issues. An individual may be competent to make some decisions, such as "I don't like rice and I won't eat it!" but incompetent to make others; for example, decisions regarding financial matters. These differences in competence require care providers to adjust their own planning to incorporate patient self-determination whenever possible, even when the person is legally incompetent. If a person truly is not capable of making decisions, the nurse should attempt to present necessary nursing actions in a way that elicits cooperation and avoids confrontation over decisions. For example, rather than asking the cognitively impaired person if she wants to take her medications, the prudent nurse simply states, "Here are your medications. It is time to take them."

Withdrawing Consent

Consent may be withdrawn after it is given. People have the right to change their minds. Therefore, if after one IV infusion a patient decides not to have a second one started, that is the patient's right. As a nurse, you have an obligation to notify the physician if the patient refuses a medical procedure or treatment.

When individuals are participating in any type of research protocol for care, they are free to withdraw from the research study at any time. When caring for individuals who are part of a research process, you have obligations to protect the patient's right to make decisions, even if they are contrary to the interests of the researcher. You would have an obligation to inform the researcher of the patient's decision.

Consent and Minors

The parent or legal guardian usually provides consent for care of a minor. You also should obtain the minor's consent when he or she is able to give it. Increasingly, courts are emphasizing that minors be allowed a voice when it concerns matters that they are capable of understanding. This is especially true for the adolescent, but this consideration should be given to any child who is 7 years of age or older. Often courts seek not consent from minors, but rather an indication that they understand the purpose of the care. For adolescents, the court may ask that negotiation with minors occur. When minors refuse care and legal guardians have authorized that care, do not proceed until legal clarification is given. Consult your nursing supervisor. This may be an issue for an ethics committee as well as for legal representation.

Minors who live apart from their parents and are financially independent, or who are married, are termed **emancipated minors**. In most (but not all) states, emancipated minors can give consent to their own treatment. Some states have specific laws relating to the **mature minor**, allowing sexually active minors to give personal consent (without also obtaining parental consent) for treatment of sexually transmitted disease or for obtaining birth control information and supplies (see Chapter 10). Be sure of the law in your state if you practice in an area where this is a concern. Most institutions have developed policies to guide employees in making correct decisions in this and other areas dealing with consent.

Advance Directives

Advance directives are legal documents stating the wishes of individuals regarding health care in situations in which they are no longer capable of giving personal informed consent. These documents are completed in advance of the situation in which they might be needed, and they direct the actions of others. There are several types of advance directives, such as a living will and a durable power of attorney for health care.

The Living Will

A **living will** or **directive to physicians** provides information on preferences regarding end-of-life issues such as types of care to provide and whether to use various resuscitation measures. The basis of a living will is an *if–then* plan. Most commonly, they declare that *if* "I am terminally ill and not expected to recover," *then* "I want this care given and do not want that care given." The *if* condition may also include that the person is in a persistent vegetative state and not expected to recover function and capacity. The condition stated as the *if* must be diagnosed by a physician. Many states require that two physicians must agree that the person is terminally ill or in a persistent vegetative state. Even when this is not the law, health care agencies often require this as a policy. The determination of the patient's condition must be documented in the legal record by the physician. Although living wills or directives were originally advisory for families and physicians as they made decisions, some states have now passed laws requiring that these documents be honored. If the physician does not agree with the decision of the patient, then the physician in that state is obligated to withdraw from care and refer the case to another physician.

If the living will requests that no resuscitation or limited resuscitation efforts be undertaken, the physician must write orders limiting resuscitation in the record. However, remember that living wills may also request that all possible resuscitation efforts be made.

Living wills or directives to the physician may address other aspects of care in addition to resuscitation efforts. For example, they may indicate whether the individual wants to be tube fed if he or she is in a persistent vegetative state, whether surgery should be used in certain instances, or whether IV fluids or ventilator support should be used. Some advance directives are several pages long, as the person addresses many different possible concerns. For more discussion and an example of a living will, see Chapter 10.

Aging With Dignity, an organization in Florida, has developed and disseminated, in conjunction with the Robert Woods Johnson Foundation, an advance directive document called the "Five Wishes." This document addresses not only life-sustaining therapies that are desired or not desired but also other aspects of end-of-life care, such as the desire for people, for touch, for music, and so forth. The five wishes that form the structure of the document are listed in Display 8-4. The Five Wishes document is an accepted legal advance directive in the majority of states. The Five Wishes Web site lists states that accept this as a legal document. In other states, the Five Wishes document may be used as an addendum to the legally accepted advance directive document to inform health care providers of personal wishes for end-of-life care.

Display 8-4   Five Wishes for End-of-Life Care

1. Which person you want to make health care decisions for you when you can't make them.
2. The kind of medical treatment you want or don't want.
3. How comfortable you want to be.
4. How you want people to treat you.
5. What you want your loved ones to know.

Aging With Dignity: *www.agingwithdignity.org/5wishes.html*

Durable Power of Attorney for Health Care

A **durable power of attorney for health care** is a document that legally designates a **substitutionary decision maker**, should the person be incapacitated. This document may also be referred to as designating a **health care proxy**. This document may be combined with a living will that contains specific advance directives, such as those discussed above. Thus, the person identifies a preferred legal decision maker if he or she is incapacitated and at the same time provides directions for that substitutionary decision maker regarding the decisions.

If an individual has designated a substitutionary decision maker for health care, this supersedes all general legal designations for decision makers. In a society where there are many different family constellations and relationships, durable powers of attorney for health care are an important personal decision. For example, individuals who live in life partnerships other than marriage must have a durable power of attorney for health care to provide that life partner with decision-making ability for emergencies or critical situations. For the adult with no living parents or spouse and multiple siblings, the designation of one person as a decision maker may diminish family conflict and facilitate the provision of the care the individual wishes. An individual may wish to designate a sibling or a trusted friend.

Physician Orders for Life-Sustaining Treatments

Limitations on resuscitation in the event of a cardiac or respiratory arrest may take many forms. These orders are generally referred to as Physician Orders for Life-Sustaining Treatments (POLST). The most comprehensive is that the order reads "Do not resuscitate" (DNR) or "No Code," meaning that no resuscitation efforts of any kind are to be made. There would be no cardiopulmonary resuscitation (CPR), no resuscitative drugs, and no mechanical ventilation. This is often the choice of the person who has a life-threatening disease and for whom resuscitation would only serve to prolong illness and discomfort. In some instances, the person may request a limited resuscitation effort, such as CPR and medications but no mechanical ventilation. Facilities may have a variety of ways to designate these limitations on resuscitative efforts and to communicate these directions to those providing care. An important understanding for nurses is that in the absence of a written order from a physician, other care providers are obligated to initiate resuscitation if an arrest occurs.

In an attempt to "effectively communicate the wishes of seriously ill patients to have or to limit medical treatment as they move from one care setting to another," the POLST organization at the Oregon Health Sciences University has developed a set of standardized orders regarding CPR, medical interventions, antibiotics, artificially administered nutrition, and a summary (POLST, 2005). See the POLST Web site for examples of this form and for specific information in relationship to the use of these forms in individual states.

An advance directive (or living will) provides information that the physician can use as a basis for deciding when an order limiting life-sustaining treatment is appropriate. In many states, there are laws that designate under what circumstances a physician might write an order limiting treatment in the absence of an advance directive. If the patient has not completed an advance directive and is not expected to recover, the physician may determine that resuscitation would be futile. **Futile** means that it would not add appreciably to life or have the potential for success. Laws or policies usually require the agreement of two physicians that resuscitation would be futile. After this medical determination, then the person who legally is the substitutionary decision maker is consulted, provided information regarding the patient's condition, and asked to consent to a DNR order. This entire process must be documented in the patient's record.

All care providers must understand that a DNR order does not limit other types of care that will be provided. Treatment of wounds to promote healing, pain management, resolution of other physical problems (such as nausea or constipation), antibiotic administration to control treatable infections, and oxygen to ease breathing are all examples of care that will still be appropriate. Even radiation therapy might be determined appropriate to reduce tumor growth and increase comfort.

In some instances, an additional order may be written that specifies "comfort care only." This order again occurs after consultation with the patient as able and family as appropriate. When this order is written, treatment of infections and other problems may not be initiated. The focus becomes maximum comfort in the face of impending death. The patient for whom comfort care only is ordered should receive the same concerted focus on end-of-life care that would occur in a hospice setting.

Nurses sometimes find themselves in situations in which they believe that the patient's condition is futile and that a DNR or comfort-care-only order would be appropriate, but the physician has not made this determination or, having made this determination, has not consulted with the family regarding a DNR order. Such situations can be difficult for nurses because they have no decision-making authority, and yet they are the ones who legally must carry out the resuscitation. Much depends on the nurse–physician working relationships and their ability to discuss difficult issues together. Some care facilities encourage care conferences where these matters can be raised for discussion. Nurses can be effective advocates for increased communication and discussion of these difficult issues.

Patient Self-Determination Act

In 1990, the U.S. Congress passed the **Patient Self-Determination Act (PSDA)**. This Act took effect in 1992 and required that, on admission to any health care service (hospital, long-term care center, or home care agency), patients be given an opportunity to determine what life-saving or life-prolonging actions they want carried out. Much of the impetus for this legislation was the belief that many individuals were having their lives prolonged in situations in which they would have preferred this not be done. The Act requires the agency to provide adequate information for the individual to make an informed decision regarding these important matters. As a result of this legislation, agencies reviewed and revised policies and protocols regarding consent. In many agencies, a nurse has the responsibility to provide the education and obtain a signature on a document indicating preferences. Some difficulties arise in this process when the person giving the information does not clearly understand that the decision about resuscitation is not based on the current situation but upon the *if* condition of a patient becoming terminally ill and not being expected to survive, *then* what does the patient want to happen. Patients may become concerned that they will be abandoned if an untoward event happens.

Information regarding the results of the PSDA is being analyzed by several government agencies to determine whether there has been a change in practice. Some have suggested that the manner in which self-determination and the possible alternatives are explained greatly influences patient choices; one suggestion has been that these matters first be discussed in the health care provider's office, before admission. When this is possible, it allows for more time to consider alternatives and consult with significant others. The final decision is then made away from the pressure of the health care environment. See Chapter 10 for a further discussion of planning for end-of-life issues.

Emergency Care

Care in emergencies has many legal repercussions; therefore, the judgment that an emergency exists is important. Certain actions may be legal in emergencies and not legal in nonemergency situations. In emergencies, the standard procedures for obtaining consent may be impossible to follow. Further, in emergencies, personnel must sometimes take on responsibilities that they would not undertake in a nonemergency situation. Critical thinking on the part of all health care professionals is essential when differentiating an emergency from a nonemergency.

Most facilities that provide emergency care have policies and procedures designed to ensure adequate support for claiming that an emergency exists. Thus, the policy will often state that at least two physicians in the emergency department must examine the patient and concur that the emergency requires immediate action, without waiting for consent. This ensures maximum legal protection for the physician and the institution.

Consent in Emergencies

If a true emergency exists, consent for care is considered to be implied. The law holds that if a reasonable person were aware that the situation was life threatening, he or she would give consent for care. An exception to this is made if the person has explicitly rejected such care in advance; an example is a Jehovah's Witness carrying a card stating his personal religion, and that he does not wish to receive blood or blood products. This is one reason why emergency department nurses should check a patient's wallet for identification and information related to care. Checking a patient's wallet should be done with another person, and a careful inventory of contents documented and signed by both. There should be little concern about liability in taking emergency action if this is completed.

Standards of Practice and Emergencies

Standards of practice in emergencies differ from those in nonemergency situations. In hospital emergencies, the nurse sometimes may be in the position of identifying an emergency and whether a needed action is one that only a physician usually performs. The hospital is expected to have a policy and procedure, which the nurse would follow, to verify and document the situation fully. This usually involves consultation with a supervisory nurse and verification of the emergency situation, as well as attempts to obtain medical assistance. Again, critical thinking by the nurse is essential to determine whether a true emergency exists. Review the information on scope of practice in Chapter 7 to help you with decision making in regard to emergency actions.

When life or limb is truly in danger, the courts have held that a nurse can do those things immediately necessary, even if they usually are considered medical functions, provided the nurse has the essential expertise to perform the actions safely and correctly. The matter of having essential expertise is crucial; this is why all members of an emergency response team must learn all aspects of the code procedure. If, for any reason, the physician were unable to respond to the code, a nurse who was prepared with this essential expertise would assume the role of the leader of the code team.

EXAMPLE

Nursing Action in a Hospital Emergency

In an orthopedic unit, it is common to care for patients with new casts. A young man with a newly applied long-leg cast is admitted through the emergency department at 6 PM. The nurse assigned to this patient's care carefully makes all the appropriate observations throughout the evening and documents his findings. The nurse notes that the leg is beginning to swell and that the edges of the cast are beginning to cut into the skin. The nurse institutes nursing actions of increasing the elevation of the leg and applying ice packs to limit swelling. At that time, the nurse notifies the supervisor that a problem is developing, and that he thinks the physician should be notified. The supervisor agrees, and the nurse begins trying to contact the physician. The nurse continues to make observations, noting increasing swelling, color changes in the exposed toes, and loss of sensation. The physician cannot be reached, and no other physician is immediately available.

The nurse follows the hospital procedure for seeking medical attention and for determining when an emergency exists. After consultation with the supervisor, the nurse decides that an emergency exists and that the cast needs to be cut open to relieve the pressure. Deciding to cut a cast open and cutting the cast are considered medical responsibilities in this hospital.

The nurse has been taught how and when to use a cast cutter in emergency situations. Thus, the nurse possesses the essential expertise. The nurse, with the supervisor's approval, cuts open the cast and secures it in place with an elastic bandage. All observations made, consultations carried out, physician notification attempted, and the final action taken are documented carefully in the patient's record. Hospital policy was followed throughout the situation to ensure that all necessary steps had been taken.

Although the action in this example went beyond usual nursing practice, it would not be considered a violation of either the nursing or the medical practice acts, because an emergency existed and the results of inaction would have been serious. Additionally, the nurse had the expertise and was prepared to carry out the necessary action safely. This emergency care usually is limited to specific technical procedures that the nurse has learned. It does not include diagnosing disease or prescribing medication, unless there are specific protocols relative to the situation.

Protocols and Emergencies

Most health care agencies have established protocols for nursing action in a variety of emergency or even urgent situations. These provide directions for nursing action that would usually be a physician's order. For example, if the patient's blood pressure drops precipitously, the protocol might indicate that the nurse would start an IV infusion with a specified fluid to maintain circulating volume and to provide IV access for emergency drugs. The administration of oxygen to a person suffering acute respiratory distress is another situation frequently covered by a protocol. When emergencies occur, nurses are protected from a charge of practicing outside the scope of the RN by following the protocol that was approved by the medical staff.

Noninstitutional Emergency Care

In many states, official emergency personnel must render all possible aid, including all resuscitative measures, when they are called to an emergency situation. This has sometimes resulted in the resuscitation of a terminally ill person who had previously stated that resuscitation was not desired. As more individuals receive terminal care in their homes, this has become an increasing concern.

Legislation allowing for patient self determination regarding emergency responders has now been passed in some states. The law usually stipulates the precise circumstances under which an individual may provide an advance directive regarding emergency procedures, and how that directive must be documented so that emergency personnel can honor it. For example, the individual may be required to wear a specific armband and the DNR order may be posted on the door of the refrigerator or other prominent position in the home. All emergency responders must be aware of their responsibilities regarding advance directives.

Fraud

Fraud is deliberate deception for the purpose of personal gain and is usually prosecuted as a crime. However, it may also serve as the basis of a civil suit. Situations of fraud in nursing are not common. One example would be trying to obtain a better position by giving incorrect information to a prospective employer. By deliberately stating (falsely) that they have completed a nurse practitioner program to obtain a position for which they would otherwise be ineligible, individuals are defrauding the employer. This may be prosecuted as a crime, because they are also placing members of the community in danger of receiving substandard care. Individuals also may commit fraud by trying to cover up a nursing error to avoid legal action. Courts tend to be harsher in decisions regarding fraud than in cases involving simple malpractice, because fraud represents a deliberate attempt to mislead others for one's own gain and could result in harm to those assigned to that individual's care.

Assault and Battery

Assault is saying or doing something to make a person genuinely afraid that he or she will be touched without consent. **Battery** involves touching a person when that individual has not consented to the action. Neither of these terms implies that harm was done; harm may or may not occur. For an assault to occur, the person must be afraid of what might happen because the individual appears to have the power to carry out the threat. "If you don't take this medication, I will have to put you in restraints" is an example of an assault. For battery to occur, the touching must occur without consent. Remember that consent may be implied rather than specifically stated. Therefore, if the patient extends an arm for an injection, he cannot later charge battery, saying that he was not asked. But if the patient agreed because of a threat (assault), the touching still would be considered battery because the consent was not freely given.

Assault and battery are crimes under the law. However, most of these cases in health care are instituted as civil suits by the injured party, rather than as criminal cases by government authorities.

Assault and battery are most commonly treated as criminal cases when they involve suspected abuse of a patient. Most of us in health care are shocked and dismayed to learn of instances in which care providers were abusive. Individuals who have difficulty with impulse control and anger may become frustrated with a patient and threaten, push, shove, or otherwise harm the individual. Another situation is when a confused patient hits or pinches a nurse. While a nurse has a right to a safe work environment, that is not justification for hitting a confused patient in response (Brooke, 2006c). Most jurisdictions have laws requiring that anyone who knows of abuse to an individual, whether a child, a developmentally delayed adult, or an elderly person, report that abuse to the proper authorities. Within an institution, there should be policies and procedures for this type of reporting. Appropriate authorities must conduct a careful investigation to ensure protection of the rights of the person accused.

False Imprisonment

Making a person stay in a place against his wishes is **false imprisonment**. The person may be forced to stay either by physical or verbal means. It is easy to understand why restraining a patient or confining a patient to a locked room could constitute false imprisonment, if proper procedures were not first carried out. Again, false imprisonment is a crime, but when it occurs in health care it is most often the basis of a civil suit rather than a criminal case.

The law is less clear about keeping a patient confined by nonphysical means. Removing patients' clothing for the express purpose of preventing them from leaving, could make a nurse liable for false imprisonment. Threatening to keep people confined with statements such as, "If you don't stay in your bed, I'll sedate you" can also constitute false imprisonment. If people need to be confined for their own safety or well-being, it is best to help them understand and agree to that course of action.

Any time patients pose a danger to themselves or others, the law requires that the least restrictive means available be used to protect patients and others. Health care providers are obligated to document the behavior of concern, problem-solve alternative actions, and then try those alternative actions before resorting to any type of restraint. Documentation of this entire process is essential. Nurses who determine the need for restraints must obtain a physician's order as soon as possible. Be sure to follow the policies of the facility.

In a conventional care setting, you cannot restrain or confine responsible adults against their wishes. All persons have the right to make decisions for themselves, regardless of the consequences. The patient with a severe heart condition who defies orders and walks to the bathroom has that right. You protect yourself by recording your efforts to teach the patient the need for restrictions and by reporting the patient's behavior to your supervisor and the physician.

In the same context, the patient cannot be forced to remain in a hospital. The patient has the right to leave a health care institution regardless of medical advice to the contrary. While this might not be in the best interests of the person's health, the patient has the right to decide to leave against medical advice. Again, document your efforts in the record and follow applicable policies to protect the facility, the physician, and yourself from liability.

False imprisonment suits are a special concern in the care of the psychiatric patient. Particular laws relate to this situation. In the psychiatric setting, you may have patients who have voluntarily sought admission. The same restrictions on restraint or confinement that apply to patients in the general care setting apply to these patients. Other patients in the psychiatric setting may have been committed involuntarily according to the laws of the state. Specific measures may be used to confine the involuntarily committed patient. Laws in terms of situation, type of restraint allowed, and the length of time restraining may be used often define these measures. If you work in a psychiatric setting, review specific policies regarding restraint to protect patients and to assist staff in functioning within the legal limits.

Medication Errors

Medication errors are one of the most common causes of adverse outcomes for hospitalized patients (Institute of Medicine [IOM], 2000). The IOM has estimated that 1.5 million preventable adverse drug events occur in health care each year (IOM, 2006). Adverse drug events have many different sources, including inappropriate medication for the condition being treated, incorrect dosage or frequency of administration of medication, wrong route of administration, failure to recognize drug interactions, lack of monitoring for drug side effects, and inadequate communication among members of the health care team and the patient.

Many health care team members may be responsible for the errors that lead to adverse events, and many team members can prevent errors. Although individuals must exercise extraordinary care and follow procedures carefully, systems for medication administration also need to be carefully scrutinized. Some errors result from drugs with similar names (for example, Zyprexa and Zyrtec); look-alike medication containers contribute to other errors; still other errors are created by poor systems for communication, in which handwriting problems may contribute to lack of clarity. Verbal orders have such a potential for error that most systems are set up to avoid them as much as possible.

Nurses are legally responsible for ensuring that the five rights of drug administration are followed. The Joint Commission requires the use to two identifiers (such as the patient's name, number, telephone number, or Social Security number). The ordered treatment or medication must be matched to the patient using the identification band information such as name and ID number and compared to the same information transcribed in the patient record or medication administration record (MAR).

Other errors occur because of the use of dangerous abbreviations, and most health care facilities now have lists of abbreviations that must be used. For example, "I.U." for international unit may be confused with "I.V." for intravenous; thus international unit must be written out.

The IOM and the Institute for Safe Medication Practice have identified specific actions that can be taken to reduce medication errors (IOM, 2006). One important action is engaging patients and families in all efforts. Patients and their family caregivers can be taught what medications they are receiving and taught to monitor what they are given. They need to feel free to ask questions, check on what they receive and keep their own careful records. The use of effective information technology and improved labeling and packaging of medications are major strategies to decrease medication errors. Computerized medication systems and computerized order entry are designed to diminish the chance of these medication errors.

When medication errors do occur, the health care professionals involved should institute corrective action immediately and communicate with the patient and family. Fiesta (1998) points out that if health care professionals are not straightforward with patients and families, fraud or intentional concealment may be charged and may contribute to the awarding of punitive damages as well as ordinary damages. Most malpractice insurance will not cover punitive damages.

FACTORS THAT CONTRIBUTE TO MALPRACTICE CLAIMS

A suit usually does not always follow the poor results or harm that may on occasion occur in the course of nursing practice. An understanding of the factors that enter into whether a suit is instituted may be helpful to you.

Consequences of the Error

When an error results in serious consequences, such as prolonged hospitalization, disability, or even death, individuals are likely to institute legal action. The aim may be to cover costs associated with the needed care, lost wages, and other direct costs associated with the error. There also may be a wish to have the individual or organization pay for the pain and suffering experienced. For example, the person who was severely burned by a cautery used incorrectly in surgery would experience lost productivity and wages due to time off for care and healing. There would also be the cost of that care to be reimbursed. And the person would experience severe pain and suffering and might have permanent scarring. That person might seek compensation for these non-monetary losses. In other situations, when no one seems to take responsibility for the error or people do not seem to care or feel regret for what happened, there may be a wish to punish those involved. Punitive damages may be awarded when the court determines that the injury reflects not just a single incident but a pattern of unsafe care.

Social Factors

Much is being written about changes in the public's attitudes toward health care personnel. Health care is big business, and patients complain increasingly of not being accepted and respected as individuals. In general, patients are more willing to bring suit against someone who is part of a large, impersonal system.

Health costs are high, and some people think hospitals and physicians have the ability to pay large settlements, whether directly or through insurance. If a patient's own income is lessened or disrupted by an illness, he or she might bring suit as a solution to economic difficulties. Increased public awareness of the size of monetary judgments that have been awarded may also be an economic incentive to initiating a suit.

Suit-Prone Patients

Some people are more likely to bring suit, for real or imagined errors. If these people are recognized as being suit-prone patients, it is possible for you to protect yourself through increased vigilance regarding care and thorough record keeping. Although it is important to guard against stereotyping, the following general descriptions may help you to avoid problems. Suit-prone patients usually are identified by overt behavior in which they are persistent fault-finders and critics of personnel and of all aspects of care. They may be uncooperative in following a plan of care and sensitive to any perceived slight.

Persons who exhibit hostile attitudes may extend their hostile feelings to the nurses and other health care persons with whom they have contact. The nurse who becomes defensive when faced with hostility only widens the breach in the nurse–patient relationship. It is necessary to pay careful attention to those principles of care learned in psychosocial nursing that deal with how to help the hostile patient. Assisting patients in solving their own problems and offering support are the best forms of protection for the nurse.

Another type of patient who appears more suit-prone is the very dependent person who uses projection to deal with anxiety and fear. These individuals tend to ascribe fault or blame for all events to others and are unable to accept personal responsibility for their own welfare. Again, meeting these patients' needs with a carefully considered plan of care is the answer.

A common error is to withdraw and become defensive when confronting a suit-prone patient; this reaction occurs partly because a situation is unpleasant and partly because a staff member feels personally threatened by the patient's behavior. This reaction increases the likelihood of a suit if a poor result occurs.

Another incorrect nursing response to the suit-prone patient is to become more directive and authoritarian. This tends to increase the patient's feeling of separation and distance from the staff and again increases the likelihood of a suit.

When staff members are helped to view the patient as a troubled person who manifests his or her problems in this manner, sometimes they find it easier to be objective. The patient is in need of all the skill that the thoughtful nurse can bring to the emotional problems. The entire health team needs to develop a careful and consistent approach, which provides security and stability to the patient and family. The suit-prone patient does not always end up suing; much depends on the response of health care personnel.

Suit-Prone Nurses

Nurses may also be suit prone. Nurses who are insensitive to the patient's complaints, who do not identify and meet the patient's emotional needs, or who fail to recognize and accept the limits of their own practice may contribute to suits instituted not only against the nurse but also against the employer and the physician. The nurse's self-awareness is critical in preventing suits (Fig. 8-3).

Staff members may contribute to a patient's distrust of care through complaining about working conditions, telling patients about problems occurring on the unit, and disparaging other health care providers. There is a distinction between informing a patient that you must meet someone else's needs, and therefore will not return for a specified period of time, and giving the patient the impression that you do not have time to attend to his or her needs.

FIGURE 8-3   Certain things can be done to prevent malpractice suits.

PREVENTING MALPRACTICE CLAIMS

A variety of things can be done to prevent malpractice claims from ever happening.

Maintaining Excellent Standards of Care

The most significant thing you can do to prevent malpractice claims is to maintain a high standard of care. To do this, work at improving your own nursing practice and also the general climate for nursing practice where you work. You can do this in many ways. An important aspect of high-standard care is excellence in communication with patients and families. Therapeutic communication skills including listening, clarifying, and problem solving are especially critical.

▦ COMMUNICATION IN *ACTION*

> ### Talking with an Upset Family
> Mr. Jenkins had been at the desk every hour demanding something for his very ill wife. Sometimes it was pain medication and at other times it was something such as a glass of water. He has said, "You people need to take better care of Mildred! If I weren't here, who knows what would happen to her?" Jennifer Tompkins approached Mr. Jenkins in his wife's room. "You seem really concerned about your wife's care," she said. "I would like to talk with both of you about it and see if together we can make some plans that help you both in this very difficult situation you are facing here."

Self-Awareness

Identify your own strengths and weaknesses in practice. When you identify a weakness, seek a means of growth. This may include education, directed experience, or discussion with colleagues. Be ready to acknowledge your limitations to supervisors, and do not accept responsibilities for which you are not prepared. For example, the nurse who has not worked in pediatrics for 10 years and accepts an assignment to a pediatric unit without orientation and education is setting the stage for an error to occur. The standard of care does not change for an inexperienced nurse (Killion & Dempski, 2000). As a professional, do not accept a position if you cannot meet the criterion of being a reasonably prudent nurse in that setting. In instances of true emergency (eg, disaster or flood), courts may be more lenient, but "we need you here today" is not an emergency.

Adapting Proposed Assignments

As discussed previously, nurses may find themselves assigned to units where they have little or no experience with the types of patient problems they will encounter. It is reasonable to be assigned to assist an overworked nurse in a special area if you can assume duties that are within your own competence and allow the specialized nurse to assume the specialized duties. It is not reasonable or safe for you to be expected to assume the specialized duties. Thus, if you were not prepared for coronary care, you might go to that unit, monitor the IV lines, take vital signs, and make observations to report to the experienced coronary care nurse; the experienced nurse then would be able to check the monitors, administer the specialized medications, and make decisions. Note that this does fragment the patient's care, and it would not be appropriate as a permanent solution, but could alleviate a temporary problem in a safe manner.

Following Policies, Procedures, and Protocols

It is your responsibility to be aware of the policies, procedures, and protocols of the institution that employs you. If they are sound, they can be an adequate defense against a claim, providing they were carefully followed. In all circumstances, avoid short-cuts and "work arounds."

For example, the medication procedure may involve checking all medications against an MAR. If you do this and there is an error in the MAR, you might not be liable for the resulting medication error because you followed all appropriate procedures and acted responsibly. The liability would rest with the person who made the error in transcribing the medication from the physician's orders to the MAR. If, however, you had not followed procedure in checking, you might also be liable because you did not do your part in preventing error. As discussed previously, policies are often designed to provide legal direction.

Changing Policies, Procedures, and Protocols

As nursing evolves, changes are needed in policies, procedures, and protocols. Part of your responsibility as a professional is to work toward keeping these up to date. Are there written policies to deal with emergency situations? Statements such as, "Oh, we've always done it this way" are not adequate substitutes for clearly written, officially accepted policies. Often facilities that are reluctant to make changes based on the suggestions of individual nurses are much more receptive to new ideas when the legal implications of outmoded practice are noted. References such as the guidelines produced by the Agency for Healthcare Research and Quality and articles with research results may provide strong support for needed changes in practice.

Documentation

Nurses' records are unique in the health care setting. They cover the entire period of hospitalization or long-term care, 24 hours a day, in a sequential pattern. Your record can be the crucial factor in avoiding litigation. Documentation in the record of observations made, decisions reached, actions taken, and the evaluation of the patient's response are considered much more solid evidence than verbal testimony, which depends on one's memory.

Because each case is determined by the facts as well as by the applicable law, clear documentation of all relevant data is important. For legal purposes, observations and actions that are not recorded may be assumed not to have occurred. Documentation needs to be factual, legible, and clearly understandable. Only use approved abbreviations. Make sure narrative notes have clear statements and correct errors according to the policy of the facility. Liquid erasing fluid, erasures, and heavy crossing out may be interpreted as attempted fraud in record keeping. Avoid any statement that implies negligence on the part of any health care provider. Nurses should be aware that their notes protect not only themselves but often other members of the health care team and the facility.

Properly kept records also may protect you from becoming liable for the error of another, by demonstrating that you did everything in your power to prevent harm, including consulting with others. These records might include a complete log of telephone calls to a physician and consultation with any relevant supervisor. Documentation should support that you followed all relevant policies and procedures when an emergency occurred. Although it is easy to become impatient with the time required by paper work and record keeping, complete and clear documentation is often the basis of a successful defense against a claim of malpractice.

One concern about problem-oriented records and charting "by exception" is that these formats may provide less-detailed information and may be less helpful in defense against litigation. This does not have to be the case. You can use any system of charting and record keeping to create appropriate and adequate documentation of care. If you identify something that needs to be recorded and cannot find a provision within your system to make that recording, you can be sure that others have experienced the same difficulty. You might begin making inquiries toward establishing a clear mechanism for the record keeping that concerns you. When nurses serve on committees to review and plan charting procedures, it is wise for them to seek consultation with the attorney for the facility. This helps to ensure that the plan for record keeping is legally sound as well as professionally useful.

ELEMENTS OF A LEGAL ACTION

Any legal action begins with the process of discovery, and then may be dropped, settled out of court, or settled by trial.

Discovery

In a civil lawsuit (one between parties for the recovery of damages), a lengthy discovery process leads up to the trial. **Discovery** involves gathering information through documents (such as previous medical records and results of mental and physical examinations), interrogatories (written questions answered under oath), and depositions (Brooke, 2006d). **Testimony** refers to an individual's verbal or written account of a situation.

A **deposition** is a formal proceeding in which each attorney has an opportunity to question a witness outside of court, and a sworn verbatim record is made by a court reporter. On occasion, the deposition may be videotaped (Killion & Dempski, 2000). Depositions in health care cases are often held in attorneys' offices or in the health care facility for the convenience of the witnesses. Sometimes depositions are taken to preserve the testimony of a witness for trial and are used in place of live testimony at trial. Most depositions in which you would participate, however, would be depositions for discovery purposes. The same guidelines that apply to testifying in court apply to giving a deposition.

Settlement Out of Court

Often cases are settled before trial because of information obtained during the discovery process. The person bringing suit may be persuaded that no malpractice occurred or that it cannot be proved, and may drop the suit. On the other hand, the persons or institutions being sued (or their insurance companies) may determine that it is in their best interests to avoid a trial and agree to pay damages; this is often done without admitting that malpractice occurred. A settlement may require that no party to the settlement reveal its terms to others. Often the cost in time and money to defend a malpractice case exceeds the cost of a settlement. However, any settlement must be reported to the National Practitioner Data Bank. This has made many health care professionals reluctant to settle a legal action for reasons of finances and convenience; however, the insurance company may have the authority to settle the case (Brooke, 2006d). Consult your policy to determine whether you would have a voice in determining any settlement.

Trials

A trial is a legal proceeding that takes place in a courtroom and is presided over by a judge. Some trials are settled before the judge (or panel of judges) alone, and others also have a jury present. In most instances, a trial is a public hearing, and anyone can attend and listen to the proceedings. The various witnesses may appear in person or, when agreed to by both sides, a deposition may be accepted in place of in-person testimony. The judge has full authority over all that takes place in the courtroom.

The **plaintiff** is the individual bringing suit. The **defendants** are all those being named in the suit. Each side presents its witnesses, who are examined (questioned) by the attorney. The attorney for the other side then is able to cross-examine (question) that witness about any of the information presented. The final decision is made by a vote of the jury meeting privately or by the judge, who considers all the information and makes a ruling. Monetary awards may be made at the time of the decision or may be established by further deliberation.

THE NURSE AS WITNESS

In the course of your practice as an RN, a time may come when you are asked to serve as a witness in a legal proceeding. Several kinds of cases may involve the nurse as a witness to fact or as an expert witness. When you become involved in any legal action, be sure that you understand both your rights and your obligations in regard to legal action. Always consult an attorney before talking to anyone about a matter in which you have been asked to testify, especially a malpractice action (Display 8-5).

The Nurse as Witness to Fact

A **witness to fact** is an individual who has firsthand knowledge of the specific situation that forms the basis of the legal action. A witness to fact testifies to the exact situation and circumstances of the event or events in question. For example, a nurse might be asked to testify as a witness to fact when a person was injured (for example, in an automobile accident) and you or your

---

Display 8-5   Guidelines for Testifying

- Listen carefully to the entire question before answering and pause to let your attorney object if appropriate.
- Answer only the questions asked and frame your answer in your mind before beginning to speak.
- Do not volunteer additional information.
- Admit if you do not remember.
- Refer to your written documentation to support your answers.
- Be brief and direct.
- Do not use medical or technical terminology unless essential—then explain your terms.
- Explain when a simple yes or no would be misleading.
- Note differences between hypothetical cases presented and the one under consideration.

organization were involved in the care of that person. Your testimony in such a case might be on behalf of the injured person, to help describe the injuries and the care received for those injuries. For example, you may be asked to testify regarding the care given in a burn center to a victim of an electrical accident who received considerable nursing care during the recovery period.

Another situation involving the nurse as a witness to fact is one in which a patient brings a lawsuit against persons or organizations who have provided health care that the patient believes was below the standard of the community. Medical malpractice is alleged in such a situation. For example, the nurse may have to give evidence regarding medical record notes or care given to the patient in the days before the alleged malpractice occurred. Sometimes a nurse is asked to provide information regarding the usual practices of the unit staff.

In both of these situations, the nurse's concern is with the specific factual details of a particular case. Nurses will testify only to what they have observed or done, not to hearsay. When nurses are asked to testify as to the facts of a situation, they sometimes believe that because they have done nothing wrong they do not need legal counsel. The law is complex, and you could jeopardize the position of an institution for which you work, or even jeopardize yourself and your professional future, with unwise statements. The person who is bringing suit may alter or amend the original complaint to involve new defendants, including you. If you have liability insurance, advise your insurance company of your role as a witness, and an attorney will be assigned to talk with you. If you are covered by an employer's policy, consult with the appropriate administrative representative immediately to obtain legal counsel. This attorney should assist you in understanding the questions in the case, your role, and how you can protect yourself in the situation (Fig. 8-4).

Every witness, is required to swear (take an oath) or affirm to tell the entire truth. Failure to tell the entire truth is **perjury**, which is a crime. As a witness, you are expected to answer the questions asked of you to the best of your ability; however, you do not have to provide an answer that would incriminate yourself, nor do you have to answer a question for which you do not

FIGURE 8-4 When testifying in court you should answer only the questions asked. Do not introduce other information.

remember or know the answer. It is perfectly permissible to state, "I do not remember" or "I do not know" if you do not.

It is helpful to use words and terms that can be understood by those who are not familiar with medical terminology, or to explain medical terminology when its use is essential. If hypothetical situations or cases are presented for your response, be sure to note the differences between the hypothetical case and the one currently under consideration before you respond.

Be brief and direct when answering questions. Answer the question asked of you. In clinical practice, nurses often use rephrasing techniques to gain information from clients. This should not be done when giving testimony (Shinn & Curtin, 2001). Do not volunteer additional information that has not been asked for by the attorney. You may open up entire areas of inquiry that would not be considered without your comments. It is the attorney's job to ask the questions to bring out the facts to which he or she wants you to testify. The opposing attorney will have an opportunity during cross-examination to ask you additional questions that the attorney believes are necessary for the facts of the case. However, be cautious about simply answering "yes" or "no." In some instances, an explanation is essential; a simple answer may sound as if you did not perform appropriately (Guido, 2001).

The Nurse as Expert Witness

A nurse also may be involved in a lawsuit as an expert witness. An **expert witness**, under Rule 702 of the Federal Rules of Evidence (accepted in the federal courts and many state courts), is defined as "a witness qualified as an expert by knowledge, skill, experience, training, or education who may testify in the form of an opinion or otherwise." An expert nurse witness may have long experience in a particular area of practice, be certified in the area, possess higher education in the area being considered, or have other evidence of special expertise. For example, in a case involving a patient's care in a critical care unit, the expert nurse witness may be certified in critical care, have a master's degree with a focus in critical care, and have worked in high-intensity critical care for 20 years.

The purpose of testimony as an expert witness is to provide information and opinion that can be used by the judge or jury to understand complex areas of care and make a decision. A nurse may provide a professional opinion, related to his or her area of expertise, on the appropriate care for a given situation. The expert witness may review the record and give an opinion as to what that record states and the meaning of the data found there.

Key Concepts

- Law includes those rules of conduct or action recognized as binding or enforced by government.
- Statutory law includes all written laws and government codes.
- Constitutional law, which has the greatest authority in any jurisdiction, is found in the U.S. Constitution and in state constitutions.
- Enacted law includes those laws passed by legislative bodies.
- Regulatory law, also referred to as administrative or executive law, includes those rules and regulations established by administrative bodies within the government.
- Common law includes judicial law, also referred to as case law, and common usage or custom.
- Civil law encompasses those laws regulating private conduct between individuals.

- Criminal law regulates actions having to do with the safety of the community as a whole.
- Violations of criminal law are considered crimes, whereas violations of civil law are considered torts.
- Legal rights are derived from constitutional guarantees and carry with them responsibilities. Other rights are ethically determined, and while not supportable by law, do govern the behavior of health care professionals.
- Malpractice actions brought against health care workers involve civil law. Nurses may be involved in cases related to intentional torts, negligence, or malpractice.
- The individual who is negligent or has committed malpractice is legally liable for the effects of that action. This means there is an obligation to the individual wronged.
- Liability may be focused on the individual, supervisor, or employer.
- Liability insurance may be purchased that transfers the cost of being sued and the cost of any settlement from the individual to a large group.
- A number of legal issues recur in nursing. Among these are the duty to report or seek medical care for a patient, protection of the patient's confidentiality and right to privacy, defamation of character, privileged information, issues related to informed consent, medication administration, and issues related to different types of emergency care.
- There are many legal issues surrounding consent by the patient or by a substitutionary decision maker. These include the provision of advance directives (orders to the physician), such as living wills, durable power of attorney for health care, and physician orders for life-sustaining treatments.
- Nurses also can be involved in criminal cases related to fraud, assault and battery, and false imprisonment. In some cases, however, a civil suit may be brought against a nurse for these issues and they may not be prosecuted as crimes.
- Many factors contribute to malpractice claims. These include seriousness of the error, social factors, characteristics of suit-prone patients, and characteristics of suit-prone nurses.
- A nurse can do many things to prevent malpractice claims. Being aware of your own practice, accepting only those assignments for which you are prepared, following policies and procedures, and properly documenting care are among the most important.
- A legal action may include a process of discovery, dropping the action, settlement out of court, or a trial.
- Nurses may be called as witnesses in trials because of personal knowledge of the case (witness to fact) or because of their expertise in a particular area (expert witness). You must understand both your rights and your obligations regarding legal action before giving a deposition or testimony.

Relevant Web Sites

Aging With Dignity: *www.agingwithdignity.org/5wishes.html*
National Council of State Boards of Nursing: *www.ncsbn.org*
Physician Orders for Life-Sustaining Treatments (POLST): *www.ohsu.edu/ethics/polst*
St. Louis University and the American Society of Law, Medicine, and Ethics:
   www.painandthelaw.org
University of Texas Medical Branch, Center for Nursing Ethics, Law, and Policy:
   www.son.utmb.edu/nursing/ethicslp/
Note: Official state Web sites with statutes are available in some jurisdictions.

References

Anonymous. (1997). Court case: A failure to communicate. *Nursing97, 27*(2), 32.

Bernzweig, E. P. (1996). *The nurse's liability for malpractice* (6th ed.). St. Louis, MO: Mosby–Year Book.

Brooke, P. S. (2006a). Legal Questions: Telephone orders: Risky chain of command. *Nursing, 36*(2), 67.

Brooke, P. S. (2006b). Legal Questions: Occurrence versus claims-made policy. *Nursing, 36*(3), 12.

Brooke, P. S. (2006c). Legal Questions: Slapping a patient: Strike one, you're out. *Nursing, 36*(7), 29.

Brooke, P. S. (2006d). So you've been named in a lawsuit. *Nursing, 36*(7), 44–48.

Curtin, L. (1997). When negligence becomes homicide. *Nursing Management, 28*(7), 7–8.

Fiesta, J. (1994). *The law and liability* (2nd ed.). New York: John Wiley & Sons.

Fiesta, J. (1998). Law for the nurse manager: Legal aspects of medication administration. *Nursing Management, 29*(1), 22–23.

Fiesta, J. (1999). Do no harm: When caregivers violate our golden rule, part 2. *Nursing Management, 30*(9), 10.

Furrow, B. R. (2001). Pain and the law. *Journal of Law, Medicine, & Ethics, 29*, 28–51 [On-line]. *www.painandthelaw.org/aslme_content/29-1/furrow.pdf.* Accessed August 18, 2002.

Guido, G. W. (2001). *Legal and ethical issues in nursing.* Upper Saddle River, NJ: Prentice Hall.

Hall, J. K. (1996). *Nursing ethics and law.* Philadelphia: WB Saunders.

Hattis, P. A., Staton, S., & Walton, J. (2004). *Understanding Charitable Immunity Legislation: A Volunteers in Health Care Guide.* Pawtucket, RI: Volunteers in Health Care.

Institute of Medicine. (2000). *To err is human: Building a safe health care system.* [On-line]. *http://books.nap.edu/books/0309068371/html/index.html.* Accessed January 22, 2003.

Institute of Medicine. (2006, July). *Preventing Medication Errors: Report Brief.* [On-line]. *www.ismp.org.* Accessed September 2, 2006.

Judson, S., & Hicks, S. (1999). *Law and ethics for medical careers* (2nd ed.). Columbus, OH: Glencoe.

Kihm, N. C. (1999). My hospital will cover me. *The Washington Nurse, 29*(4), 32–33.

Killion, S. W., & Dempski, K. M. (2000). *Legal and ethical issues.* Thorofare, NJ: Slack, Inc.

'Lectric Law Library. (2006). *Gross negligence.* [On-line]. *www.lectlaw.com/def/g020.htm.* Accessed September 24, 2006.

National Conference of State Legislatures. (2006). *State laws on heart attacks, cardiac arrest & defibrillators.* [On-line]. *www.ncsl.org/programs/health/aed.htm.* Accessed September 23, 2006.

Needleman, J., Buerhaus, P., Mattke, S., Stewart, M., & Zelevinsky, K. (2002). Nurse staffing levels and the quality of care in hospitals. *New England Journal of Medicine, 346*(22), 1715–1722.

Non-Profit Coordinating Committee of New York. (1998). Volunteer Protection Act of 1997. [On-line]. *www.npccny.org/info/gti2.htm.* Accessed September 23, 2006.

Physician Orders for Life-Sustaining Treatments. (2005). *POLST is about choices, your choices.* [On-line]. *www.ohsu.edu/ethics/polst.* Accessed September 24, 2006.

Search and Rescue Society of British Columbia. (1995). *The risk of rescue: The plight of the Good Samaritan.* [On-line]. *www.islandnet.com/sarbc/sarbc/goodsam.html.* Accessed September 23, 2006.

Shinn, L. J., & Curtin, L. L. (2001). *What to do if you are sued. In The ANA nursing risk management series I: An overview of risk management.* (pp. 13–31). [On-line]. *http://nursingworld.org/mods/mod310/cerm1ful.htm.* Accessed November 13, 2005.

9

Ethical Concerns in Nursing Practice

LEARNING OUTCOMES

After completing this chapter, you should be able to:

1. Discuss the concepts of ethics and morality and their application in the health care field.
2. Describe four ethical theories that may be used to guide ethical decision making and give an example of each applied to a nursing situation.
3. Explain how personal religious and philosophic viewpoints, the Codes for Nurses, and documents addressing patients' rights are used as a basis for ethical decision making.
4. Analyze ways in which sociocultural and occupational factors affect ethical decision making for nurses.
5. Outline a framework for ethical decision making.
6. Discuss how ethics relate to commitment to the patient, commitment to personal excellence, and commitment to nursing as a profession.
7. Analyze how ethics affect specific work situations, such as your obligations related to a chemically impaired nursing colleague.
8. Discuss the importance of recognizing and adhering to boundaries with clients.

KEY TERMS

Autonomy	Ethical dilemma	Right
Beneficence	Ethics	Standard of best interest
Boundary violations	Fidelity	Theory of social justice
Chemically impaired professional	Futile	Utilitarianism
	Justice	Values
Code of ethics	Morals	Values clarification
Cultural relativism	Moral distress	Values conflict
Deontology	Nonmaleficence	Veracity
Distributive justice	Paternalism	Whistleblowing

Have you ever been nearby when a physician discussed with a patient's family whether to start an elderly comatose patient on a series of antibiotics to treat possible pneumonia? Or have you been present at a nurses' conference while attendees discussed an order to stop enteral therapy on a patient who has shown no response to stimuli? Or perhaps you have observed a staff nurse leaving the unit after completing the shift with a pocket full of pens, bandaids, and tape. These are examples of situations that involve moral and ethical judgments—judgments as to what is right, what is wrong, and what one ought to do in a given situation.

In nursing today, it is impossible to escape situations that call for judgments requiring serious consideration of what is right or best for our clients, their families, and the community. Although some of these decisions can be based on the clinical knowledge that you have been developing, many will require additional expertise in the realm of ethical and moral decision making.

Fortunately, there are guiding principles to assist us in the process. As you work at the process of applying critical thinking to your ethical nursing decisions, look seriously at the assumptions that have been made. Assumptions are often based on ethical and moral values. All of these are good reasons why, as nurses, we need knowledge of ethics, morality, and the process of ethical decision making.

It is not possible in this text to explore the topic of ethics in depth; however, we provide an overview of the topic in this chapter. To assist you in understanding some of the terminology used in the discussion of ethics (and as a point of reference), we have provided a list of definitions in Table 9-1. Some of these terms are fully explained in the text of this chapter; others are not. We discuss some of the approaches to ethical decision making and give examples of its application in health care. We also provide some direct application to your performance as a nurse and to personal decision making. As you read about ethical issues and conflicts, and discuss them in your classroom or with a classmate, respect others by listening carefully to what they have to say and honestly attempting to understand their positions and their accompanying values and beliefs. Only by considering all aspects of an issue can we seek and find understanding for ourselves.

UNDERSTANDING THE CONCEPT OF ETHICS

Since the time of Socrates and the Golden Age of Greece, philosophers have attempted to provide a logical approach to the questions of human conduct that arise in our lives. Why do we act the way we do? What constitutes good and evil, ethical and unethical? What are the factors that result in various cultures embracing different values? How are we to be guided in our decision making? How will the ethics of care affect our professional performance? We continue to search for answers to these questions.

When we talk about **morals**, we are referring to the basic standards for what we consider right and wrong. If we are of good moral character, we would not steal from a neighbor or cheat on an examination. This word, derived from the Latin *mores*, means custom or habit. Morals or standards typically are based on religious beliefs, social influences (including education), group norms, culture, and life experiences.

In the formal sense, **ethics** is a branch of philosophy (the study of beliefs and assumptions) referred to as moral philosophy. The word *ethics* is derived from the Greek term *ethos*, which

TABLE 9-1	TERMINOLOGY RELATED TO ETHICS
TERM	**DEFINITION**
Absolutism	View that there is only one correct moral principle or code for which there are no exceptions
Altruism	Behavior motivated by concern for the well-being of others and that is intended to benefit others
Amoral	State or quality of being indifferent to morality
Categorical imperative	From Immanuel Kant's ethics, the view that for an act to be moral, it must be able to be applied to everyone
Cultural relativism	View that there is enormous variety in the mores and morals of people in different cultures and times, and no single cultural position is correct
Descriptive ethics	Focuses on what people actually do in given situations
Ethics	Specific area of study of morality that concentrates on human conduct and human values (from the Greek ethos, meaning character, habitual uses, customs)
Ethical/Moral egoism	When one considers only his or her own good or self-interest
Ethical/Moral nihilism	View that no universally valid or true moral principles exist
Ethical/Moral objectivism	View that universally valid and true moral principles exist
Ethical/Moral relativism	View that no universally valid or true moral principles exist but, rather, that all moral principles are valid relative to culture or individual choice
Ethical/Moral skepticism	View that we cannot know whether there are universally valid moral principles
Ethics of care	Focuses on those traits valued in intimate personal relationships, such as compassion, love, sympathy, and trust
Hedonism	View that good can be defined as that which is pleasurable
Meta-ethics	Deals with the extent to which moral judgments are reasonable or justifiable
Moral	Generally accepted as dealing with what is good and what is bad, what is right and what is wrong
Moral agent	Person capable of making distinctions between what is right and what is wrong
Moral philosophy	Branch of philosophy that examines beliefs and assumptions about the nature of certain human values
Moral thought	Individual cognitive evaluation of right and wrong, good and bad
Naturalism	View of moral judgment that regards ethics as dependent on human nature and psychology
Normative ethics	Examines individual rights and obligations as well as common good
Philosophy	Intense and critical examination of beliefs and assumptions (from the Greek words philia, meaning love or friendship, and sophia, meaning wisdom)
Practical ethics	Use of ethical theory and analysis to examine commonly occurring moral problems
Situational ethics	View that one's actions are governed entirely by the situation rather than by principles or rules
Subjectivism	View that moral principles are applicable to the agent alone, that what is right for one might not be right for another
Virtue ethics	Places emphasis on the agents or people who make choices and take actions

means customs, habitual usage, conduct, and character. Ethics offers a formal process for answering the question about what one ought to do in a given situation. Understanding some of the basic ethical principles and guidelines assists us in making logical and consistent decisions. It helps us identify the motives for action and define relationships between human beings.

As we work at sorting out those behaviors that we typically describe as good, right, desirable, honorable, fitting, or proper (or the direct opposite), we also are dealing with values. Perceptions are based on **values**, and each of us (and each society) has a differing set of values. Videbeck (2006, p. 89) states, " . . . values are abstract standards that give a person a sense of what is right and wrong and establish a code of conduct for living." Some examples could include the values seen in hard work, honesty, sincerity, genuineness, and being clean. Values are most commonly derived from societal norms, religion, and family orientation, and they provide the framework for making decisions about the actions we take every day. For example, if you were born in the United States, you may have been raised to believe it is unethical to restrict women's right to vote. Those in other societies may have been raised to believe that this is the ethical (and logical) way to structure public life.

We all have been in a situation in which we experienced a **values conflict**. This occurs when we must choose between two things, both of which are important to us. For example, if you are a new mother, you probably value caring for your child on a full-time basis; however, if you also must help provide support for the family and your values support the concept that this is your responsibility, leaving your child to go to work results in a values conflict.

Most of the time we don't think about our values—we just accept them. We are most likely to think about them when we have a difficult decision to make, when something goes wrong, or when we find ourselves in a conflict because of differing values. In nursing, we work with a diverse patient population and therefore are exposed to a variety of values and ethical standards. The need to give conscientious care to all patients often forces us to examine our own values.

The process of becoming more conscious of and naming what one values or considers worthy is known as **values clarification**, which Videbeck (2006) outlines as a three-step process: (a) choosing the value that feels right, (b) prizing the value or cherishing it (making it one's own), and (c) acting on the value. We examine what we believe is good, bad, beautiful, worthy, meaningful, and so forth, and explore the process of determining our personal values. This increases our self-awareness or understanding of ourselves and assists us in making choices. It facilitates decision making, because we have a better grasp of our own value systems.

Having a good understanding of yourself will be helpful when you are faced with an ethical dilemma. An **ethical dilemma** occurs when an individual must choose between two unfavorable alternatives. For example, assisted suicide may provide an ethical dilemma for those having to face the situation. Although they certainly are opposed to seeing a loved one spend the last months of life in great pain and suffering, they may be equally opposed to assisting with an earlier death. Ethical dilemmas usually have no perfect solution, and those making decisions may find themselves in the position of having to defend their decisions. Although there are times when a difference in values and decisions can be accepted, there are also times when differences put people into direct conflict. Should you experience such a situation, be constructive (rather than destructive) in the methods you choose to work toward resolving the differences. Listen carefully without interrupting and be willing to hear what others have to say. Seek clarification using gentle questioning. Respect cultural differences and be attentive to body language. Explain the context of your point of view and try to picture the other person's perspective of what you are saying.

Critical Thinking Activity

Identify situations you might confront in nursing in which your personal religious or philosophic values would be involved. What would be the consequences of following the dictates of your value system? Do conflicts exist between your value system and actions required by the situation? If so, how will you recognize the differences and how will you deal with them? Are there any other alternatives? What might they be?

BASIC ETHICAL CONCEPTS

Various authors and theorists identify different concepts as basic to ethics. Those concepts that are most frequently addressed include autonomy, beneficence, nonmaleficence, justice, fidelity, and veracity. Identifying how they apply to a particular situation and balancing their competing claims often present a challenge.

Autonomy

Autonomy involves the right of self-determination or choice, independence, and freedom. It comes from the Latin *auto*, meaning "self," and *nomy*, which means "control." Some refer to autonomy as respect for the individual and include the expectations that each individual will be treated as unique and as an equal to every other individual (Davis, Aroskar, Liaschenko, & Drought, 1997). Writers may refer to it as the Principle of Individual Freedom (Thiroux & Johnson, 2006). Other words often associated with autonomy include dignity, inherent worth, self-reliance, individualism, and power.

When we consider an individual's autonomy, the way we approach a problem may result in the decision-making process becoming more time-consuming. It is closely tied to informed consent (see Chapters 8 and 10), which requires that clients be provided clear and sufficient information about their situation to make a rational decision for themselves. Giving consideration to an individual's autonomy also requires that justification be provided for why the patient is not participating in decision making, if that is the case. In today's health care delivery system, it is important to respect patients' rights to make decisions about and for themselves, even when we do not agree with those decisions (rights are discussed later in this chapter). For example, you may have difficulty supporting the decision of a new mother, who is a Jehovah's Witness and whose life is in danger because of blood loss, to refuse to have a blood transfusion.

As with most other rights, there may be restrictions on the right to choose—autonomy does not mean that individuals can do anything they want. When one person's autonomy interferes with another individual's rights, health, or well-being, limitations may be imposed. Does a patient's right to self-determination allow that individual to choose a certain expensive treatment if that choice would unjustly deny money to another person for another treatment? What if a patient demands a bone marrow transplant when the physician does not believe the outcome is a realistic chance of success? What if the patient demands the newest brand-name drug when the public clinic provides only a generic drug? Does the autonomy of a patient with a highly communicable disease take precedence over the right of the community not to be exposed to the disease? If there are to be limitations, what should they be? In what instances should the legal system interfere with personal decision making?

For some individuals, autonomy may be less important than values related to the family and community. Is this acceptable? Who decides how much autonomy is enough? Once again, we must consider the idea that autonomy is predominantly a Western value. For example, tribal life occurs under more strenuous circumstances than we normally encounter; it requires more cooperation and less variation from the norm. The individual's freedom to do things is far more limited because decisions are directed toward the common good of the community. Many cultures have deeply held values about the family, rather than the individual, as decision maker. So what happens when the family decision is not what health providers think is best for the patient?

■■ COMMUNICATION IN *ACTION*
■■

Exercising Autonomy

Joan Wagner often studied with a group of classmates as they prepared for examinations. An examination on medications and dosages was scheduled and Joan believed she would profit most from studying independently because study sessions often strayed from the content being studied. Additionally her time was very limited the evening study was planned. As the group discussed study plans Joan said, "I really appreciate the opportunity to study with you, but I believe I need to approach this material individually. I need to be sure I can independently master some of the areas related to dosage. Perhaps we can study together later for the content of our next unit." In addressing her own needs, Joan expressed autonomy.

Beneficence and Nonmaleficence

Beneficence refers to the obligation to do good, not harm, to other people. It also maintains that we should prevent evil or harm (Burkhardt & Nathaniel, 2001). Thus, the concept of beneficence extends from promoting good to **nonmaleficence** (the prohibition of intentional harm). As far back as Hippocrates, physicians were entreated to do no harm. Florence Nightingale stated that the patient should be no worse for having been nursed. The *Code for Nurses with Interpretive Statements* (ANA, 2001) addresses this issue when it clearly delineates the steps to be taken to remove harm or evil. Some examples include reporting unethical practice of a colleague to appropriate authorities or expressing concern to the individual who is engaged in practices that result in substandard practice.

In health care, we recognize that sometimes we unintentionally do harm to individuals. Nosocomial infections, adverse drug reactions, and the side effects of such treatments as irradiation and chemotherapy for cancer are certainly harmful to the individuals who experience them. In some cases, given the alternatives, a patient will opt to have the treatment (eg, irradiation) in spite of the harm that may occur. The ethical mandate is that we refrain from intentionally inflicting harm. Sometimes it is difficult to accept that a side effect of a particular treatment might result in harm to a patient. Concern for the possible although rare reaction to vaccination for pertussis (whooping cough) is but one example.

Even more problematic is the continued use of medical therapies when they are **futile**, that is, do not have the potential for creating a positive outcome but clearly have the potential for adverse outcomes. Additional chemotherapy in the patient with terminal cancer may fall into this category. Deciding when a treatment is medically futile is a physician's decision, but there are many areas of gray in which one physician might identify a treatment as futile and another suggest that there is at least some possibility of effectiveness.

Good is a general term of approval or commendation, and may be defined as that which is "of a favorable character or tendency" (Merriam-Webster, 2006). Thus, we tend to think of it as that which promotes life, development, and fulfillment. We view it as good when a friend makes a quick recovery from surgery, when a child graduates from high school or college, or when aging parents are able to take that long-awaited trip they have been planning for years.

It is sometimes difficult to decide who will determine what is good for a specific person in a specific situation. In most instances, we expect that people will make their own decisions about what is good for them. But who decides for the infant regarding procedures such as immunizations that inflict some degree of pain, but have long-lasting and positive benefits? Who decides for the individual who is unconscious or mentally incompetent?

Another problem centers on how we identify what is good. Is all life good, or are there situations in which not living is better than life? Is it better to sustain life in the face of suffering, or is it better to allow a person to die and have suffering end? If giving good care to one patient means that lesser care will be given to another (a situation encountered more frequently in today's health care environment), how can we defend such an action? What if giving good care means violating good nursing economics (ie, cost containment)? There are no simple answers, and the answers are not the same for everyone.

The issue of sanctity of life is of major concern in the health care arena. Some would argue that all life is good. Others would adamantly assert that life is not good when the quality of life is greatly diminished; this latter belief has led to serious discussions regarding euthanasia and assisted suicide, supported the establishment of such groups as the Hemlock Society, and has resulted in one state (Oregon) legally permitting assisted suicide. Many people, particularly physicians, believe that the principles of respect for the patient and relief from suffering that are the basis for approving of assisted suicide, fail to do justice to the internal values, professional integrity, and norms of medicine (Boyd, 2006). Another example of a situation in which quality-of-life issues emerge can be seen in an instance in which parents are advised that a fetus has a life-compromising condition such as meningomyelocele. The parents must weigh the quality of the life against the complications inherent in the meningomyelocele if the pregnancy is allowed to go to term. Surrounding all issues dealing with the sanctity of life are religious views and values, particularly those maintaining that all life is sacred. Certainly arguments regarding the sanctity of life play a major role in discussions regarding abortion, whether supported by religious beliefs or personal value systems. The sanctity of life also affects our personal beliefs about capital punishment.

Closely aligned to the issue of sanctity of life is the concept of medical futility. Medical futility is a term applied to situations in which interventions are judged to have no medical benefit or in which the chance for success is low (Burkhardt & Nathaniel, 2001). This concept is often applied to cardiopulmonary resuscitation and to do not resuscitate orders but also relates to situations in which a patient exists in a persistent vegetative state (see Chapter 10). The issue is further complicated by the fact that no set definition of the concept exists and that personal values affect the determination of futility. Should the decision regarding futility of treatment be different for a young child than for an elderly client? Should the cost or the effectiveness of the treatment affect the answer? Should an individual's ability to pay be considered?

Thus it can be said that although the topics of the sanctity of life and medical futility are widely discussed, there exists little consensus about them. As a nurse, you will often encounter difficult situations in the care of your patients in which opposing values play against one another. Understanding your own values, which may change over time, is important in these situations.

COMMUNICATION IN *ACTION*

A Case of Unwashed Hands

You entered the women's lounge and noticed a fellow worker also there. After using the toilet, that individual walked to the door to leave the area without first washing her hands. You said, "Hey, Judy! You must have a lot on your mind this morning. You were heading out without washing your hands before returning to work. I know you know how important proper hand washing is and would want to be reminded." Preventing harm through speaking up reflects an ethical value.

Critical Thinking Activity

Identify ways in which the concept of beneficence has shaped medical and nursing care provided to patients. Do you believe this is a concept that will have the same impact in years to come? What assumptions are you making? Are your data accurate? What are the implications for the future?

Justice

Justice, sometimes referred to as fairness, refers to the obligation to treat like cases similarly. It looks at the concepts of fairness, justice, and entitlements (Edge & Groves, 1999). We must ask, "How is fairness defined?" Does fairness mean that people should always be treated the same? In terms of access to health care, is it "just" for one person to receive more resources than another receives? If so, what makes it just, and how does that relate to the distribution of scarce medical resources? Does age make a difference in what we consider just? Should it? Does justice imply that the government should provide the resources or services individuals are unable to provide for themselves? Can we measure fairness in any objective sense? What should occur when one person's rights interfere with the rights of another? These issues will be discussed in greater detail in Chapter 10.

The concept of **distributive justice** requires the fair distribution of limited resources relative to demand (Lamont, 2003). The expectation is that all individuals have an equal opportunity to access scarce resources and requires health care organizations and health plans to provide to individual recipients the care and service each is due. This would include the frail elderly, poor, disabled, and homeless. Providers, managers, and policy makers struggle with complicated and complex rules that fail to provide guidance in difficult or ambiguous situations (Maddox, 1998).

Armstrong and Whitlock (1998) cite six criteria that are often used to define the just distribution of limited resources: need, equity, societal contribution, ability to pay, effort, and merit. The use of these criteria is controversial. Need involves known medical need, not elective procedures. Equity addresses trying to distribute equally to all in need. Contribution considers what an individual might be expected to give to society at a future date. This approach has met with concern over labeling those who are disabled or unable to contribute as less worthy and thus can be discriminated against. Ability to pay is self-explanatory, but to deny needed health services because an individual cannot pay contradicts the concepts of charitableness that exist in our society. Patient effort deals with a patient's compliance or noncompliance with medical advice. While some might find this reasonable in the case of the person who does not follow advice to quit smoking, would they also find this acceptable for the person who does not eat as prescribed or fails to engage in daily exercise? Where would the line be drawn? Merit addresses the potential that exists for benefit from the additional investment of limited health resources. Who will decide about the future potential for a current investment? These six criteria have not always provided a strong basis for decision making, and the ethical issues related to allocation of scarce resources promise to become more complex in the coming years.

Fidelity

Fidelity refers to the obligation to be faithful to the agreements, commitments, and responsibilities that one has made to oneself and others, both implicitly and explicitly. Interestingly, it is one of the ethical concepts not addressed specifically in some textbooks of nursing ethics. Fidelity is the foundation of the concept of accountability that we hear about so often in nursing today. What are the responsibilities of health care personnel to individuals, employers, the government, society, and each other? When these responsibilities conflict, which should take priority? In reality, which do take priority? Are nurses obligated to provide care to all patients? Under what circumstances, if any, might this be challenged? What are the nurse's promises to society? Would it also cover areas such as competence? Abiding by institutional policies? Operating within the profession's code of ethics?

Chaffee (2006) illustrates the conflict nurses may experience with this concept in a discussion of situations in which duties clash—as in a disaster where there is a clash between obligations to one's family (particularly if small children or elderly adults are involved) and to a professional obligation to report to work. She points out that the American Nurses Association's (ANA) *Code of Ethics for Nurses with Interpretive Statements* (2001) offers conflicting guidance: on the one hand stating that the nurse's primary commitment is to the patient and on the other that the nurse owes the same duties to self as to others. She suggests the following be considered when deciding whether to report for work in the event of a disaster: the nurse's safety, the prioritization of relationships of responsibility, the nurse's expertise, the benefits to be gained over the risks, consideration of the harm that would occur if the nurse fails to report for work, and consideration of the good that would come from reporting versus the good that would come from not reporting for work.

Another situation that often challenges us in health care is that of confidentiality. Is maintaining confidentiality one of the promises that nurses make to clients? Is maintaining confidentiality a moral/ethical issue as well as a legal issue? Are there any instances when it is acceptable to violate the principle of confidentiality? If you are working with an impaired colleague, is it appropriate and ethical to violate a confidential situation in the interest of patient well-being? We discuss this issue in detail later in the chapter.

Veracity

Veracity refers to telling the truth or not intentionally deceiving or misleading patients. From childhood, we are all admonished to tell the truth and to avoid lying. When we are children, this seems straightforward. As we become adults, we see more instances in which the choices are less clear. For example, do you tell the truth (veracity) when you know the truth will cause harm to an individual (maleficence vs. nonmaleficence)? Do you tell a lie when it would make someone less anxious and afraid? You might see this as beneficence (doing good), but then you have abandoned the principle of veracity. Edge and Groves (1999) refer to the lack of truth telling as leading to a slippery slope, because when we conceal the truth from a patient, it teaches all others involved (eg, family members, friends, nursing assistants, housekeeping staff) that health practitioners lie. This deception is later remembered, and the concept that one cannot rely on health professionals pervades. In other words, it diminishes one's esteem and reliability and erodes trust, which is an essential element of the nurse-patient relationship. Lying also diminishes oneself. Lying can change your concept of yourself as an honest person and may adversely affect future behavior if practice in lying makes it easier to lie in the future. Not all societies value telling the truth to the ill person. In some societies, such as Japan, the patient is to be protected from bad news or information that would provoke anxiety. Therefore, to lie and provide false reassurance may be considered doing good (beneficence) and avoiding harm (nonmaleficence.) When health professionals relate to families with a different view of truth telling to the ill person, their values may come in conflict.

■■■ COMMUNICATION IN *ACTION*
■■

To Tell or Not to Tell
You assessed your patient every hour because of elevated blood pressure. The fourth time you checked it during your shift, you noted that the reading was 195/105, more elevated than previously. The patient asked you, "How was the reading this time?" You replied, "This time I got a reading higher than before. I am going to check it again in 15 minutes and, in the mean time, notify your physician of my findings. I will return in just a few minutes." The choice of the nurse was to tell the truth to the patient even if it caused anxiety. The nurse also knew that the patient's anxiety may have been increased by feeling that information was being denied to him or by the uncertainty of not knowing.

🌐 ETHICAL THEORIES

It is not our intent to delve with any depth into the writings of early philosophers. However, because ethical theories are mentioned frequently in the literature that deals with bioethical issues, some background seems appropriate.

An ethical theory is a moral principle or a set of ethical concepts and moral principles that can be used to assess what is morally right or morally wrong in a given situation. Over the years, many people have called on the theories of philosophers to guide in decision making. The most widely used theories are presented in Table 9-2. You are encouraged to consider various ethical approaches and discuss with your classmates when each might be used appropriately.

An application of **utilitarianism** (or consequentialism) as seen in the health care industry would be the justification of capitation in the managed care organization (MCO). Because the MCO pays a certain amount of money per member per month to a contracted provider, the MCO would argue that it has provided the greatest good for the greatest number of members. In public life, it would illustrated by the public health department fully funding immunizations and providing only limited funding for episodic care of illness. Preventing communicable disease will benefit many more people in the community than will caring for individual illnesses.

An example of **deontology** might be applied to a situation in which all persons involved in a research study have a complete understanding (informed consent) of the study and its purposes. The participant is treated as a moral being with freedom of decision making and not simply a

TABLE 9-2	MAJOR ETHICAL THEORIES AND THEORISTS	
TITLE OF THEORY (OTHER NAMES)	**THEORIST ASSOCIATED WITH WORK**	**BASIC PRINCIPLES OF THEORY**
Natural Law (Objectivism)	St. Thomas Aquinas (1225–1274)	Actions are morally right when they are in accord with our nature and end as human beings. Good should be promoted, evil avoided, and ethics grounded in our concern for human good.
Deontology (formalistic system, the principal system of ethics, or duty-based ethics)	Immanuel Kant (1724–1804)	Ethical decision making is based on moral rules and unchanging principles (or motivations that are derived from universal values), considered separately from the consequences. The fundamental principle is called the categorical imperative, unconditional commands that must be applied similarly in all situations without exception.
Utilitarianism (often referred to as teleology, consequentialism or situation ethics, although there are some differences)	Jeremy Bentham (1748–1832) and John Stuart Mill (1806–1873)	An act is right when it is useful in bringing about a desirable or good end. A second principle allows the end to justify the means. Fits well into Western society's values regarding work ethic and the behavioristic approach to education, philosophy, and life. Applicable to research.
Social Equity and Justice	John Rawls (1921–2002)	Sets forth principles of justice developed in 1971. Allows social and economic positions to be to everyone's advantage and open to all. Introduces a "veil of ignorance" whereby persons making choices would not have any specific information regarding those involved thus choosing the alternative that supported the most disadvantaged person. Supports justice and equal rights for everyone.
Ideal Observer	Raymond W. Firth (1901–2002)	Requires that decisions be made from a dispassionate, disinterested, and consistent viewpoint with full information about the situation and the consequences available.

means to an end. The individual participant who has a bad result might be immediately dropped from the study because the well-being of the individual participant is considered more important than the study itself.

In applying Rawls' (1971) **theory of social justice**, one could not ethically justify using income inequalities or the ability to pay to determine a patient's eligibility for access to health care. According to social justice the most disadvantaged person should receive the preferential benefit.

Critical Thinking Activity

Of the ethical theories provided in this chapter, select the one that is of greatest interest to you and describe the aspects of the theory that make it most attractive. Examine factors that bring you to this point of view. What are your biases? What are the consequences of supporting this ethical theory on your professional practice?

APPLYING BASIC CONCEPTS

The basic ethical concepts discussed so far have many applications to the way we live our daily lives and how we interact with others, as well as how we perform as professional nurses. A major application of these concepts is seen in how we view the rights of an individual, a concept tied to the concept of autonomy.

Rights

The discussion of ethical concepts is founded on the belief that people are entitled to certain rights or privileges. Typically, we think of a **right** as a just claim or entitlement, or as something that is owed to an individual on a legal, moral, or ethical basis. Most rights are based in the concept of autonomy of the individual. In common usage, this is often extended to include privileges, concessions, and freedoms. Rights are associated with many different areas of our lives. We tend to think of ourselves as having civil and political rights such as the right to assembly, to vote, to own property, and to speak freely. We have economic, social, and cultural rights, such as the right to health care, the right to education, and the right to work. Rights form the basis of most professional codes and legal judgments (see Chapter 8 for more discussion of rights as used in the legal sense). Legal rights include the right to due process and trial. And we have personal rights, such as the right of an individual to self-determination and privacy. Problems occur when one individual's rights come in conflict with the values of others. For example, if a patient is admitted to a hospital and refuses treatment, and there is a strong indication that the patient could recover, should the physicians and nurses respect the patient's right to self-determination? The conflict of rights provides us with many challenges and dilemmas. Although it is not within the confines of this text to discuss all of the circumstances, consider some of the major areas in which you may deal with rights in your role as a nurse.

Right to Self-Determination

Federal legislation has been passed to ensure that individual rights are respected. The Patient Self-Determination Act, also known as the Danforth amendment, is discussed in Chapters 8 and 10. This act was created because of our society's fundamental belief in the individual's right to decide. However, this act does little to recognize cultural diversity and sensibility to groups such as Chinese-Americans, who have a unique set of values and well-defined role relationships, in which the role of family in making health care decisions is strongly valued.

Rights and Cultural Relativism

Although the concept of rights is almost taken for granted in our Western culture, there are some who suggest that the validity of all moral judgments is culturally relative. **Cultural relativism** is the principle that what an individual believes and does make sense in terms of his or her own culture. Cultural relativism embraces the notion that groups and individuals hold different sets of values that must be respected. The principle was made popular by anthropologists who wanted to compare and contrast a wide range of cultures in a systematic and even-handed manner. It gained greater popularity when the Commission of Human Rights of the United Nations began preparing the Universal Declaration of Human Rights. The Commission struggled to formulate a statement of human rights that would take into account the individual as a member of a social group of which he or she was a part.

Those of us raised in the Western culture have difficulty imagining the prospect of performing as a suicide bomber, as witnessed in news broadcasts from the Mideast where such behaviors are viewed as heroic by some groups. This is also an interesting concept to consider in relationship to health care practices with which we, in the Western culture, have great difficulty accepting, such as female circumcision. Although it is appalling to us, in some non-Western cultures, concerns about virginity, ability to attract a husband, the husband's sexual pleasure, and religious beliefs dictate that female children be circumcised. Such beliefs challenge our comprehension of others' values.

Rights of the Unborn

There are many times when we grapple with whose rights should be respected. The most obvious example of this situation occurs when we consider the rights of the unborn to life versus the right of the mother to make choices regarding her own body. This issue is one that has continued to divide members of our society and is often an issue brought forth when candidates run for election or when appointments are made to the Supreme Court. The concern becomes even more contradictory, paradoxical, and convoluted when we consider that some states will permit a late-term abortion; however, in that same state, if an automobile accident occurs in which a pregnant woman is killed (thus also killing the fetus she is carrying), the offending driver can be charged with two cases of manslaughter—both the mother and the unborn child.

Right to Privacy and Right of Confidentiality

An area receiving much attention today is that of the rights of the patient to privacy and the confidentiality of medical information. Privacy may be thought of as the right to be left alone or free from intrusion. It also includes the right to select desired care based on personal values and beliefs and to have control over how sensitive information is shared.

Confidentiality deals with not sharing information. This has surfaced as a major concern, because sensitive health records are now computerized and can be e-mailed, telecommunicated, faxed, or copied to various individuals or groups who may have an interest in the information. This information, which could include individually identifiable health data, might be readily available to anyone who walks by a fax machine or logs on to a computer. People are concerned that exposure to personal health information, especially that related to genetic tests or communicable illnesses such as sexually transmitted diseases or HIV, could result in loss of or denial of health insurance, or could result in embarrassment or discrimination in the work environment.

In 1996, Congress passed legislation in the Health Insurance Portability and Accountability Act. It required that steps be taken or legislation passed to ensure the privacy of individually identifiable health information.

The ANA has been concerned about this issue for some time. In 1995, the ANA's House of Delegates approved a policy called "Privacy and Confidentiality Related to Access to Electronic Data." In 1998, its Board of Directors endorsed the "Core Principles of Telehealth," intended to regulate telecommunication technologies used to provide long-distance care, education, and patient data. In 1999, it developed a position statement, *Privacy and Confidentiality*, which, at this writing, is pending review and update. In addition to maintaining a patient's right to privacy with respect to individually identifiable health information, it supports patients' right to access their own health information and to supplement such information to correct any discrepancies they may perceive. The organization continues to work with other national groups on the issue of privacy and confidentiality. The ANA *Code of Ethics for Nurses with Interpretive Statements* (2001) and the International Council of Nurses Code of Ethics for Nurses (2006) both address the issue of patient confidentiality. As a student and future nurse, remain ever mindful of your responsibility to maintain patient privacy and confidentiality in all matters.

The Standard of Best Interest

When a decision must be made about a patient's health care and the patient is unable to make an informed decision, the decision may be made based on the **standard of best interest**. As the name implies, it is based on what the health care providers or family believes is best for that individual, taking into account tangible factors such as how the patient may be harmed, how the patient may benefit, and any physical and fiscal risks. This is an application of the concepts of beneficence and nonmaleficence. Such decisions may be based on the individual's expressed wishes and preferences as noted in verbal statements, or by written documents such as living wills if they are available. Health care professionals strive to avoid unilateral decisions made by a health care provider. Unilateral decisions often imply that the decision maker knows what is best for the patient. This is referred to as **paternalism**, or the deliberate treatment of people in a fatherly manner, especially by caring for them but not allowing them to have rights or responsibilities. In instances where parents have denied their children lifesaving care, the courts have, on occasion, overturned the parent's decision on the best-interest standard.

Ethics and Financial Compensation

Another issue receiving attention, discussion, and review is the practice of rewarding physicians (monetarily or not) for limiting care. This process was first seen in the advent of diagnosis-related groups under Medicare that established limits for payment for services (Silva, 1998). Recently, health maintenance organizations have come under fire for rewarding physicians who maintain lower costs of care or for penalizing those who do not. What impact might this have on nurses who are involved in the care of clients perceived to be receiving less than adequate treatment? How does this affect the nurse's obligation to serve as an advocate for the patient? These and similar issues are yet to be played out in the health care environment, but certainly emphasize the importance of all nurses understanding ethics and ethical principles.

FACTORS THAT INFLUENCE ETHICAL DECISION MAKING

Ethical decisions are not made in a vacuum. Many factors influence us as we seek appropriate answers to the dilemmas that we face. As change continues, the realities and new problems confronting us today challenge yesterday's answers.

In determining their own bases for making ethical decisions, some individuals rely on formal philosophic or religious beliefs that define matters in relation to what is believed to be the truth or good or evil. Others make decisions based on personal life experiences or on the experiences of those close to them. Still others rely on professional codes of ethics to give guidance on ethical issues. In reality, ethical decision making often involves a combination of all of these factors.

In studying ethical issues, it is important for you to understand the many forces that are operating simultaneously in our society. These forces are not independent or mutually exclusive, but act and react with one another in a constantly changing milieu, causing evolutionary changes

FIGURE 9-1   Decisions made in relation to one aspect of an ethical situation will affect all other aspects of the problem.

in all segments of society (Fig. 9-1). The following is a discussion of some of the factors that affect ethical decision making in the health care environment.

Codes for Nurses

Through their professional organizations, nurses have developed some common guidelines to use in making ethical decisions. They are contained in the ANA's code for nurses, the International Council of Nurses' code for nurses, and the National Association for Practical Nurse Education and Service's (NAPNES) Standards of Practice for licensed practical/vocational nurses. Each attempts to outline the nurse's responsibilities to the patient and to the profession of nursing.

The ANA code is unique among professional codes because it addresses specific issues and does not confine itself to matters of etiquette or broad general statements. Nurses presented tentative codes in the 1920s, 1930s, and 1940s. Finally, in 1950, a **code of ethics** was adopted. It has been revised several times since then (Table 9-3). Early versions stated that a nurse had an obligation to carry out a physician's orders; later versions, however, stress the nurse's obligation to the patient. This includes protecting the patient from incompetent, unethical, or illegal practice. The nine primary provisions of the code for nurses without explanatory provisions are presented in Display 9-1. You can view the entire code, including the preface, by accessing it on the ANA Web site, *http://nursingworld.org/ethics/chcode.htm* and clicking on "View The Code Online."

The International Council of Nurses (ICN) first adopted a code in 1953, and the code has been revised and reaffirmed several times since then. The most recent revisions occurred in 2005. The preamble of this code addresses the general responsibilities of the nursing profession. Four sections follow, dealing with the more specific concerns of people, practice, the profession, and

TABLE 9-3	CHRONOLOGY OF THE DEVELOPMENT OF CODE FOR NURSES AND DISTINGUISHING CHARACTERISTICS
DATE	**CHARACTERISTICS**
1896	The Nurses' Association Alumnae of the United States and Canada identify their purposes—the first is to establish and maintain a code of ethics
1921	The National League for Nursing Education appoints an advisory Committee on Ethical Standards. Development of a statement recommended.
1923	Task of developing a Code of Ethics shifted to the American Nurses Association (ANA)
1926	"A Suggested Code" published in August issue of AJN to solicit input. Rhetorical and effusive in style; never formally adopted; discussed moral duties of the nurse and ideal of service.
1940	"A Tentative Code" published, expressing more overt concern for the profession of nursing; input sought from AJN readers.
1950	The Code for Professional Nurses unanimously adopted at ANA House of Delegates. The Code had a preamble and listed 17 provisions; several related to personal ethics of the nurse. Response solicited.
1960	Code revised to reflect social context of increasing assertiveness of nurses and increasing sense of nurse's participation in the care of patients (as opposed to subordination).
1968	Code revised. Preamble deleted and provisions reduced to 10. Omits for the first time any reference to the private behavior of the nurse.
1976	Code revised, with greater emphasis on patients participating in their care. Published with Interpretive Statements. Changed the word "patient" to "client."
1985	Code remained basically the same but Interpretive Statements revised to reflect concerns of the day— bioethics, legal language, societal discrimination, effects on the person of technological advances in medicine.
1996	ANA convened a task force to examine the Code. Task force recommended revision of both the Code and the Interpretive Statements.
1998	Revised draft of code presented to the ANA House of Delegates.
2001	Revised code adopted.

Adapted from Fowler, M. (1997).

coworkers. In addition, the ICN provides suggestions for use of its code and a chart to assist nurses in translating the standards into action. The four elements of the ICN code are presented in Display 9-2. The full document is available at the ICN Web site, *www.icn.ch/ethics.htm.*

Critical Thinking Activity

Compare and contrast the value statements found in the ANA Code of Ethics for Nurses with Interpretive Statements and the ICN Code of Ethics for Nurses. What topics are included in each? Which are not? What does the inclusion of similar topics signify to the profession of nursing? How do you account for topics that are not included in both?

Since 1941, NAPNES has set standards for nursing practice of LPNs; they were last published in 2004. These standards (presented in Display 9-3) also incorporate moral, ethical, and legal components to guide the practice of the practical nurse.

Display 9-1   Primary Provisions of the ANA Code for Nurses

1. The nurse, in all professional relationships, practices with compassion and respect for the inherent dignity, worth, and uniqueness of every individual, unrestricted by considerations of social or economic status, personal attributes, or the nature of health problems.
2. The nurse's primary commitment is to the patient, whether an individual, family, group, or community.
3. The nurse promotes, advocates for, and strives to protect the health, safety, and rights of the patient.
4. The nurse is responsible and accountable for individual nursing practice and determines the appropriate delegation of tasks consistent with the nurse's obligation to provide optimum patient care.
5. The nurse owes the same duties to self as to others, including the responsibility to preserve integrity and safety, to maintain competence, and to continue personal and professional growth.
6. The nurse participates in establishing, maintaining, and improving health care environments, and conditions of employment conducive to the provision of quality health care and consistent with the values of the profession, through individual and collective action.
7. The nurse participates in the advancement of the profession through contributions to practice, education, administration, and knowledge development.
8. The nurse collaborates with other health professionals and the public in promoting community, national, and international efforts to meet health needs.
9. The profession of nursing, as represented by associations and their members, is responsible for articulating nursing values, for maintaining the integrity of the profession and its practice, and for shaping social policy.

Source: Reprinted with permission from American Nurses Association. (2001). *Code of Ethics for Nurses with Interpretive Statements.* American Nurses Publishing, American Nurses Association, Washington, DC.

The Patient's Rights

The patient's rights, as discussed earlier, are another consideration in decision making. Ideally, we have always recognized them in some way. As early as 1959, the National League for Nursing formulated a statement regarding patient rights. For many years, however, health care professionals assumed that they knew what was best for patients and made many decisions without consulting or considering the rights of the patient. For example, a patient with a specific disease was not offered information about possible treatment alternatives, even when valid alternatives did exist. The patient's physician decided which treatment method was preferable, and that was the only one presented to the patient. This is another example of paternalism, discussed earlier in this chapter.

As the health consumer movement became more active, greater attention was paid to the rights of the patient. Today patients may expect to be informed of all alternatives for treatment and often want to participate in choosing a type of treatment, weighing the possible benefits and risks of the treatment methods presented. Many research their health problems on the Internet and come to the physician with questions about specific therapies and approaches to treatment. The law also has supported the right to informed decision making. Despite these efforts, a recent study of 1,057 audiotaped encounters during routine office visits involving 59 primary care physicians and 65 general and orthopedic surgeons found that informed decision making was often incomplete (Braddock, Edwards, Hasenberg, Laidley, & Levinson, 1999).

Display 9-2   International Council of Nurses Code for Nurses—Elements of the Code (2006)

Nurses and People

The nurse's primary responsibility is to people requiring nursing care.

In providing care, the nurse promotes an environment in which the human rights, values, customs and spiritual beliefs of the individual, family and community are respected.

The nurse ensures that the individual receives sufficient information on which to base consent for care and related treatment.

The nurse holds in confidence personal information and uses judgment in sharing this information.

The nurse shares with society the responsibility for initiating and supporting action to meet the health and social needs of the public, in particular those of vulnerable populations.

The nurse also shares responsibility to sustain and protect the natural environment from depletion, pollution, degradation and destruction.

Nurses and Practice

The nurse carries personal responsibility and accountability for nursing practice and for maintaining competence by continual learning.

The nurse maintains a standard of personal health such that the ability to provide care is not compromised.

The nurse uses judgment regarding individual competence when accepting and delegating responsibility.

The nurse at all times maintains standards of personal conduct that reflect well on the profession and enhance public confidence.

The nurse, in providing care, ensures that use of technology and scientific advances are compatible with the safety, dignity and rights of people.

Nurses and the Profession

The nurse assumes the major role in determining and implementing acceptable standards of clinical nursing practice, management, research and education.

The nurse is active in developing a core of research-based professional knowledge.

The nurse, acting through the professional organization, participates in creating and maintaining equitable social and economic working conditions in nursing.

Nurses and Co-workers

The nurse sustains a cooperative relationship with co-workers in nursing and other fields.

The nurse takes appropriate action to safeguard individuals, families and communities when their care is endangered by a co-worker or any other person.

Copyright © 2006 by ICN-International Council of Nurses, 3, Place Jean-Marteau, CH-1201 Geneva (Switzerland) ⵌ

In 1973, the American Hospital Association (AHA) published *A Patient's Bill of Rights* (AHA, 1992), which outlined the rights of the hospital patient and served as a basis for making decisions about hospitalized patients. Some criticized this document, saying it is rather innocuous because it simply reminded patients of their rights (such as privacy, confidentiality, and informed consent) but said nothing of hospitals that fail to act in accordance with these rights. The AHA revised this document in 1992 to speak more forcefully to the hospital's responsibility for providing medically indicated care and services and to emphasize the collaborative nature of

LP/VNs Provide Individual and Family-Centered Nursing Care by:

A. Utilizing appropriate knowledge, skills and abilities.

B. Utilizing principles of the nursing process in meeting specific patient needs in diversified health care settings.

C. Maintaining appropriate written documentation and utilizing effective communication skills with patients, family, significant others and members of the health team.

D. Executing principles of crisis intervention to maintain safety.

E. Providing appropriate education to patients, family, and significant others to promote health, facilitate rehabilitation and maintain wellness.

F. Serving as a patient advocate to protect patient rights.

The LP/VN Fulfills the Professional Responsibilities of the Practical/Vocational Nurse by:

A. Applying the ethical principles underlying the profession.

B. Following legal requirements.

C. Following the policies and procedures of the employing facility.

D. Cooperating and collaborating with all members of the health-care team to meet the needs of family-centered nursing care.

E. Assuming accountability for his/her nursing actions.

F. Seeking educational opportunities to improve knowledge and skills.

G. Building post-licensure skills to assure and in-crease continuing competence.

Code of Ethics
The Licensed Practical/Vocational Nurse Shall:

1. Consider as a basic obligation the conservation of life and the prevention of disease.
2. Promote and protect the physical, mental, emotional and spiritual health of the patient and his family.
3. Fulfill all duties faithfully and efficiently.
4. Function within established legal guidelines.
5. Accept personal responsibility (for his/her acts) and seek to merit the respect and confidence of all members of the health team.
6. Hold in confidence all matters coming to his/her knowledge, in the practice of his/her profession, and in no way and at no time violate this confidence.
7. Give conscientious service and charge just remuneration.
8. Learn and respect the religious and cultural beliefs of his/her patient and of all people.
9. Meet his/her obligation to the patient by keeping abreast of current trends in health care through reading and continuing education.
10. As a citizen of the United States of America, uphold the laws of the land and seek to promote legislation that will meet the health needs of its people.

Display 9-4   The Patient Care Partnership: Understanding Expectations, Rights, and Responsibilities

When you need hospital care, your doctor and the nurses and other professionals at our hospital are committed to working with you and your family to meet your health care needs. Our dedicated doctors and staff serve the community in all its ethnic, religious, and economic diversity. Our goal is for you and your family to have the same care and attention we would want for our families and ourselves.

The sections below explain some of the basics about how you can expect to be treated during your hospital stay. They also cover what we will need from you to care for you better. If you have questions at any time, please ask them. Unasked or unanswered questions can add to the stress of being in the hospital. Your comfort and confidence in your care are very important to us.

What to Expect During Your Hospital Stay

- **High quality hospital care.** Our first priority is to provide you the care you need, when you need it, with skill, compassion, and respect. Tell your caregivers if you have concerns about your care or if you have pain. You have the right to know the identity of doctors, nurses, and others involved in your care, as well as when they are students, residents, or other trainees.
- **A clean and safe environment.** Our hospital works hard to keep you safe. We use special policies and procedures to avoid mistakes in your care and keep you free from abuse or neglect. If anything unexpected and significant happens during your hospital stay, you will be told what happened, and any resulting changes in your care will be discussed with you.
- **Involvement in your care.** You and your doctor often make decisions about your care before you go to the hospital. Other times, especially in emergencies, those decisions are made during your hospital stay. When they take place, making decisions should include:
  - *Discussing your medical condition and information about medically appropriate treatment choices.* To make informed decisions with your doctor, you need to understand several things:
    - The benefits and risks of each treatment.
    - Whether it is experimental or part of a research study.
    - What you can reasonably expect from your treatment and any long-term effects it might have on your quality of life.
    - What you and your family will need to do after you leave the hospital.
    - The financial consequences of using uncovered services or out-of-network providers.
      Please tell your caregivers if you need more information about treatment choices.
  - *Discussing your treatment plan.* When you enter the hospital, you sign a general consent to treatment. In some cases, such as surgery or experimental treatment, you may be asked to confirm in writing that you understand what is planned and agree to it. This process protects your right to consent to or refuse a treatment. Your doctor will explain the medical consequences of refusing recommended treatment. It also protects your right to decide if you want to participate in a research study.
  - *Getting information from you.* Your caregivers need complete and correct information about your health and coverage so that they can make good decisions about your care. That includes:
    - Past illnesses, surgeries, or hospital stays.
    - Past allergic reactions.
    - Any medicines or diet supplements (such as vitamins and herbs) that you are taking.
    - Any network or admission requirements under your health plan.

Display 9-4   The Patient Care Partnership: Understanding Expectations, Rights, and Responsibilities (*continued*)

- *Understanding your health care goals and values.* You may have health care goals and values or spiritual beliefs that are important to your well-being. They will be taken into account as much as possible throughout your hospital stay. Make sure your doctor, your family, and your care team know your wishes.
- *Understanding who should make decisions when you cannot.* If you have signed a health care power of attorney stating who should speak for you if you become unable to make health care decisions for yourself, or a "living will" or "advance directive" that states your wishes about end-of-life care, give copies to your doctor, your family, and your care team. If you or your family need help making difficult decisions, counselors, chaplains, and others are available to help.
- **Protection of your privacy.** We respect the confidentiality of your relationship with your doctor and other caregivers, and the sensitive information about your health and health care that are part of that relationship. State and federal laws and hospital operating policies protect the privacy of your medical information. You will receive a Notice of Privacy Practices that describes the ways that we use, disclose, and safeguard patient information and that explains how you can obtain a copy of information from our records about your care.
- **Help preparing you and your family for when you leave the hospital.** Your doctor works with hospital staff and professionals in your community. You and your family also play an important role. The success of your treatment often depends on your efforts to follow medication, diet, and therapy plans. Your family may need to help care for you at home.

  You can expect us to help you identify sources of follow-up care and to let you know if our hospital has a financial interest in any referrals. As long as you agree we can share information about your care with them, we will coordinate our activities with your caregivers outside the hospital. You can also expect to receive information and, where possible, training about the self-care you will need when you go home.
- **Help with your bill and filing insurance claims.** Our staff will file claims for you with health care insurers or other programs such as Medicare and Medicaid. They will also help your doctor with needed documentation. Hospital bills and insurance coverage are often confusing. If you have questions about your bill, contact our business office. If you need help understanding your insurance coverage or health plan, start with your insurance company or health benefits manager. If you do not have health coverage, we will try to help you and your family find financial help or make other arrangements. We need your help with collecting needed information and other requirements to obtain coverage or assistance.

While you are here, you will receive more detailed notices about some of the rights you have as a hospital patient and how to exercise them. We are always interested in improving. If you have questions, comments, or concerns, please contact _____.

_____

health maintenance. In April 2003, the bill of rights was updated with a version titled, *The Patient Care Partnership*. This document outlines what patients may expect during a hospital stay and encourages patients to ask questions if they have concerns. *The Patient Care Partnership* is presented in Display 9-4.

Some groups, nurses associations among them, also have formulated statements regarding the rights of the health care consumer. In some states, the rights of the health care consumer are being formalized into legal statements.

Social and Cultural Factors

Changes in the attitudes of society as a whole profoundly influence each of its segments. For example, the changing roles of women, the shifting attitudes toward marriage and the family, and the increasing emphasis on culturally competent care have all required nurses to reexamine their personal feelings and alter their approach to providing nursing care.

Ethical concerns are the by-products of many factors at work in our society today, including the role of the individual and the family. In the health care field, this is most pointedly illustrated by the use of the terminology "health care" as opposed to "medical care." Health care suggests much greater involvement of others and places the patient in the center of the activity, whereas medical care places the physician in the key role. We see similar language being applied to "tele-health" as opposed to "telemedicine." The meaning of "consumer unit" is shifting from an individual to a whole family or even a whole community. The focus of care also has shifted from disease to prevention and wellness, even when encountering chronicity.

The size of the group being affected by ethical decisions has a bearing on the decision-making process. The smaller the group, organization, or society involved in or affected by the decision making, the easier the process of arriving at an acceptable alternative. In 1994, for example, the Oregon Health Plan limited Medicaid coverage for HIV-infected people based on the reasoning that their average life expectancy is short (Hall, 1996). It is unlikely that this decision could have been made if the state had a large population of people who were HIV-infected. The larger the group affected by a decision, the more complex it becomes and the more divergent views encountered. Many of our ethical considerations now involve our society as a whole or, in some cases, the world; therefore, solutions are difficult.

The value a society places on the individual or the family directly influences the standard of care (Fig. 9-2). In Western society, we believe in each person's right to exercise choice based on individual beliefs and conscience. We also place high value on preserving individual life; therefore, we often use tremendous resources to try to achieve additional years, months, or even days of life, for example, in the case of heart transplantation. A society that placed greater emphasis on the community good than on the individual might not choose to use resources in that way. The standard of care might aim for comfort without the use of expensive treatment modalities.

A culture's religious values and belief in an afterlife directly affect ethical issues. The Hindu belief in rebirth after death and the immutability of fate affects decisions about using health care resources. Those who believe that an outcome is predetermined by fate will not choose to commit major resources and efforts toward altering that outcome.

The population, or, more accurately, the overpopulation, of a country relative to its resources also may have a direct bearing on the value placed on life. The material resources to provide many health services may not be available. Decisions may be made to eliminate certain costly health care procedures even though they are known to be effective and desired by individuals.

Critical Thinking Activity

Identify two sociocultural factors with which you have had personal experience that could affect ethical decision making. How is your view of this different than it might have been 5 years ago? In what ways have your views remained the same? Why do you think your views have changed or remained the same? What implications does this have for the way you will view things in the future?

FIGURE 9-2   In providing care, the nurse respects the beliefs, values, and customs of the individual.

Science and Technology

Scientific advancement and technology have left us wrestling with concerns that would have been considered science fiction 50 years ago. Before the development of kidney dialysis, we accepted the fact that people with nonfunctioning kidneys would soon die. After machines that could filter body wastes were invented, a genuine dilemma arose over who would have dialysis and who would not; the number of people needing treatment far exceeded the personnel, time, and equipment available to treat them. As the technology increased the availability of equipment to treat those needing it, the ethical questions refocused on decisions to end treatment rather than on issues related to initiating treatment.

Other technology has had similar effects. The advent of machines that could artificially breathe for someone challenged the medical and legal professions to examine their definitions of life, and brought into focus problems of whether and when to turn off a ventilator. Heart and lung machines that could adequately perfuse the body while the heart was stopped for surgical procedures enabled operations to be performed that could not be considered in times past. Fetal monitors, which can be attached to women in labor, provide a continuous readout of the status of the fetus. Such monitoring has resulted in a greater number of infants delivered by cesarean section. The transplantation of organs from one individual to another has created untold ethical dilemmas. Stem cell research using embryos challenges us at a national level. Individuals with AIDS have a shortened life expectancy even with the best of health care. Should they be encouraged to participate in research that is sometimes risky in an effort to advance scientific knowledge and the possibility of future benefit to others? How far should experimentation go? Advances in science and technology continue to offer us some of the greatest challenges.

Legislation

Social change and legislation interact constantly. Legislation may follow changes in society's attitudes, converting new ideas into law. For example, a greater acceptance of infants born to single mothers has resulted in legislation that changed the wording of birth certificates and dropped the word "illegitimate." Similarly, attitudes are being challenged regarding parenting by lesbian and gay couples, either through artificial insemination or adoption. Some individuals who disagree with these actions seek legislation to prohibit them.

When social change is desired, legislation may be actively sought to require people to behave in new ways. This was true for civil rights legislation. A change in society was desired, and supporters of civil rights sought legislation as one step toward change. Recent legislative action that addresses the needs and opportunities available to the disabled has brought about changes in public policies, procedures, and even architecture.

Judicial Decisions

The judicial system provides a major avenue for debating and trying to solve ethical problems. More issues are being taken to court, and judicial decisions are used more often as the basis for determining appropriate action. As you continue to study this topic, note that we have cited landmark decisions regarding ethical issues. The process does not stop there, however. Some people may disagree with a judicial decision and continue to oppose it, appealing the decision to a higher court. Higher courts may overturn judicial decisions. Meanwhile, the questions regarding the individual's role in carrying out a judicial decision remain. For example, although the law in the past forbade abortions, some physicians believed strongly in the right of the individual to have the procedure done. These physicians were upset by the results of abortions performed by individuals who lacked the necessary education and skill to do it safely, and therefore were willing to perform abortions despite the law prohibiting the procedure. These physicians were, of course, liable to prosecution if it were discovered they were performing illegal abortions, and some were prosecuted. The issues of abortion and government funding of the procedure are still controversial. It is not likely that these issues will be resolved in a way that is satisfactory to everyone.

Funding

The financing of health care represents a major area of conflict that has ethical dimensions. The government has become increasingly involved in providing funds for health care. Some people are asking how much time, money, and energy we should allocate to health care, and how those resources should be divided. How obligated are we as a society to make some form of health care available to all? Should that care be provided to illegal immigrants who live in this country as well as to legal residents? What is it that health care can and cannot provide? Which is more important, prevention or cure? Health care includes controversial procedures as well as high-cost options, such as abortion, sterilization, transplantation, and gene therapy. This challenges the basic values of some taxpayers who do not ethically sanction these procedures and do not want their tax dollars used to fund them.

Personal Religious and Philosophic Viewpoints and Ethical Decision Making

Religious beliefs form the basis for ethical decision making for most people; however, a person who is a member of a particular religious group may not ascribe to all of the beliefs of that group.

Some individuals make their own decisions regarding each situation, which, in some cases, may not parallel the doctrines of their religious group. For example, some Muslims maintain that women should be completely separated from men and wear veils when in the presence of men. They would find any health care setting that did not respect this belief to be in conflict with their basic values. Other Muslims do not adhere to this strict interpretation of Islamic law, and believe women should wear modest clothing but need not wear veils. They would be more comfortable in most Western health care settings because they would not feel a conflict with their personal values.

Your personal viewpoint certainly will be a major factor influencing your ethical decision making. Achieving self-understanding in values is a lifelong learning task, and undoubtedly your position on various issues will change as you move through life. Values are the product of our life experiences and are influenced by family, friends, religion, culture, environment, education, and many other factors.

RECOGNIZING THE IMPACT OF PERSONAL VALUES

Nursing offers a variety of job opportunities to the new graduate, and you will want to consider your personal values when choosing a position after graduation. You certainly cannot expect to avoid all conflict or problem situations, but you will want to avoid working in an area in which conflict is constant. Before you accept a position, consider whether it has the potential to conflict with your basic beliefs. For example, if you believe that no individual should be denied life-saving techniques, you might be unhappy working in a research institution where the effects of treatment or no treatment are studied. In this situation, making your views known and refusing certain assignments after you begin employment might result in termination, because the employer may justifiably assert that you agreed to fulfill all the responsibilities of the position when you accepted employment.

Similarly, you might choose to work in an area that supports your personal value system or strong ethical commitment. For example, religious groups that saw value in the life of the dying person began the hospices for the dying in England. Their religious beliefs were and have continued to be part of their approach to care. If you strongly value your own ethnic or cultural approach to health care, you might choose to work in a health care setting where that approach is part of the philosophy.

FACTORS IN THE WORK ENVIRONMENT THAT AFFECT ETHICAL DECISION MAKING

By virtue of the positions they hold in the health care system, nurses experience special pressures as they try to make decisions. An awareness of these factors may help you as you grapple with personal problems in decision making.

Status as an Employee

Most nurses are not in independent practice, but are employed by hospitals, nursing homes, community agencies, or outpatient facilities. Pressures divide the nurse's loyalty among patient, employer, and self. You will notice that codes do not speak of responsibilities to the employer, yet, from an ethical standpoint, you have certain loyalties and obligations to the employer who pays your salary and makes decisions regarding your work. It is not unusual for an ethical decision to involve conflict between the best interests of the employer and the patient.

When discussing ethical decisions in the abstract, most people say that, of course, the patient's best interest should be the only priority. In real situations, however, the issues often are not so clearly defined. If a nurse's decision affects the employer adversely, the result may be job loss, poor references, and a severely curtailed economic and career future. For example, one physician was known to routinely require his patients to sign blank surgical permits on admission to the hospital; a staff nurse became upset with this procedure after learning that the patients often did not understand what was being planned. Eventually, she discussed the matter with the physician, pointing out that she did not believe it was ethical to require the patients to sign the blank documents, especially because they were not informed of alternative methods of treatment. The physician became angry and complained to the hospital administration, threatening to take his surgeries elsewhere. This might have created a considerable economic loss for the hospital, and, depending on the action of the hospital administrator, the nurse might have been labeled a troublemaker and discharged to placate the physician.

When nurses are consistently faced with situations such as the one described above, it is referred to as the human condition of **moral distress**. Jameton (1984, p. 6) defines moral distress as the situation that occurs "when one knows the right thing to do, but institutional constraints make it nearly impossible to pursue the right course of action." Wilkinson (1987–1988) further stated that nurses experience moral distress when they participate in actions they have judged to be morally wrong. Situations in which the patient or family make decisions that the nurse does not agree with and yet require the nurse's participation fall into this category. We will discuss this in greater depth in Chapter 11. Moral distress may be a significant factor in nurses' feelings of loss of integrity and job dissatisfaction (Nathaniel, 2002).

Collective Bargaining Contracts

Collective bargaining contracts can protect nurses in making ethical decisions. By formalizing reasons and procedures for termination of employment, and outlining grievance measures to provide a mechanism by which the individual nurse can be protected, a contract may provide greater freedom. Others believe that contracts hamper individual freedom because of the lengthy processes that are required. See Chapter 11 for more discussion of collective bargaining and grievance measures.

Collegial Relationships

An excellent climate for ethical decision making can be provided when nurses who work together support one another, share in decision making, and present a unified approach to others. All too often, such relationships are lacking in health care institutions. Nurses feel alone and are not experienced in seeking and providing support to one another. Greater effort on the part of all nurses in this area might be rewarding and is certainly long overdue. This will be discussed in greater detail in Chapter 13.

Authoritarian and Paternalistic Backgrounds

The historically authoritarian and paternalistic (sometimes also referred to as maternalistic) attitudes of physicians and hospitals often have relegated nurses, most of whom are women, to dependent and subservient roles. These role differentiations have discouraged nurses from taking independent stands on issues and continue to affect relationships in the health care field. In some settings, ethical decisions are made without the participation of nurses, yet nurses are expected to implement the decisions.

More nurses are speaking out against an approach that leaves them out of the decision-making process. Nurses today might expect a physician to discuss the possibly futile treatment of a critically ill patient with the patient, family, and nursing staff. The patient would be encouraged to express personal needs, the family's views would be included, and the nurses' input would be part of the decision-making process regarding the medical plan of care. The advent of ethics committees, in which nurses have a voice, has created a positive environment for discussions in many institutions.

Institutional Supports for Ethical Behavior

An institution or organization that recognizes the individuality of all employees and treats them with respect in regard to decisions may provide a working climate that supports ethical behavior. When nurses are respected and there is no fear of reprisal or adverse response, ethical concerns can be voiced and issues raised.

For years, many hospitals have had ethics committees composed of physicians. With a major goal of monitoring physician behavior, they acted when a physician's inappropriate behavior, such as arriving at the hospital intoxicated, was reported to them. Today the scope of ethics committees has enlarged considerably. Membership has grown, and representatives of the hospital administration, the community, and a variety of health care disciplines are being included. An ethicist may serve as a consultant or as a member of the committee. If nurses participate, their membership and attendance allow them to share in decision making.

With their expertise and experience, the members of ethics committees help individuals who must make ethical decisions to identify whether they have all the relevant information, to determine other options they have not considered, and to compare the situation with basic ethical principles and theories. Often the committee acts in an advisory capacity to medical staff members and families struggling with difficult decisions. Ethics committees also may help institutions establish policies regarding ethical concerns that tend to recur in that setting.

Consumer Involvement in Health Care

With consumer involvement in health care, nurses again may face situations in which they are expected to take action based on the conclusions of others. Many nurses may find this problematic. For example, an elderly diabetic who has gangrene of the foot may refuse amputation, saying, "If I'm going to die, I'm going to die whole." The nurse, recognizing the life-saving benefit of the amputation, may have difficulty maintaining effective communication and rapport with the patient and family because of his or her own conviction that an amputation is the best treatment. Mental health is another area in health care in which nurses may struggle. Patients may refuse to comply with the recommended treatment and, as a result, live in a homeless, psychiatrically unhealthy situation. This also is very difficult for family members.

A FRAMEWORK FOR ETHICAL DECISION MAKING

When faced with ethical decisions, most of us hope to find the right answers. Unfortunately, a right answer may not exist for everyone or every situation; such is the nature of dilemmas. However, you can proceed from a basic framework that encourages you to look beyond your first thoughts or feelings to basic issues. A great deal has been written about the decision-making process in the past two decades—more in recent years than before. Along with this, several models have been developed to assist us when ethics are involved (Curtin, 1978; Jameton, 1984; Milner, 1993; Thompson & Thompson, 1981). The steps about to be identified, gleaned from various approaches, offer a process you can use as a guide. In studying it, you will recognize a similarity to the steps of the nursing process with which you are already familiar. When patients and families must make ethical decisions, you may assist them in working through this process within the framework of their own values.

Identify and Clarify the Ethical Problem

To define the ethical concern, the situation needs to be reviewed so as to gain as clear a perception of the problem as possible. Is there something wrong? How deep does the issue go? Are there legal or institutional concerns? What is the decision to be made? If there are questions about the information, they need to be answered. Consider what ethical principles might be involved. Are those principles in conflict? Who are the relevant parties to this decision? What are their values? What is your role and relationship to the problem? Who should assume responsibility for this decision? Is this an individual's decision or is it one in which a collaborative decision must be made? Are there time constraints on making this decision? What other factors influence the decision? Once a clear picture of the problem has been achieved, more information can be gathered about the situation.

Gather Data

It is important to have as much information about the unique situation as possible. The facts of the situation make a difference in what options are possible. Remember that there is no magic pattern or formula to facts in most situations; they are screened through each person's background and experience. What clearly appears to be a true fact to one person may seem to be opinion to another or perhaps even a falsehood. Therefore, seeking other viewpoints may help everyone involved to see the situation more clearly. Who are the relevant people in the situation and what are their concerns and perspectives? Consider whether legal cases might affect decision making in this case.

Identify Options

Most ethical problems have more than one possible solution. If only one solution existed, there would be no ethical dilemma because there would be no choice. In some cases, more than one solution may be satisfactory; in others, none of the options will seem satisfactory. The more options identified, the more likely those involved will find one they can support. What is the range of actions that could be taken? What would be the anticipated outcome of those actions?

For each option, consider its impact on each person involved. Also think about the impact on society as a whole if this option were chosen. Consider the ethical theories presented and explore how each option compares with the basic principles of each theory. In this way, it might be determined that one option is basically a utilitarian approach (seeking the greatest good for the greatest number), whereas another clearly supports a deontologic position of doing one's duty. Which option does the greatest good while at the same time doing the least harm? Which option respects the rights and dignity of all persons involved? Is one approach more appropriate than another in this situation? Is this approach in keeping with your own moral and ethical position? Helping others to explore these questions (without necessarily using the terminology of formal ethical theories) requires personal involvement and interpersonal skill.

Make a Decision

At some point, a decision must be made. Patients and families, as well as care providers, may find this difficult and, in some instances, painful. However, to not make a decision is, in fact, making a decision. There will never be enough time, data, or alternatives in some situations. No matter how thorough the analysis or how carefully people weigh all competing claims, there may still be uncomfortable feelings. When dealing with these feelings, it is helpful to plan ahead to the action that will be taken. What would a respected and admired individual say? This strategy may be helpful to you as well as to patients and families.

Act and Assess

Once a course of action is chosen, it must be carried out. This may involve working with others or personally carrying out plans. Patients and families need ongoing support as they carry out their decisions. Assess the outcomes as the processes go forward. Unforeseen outcomes are common in ethical situations. Share your thoughts and concerns with others as you proceed, and continue to seek new insights into the situation.

As you assess the outcome in any particular situation, consider its relevance for a wider range of situations and concerns. Use this situation as a foundation from which to grow and develop. Ask yourself, "What have I learned from this experience that will be useful in the future?" "What would I do in another situation?" "What would I change?"

SPECIFIC ETHICAL ISSUES RELATED TO THE PROFESSION OF NURSING

Some ethical issues of concern to nurses relate specifically to the nursing profession; others relate to bioethical issues confronting all of society. In this section, we discuss the issues facing nurses through commitment to the patient, commitment to personal excellence, and commitment to the nursing profession as a whole. Bioethical issues that relate to the whole society are discussed in Chapter 10. We present a definite viewpoint regarding ethics in the nursing profession. We feel strongly about the individual nurse's responsibility for nursing practice and place high value on personal integrity in professional relationships.

Commitment to the Patient

Nursing has a strong history of being committed to the well-being of patients who need care. Both codes of ethics—from the ANA and ICN—clearly point out the nurse's obligation to fulfill this commitment. In the past, this obligation has been used to try to persuade nurses that they must not be concerned for themselves, their working conditions, their salaries, or other aspects of their employment. However, rejection of the handmaiden philosophy and the adoption of more nurse autonomy does not require rejection of a basic philosophy that nursing is focused on providing patients and their families with support for growth toward maximum health and well-being. Patients can never become the objects of nursing care, but must be approached as unique individuals who deserve concern, respect, and culturally competent care.

Commitment to Your Employer

Once you have accepted a position in a health care organization, you also have accepted the responsibilities that the position encompasses. Some of these responsibilities may be spelled out in the contract, if a formal contract exists between the employer and the employee. Others are more or less taken for granted. It is these latter responsibilities than can present problems.

Responsible Work Ethic

First, it is understood that you will arrive at work on time. When you arrive late, you obligate others to remain overtime to ensure continuous patient care. If you find yourself in an emergency situation that is going to cause you to be delayed, it is important that you notify your supervisor that you are going to be late.

Second, it is also expected that you will not abuse breaks or sick leave. When one extends a break beyond the usual time allowed, it jeopardizes the opportunity for others to have a full break. Your patients also receive less than optimum care if you are unavailable. Likewise, the fact that you have a given number of paid sick days each year does not mean that you are entitled to that many more days off. They are intended for use if you are ill. Often, it is difficult to find replacements when staff members do not report for work. This means that others must pick up additional work assignments and that the quality of care provided that day may be less than desired.

Many health care facilities operate 24 hours a day, 7 days a week. This means that there are at least two or three shifts to be covered, as well as weekends and holidays. Be prepared to take your share of weekend and holiday shifts, as well as evening and night rotations, without grumbling if this is part of the staffing pattern. Most employers have developed some system of rotation, with employees able to make requests for the time that works best for them. Some employees for whom the holiday carries less significance may prefer to work, especially if there is additional pay for those days.

If you work in an area where you have a fair amount of privacy, remember that you should not conduct personal business during your work shift. Scheduling appointments, telephoning friends or business associates, writing notes, and similar activities should occur during your break or after you have finished your shift.

When you decide to terminate your employment, it is expected that you will give appropriate notice. Please refer to Chapter 15 for further discussion regarding resignation.

Responsible Use of Supplies

Pilfering includes stealing in small amounts or stealing objects of little value. Many people who are scrupulously honest in other aspects of their lives do not recognize that taking small items from a place of employment is indeed theft. Employees often take home adhesive bandage strips, pens, and other such objects so routinely that they do not even consider whether this is right or wrong. This constant petty theft may total thousands of dollars, the cost of which must be passed on to those who pay the bills—the patients. As a leader in the care setting, the registered nurse (RN) is often in a position to communicate clearly to all employees that pilfering is unacceptable. The nurse can set an example of careful stewardship of the hospital supplies.

Sometimes removing supplies is an oversight rather than a planned action (Fig. 9-3). To make efficient use of time, nurses commonly place many small items such as alcohol wipes, extra needles, and pens in their pockets. One hospital unit found that its yearly supply budget for black pens was almost exhausted in the first 6 months of the year. The simple action of placing a basket in the lounge into which nurses dropped everything from their pockets before leaving cut the pen costs dramatically. Perhaps you can be equally creative in helping to solve such problems in your work setting.

FIGURE 9-3 Many people who are otherwise scrupulously honest do not recognize that taking small items from a place of employment is theft.

As the costs of health care soar, it is important that everyone associated with health care be mindful of the use of resources. You can help reduce costs by being judicious in your use of resources. For example, supplies that will not be used should not be taken into patient rooms, only to be discarded later. Using extra linens such as bath towels to clean up spills adds to costs. Determining that a clean glove is acceptable rather than reaching for sterile gloves reduces costs. Ensuring that all charges are processed for supplies that are used is also important. Operating equipment in a knowledgeable manner to reduce breakage or repairs is the responsibility of all workers. When all persons do their part, the cumulative effect can be significant.

Commitment to Your Colleagues

It has been suggested that a strategy to improve the nurse shortage is to improve the quality of the work environment (Bates, 2002). Many factors influence the climate of the work environment. One of the most noteworthy is our relationship with colleagues. As a new graduate, how do you affect this area?

One approach is to model those behaviors that you wish to see in others. Develop a collaborative approach. Maintain a positive attitude; respond to others in a pleasant, courteous manner; be sensitive to others; and be a positive ambassador for nursing. Be supportive of others and avoid opportunities to gossip about your colleagues and their activities. Compliment others on things they do well and provide assistance with things they are still learning. This is especially important as you become a more seasoned employee and have responsibility for helping to orient others. Give new employees time to learn skills that are new to them and to become efficient in their execution. Show care and compassion to fellow workers as well as to your clients.

Commitment to Personal Excellence

Nurses must be committed to personal excellence and assume responsibility for maintaining competence. They must be willing to engage in genuine self-evaluation in the work setting. You are

Display 9-5   Self-Evaluation Plan

Assessment of Patients
- Do I gather enough data about patients and families, including both strengths and deficits?
- Is there sufficient depth and breadth in the data I gather?
- Do I listen closely to the patient and attend to what is being said?
- Do I regularly use all available sources for information about my patients (eg, patient, family, other staff, chart, Kardex)?
- Have I recognized problems quickly so that they did not become worse through inattention?
- Do I recognize physiologic, social, and psychological problems?
- Is my assessment free of personal biases and viewpoints?
- Do I separate relevant from irrelevant data?

Planning for Patient Care
- Do I routinely seek more information on which to base decisions about patient care?
- Are my assumptions correct?
- Do I include the patient in decision making whenever possible?
- Do I consult with others on the health care team when planning?
- Are my written plans clear, concise, and reasonable to carry out?
- Do I take into account the realities of the situation when planning care?
- Are my plans for care sound and appropriate to the individual patient?
- Do I employ principles from the biologic and social sciences in planning?
- Have I considered all alternatives?

Intervention
- Is my work organized and finished on time?
- Do I maintain optimum safe working habits?
- Do I perform technical skills in an efficient and safe manner?
- Do I communicate clearly and effectively with patients, family, and staff?
- Do I use therapeutic communication techniques appropriately and effectively?
- Do I use teaching approaches appropriate to the individual patient and family?
- Do I keep accurate and complete written records?
- Do I understand and perform any administrative tasks that are my responsibility (eg, ordering supplies, planning for laboratory tests)?
- Do I make the effort to learn about new techniques and procedures?
- Do I function as a team player?
- Do I incorporate critical thinking into all of my activities?

Evaluation
- Do I routinely evaluate the effectiveness of the nursing care I give?
- Do I effectively assist in evaluation of the patient's response to medical care and to ordered therapies?
- Do I encourage the patient to participate in evaluating both the process and the outcome of care?
- Have I evaluated all aspects of care fair-mindedly?

Display 9-5   Self-Evaluation Plan (*continued*)

Personal Growth and Relationships

- Have I established a sound trust and working relationship with coworkers?
- Do I support and assist my co-workers when possible?
- Do I communicate effectively with others on the health care team?
- Do I seek answers to questions for which I have no answer?
- Have I sought opportunities for learning and personal growth?
- Is my attitude helpful and productive?
- Do I have sound working habits (eg, appearing on time, limiting coffee and lunch breaks to the correct time)?
- Is my appearance appropriate to the working environment?
- Do I use appropriate channels of communication within the institution?
- Do I handle criticism constructively?
- Do personal biases interfere with the care that I provide or my relationship with colleagues?
- Am I doing my share in overall professional activities (eg, serving on committees, assisting with development projects)?
- Am I honest with myself, being neither too harsh nor too easy on myself?
- Do I have personal values and beliefs that interfere with providing quality nursing care?

the one who is best able to identify your weaknesses and practice deficits as well as your strengths. Your careful self-evaluation is the patient's best protection against poor or inadequate care.

When we are truly honest with ourselves in the self-evaluation process, we often uncover areas we wish were not there. These weaknesses, once identified, provide the greatest opportunity for growth and improvement. It is helpful to remember one of the beauties of self-evaluation: When it is done informally, these weaknesses do not have to be shared with anyone. On the other hand, do not hesitate to ask for assistance if you think you need it.

Many institutions now include self-evaluation and the establishment of personal goals in the formal evaluation of employees. In this process, you might be asked to prepare a written self-evaluation that will be shared with your immediate supervisor and may be incorporated into your records.

So how do you proceed? One approach to self-evaluation is the use of the nursing process format. Begin with a thorough personal assessment, objectively gathering data about your own performance. After outlining areas in which you want to gather data, actually keep notes on yourself. For example, if you want to increase your efficiency in carrying out treatments, you may want to time yourself on several occasions to determine how long you are taking and whether you improved with performance.

After data have been collected, give yourself time to analyze it thoroughly. The self-assessment outline includes questions you should ask yourself (Display 9-5); however, the criteria that you use to determine whether your answers reflect the quality of performance you want to attain are not included. Those specific criteria must be individualized to the setting in which you work and the nature of your role in that setting. The breadth of data that represent excellent practice for the nurse in the emergency department differs from what would represent excellence for the nurse working in a rehabilitation setting. The degree to which a patient participates in decisions regarding care differs between the postanesthesia recovery room and the outpatient clinic. Thus, criteria specific to your work situation are needed.

Your analysis can reveal strengths, weaknesses, and areas for growth or improvement. Congratulate yourself on the strengths identified and then clearly delineate those areas in which you want to change or to improve. Identifying and stating the problems or growth needed helps you to plan more effectively, just as it has in nursing care planning.

Next establish a plan of action. The plan will be more helpful to you if it contains clearly defined goals. What is a realistic expectation? How long should it take to reach that expectation? Once the goals are set, you will be better able to plan appropriate action to meet them. You might consider such things as requesting in-service education, taking continuing education courses, consulting with colleagues, and doing independent reading and study. Some plans need to include specific things related to your daily nursing care. To do this, you may want to request assignments that provide opportunities for practice of the desired skills. Perhaps you are interested in transferring to a specialty area of care. This will involve communication with your immediate supervisor and may involve enrolling in special classes.

Implementing this plan will require you to remain focused on what you are trying to accomplish. Keeping records on your progress is often helpful. It also provides positive reinforcement when you realize that some of your goals have been met.

Periodic evaluation of your progress is necessary so that you do not become discouraged. Sometimes it is hard to identify gradual change. Any records you have kept are valuable for this purpose. You might even plan rewards for yourself for improvement that occurs. Try not to become discouraged if you do not see the improvement you desire. Remember that just as a reassessment and a new plan are often necessary in patient care planning, a revised plan also may be needed in the self-evaluation process. Keep in mind that your overall goal is personal excellence in nursing practice.

Commitment to the Nursing Profession

Commitment to the nursing profession requires that each individual nurse be concerned not only about personal performance, but also about how nursing is practiced. This involves participation in formal and informal evaluation of nursing care, dealing with poor care, and identifying the impaired nurse. Nurses always have evaluated one another in both formal and informal ways. Some people think that evaluation implies noting error or deficiency. Good evaluation is much broader than this. The main purpose of peer evaluation is to maintain consistent high-quality nursing care. This is an ethical, professional obligation.

Formal Evaluation

Formal evaluation of nursing care occurs in most settings under the title of quality assurance and quality improvement. Quality assurance is a planned program of evaluation that includes ongoing monitoring of the care given and outcomes of care. It includes a mechanism for instituting change when problems or opportunities for improvement are identified. Quality assurance programs are required by The Joint Commission (see Chapter 1). Special nursing projects such as the work done on nursing outcomes (see Chapter 5) have a focus on the quality of care provided.

All types of evaluation first call for establishing specific criteria to be used in the evaluation. These criteria may refer to process, outcome, or both. The creation of the criteria is a professional nursing responsibility.

The process begins by determining whether the nursing actions taken are complete and appropriate. Criteria developed to evaluate this aspect are called process criteria. One basis for developing process criteria is *Nursing: Scope and Standards of Practice*, published by the ANA (2004), which is a revised version of *Standards of Clinical Nursing Practice*, published in 1991 and again in 1998. General standards refer to all settings; more specific ones exist for some 21 specialty areas of nursing. Some specialty organizations, such as the Intravenous Nurses' Society, also have published standards that refer to their specialty.

Another basis for formal evaluation is the use of outcome criteria for patient care. Outcome criteria are specific, observable patient behaviors or clinical manifestations that are the desired results of care. *Nursing: Scope and Standards of Practice* identifies six standards of nursing practice, one of which is outcomes identification (ANA, 2004).

Typically, nurses working in groups develop the criteria. They consult nursing literature so that they establish the appropriate criteria. Several methods have been used to evaluate both the process and the outcomes of nursing care. These may include conferences designed to discuss the matter to be evaluated, interviews with patients or staff, or direct observation of patients. The method that is gaining wider acceptance in nursing is the audit based on review of the patient's record. This chart review involves comparing the patient record with the criteria and is often completed by medical records personnel. The accuracy of the review depends on the adequacy (that is, the completeness) of the charting. If information does not appear in the record (other than situations in which "charting by exception" are employed), then, for the purposes of the audit, the appropriate observations were not made or the actions were not taken.

This is just one of the reasons why you must recognize the importance of your charting and make sure that you maintain a high standard in written records. If audits are being done at your institution, you should become familiar with the criteria being used, which can serve as guidelines in evaluating your own care and record keeping. The chart review has raised serious concerns, which have resulted in greater attention to documentation and even revision of record systems. Nurses then have taken the initiative to determine the meaning of the data in relationship to enhanced patient well-being. Changes in policies and procedures and in-service education classes often occur. Once remedial action has been taken, re-evaluation is done to determine its effectiveness.

Informal Evaluation

An important day-to-day evaluation of patient care occurs informally as peers observe the performance of others. Watching other nurses also helps you to grow in your own practice. When you observe coworkers, strive for objectivity. A common mistake is to let personal feelings influence what we see, viewing a close friend in a positive light and seeing only the negative aspects of a nurse with whom we have a poor relationship. Remember to examine the results or outcomes of care. Two nurses may use different approaches or techniques in similar situations, but both may achieve positive results. In most instances, you will see good care. Do not hesitate to commend others and share your positive feelings. Everyone benefits from positive reinforcement of skill; it helps nurses to create a good climate for personal growth and sharing.

Addressing Substandard Care

Concern for the welfare of patients requires that nurses acknowledge the existence of substandard care and work toward improving that situation. It is not a matter of whether the nurse should become involved, but rather how to most effectively accomplish the goals of better care.

If faced with a situation where patient care is less than desired, consider whose care you are criticizing. If it is the care of another nurse, or a care provider with less educational preparation than you possess, the situation is more straightforward. If you have questions about medical care delivered or the action of a physician, it becomes more difficult, because medical actions are outside the scope of practice of nursing. Be careful about how you proceed, referring to hospital policy manuals, trusted colleagues, your supervisor, or possibly the chief of the medical staff for advice before taking action.

When you observe a colleague practicing what you think is poor patient care, such as poor sterile technique, it is not as difficult. The action you choose to take will depend on the seriousness of the situation you have observed.

Suppose you observed a break in sterile technique during a dressing change. Usually the simplest and most effective solution is to go directly to the person involved and to say, "I observed this specific incident, and it seemed to me that it was not in the best interest of the patient because . . . What is your perception of the situation?" This approach allows the nurse to give a rationale for the action taken. When you understand the situation more fully, you may have a different point of view. If you disagree with your colleague and the situation is not critical, you might want to state simply that you disagree. If the situation is critical, the two of you will want to seek resources that will outline the best approach. If you observe poor care a second time, and it has been determined that your colleague's care is substandard, you should again approach the person. State what you have seen and note that it is the second time. If the person still disagrees that a problem exists, state that you feel obligated to discuss this with your immediate superior because it is not in the best interest of the patient. You should then follow through on this.

If you have a reputation on the unit for maintaining a focus that enhances the welfare of patients, and you have been quick to praise the good care provided by others, your action in response to poor care will be more readily accepted. Remember that your attitude when approaching another nurse is crucial. Facial expressions and tone of voice, as well as words, need to be considered. If you are perceived as friendly and caring, your comments probably will be accepted in a far different manner than if you are seen as being negative and critical.

However, you cannot always count on this reaction. Many nurses feel threatened by the idea of evaluation, or have had bad experiences in which evaluation only involved pointing out deficiencies. These nurses may be angry and upset with any colleague who considers evaluation part of the colleague role. Therefore, it is wise to have thought out how you will proceed.

A Basic Pattern for Action. The first step to be taken in any situation in which you believe substandard care exists is to collect adequate, valid information on behavior that you have personally observed. Do not make decisions based on gossip, hearsay, or an isolated instance, unless the single incident was very serious. If this is the case, be certain of your facts before taking action.

Also be certain you understand both the formal and the informal systems of authority and responsibility within your facility and the laws of the state in which you practice. In some states, laws exist requiring that poor practice be reported directly to the relevant licensing board. In others, reporting to your supervisor is considered adequate reporting. You need to know which people have the authority to make decisions and changes, what the official prescribed route of change is, and what the hidden priorities of the institution might be. It is most commonly recommended that once you are certain of your data and know how the system works in your organization, you should take concerns to your immediate supervisor, who would forward the concern until it reached the individual or body with the authority and duty to act. Many people believe that reporting to a supervisor fulfills your ethical responsibility as well as your legal responsibility.

When you approach a supervisor, give specific information that includes the dates, the situations, and the action you took. Do not indulge in generalities or sweeping statements; stick to specific observed instances by simply describing what you saw. Let the supervisor know that you have talked with the person under discussion and have informed the person that you would speak with the supervisor. It is important to specify the action you would like to see occur. You might ask the supervisor to discuss the matter with both of you, or you might ask the supervisor to discuss the matter with the other nurse or observe the nurse. It is also important to remember that once you have initiated this action, you may or may not be involved in some follow-up. You may never learn what was done, even when positive action was taken, because of the constraints of confidentiality for the affected employee. If the manager decides to observe and take corrective action, that will be confidential for the employee involved and you may never learn the outcome of your action. Occasionally, results emerge only much later, when a change in procedure and policy occurs.

If you observe an incident that has the potential to cause a patient danger (eg, an unreported medication error) or one that has legal ramifications (eg, the falsifying of narcotic records), you have a legal as well as an ethical responsibility to go immediately to a supervisor with your information. In a situation that has the potential for legal involvement, keep an exact personal record of your observations and actions. Include in the record the times and dates of incidents and of your reporting efforts (see Chapter 8).

Alternative Approaches for Action. At times, the system does not always work as expected. Your concern regarding what you perceive as poor practice may be dropped or ignored at any one of many points.

Often there are good reasons for this. Perhaps the persons in authority want to collect more specific data about a situation, with as little general discussion as possible. Sometimes there are aspects of a legal contract or a collective bargaining contract of which you are unaware that must be considered in the actions that are taken. Other times, professional confidentiality may make it seem that nothing is being done, when, in fact, steps have been taken to correct a situation. It is easy as a newcomer to the health care scene to see only part of a picture. Simply checking back with a manager, acknowledging that information may be confidential, and asking for reassurance that the matter is being addressed may be an appropriate action.

If your initial approach is not effective, a formal route for seeking further change would lead you through the official lines of authority within your facility. After discussing your concern with your immediate supervisor and receiving no satisfactory response, tell the supervisor formally that you intend to carry your concern to the next higher authority. Technically, you could proceed in this manner until you reached the administrator or even the board of directors, although it is unlikely that this would occur. Informing your supervisor of your plans should help to avoid problems, but be prepared to listen to some words of warning from the supervisor or efforts to discourage you from taking action. There are reasons this individual has chosen not to pursue the issue; some of these may be valid.

However, there are times when an alternative approach is more appropriate than formal action. Another route for seeking further change is through designated committees or procedures within your facility. As hospitals move into models of shared governance, this may be your best alternative. Discussing or sharing a problem with a particular committee might require a carefully written and documented report explaining your concern. You then might be called to answer questions that the committee believes are important.

You may volunteer to serve on committees that deal with peer review. If there are no such committees, you may work to have them established, perhaps through a bargaining unit. This route of action will require a considerable investment of your own time and effort, a factor you need to consider.

Another alternative approach is to use the informal system within the facility. You may discuss your concern with a trusted person (or mentor) who has influence within the system. You may learn that you are not alone in your concerns, that efforts toward change are being made, and that your input of data is welcomed. Another approach would be to seek the assistance of another individual with power within the organization. However, we must caution you about using informal systems, as they can backfire. Therefore, we suggest that you use these alternative approaches only when the ones suggested earlier have failed to bring about the desired results.

A final alternative to a problem in your work setting is to offer your resignation if a change is not made. Continuing to work in an environment in which poor practice exists may place you in conflict with your ethical standards and values. If you find it necessary to do this, be careful that you do not jeopardize your own future with angry letters or intemperate remarks. Render your resignation in a polite and professional manner, even when expressing dissatisfaction with the system.

Reporting directly to a state licensing board or professional organization's disciplinary committee is an avenue of action outside of the employment setting. The licensing board exists to assure the public of safe practice; therefore, these organizations and agencies usually deal with serious problems that represent a breach of the public trust or serious harm. They may not have the capacity or desire to pursue minor (though still important) problems. The same constraints apply when reporting to these organizations. Remember that their investigation and decisions may be done in a judicial or legal manner. This may involve the requirement that you provide legal testimony regarding your complaints.

Personal Risks in Reporting. If you decide to pursue any of these routes, be fully aware of the possible consequences. You may be labeled a troublemaker, or worse. You may lose the opportunity to be promoted because you are seen as being antagonistic to the system. Although officially it should not happen, it is even possible that you could lose your job for raising too many issues. We do not mean to be unduly discouraging, but we want to warn you that the role of change agent is not easy, and you should be aware of the consequences and weigh them before you decide to act. And above all, be certain that your perceptions are correct and that your concerns are well grounded.

Whistleblowing. The ultimate step one might take in a situation in which negligence or maltreatment are allowed to persist would be whistleblowing. **Whistleblowing** involves going public or speaking out to one's professional organization or to the media in order to protect the welfare of patients because of a perceived wrongdoing on the part of others. In the business world, whistleblowing resulting in high-profile cases involving manipulation of gas prices, breast implants, accounting fraud, and insider trading has alerted the public to ethical wrong-doing. Although some question its application to nursing, Hook (2001) defends whistleblowing in nursing on the basis of patient advocacy, citing the *Code of Ethics for Nurses with Interpretive Statements—Provision 3* as justification for such action.

If a situation is one that you consider serious enough to take such action, do so only after thoughtful consideration, because exposing unethical and incompetent health care providers is not without risk. The worst case scenario might be legal retaliation, but there may less serious reactions from coworkers or you may place your job in jeopardy. In one instance in California, a convalescent home nurse committed suicide as a result of the fury directed toward her by her supervisors after she reported a case in which a nurse's aide hit an 81-year-old who suffered from dementia ("Legislation helps nurses 'blow the whistle' on patient neglect and abuse," 2001). Some states have enacted legislation that protects nurses and other health care staff members from retaliation when they report a case, but others have not. There is no federal legislation that specifically protects nurses.

Because there can be serious ramifications to whistleblowing, do not go public until all the avenues to address concerns through the system have been exhausted, with no response. As Wilmot (2000, p. 1053) points out, "Exposure of abuse or poor care does not necessarily lead straight to the achievement of good care." The following should guide your activities:

- Consider contacting an attorney before taking any steps.
- Learn as much as you can about your state's policies by contacting your state nurses association or the ANA.
- Be certain on your facts and have them well documented. Be confident that a wrong-doing has occurred.
- As you pursue your concern within the system, follow the health care organization's chain of command.
- Be professional when dealing with others.

Recommending A Care Provider

Patients and acquaintances may ask you to recommend a physician or other care provider because they believe that, as a nurse, you have special knowledge and insight in such matters. If you have no personal knowledge about the requested information, then honestly tell the individual requesting information that you have no personal or professional knowledge regarding a particular care provider. However, if you do have knowledge, you could recommend several competent persons, pointing out characteristics of each that might be factors in personal choice. For example, if you were asked to recommend an obstetrician, you might recommend three. You then could state further that Drs. A, B, and C are all board-certified specialists in obstetrics. You might add some information about their practices: Dr. A is an older physician with a more traditional approach to childbirth; Dr. B is a young and innovative physician who strongly advocates partner participation and the Lamaze natural childbirth method; Dr. C is new in the community, but appears to allow patients a great deal of choice in their approach to childbirth. From this, the patient can further research these physicians and make a personal choice.

If you are asked specifically about a physician whose care you believe to be less than satisfactory, you are faced with a different dilemma. Making severely critical statements might leave you open to a legal charge of slander by the physician (see Chapter 8). However, saying nothing is ethically a problem because you are not acting to protect the patient. A safe approach is to state, "I personally would not choose Dr. X as my physician. Instead, I would prefer to see Dr. N or Dr. O." If pressed to give reasons, you are legally more secure if you say that you would prefer not to discuss specifics.

Be careful that any recommendations are not based on hearsay or gossip. If you do not have solid information on which to base a referral, do not be drawn into making one. Being a nurse does not obligate you to be an expert on all health care questions.

THE CHEMICALLY IMPAIRED PROFESSIONAL

Chemically impaired professional is a term used to describe that person whose practice has deteriorated because of chemical abuse, specifically, the use of alcohol and drugs. The terms addiction, drug addiction, alcoholism, chemical dependency, and chemical impairment are all names that we associate with the dependence on alcohol, drugs or other behaviors. Addiction has been defined as "the compulsive need for and use of something that is psychologically or physically habit-forming, characterized by tolerance and by well-defined physiological symptoms upon withdrawal" (Addiction Intervention Resources, 2006, para. 2). Dependency refers to the strong desire and impaired control over the use of a substance despite the consequences associated with continued use (Wood, 2006). There is a strong possibility that if you remain active in the profession, at some time will find yourself working with a chemically impaired colleague; perhaps you already have.

Chemical Impairment in Health Care Professionals

One would like to believe that nurses, who have studied the physiologic effects of alcohol and drugs on the system, would avoid such abuse. However, this is not the case. As a result of increasing concern about the problem, in the 1980s, nurses began to collect data on the topic (Bissell & Haberman, 1984; Bissell & Skorina, 1987; Sullivan, Bissell, & Williams, 1988). Sullivan and colleagues conclude that the percentage of chemically dependent nurses is at least as great as the percentage of chemically dependent people in the general population, and it may be that there is a greater percentage in the nursing population, based on accessibility of drugs.

Studies conducted in the 1990s have assessed probable alcoholism among nursing students. Marion and colleagues (1996) reported that the use of alcohol by nursing students paralleled the alcohol consumption of other college students, an age group recognized as demonstrating high usage. Their findings indicate significant drinking problems among the students sampled. Campbell and Polk (1992) also have expressed concern about substance abuse among students, and have encouraged nurse educators to identify students suspected of abuse and to educate students about the problem. Sullivan, Bissell, and Leffler (1990) reported that the addiction process may begin earlier, even before nursing school, and that younger nurses were more likely to use narcotics, resulting in serious problems in job performance. Trinkoff, Eaton, and Anthony (1991) stated that nurses reported substance abuse behaviors less often and in lesser amounts than did their non-nurse counterparts. Trinkoff and Storr (1998) conducted an anonymous mailed survey of RNs (n = 4438) regarding their use of marijuana, cocaine, prescription-type drugs, cigarette smoking, and binge drinking. The prevalence of use of all substances was 32%, with emergency nurses 3.5 times as likely to use marijuana or cocaine; oncology and administration nurses twice as likely to engage in binge drinking; and psychiatric nurses most likely to smoke.

Why are nurses affected by this problem? Factors that lead to chemical dependency include the stress of the nursing profession, particularly in intensive care units and emergency departments. Frequent shift changes and staffing shortages add to the situation. Unrealistic personal expectations, frustration, powerlessness, anxiety, and depression contribute to the problem. Once the problem exists, denial is a big part of the disease.

All areas of the profession are affected by the problem of chemical dependency in nursing. A significant financial impact, in the forms of sickness, absenteeism, tardiness, accidents, errors, decreased productivity, and staff turnover, is realized by institutions that employ nurses with dependency problems. Problems related to drug abuse are complicated by the fact that the nurse often obtains drugs from the supply available on the hospital unit and is therefore in violation of the Controlled Substances Act. As with other health care conditions, early recognition and treatment have been recommended to help offset this problem.

In 1981, the ANA appointed a Nursing Task Force on Addiction and Psychological Disturbance to develop guidelines for state associations in the treatment and assistance of nurses whose practice was impaired by alcoholism, drug abuse, or psychological dysfunction. These guidelines approached chemical dependency in nursing from a treatment and rehabilitation viewpoint rather than from a punishment viewpoint. In 1990, the ANA developed suggested state legislation to respond to the problems of chemical dependency and drug diversion in nurses that emphasized voluntary treatment and monitoring programs rather than traditional legal proceedings (ANA, 1990). Since that time, many states have established treatment and monitoring programs as their first approach for chemically dependent health professions.

Recognizing the Chemically Impaired Nurse

The concerns about the chemically impaired nurse are twofold. The first is a personal concern for the nurse who is afflicted: The illness may go undetected and untreated for years. The second concern is for the patient, whose care is jeopardized by the nurse whose judgment and skills are weakened.

The major avenue for identifying impaired nurses is through nonimpaired coworkers. However, nurses, by virtue of their education, are socialized into caring roles and have not always dealt with the problem in a straightforward fashion. Beckstead (2002) reports that only 37% of nurses who have had experiences working with impaired colleagues reported them to supervisors. The impaired nurse was often protected, transferred, ignored, and, in some instances, promoted. None of these actions helped solve the problem. As you enter the nursing field, be aware of the following characteristics, which are commonly seen in impaired health care practitioners:

- Mood swings
- Inappropriate behavior
- Frequent days off for implausible reasons
- Noncompliance with acceptable policies and procedures
- Deteriorating appearance
- Inconsistent job performance
- Inadequate documentation
- Unusual prescribing practices
- Alcohol on breath

- Poor judgment, concentration
- Dishonesty
- Missed appointments
- Boundary violations

(Washington Health Professional Services, 2006)

Reporting the Chemically Impaired Colleague

As an RN, what should you do if you suspect that a colleague has a chemical dependency problem? First of all, you need to know what the law in your state requires of you. In many states, every professional is legally obligated to report a chemically dependent health care professional. This reporting most commonly is done through channels at the place of employment, but also may be done directly to the state board of nursing. If you do not know the requirements, you should immediately learn what they are. In some states, failure to report can result in disciplinary action toward you.

When planning to report, you do not have to be sure beyond any doubt that a problem exists. You need to have enough data to present a reasonable concern. The investigation to clearly establish the problem is the responsibility of the employing agency or the state board.

To establish reasonable concern, collect and document data, including objective facts, dates, and times when the situation occurred. For several good reasons, you should not confront the person whom you suspect at this time.

First, the person may become more secretive about the behavior because of the danger of being caught. This will make collection of data difficult, if not impossible. Personal defenses and denial may become stronger. The suspected person may ask for a transfer to another shift or to a different part of the facility, or, if truly feeling threatened, may seek employment in another facility.

Second, the person may feel attacked and rejected. To ensure that it will not end in a disaster, a confrontation needs the support of an appropriate and knowledgeable health care professional to ensure that the individual is guided to appropriate choices for treatment and rehabilitation. If the person is someone you know well, who confides in you regarding personal problems, you might use those occasions to refer the individual to appropriate resources for personal assistance and counseling.

Another reason why you should not confront the suspected person at this time is that you are still collecting data and documenting it. You cannot be sure from a single observation that a problem exists. There are often reasons why things are not what we initially perceived them to be.

Once you feel you have data to support a realistic concern, report them to a supervisor to validate your observations. Usually, once you have notified your supervisor, he or she will assume responsibility for the problem, but may ask for your continued assistance with data collection or with confrontation (see earlier discussion on reporting to your supervisor).

Once adequate information has been gathered, agency administrative personnel will notify the state board of nursing. In addition, they usually must notify the state board of pharmacy if drugs are involved. More investigation will be carried out; records will be examined. If a problem exists, actions appropriate to the situation will be taken. These usually include a carefully planned confrontation by an intervention team, a requirement that treatment be sought, and a presentation of the consequences of not seeking treatment.

The worst thing you can do if you suspect a problem is to ignore it or help a colleague cover for inadequacies. The colleague will not get better if the problem is not recognized and treated. The longer the delay, the greater the chance that an innocent patient will be placed in jeopardy.

Fortunately, help and rehabilitation are being made available to those who need it through state nurses associations and state licensing authorities. These programs usually provide a specific contractual agreement regarding professional practice during the treatment and monitoring period. This is often done without formal disciplinary proceedings. The goal of this process is restoration of the individual to effective functioning.

In some states, the licensing boards may institute formal disciplinary proceedings to suspend a license or issue a license with limitations on practice, and to provide monitoring and supervision while the individual seeks treatment. When treatment is completed, the board may reinstate the license with temporary limitations and continued monitoring and support. The goal is the eventual full rehabilitation of the health care professional to the service of the community. Baldwin and Smith (1994) reported a much higher treatment success rate in nurses than in the general population. These researchers further identified that successful recovery was most likely in those nurses who retained their employment during treatment. Therefore, reporting a chemically dependent colleague may be the most caring action you can take.

If, as a nursing student, you suspect that a fellow classmate (or worse yet, an instructor) has a problem with chemical abuse, you would be wise to discuss your concerns with your instructor (or with the director of the program if you suspect an instructor). Because such problems typically worsen with time, the earlier they are addressed and corrected, the better it is for everyone. Again, it is important that you have accurate information to report, along with times, dates, and examples of the behavior that caused your concern.

Critical Thinking Activity

Assume that you have serious concerns that a colleague is delivering poor patient care because of problems with chemical dependency. Where would you begin? What is your personal responsibility? What is your responsibility to your colleague? What is your responsibility to the patients? What steps should you take? Do you have a personal liability in the situation?

BOUNDARY VIOLATIONS

The term **boundary violations** is used to refer to situations in which nurses move beyond a professional relationship and become personally involved with a patient and the patient's life. It is of particular concern because it represents a violation of the trust relationship that exists between the patient and the nurse. In nurse–patient relationships, the nurse necessarily holds power, creating a vulnerable situation for the patient. The nurse also has access to confidential and privileged information about patients and their families. It is the nurse's responsibility to define the boundaries of the relationships and ensure that they are maintained. The nurse must be warm and empathetic but should not try to be friends with the patient (Fig. 9-4).

Perhaps the most extreme boundary violation is professional sexual misconduct. Professional sexual misconduct has been defined as "any expression by a nurse or other health care

NON-PROFESSIONALISM
- Overinvolvement with patient
- Exploitation
- Excessive self-disclosure
- Abuse of power
- Secretiveness

PROFESSIONALISM
- Patient safety & welfare first
- Helpfulness
- Professional distance
- Respect for patient & family
- Professional behavior

NO LOITERING

FIGURE 9-4   Everyone benefits when boundaries are clearly established and maintained.

provider of erotic or romantic thoughts, feelings, or gestures that are sexual or may be reasonably construed by the patient as sexual" (Smith, Taylor, Keys, & Gornto, 1997). At present, there is no official reporting of the violation of sexual boundaries; however, it is the topic of focus groups and workshops conducted by the National Council of State Boards of Nursing.

Although sexual misconduct is the major focus of this concern, boundary violations expand into other areas of conduct, such as overidentifying with a particular family member or moving into pseudofamily relationships with the patient's family. If this happens, the family may question the nurse's motives, wondering whether the nurse is looking for a bequest in a will or other tangible benefit. Such overinvolvement will interfere with the nurse's personal life and even could result in legal actions on the part of the family.

Some early indications that boundaries are beginning to break down include situations in which the nurse spends extended time with a patient beyond assigned duties or visits the patient when not on duty. Showing favoritism or possessiveness of a patient, meeting patients in isolated areas in a manner that has nothing to do with direct patient care, or personal disclosure by the care provider are other indicators that boundaries are being violated (Ellis & Hartley, 2005).

It is important that you are able to recognize situations in which a colleague may cross sexual boundaries. If you believe sexual misconduct is occurring on the unit where you are employed, the steps you would follow are similar to those you learned to use in dealing with chemical abuse. It is extremely important that you document the behavior carefully, noting dates, times, and the names of the individuals involved. Keep your documentation focused on factual information and objective data. You would then share this information with your immediate supervisor.

Key Concepts

- Ethics is a branch of philosophy referred to as moral philosophy. It seeks to provide answers to some of the questions of human conduct that arise in our life, and attempts to determine what is right or good.

- Inherent in the study of ethics is an appreciation of individual values that are derived from societal norms, religion, and family orientation. We can get in better touch with our own value system through the process of values clarification.

- The basic ethical concepts of beneficence, nonmaleficence, autonomy, justice, fidelity, veracity, and the standard of best interest underlie ethical decision making and may be in conflict in an individual situation.

- The ethical theories of utilitarianism, deontology, natural law, and social equity and justice may be used to examine the implications of ethical decisions.

- The concept of justice has been expanded to include distributive justice that is applied in situations requiring the allocation of scarce resources. The problems associated with the allocation of scarce resources are expected to increase in the near future.

- Ethical decision making may be based on personal religious and philosophic viewpoints, but must always be grounded in professional standards seen in the Codes for Nurses and the statements of patient rights.

- A variety of social and cultural factors including attitudes, science and technology, legislation, judicial decisions, and funding all influence ethical decision making.

- The nurse's status as an employee, collective bargaining contracts, collegial relationships, the authoritarian and paternalistic backgrounds of health care, deliberations of ethics committees, and consumer involvement create pressures regarding ethical decision making.

- A basic framework for ethical decision making emphasizes identifying and clarifying the problem, gathering data, identifying options, making a decision, acting, and assessing.

- Nurses have ethical obligations to the patient and to the employer, and must maintain an objective stance regarding other health care providers, and when confronting substandard care. Commitment to personal excellence and to the profession of nursing are also desired characteristics of the professional nurse.

- In serious situations, when using the chain of command doesn't invoke response to voiced concerns, one might use whistleblowing to bring attention to the circumstances. This should be used as a last resort because of the possible ramifications to the individual blowing the whistle.

- The chemically impaired nurse is a concern to the profession and a danger to patients. All nurses have an obligation to report those who demonstrate chemical impairment and to assist impaired colleagues in finding treatment and rehabilitation.

- Boundary violations, a situation in which the nurse moves beyond a professional relationship and becomes involved with patients and their families, has become a concern in nursing. Educational programs to increase understanding of this problem and to help avoid its occurrence are being conducted.

Relevant Web Sites

The American Nurses Organization: *http://nursingworld.org* (Click on "Ethics" and go to the "Center for Ethics and Human Rights")

Boston College, Nursing Ethics Network: *www/bc.edu/nursing.ethics*

International Council of Nurses: *www.icn.ch/ethics.htm*

John Hopkins University, Bioethics Institute: *www.med.jhu.edu/bioethics_institute*

Midwest Bioethics Center: *www.midbio.org*

National Catholic Bioethics Center: *www.ncbcenter.org*

National Reference Center for Bioethics Literature: *http://bioethics.georgetown.edu/nrc/index.htm*

University of British Columbia, The W. Maurice Young Center for Applied Ethics: *www.ethics.ubc.ca*

References

Addiction Intervention Resources. (2006). *What is addiction?* [On-line]. *www.addictionintervention.com/addition/index.asp.* Accessed September 13, 2006.

American Hospital Association. (1992). *A patient's bill of rights.* Chicago: Author.

American Nurses Association. (1990). Suggested state legislation: Nursing Practice Act, Nursing Disciplinary Diversion Act, Prescriptive Authority Act (Pub. No. NP-78). Washington, DC: Author.

American Nurses Association. (2004). *Nursing: Scope and standards of nursing practice.* Washington, DC: Author.

American Nurses Association. (2001). *Code for nurses with interpretive statements.* Silver Spring, MD: Nursesbooks.org.

Armstrong, C. R., & Whitlock, R. (1998). The cost of care: Two troublesome cases in health care ethics. *The Physician Executive, 24*(6), 32–35.

Baldwin, L., & Smith, V. (1994). Relapse in chemically dependent nurses: Relevance and contributing factors. *Issues, 15*(1), 1, 4–5.

Bates, T. J. (2002, October 14). Letters of advice. *Mountain West Nurse Week, 3*(14), 7.

Beckstead, J. W. (2002). Modeling attitudinal antecedents of nurses' decisions to report impaired colleagues. *Western Journal of Nursing Research, 24*(5), 537–551.

Bissell, L., & Haberman, P. W. (1984). *Alcoholism in the professions.* New York: Oxford University Press.

Bissell, L., & Skorina, J. (1987). 100 alcoholic women in medicine. *Journal of the American Medical Association, 257*(2), 939–944.

Boyd, A. D. (2006). *Physician-assisted suicide: For and against.* [On-line]. *www.amas.org/bio/pas.ctm.* Accessed September 12, 2006.

Braddock, C. H., Edwards, K. A., Hasenberg, N. M., Laidley, T. L., & Levinson, W. (1999). Informed decision making in outpatient practice: Time to get back to the basics. *Journal of the American Medical Association, 282*(24), 2313–2320.

Burkhardt, M. A., & Nathaniel, A. K. (2001). *Ethics & issues in contemporary nursing.* Albany, NY: Delmar Publishers.

Campbell, A. R., & Polk, E. (1992). *Legal and ethical issues of alcohol and other substance abuse in nursing education.* Atlanta, GA: Southern Council on Collegiate Education for Nursing.

Chaffee, M. W. (2006). Making the Decision to Report to Work in a Disaster. *American Journal of Nursing, 106*(9), 54–57.

Curtin, L. (1978). A proposed model for critical ethical analysis. *Nursing Forum, 17*(1), 12–17.

Davis, A. J., Arokar, M. A., Liaschenko, J., & Drought, T. S. (1997). *Ethical dilemmas in nursing and nursing practice* (4th ed.). Stamford, CT: Appleton & Lange.

Edge, R. S., & Groves, J. R. (1999). *Ethics of health care: A guide for clinical practice* (2nd ed.). Albany, NY: Delmar.

Ellis, J. R., & Hartley, C. L. (2005). *Managing and coordinating nursing care* (4th ed.). Philadelphia: Lippincott Williams & Wilkins.

Fowler, M. (1997). Nursing ethics. In A. J. Davis, M. A. Aroskar, J. Liaschenko, & T. S. Drought, *Ethical dilemmas & nursing practice* (4th ed.) (pp. 17–34). Stamford, CT: Appleton & Lange.

Hall, J. K. (1996). *Nursing ethics and law.* Philadelphia: W.B. Saunders.

Hook, K. (2001, fall). Toward an ethical defense of whistleblowing. *Ethics Update, 1*(2). [On-line]. *http://nursingworld.org/ethics/update/vol1no2a.htm.* Accessed October 19, 2005.

International Code for Nurses. (2006). *The Code of Ethics for Nurses.* Geneva (Switzerland): Author.

Jameton, A. (1984). *Nursing practice: The ethical issues.* Englewood Cliffs, NJ: Prentice-Hall.

Jefferson, L. V., & Ensor, B. E. (1982). Confronting a chemically impaired colleague. *American Journal of Nursing, 82*(4), 574.

Lamont, J. (2003). *Distributive justice.* [On-line]. *http://plato.stanford.edu/entries/justice-distributive.* Accessed September 12, 2006.

Legislation helps nurses 'blow the whistle' on patient neglect and abuse. (2001). [On-line]. *www.nursezone.com.* In search box type in "patient neglect", choose from articles listed. Accessed May 25, 2007.

Maddox, P. J. (1998). Administrative ethics and the allocation of scarce resources. *Online Journal of Issues in Nursing*. [On-line]. *http://nursingworld.org/ojin/topic8/topic8_5.htm*. Accessed September 13, 2006.

Marion, L. N., Fuller, S. G., Johnson, N. P., Michels, P. J., & Diniz, C. (1996). Drinking problems of nursing students. *Journal of Nursing Education, 35*(5), 196–203.

Merriam-Webster Online Dictionary. (2006). [On-line]. *www.m-w.com/dictionary*. Accessed September 12, 2006.

Milner, S. (1993). An ethical nursing practice model. *Journal of Nursing Administration, 23*(3), 22–25.

National Association of Practical Nurse Education and Service. (2004). *NAPNES Standards of Practice for Licensed Practical/ Vocational Nurses*. Falls Church, Virginia: Author.

Nathaniel, A. (2002). Moral Distress Among Nurses. *The American Nurses Association Ethic & Human Rights ISSUES UPDATE, 1*(3) Spring, 2002 [on-line]. *http://nursingworld.org/ethics/update/vol1no.3.htm moral*. Accessed May 24, 2007.

Rawls, J. A. (1971). *Theory of justice*. Cambridge, MA: Harvard University Press.

Silva, M.C. (1998). Financial compensation and ethical issues in health care. *Online Journal of Issues in Nursing*. [On-line]. *http://nursingworld.org/ojin/tpc6/tpc6_4.htm*. Accessed September 13, 2006.

Smith, L. L., Taylor, B. B., Keys, A. T., & Gornto, S. B. (1997). Nurse-patient boundaries: Crossing the line. *American Journal of Nursing, 97*(12), 26–31.

Sullivan, E., Bissell, L., & Leffler, D. (1990). Drug use and disciplinary actions among 300 nurses. *International Journal of the Addictions, 25*(4), 375–391.

Sullivan, E., Bissell, L., & Williams, E. (1988). *Chemical dependency in nursing: The deadly diversion*. Menlo Park, CA: Addison-Wesley.

Thiroux, J., & Johnson, C. E. (2006). *Ethics: Theory and practice* (9th ed.). Upper Saddle Drive, NJ: Prentice Hall.

Thompson, J., & Thompson, H. (1981). *Ethics in nursing*. New York: Macmillan.

Trinkoff, A. M., Eaton, W. W., & Antony, J. C. (1991). The prevalence of substance abuse among registered nurse. *Nursing Research, 40*(3), 172–175.

Trinkoff, A. M., & Storr, C. L. (1998) Substance use among nurses: Differences between specialties. *American Journal of Public Health, 88*, 581–585.

Videbeck, S. L. (2006). *Psychiatric mental health nursing*. (3rd ed.) Philadelphia: Lippincott Williams & Wilkins.

Washington Health Professional Services. (2006). *Symptoms*. [On-line]. *http://fortress.wa.gov/doh/hpqa1hps2/WHPS/Symptoms.htm*. Accessed September 13, 2006.

Wilkinson, J. M. (1987–1988). Moral distress in nursing practice: Experience and effect. *Nursing Forum, 23*(1), 16–29.

Wilmot, S. (2000). Nurses and whistleblowing: the ethical issues. *Journal of Advanced Nursing, 32*(5), 1051–1057.

Wood, D. A. (2006). Nurses poised to assess patients' alcohol use. *Nurse Week: Mountain West Edition, 7*(17), 22.

Bioethical Issues in Health Care

After completing this chapter, you should be able to:

1. Explain why nurses need an understanding of bioethical issues.
2. Outline the history of family planning in the United States and discuss how various value systems and beliefs have affected it.
3. List some of the ethical and legal problems associated with artificial insemination, surrogate motherhood, and in vitro fertilization.
4. Discuss the problems associated with determining when death has occurred and outline ways in which it affects decisions regarding health care.
5. Analyze the multiple factors in right-to-die issues, including assisted suicide and the difference between active and passive euthanasia.
6. Analyze the various points of view related to withholding and withdrawing treatment.

7. Discuss the ethics that establish the foundation for providing clients with informed consent and involving them in decisions regarding treatment.
8. Identify the major issues associated with organ transplantation.
9. Discuss the purposes of the Human Genome Project and identify possible bioethical issues that could evolve from it.
10. Describe the arguments for and against gene therapy and identify related bioethical concerns.
11. Analyze the reasons that controversy surrounds stem cell research and outline the positive and negative outcomes that could result from that research.
12. Discuss the multiple concerns that affect decisions regarding the treatment of the mentally ill.
13. Outline concerns related to the rationing of health care.

Abortion (spontaneous, therapeutic, elective)
Advance directive
Age of consent
Amniocentesis
Artificial insemination
Assisted suicide

Behavior control
Bioethics
Chorionic villus sampling (CVS)
Durable power of attorney for health care
Emancipated minor

Eugenics
Euthanasia—negative and positive
Family planning
Fatal pathology
Futile treatment
Gene therapy

Genetic screening	Organ transplantation	Sonogram
Genome	Patient Self-Determination Act	Stem cell
Human Genome Project	(PSDA)	Sterilization
(HGP)	Pre-implantation Genetic	Surrogate mother
Informed consent	Diagnosis (PGD)	Withdrawing/withholding
In vitro fertilization (IVF)	Property rights	treatment
Living will	Rationing of health care	Wrongful birth
Mature minors	Right-to-die	Xenotransplantation
Organ procurement	Right to refuse treatment	

Bioethics is the study of ethical issues that result from technologic and scientific advances, especially as they are used in biology and medicine. This area of study is also called biomedical ethics because of its association with medical practice. It is a subdiscipline within the larger discipline of ethics, which (as discussed in Chapter 9) is the philosophic study of morality, or what is right and what is wrong. Dr. Edmund D. Pelligrino, Chairman of the President's Council on Bioethics has stated, "To advance human good and avoid harm, biotechnology must be used with ethical constraints. It is the task of bioethics to help society develop those constraints and bioethics, therefore, must be of concern to all of us" (Pelligrino, 2005).

Today more than ever, nurses and their patients need to keep pace with the technologic changes occurring in health care. Murray (2003) states that two distinct sorts of challenges will be important in the near future. The first he identifies as the responsible use of the power conferred by science and technology; the second deals with important problems of access, distribution, and justice.

This chapter discusses some of the choices with which nurses and their clients must grapple. It should be read, studied, and discussed within the framework of the information concerning ethical decision making that was provided earlier. The content of the chapter should provide a basis with which you can look at judicial rulings, legal mandates, and social standards and understand how they can be used to assist in resolving concerns that face us in health care delivery. You have had some experience in looking at what is right or wrong regarding your personal professional practice. This chapter examines more specifically the issues that apply to the bioethics of patient care.

MAJOR AREAS WHERE BIOETHICS ARE APPLIED

The bioethical issues surrounding the delivery of health care grow in number each year, constantly changing and taking on new scope and proportions. For years we have debated issues related to birth and death; today those topics represent just the tip of the iceberg. Of equal or greater concern are such matters as universal access to health care and insurance for all, rationing of health care, cost containment and quality of care, where and how federal dollars should be spent with regard to the nation's health, and the obligation of others to assist the homeless. Our media thrive on issues created by recent biomedical research, such as concerns regarding the

Human Genome Project (HGP), gene therapy, and stem cell research, with one area blurring into another. Biotechnology opens many doors, and as more and more possibilities become reality, new issues must be addressed. How far should a society go in memory boosting or its suppression? Is it appropriate to carry out sex selection? What about cloning? Should assisted reproduction be regulated? To what extent should drugs be used on children to control their behavior? Should we extend life through age-retardation? These are but a few of the questions for which our society must find answers.

Each year, the percentage of America's gross domestic product (GDP) spent on health care increases. In 2003 (the latest figures available), the United States spent 15.3% on health care, as spending reached $1.7 trillion (National Coalition on Health Care, 2005). It is projected to reach $3.4 trillion in 2013 to represent 18.4 percent of the GDP (Centers for Medicare & Medicaid Services, 2004).

Because of lifestyle changes and medical breakthroughs, more people today live to reach old age, thus placing a greater burden on an already stressed system. Life expectancy has increased 1 to 2 years in each recent decade. In the United States, the life expectancy for females born today is 79.5 years, and for males it is 74.1, compared with 47 years at the beginning of the 20th century. Diseases such as Alzheimer's and AIDS, for which cures are still being sought, have increased in prevalence. With globalization have come new threats to our well-being, such as that created by the West Nile virus.

New technologies have led to treatments that were not available even 5 years ago. But rather than decreasing health care needs, the new technologies have resulted in increased needs because these specialized services are in high demand. Many treatments require use of technologies so expensive that they are priced beyond what an individual or family can afford without help from third-party payers. Finding new and better ways to treat life-threatening conditions challenges medical researchers, and the treatments that become available often invite debate among bioethicists. For example, stem cell research is forcing our society to make distinctions about life's beginnings that have enormous scientific and religious implications.

Some would argue that the birth of bioethics occurred with the publication of a magazine article in *Life* titled "They Decide Who Lives, Who Dies" (November 9, 1962). This article told the story of a group of individuals in Seattle whose duty it was to select patients for the first hemodialysis program to treat chronic renal failure. Many more patients needed treatment than could be accommodated; those not selected would likely die. This event was followed several years later by an article about the ethics of medical research that provided the impetus for examining these issues.

Soon after, centers for research in bioethics emerged, most notably the Institute of Society, Ethics, and the Life Sciences, located in Hastings-on-Hudson, New York (often called The Hastings Center), which was founded in 1969, and the Kennedy Institute of Ethics, located at Georgetown University in Washington, DC. The Kennedy Institute of Ethics, founded in 1971 by Joseph and Rose Kennedy, is a teaching and research center that provides ethical perspectives on major policy issues. It boasts the largest university-based faculty in the world devoted to research and teaching biomedical ethics. Journals such as the *Hastings Center Report* and the *Journal of Medicine and Philosophy* have come into being, and an encyclopedia, *The Encyclopedia of Bioethics*, has been published. Web sites devoted to the topic of bioethics are so numerous that they cannot be listed in the confines of this textbook. Today, bioethicists are included in many important task forces and special committees.

Entire textbooks have been devoted to bioethical considerations. Initially, most of these were written for medical students, but now just as many are written for nursing students. Some nursing programs include a course in ethics and bioethics in the curriculum. This chapter can only introduce the topic and, we hope, broaden your perspective and deepen your interest. You are encouraged to read about and study these issues further as they affect your nursing practice.

As we mentioned earlier, most of the bioethical issues have evolved as a product of the technologic advances occurring in medical practice and research and were not a concern 25 years ago. Table 10-1 lists some of the significant medical milestones that have occurred since 1920, some of which we have come to take for granted (eg, antibiotics and DNA). You readily can see that in 1960 there was no quest for human organs or critical decisions regarding the life status of a possible donor. We were not able to fertilize ova outside the human body and transfer the fertilized eggs in a woman's uterus until 1978. Certain life-saving machines (eg, ventilators) and miracle drugs (eg, some of the chemotherapeutic agents used today) were not available to offer extension of life. Technologies such as magnetic resonance imaging, which gives us information about the structure of tissues and allows for early diagnosis and treatment, were not available. Positron Emission Tomography was to follow. As advances occur in medical practice, we must challenge ourselves to think through our own beliefs and feelings about these practices, especially as they relate to quality of life and patients' choices.

BIOETHICAL ISSUES RELATED TO THE BEGINNING OF LIFE

Many bioethical issues with which we wrestle are focused on the process by which conception occurs, the products of conception, and the beginning of life, including whether it should occur. Much of the early debate related to family planning and conception.

Family Planning

Family planning refers to the various methods used to control the size of one's family or to space births. Although we often think of it as synonymous with contraception, in reality it is much broader. For some it could include abortion, for others it might involve adoption. It can employ natural methods, pharmaceutical preparations, or barriers. The religious beliefs and personal values of individuals usually influence the methods and approaches used.

In 1798, in an essay titled, "On Population," Thomas Malthus, a minister in the Church of England, expressed deep concern about a population that was growing faster than were the resources to support it. To offset this problem, he advocated late marriage, no marriage, or sexual abstinence in marriage. No forms of contraception as we know them today were available, although women sometimes developed homemade devices in an effort to prevent pregnancy, such as pessaries inserted vaginally.

In 1873, the U.S. Congress passed the Comstock Act, prohibiting the selling, mailing, or importing of "obscene literature and articles for immoral acts." All contraceptives and any material teaching about sexuality or birth control were included in this prohibition. Those who continued to import and distribute birth control literature or contraceptives were breaking the law. You may have read about Margaret Sanger (1883–1966), a nurse who championed for contraceptive practices in the early 1900s. Although charged and sentenced for disseminating information

TABLE 10-1	SOME MEDICAL MILESTONES OF THE 1900s	
WHEN	**WHO**	**WHAT**
1928	Alexander Fleming	This British bacteriologist noticed that one of his culture plates had grown a fungus and the colonies of staphylococci around the edge of the mold had been destroyed. Because this fungus was a member of the *Penicillium* group, he named it penicillin.
1938	Howard Florey & Ernst Chain	These two pathologists took up the work of Fleming and demonstrated the efficacy of penicillin in treating infection. In 1945, the three were jointly awarded the Nobel Prize for Physiology of Medicine.
1951	Forrest Bird	The first Bird breathing device was developed (Bird Mark 7) and breathing treatment machines were introduced. Inhalation (respiratory) therapy rapidly developed as a health profession (Pilbeam, 1998).
1953	James Watson & Francis Crick	These two geneticists deciphered DNA's double-helix structure. Researchers began to focus on the internal functioning of the cell and molecular biology developed as a specialty.
1954	Physicians in Boston	Transplanted the kidney from one twin to the other, thus moving kidney transplantation from the experimental stage it had occupied since 1902. Kidney transplantations have been the most successful of transplantations (Congressional Kidney Cancus, 2002).
1955	Jonas Salk	Public health officials began immunizing children against polio with Dr. Salk's vaccine, which contained dead virus.
1957	Albert Sabin	A polio vaccine was developed, which was based on weakened live virus, that could be administered orally.
1967	Christiaan Barnard	This South African surgeon performed the first human-heart transplant.
1972	British engineers	The computed tomography (CT) scanner, which assembles thousands of x-ray images into a highly detailed picture of the brain, was developed in England. It was later expanded to provide scans of the entire body.
1978	English physicians	The process of in vitro fertilization was developed. Louise Brown became the first person to be conceived in a test tube, then implanted into the mother's uterus.
1979	World Health Organization	This group declared that smallpox had been eradicated 2 years after the last known case was identified. This occurred because of world-wide immunization against the disease.
1981	Physicians in San Francisco and New York	Doctors from these two cities reported the first cases of what would later become known as acquired immunodeficiency syndrome (AIDS). To date, no cure exists.
1982	The U.S. Food and Drug Administration	The first drug developed with recombinant-DNA was approved by this group. It was a form of human insulin; its availability saves thousands of lives.
1995	Duke University surgeons	Hearts from genetically altered pigs were transplanted into baboons, proving that cross-species transplantations can be done. Transmission of animal viruses to humans emerges as a serious concern.
1998	James Thomas and Scientists from University of Wisconsin—Madison	Culture embryonic stem cells (cells that are the parent cells of all body tissues) from donated human blastocysts, opening the door to potential repair or replacement of diseased tissues or organs (DHHS, 2001).

*Much of the material for this table was gathered from an article by Sherwin B. Nuland, *Time Special Issue*, Fall 1996.

about birth control, she went on to establish the National Committee on Federal Legislation for Birth Control, the forerunner of the Planned Parenthood Federation. In 1938, in Sanger's landmark case, a federal judge dismissed this federal law as unconstitutional, thus ending the federal ban on contraceptives.

Although some states were more liberal than others, and some changed sooner than others, the state that had prohibitions against contraceptives for the longest time was Connecticut. It was not until 1965, in the case of *Griswold and Buxton vs. the State of Connecticut*, that the Supreme Court of the United States overrode the state law forbidding sale or teaching about contraception and established the right of the individual to obtain medical contraceptive advice and counseling (*http://womenshistory.about.com/library/ency/blwh_comstock.htm*).

Much of the controversy over birth control is related to the theological teachings of some religious groups, who believe interference with procreative powers is wrong. The Roman Catholic Church has strongly advocated that the natural purpose of sexual activity is to create new life and nothing should try to interfere with that potential.

The members of the Church of Jesus Christ of Latter Day Saints (Mormons), although less adamant in their teachings, also discourage the use of artificial birth control under normal circumstances. Some conservative Protestant Christians and conservative Muslims also advocate allowing God to plan families and do not use birth control methods. Orthodox Judaism has specific rules about when sexual intercourse may or may not occur; these rules have the effect of supporting sexual activity when a woman is fertile. The Orthodox Jewish population is so small in proportion to other groups that the impact is not significant.

The opposite end of the spectrum is found in those who are strong advocates of zero population growth and encourage individuals to limit families to one or two children in all instances. Others are so concerned about population growth and the state of the world that they decide to not have children.

During your career as a nurse, you will care for patients who represent many differing viewpoints. When caring for individuals whose personal beliefs prohibit the use of artificial birth control, you must be knowledgeable about natural methods of family spacing, such as fertility awareness methods, that will meet the patient's needs. If your personal views regarding contraception differ, your values must be set aside as you focus on assisting the patient in selecting a method that is compatible with the patient's personal values and beliefs. If you are unable to do this, find a colleague who can provide answers to the questions and supply the needed information.

Among the methods of birth control available to those who have no religious sanction against their use, not all methods are acceptable to all people. For example, some find the intrauterine device unacceptable because they believe that interfering with a fertilized egg should be viewed as abortion (researchers are not entirely sure how the intrauterine device works, but some suggest that it prevents the fertilized egg from implanting in the wall of the uterus). Those who find abortion an acceptable method of coping with an unwanted pregnancy represent another set of values.

Central to all discussions of contraception is the issue of freedom of a woman to control her own body. This immediately raises a second question: Who has that right? Is it the woman's right because it is her body? What if the partners disagree about family planning practices? Does one have more say than the other? What if one partner wants to have a family and the other does not?

EXAMPLE

Abortion

In Pennsylvania in August 2002, a temporary injunction blocked a young single woman from securing an abortion. The injunction was issued in response to a lawsuit filed by her boyfriend (from whom she was estranged), who wanted the pregnancy continued. Appeals were filed. A week later, a judge dismissed the injunction and was critical of the fact that the young woman had experienced emotional distress and possible risk because of the delay. She miscarried (aborted spontaneously) the afternoon of this ruling.

Problems of Consent and Family Planning

The ability to have children precedes what is generally considered legal age; therefore, we find ourselves grappling with problems related to age of consent, its definition, and the role of the parents and the family. In legal terms, the **age of consent** is the age at which one is capable of giving deliberate and voluntary agreement. This implies physical and mental ability and the freedom to act and make decisions. The age of consent is established state by state and varies from age 14 to age 18 and may be different for males and females. Most states have established age 16 as the age of consent (Legal Age of Consent, 2005).

Until children reach the age of consent, parents are required to give consent for the care of their children. Implicit in this is the assumption that the parents have the best interests of the child at heart and that they are better qualified than the child to make decisions in the child's best interest. Generally speaking, the parents are responsible for the care (including medical costs) and education of the minor. However, today's trends cloud the issue, as we struggle with individual rights.

With regard to research, federal guidelines required that children with a mental age of 7 years or older be informed about proposed treatment or research and agree or concur with the decision made by the parent or guardian. This is referred to as *assent.*

Another example is the concept of the **emancipated minor**. As previously discussed, emancipated minors (an individual legally under the age of majority), who are financially independent, married, or in the military, may give consent for medical treatment, including all treatment for sexually transmitted diseases (STDs), contraception, and pregnancy-related concerns, regardless of their parent's or legal guardian's knowledge or agreement. Most states recognize some form of emancipation of minors.

The term **mature minors** is generally applied to individuals in their mid- to late teens who are considered mature enough to understand the treatment being recommended and provide **informed consent**. Under this definition, most states allow mature minors to seek treatment for STDs, drug or alcohol abuse, contraception, and pregnancy care without the consent of a parent or guardian. The most liberal legislation applies to the treatment of STDs and is endorsed by most states. Minors of any age can consent to diagnosis and care for STDs. However, the definition of the word "mature" varies from state to state, so some ambiguity continues to affect this area of care. For more discussion of age of consent and informed consent, see Chapter 8.

In some instances, this autonomy of the mature minor may bring health providers into a conflict between two laws. Although the mature minor may be able to consent to treatment for an STD, if the health provider believes it to have been contracted through sexual abuse of the minor, the provider is required to report that abuse. Most authorities direct that child abuse laws take precedence over privacy laws.

Certainly, there are times when a health care provider's ethical and moral convictions prevent them from complying with adolescents' requests for care. This occurs most commonly in response to requests for contraceptive pills and abortions. In such cases, the care provider often discusses his or her beliefs with the adolescent, and refers the patient to another provider for assistance.

A major controversy exists around the role of the school in the sex education of high school students and the dispensing of contraceptives through high school health clinics. Those who are concerned about the high incidence of teenage pregnancies and STDs argue that the information must be disseminated, regardless of who does it. Others believe that this promotes erosion of the role of the family and worry that dispensing contraceptives encourages promiscuity among teenagers. Concern about the spread of AIDS has done much to alter thinking, particularly regarding the dispensing of condoms.

The advent of emergency contraception in the form of birth control pills taken in high dose for a limited time after intercourse has added another dimension to these ethical issues about birth control. In some states, emergency contraception is available directly from a pharmacy without a physician's prescription. The pharmacist, therefore, is drawn into the decision-making web. Some pharmacists have refused to fill birth-control prescriptions for college students, and others have refused to fill prescriptions for emergency contraception. In Illinois in July 2005, an emergency order was filed requiring all pharmacies—not all pharmacists—to fill prescriptions for emergency contraception. The regulation became permanent in mid-August (Jacobson, 2005). Although many believe that people should not be compelled to engage in work they regard as unethical, others view this position as one of dispensing morality. Nurses working in emergency departments, student health services, family planning clinics, and similar environments find themselves in a comparable dilemma when it comes to administering these medications or counseling about their availability. If the nurse is the only care provider available, this would leave the patient without care and could constitute patient abandonment. With this in mind, some nurses choose not to apply for or accept positions where such care is required. In other instances, as long as there is another care provider present who can administer or dispense the medication the concern is resolved.

Abortion

What has been said about contraception becomes an even greater issue when related to abortion. In medical terms, **abortion** is the termination of pregnancy before the viability of the fetus—that is, any time before the end of the 6th month of gestation. An abortion may occur spontaneously as a result of natural causes (**spontaneous abortion**). A pregnancy may be interrupted deliberately for medical reasons (**therapeutic abortion**) or for personal reasons (**elective abortion**). It is the latter two classifications (especially the last) that induce bioethical debate. Ethically, the entire debate revolves around the definition of human life and when the fetus should be considered a human being. There are two major schools of thought about the nature of the fetus: One supports the belief that new life occurs at the moment of conception; the other contends that human life does not exist until the fetus is sufficiently developed biologically to sustain itself outside the uterus.

The legal aspects of abortion were set forth January 22, 1973, when the U.S. Supreme Court ruled in the case of *Roe vs. Wade* that any state laws that prohibited or restricted a woman's right to obtain an abortion during the first 3 months of pregnancy were unconstitutional. In this case, the Supreme Court identified that, during the first trimester of pregnancy, a privacy right exists that allows an individual woman to make the final decision with regard to what happens to her own body (*Roe vs. Wade*, 1973). Certain time limitations as to when an abortion can be performed were determined to be necessary because of the state's interest in protecting potential life. At the period of viability, the state's interest took precedence over the mother's desire for an abortion. Supreme Court Justice Blackmun, in writing an opinion that met with agreement from six other justices in *Roe vs. Wade*, decided that a woman's decision to terminate a pregnancy was encompassed by the right to privacy, up to a certain point in the development of the fetus (Blackmun, 1981). It was established that this lasted until the end of the first trimester. Thus, the courts ruled that the state could not prevent abortions during the first trimester, but could regulate abortions during the second and third trimesters of pregnancy, at which point the interests of the fetus took precedence over those of the mother. In 1992, the Court reaffirmed the basic principles of the 1973 decision.

Despite these rulings, the issue of abortion continues to surface, with new legislation and rulings being considered each year and the issue being debated before each presidential election. In 1977, Congress barred the use of Medicaid funds for abortion, with the exception of those done for therapeutic reasons and in other specific circumstances. However, the legal positions do little to help us deal with bioethical concerns. Many people view termination of life at any point after conception as murder. The Roman Catholic Church firmly upholds its traditional position on abortion. Many conservative Protestant Christian groups also are active in opposing abortion.

Some believe that although abortion is not desirable, under certain circumstances it would be justifiable—for example, in cases of rape or incest, or in instances where amniocentesis indicates that a fetus would be born retarded or genetically defective. Others think that early termination of a pregnancy might be acceptable, but that termination after the 4th month would not be appropriate.

Those who support abortion without restriction usually do so because they believe that women should have control over their own bodies, which is tied to issues of privacy. They further argue that the quality of life of an unwanted child, or a child born with a deformity or genetic defect, may be minimal. Interesting and challenging cases have emerged with respect to this concept. These are generally known as **wrongful birth** cases, and they are based on the principle that it is wrong to give birth to children (such as those with birth defects or limitations that can be diagnosed or anticipated before birth) who will not have the same quality of life as other children.

As a nurse, these issues present difficult questions you will need to answer. To what extent do you believe you can personally participate in the abortion procedure? Would the stage of pregnancy and type of procedure make a difference? As a nurse, you have the right to refuse, based on your own ethical beliefs, to be involved in abortion procedures or the care of patients seeking abortion. Employment in certain areas (eg, labor and delivery rooms), however, may rest on the nurse's willingness and ability to assist with abortions and to give conscientious care to the patient who has had an abortion. Some religiously affiliated hospitals have elected to close their labor and delivery services rather than perform abortions.

Although textbooks traditionally have defined the age of viability (the earliest age at which fetuses could survive outside the uterus if they were born at that time) as 20- to 24-weeks' gestation, technology has increased the ability to enable very–low-birth-weight and premature babies to survive. The age of viability is less clear than it once seemed. Attention has been focused on incidents in which an abortion was attempted toward the end of the 5th or 6th month of gestation, and the fetus was born showing signs of life. Is the doctor or nurse obligated to try to keep the infant alive? Is the doctor or nurse guilty of malpractice, or even murder, if he or she does anything to hasten the infant's death? Should this infant be considered a human being? Does the infant have rights? Does the mother have legal possession of and responsibility for the child if, in fact, she attempted to abort the fetus? This issue, like so many others, probably will be settled in a court of law while we continue to debate it ethically.

The abortion issue also is complicated by consent problems. Many states have recognized the special problems related to parental consent for teenagers and to health care involving pregnancy and have legislated special exceptions. Nurses practicing in areas that provide abortions to minors must be concerned about parental consent and counseling issues because of the wide variations in state statutes governing abortions (Killion & Dempski, 2000).

In the past few years, the abortion issue has been made more complex by research that would use the fetal tissue resulting from an abortion for stem cell research and therapeutic purposes. We will discuss stem cell research later in this chapter.

As a society, it seems likely that we will continue to debate the issue of abortion. Ultimately, the decision rests with the individual who must make the choice. Certainly the legal entanglements become more complex with each court ruling, and will be limited only by our willingness to challenge other aspects of the question.

Critical Thinking Activity

Select one of the positions taken regarding abortion. Defend your position, providing a strong rationale for your thinking. Examine your thinking for biases. Why did you develop those biases? Discuss the topic of abortion with a classmate who holds a different position, remembering that all persons are entitled to their own viewpoints.

Prenatal Testing

The ability to identify birth defects and genetic disorders of the fetus has created a different dimension in the abortion debates. A major breakthrough in our ability to detect genetic abnormalities in the fetus occurred in the 1970s with the development of techniques to carry out amniocentesis. **Amniocentesis** is performed between 14 and 20 weeks after the woman's last menstrual period. Amniotic fluid is aspirated and analyzed. From these cells, many genetic problems of the fetus can be diagnosed prenatally, including such conditions as Down syndrome (which accounts for about one third of the cases of mental retardation in Western countries), hemophilia, Duchenne's muscular dystrophy, Tay-Sachs disease, and problems related to the brain and spinal column (eg, anencephaly and spina bifida).

The potential for Down syndrome, a condition occurring with higher frequency in mothers in their early 40s and older, is the most common reason for seeking amniocentesis. When amniocentesis reveals a genetic disease, a woman will often choose to have an abortion. Some of the diseases that have resulted in the parents choosing the alternative of an abortion include muscular dystrophy, cystic fibrosis, alpha and beta thalassemia, hemophilia, and sickle cell anemia, as well as congenital and genetic defects. Some couples request amniocentesis if they are in an at-risk group, but state that they would not abort the fetus under any circumstances; instead, they believe that an additional 5 months will give them time to adjust to the presence of a serious condition before the baby is born. Usually doctors are reluctant to do an amniocentesis under these circumstances, because the risk of performing the procedure, although small, does not seem justified.

Chorionic villus sampling (CVS) involves securing a sample of chorionic villi from the developing placenta. A sample of the placenta is obtained either vaginally or percutaneously and then analyzed genetically. Like amniocentesis, these tests can predict birth defects and certain diseases. CVS can be performed earlier than an amniocentesis, usually in the 10th or 11th week of pregnancy, but carries with it a risk to the developing fetus that increases the miscarriage rate.

Today almost all pregnant women have a **sonogram** (ultrasound). It is used for fetal assessment at least once in a normal pregnancy, more often in those who have a risk factor. The sonogram can detect abnormal conditions that are manifested in abnormal anatomy in addition to ensuring that the pregnancy is progressing normally.

The advent of amniocentesis, CVS, and ultrasound heralded the development of yet another medical specialty: prenatal surgery. Although the specialty is still new, some corrective surgery is being performed on infants while they are in their intrauterine environment.

Some people are concerned about prenatal testing because of where it might lead. Is mass genetic screening a possibility? **Genetic screening** makes it possible to determine whether persons are predisposed to certain diseases and whether a couple might have the possibility of giving birth to a genetically impaired child. Ethicists have expressed concern about the possibility that the government may make diagnostic amniocentesis and abortion of all defective fetuses mandatory. Others argue against genetic screening, counseling, and amniocentesis because of the stress it places on a couple and because of the guilt placed on the partner carrying the defective gene (when that can be determined). They argue that there are some things we are better off not knowing. Genetic screening also may result in at least one of the partners (often the carrier) seeking voluntary sterilization to prevent pregnancies with less-than-favorable outcomes. Despite concerns, amniocentesis has become a fairly common test offered to mothers who are in an at-risk group. One argument in favor of amniocentesis is that information from the amniocentesis will reduce stress if the news is good; if it is not, the parents will have the option of aborting the pregnancy or preparing for the child's condition.

As genetic screening of a fetus becomes more available, the tests may also be used to identify gender. China, India, and Asia have traditional societies in which sons are highly prized and daughters are an economic liability. As gender identification has become more widespread, the ratio of boys to girls born in those countries is changing as couples choose to abort female fetuses (Bardia, Paul, Kapoor, & Anand, 2004; Miller, 2001). The long-term effects of this on a society are very troubling, as is the low value placed on female children. In the United States and Europe, most providers do not include this as a valid reason for termination of pregnancy.

As a nurse, you may care for clients with varying viewpoints regarding prenatal screening and abortion, and you will also have your own values to consider. Will your values conflict with those of your clients? Are you obligated to advocate for a client when the client's request is squarely in opposition to what you believe to be right? Should you try to sway a woman who is indecisive toward either decision?

■■ COMMUNICATION IN *ACTION*
■■

> **When Others Seek Advice**
>
> Your cousin Edwina, age 37, learned that she was pregnant. Because of her age, it was
> recommended that she have an amniocentesis. Because you are in nursing, she asked
> what you think she should do. You sat with her and said, "It is not uncommon for women
> who become pregnant after age 35 to have an amniocentesis. Perhaps, to help you to
> decide if this is something you want to have done, you should make two lists—one listing
> the advantages to you of having this done and the other listing the disadvantages. This
> might also help you develop a list of questions you would want to discuss with your
> obstetrician."

Sterilization

For years, surgical operations resulting in permanent **sterilization**, such as the removal of reproductive organs to halt the spread of cancer, have been performed for therapeutic purposes.
Although problems may arise for the patient and family as a result of such surgeries, usually they
are resolved without serious ethical debate, depending on the family's religious values, the
patient's body concept, family plans, and personal values.

With increasing frequency, voluntary sterilization has been requested by individuals to terminate reproductive ability. In 1990, 42.1% of all contraceptive users in the United States were
protected by sterilization—29.5% by female sterilization and 12.6% by vasectomy (Law, 1998).
Although sometimes reversible, patients are counseled that these surgical procedures, whether
performed on men or women, should be considered permanent and irreversible. Many people see
it as the prerogative of an individual; others find any type of sterilization in conflict with their
religious and moral beliefs. Sterilization may pose few problems for those who are satisfied with
the number of children they have had or who are adults who have determined that they do not
want to have children. People may decide not to have children for a variety of reasons, including
personal health status, familial genetic disorders, or simply not wishing to parent. Full and
informed consent is required of the person being sterilized; however, health care providers often
prefer to also obtain assent from the spouse if the person is married to avoid subsequent emotional and family problems. Some people question whether a man or woman should be free to
make such a decision without consulting the partner, but doing so is completely legal. A few
states still have laws forbidding voluntary sterilization for contraceptive purposes, but these laws
may not be enforced. In 1935, Oklahoma passed a law that was not struck down by the U. S.
Supreme Court until 1942. It resulted in 13 states establishing laws specifically permitting sterilization of repeat criminals (Lombardo, 2002).

Chemical sterilization, sometimes called chemical castration, refers to providing drugs that
decrease libido, sperm production, and sexual ability. This approach has been used in individuals with a history of repeated rape, who are often incarcerated during the time they are receiving
chemical sterilization. In some instances, this has been recommended or even requested by those
individuals who were convicted of repeated sexual offenses, particularly those against children.
Despite the criminal history, some challenge the ethics of this action.

Because sex crimes are related to power and aggression, and not just to sex drive, this
remains a controversial issue.

Eugenics

Eugenics is a term that has had different meanings in different eras, but is generally thought of as the study of methods to improve inherited human characteristics. The idea of improving the quality of the human race is at least as old as Plato, who wrote on the topic in his *Republic*. The philosophic beliefs of certain 18th-century thinkers about the notion of human perfectibility were central to the eugenics movement, which is thought to have started in the 19th century. Charles Darwin's cousin, Francis Galton, who created the term "eugenics," based his work on Darwin's theory of evolution. When Mendel's law provided a framework for explaining the transmission and distribution of traits from one generation to another, the eugenics movement took hold. Organizations focusing on eugenics were created around the world.

The center of the eugenics movement in the United States was the Eugenics Record Office in Cold Spring Harbor, New York, and its leader was geneticist Charles Davenport. Until the early 1930s, the eugenics movement grew. Eugenicists presented a two-part policy. Positive eugenics encouraged increasing the desirable traits in the population by urging "worthy" couples to procreate. "Superior" couples were encouraged to have more children. Negative eugenics advocated the elimination of unwanted characteristics from the nation by discouraging "unworthy" couples from procreating.

Negative eugenics included a variety of approaches, such as marriage restriction, sterilization, and permanent custody of "defectives." Many eugenicists were actively involved in other issues of the day, including prohibition, birth control, and legislation that would outlaw miscegenation (ie, marriage between two persons of different races, especially between white and black people in the United States). Indiana enacted the first law permitting sterilization on eugenic grounds in 1907; Connecticut followed soon after. In 1914, Harry Laughlin, who worked at the Eugenics Record Office, published a Model Eugenical Sterilization Law that proposed sterilization of the "socially inadequate," a group that included "feebleminded, insane, criminalistic, epileptic, inebriate, diseased, blind, deaf, deformed and dependent," including "orphans, ne'er-do-wells, tramps, the homeless and paupers." By the time the law was published in 1914, 12 states had enacted sterilization laws; by 1937, 31 of the 48 states had compulsory laws. By 1924, approximately 3,000 people in America had been involuntarily sterilized (Lombardo, 2002). By 1979, this number increased to more than 60,000. The Immigration Restriction Act of 1924 also was passed at this time, dramatically limiting the immigration of people from southern and eastern Europe on the grounds that they were "biologically inferior." The trend in recent times has been for states to modify, repeal, or ignore sterilization laws.

The eugenics movement also grew in Germany. In 1933, Hitler sanctioned the Hereditary Health Law, or the Eugenic Sterilization Law, thus ensuring that the "less worthy" members of the Third Reich did not pass on their genes. This action resulted in the sterilization of several hundred thousand people and helped lead to the death camps. By the late 1930s, eugenics in the United States began a tremendous decline. Americans became concerned about the concept of a "master race."

When the eugenic movement was rekindled in the 1960s, it had a different focus—one related to genetic counseling and genetic research. Today, a couple giving birth to a child with a congenital anomaly (or who realize that one of them is carrying a genetic trait that could cause a child to have a congenital anomaly) might voluntarily seek genetic counseling, and possibly opt for the sterilization of one of the partners. Again, this approach offends the religious and moral values of some, but generally it is viewed as the couple's prerogative.

In states that permit sterilization of a person who is not competent to give consent, questions can be raised about who may request sterilization, who may sign the consent, and who must fund the procedure as in the case of a parent requesting surgical sterilization of a mentally retarded adolescent. Some states allow a guardian to make such a decision, but other states specifically prohibit guardians from consenting to sterilization. As the result of a court decision, federal dollars may not be used for sterilization of a person who cannot give personal consent. However, the taxpayer contributes to the cost of institutionalizing people who are not capable of living independently in today's society, and caring for those with severe illnesses and disabilities. The question must be raised regarding the ability of two individuals who are mentally retarded to care for children they may parent. Therefore, it is not only a personal concern, but also society's concern.

The use of prenatal testing to determine characteristics of a child and to abort children without desired characteristics is a matter of concern to those who are skeptical of the use of this high technology. The practice of sex-selective abortion of a female fetus among some Asian cultures that place a high value on the birth of males is another example that presents distress to many. Where should lines be drawn between what is an acceptable variation and what is not? What happens to a society that suggests that those who do not conform to a "norm" should not live?

In Vitro Fertilization

In 1978 in England, much attention focused on the birth of the first child who was conceived in a test tube, a process we refer to as **in vitro fertilization (IVF)**. Due to a blockage in the mother's fallopian tubes, conception in her tubes was impossible. The ovum was removed from the mother, united with the father's sperm in a laboratory setting, and then implanted in the mother's uterus, where it grew to term and was delivered by cesarean section. Today ova for IVF may be gathered from the mother or from a donor, sometimes a family member. IVF and similar procedures (Table 10-2) help many infertile couples.

Many herald this as one of medical science's great advances. For others, it raises many concerns. Several fertilized ova are usually returned to the uterus to ensure that at least one will survive. If more than one implants successfully, it is possible for the mother to have multiple births. Multiple births seldom go full term, resulting in financial and emotional costs. When the number of implanted embryos is too great, consideration is given to aborting several of them to improve the chances of full development for the remaining ones; this creates additional ethical dilemmas for the family.

What should be done with fertilized ova that are not returned to the uterus? (There are an estimated 100,000 to 200,000 such embryos in the United States.) Should they be thrown away? Given to a donor? Used for research? Should tax dollars be used to fund this type of research? If frozen, how long should they remain frozen? What should be done with them at the end of that time? Is discarding the embryos the moral equivalent to having an abortion?

Some couples with embryos to spare have chosen to give the embryos to another infertile couple. The fertilized ovum is implanted into the uterus of the infertile female and often results in a full-term pregnancy. Recently, a $1-million federal program was funded to promote the practice. Although opponents of abortion rights may view this as a better alternative than stem-cell research, in which embryos are destroyed, the moral and legal implications comprise a gray area.

TABLE 10-2	TYPES OF ASSISTED REPRODUCTIVE TECHNIQUES		
NAME	**INITIALS**	**DESCRIPTION**	**FIRST USED WITH HUMANS**
Artificial Insemination: Homologous	AIH	Husband's semen is collected and then deposited at the cervical os or in the wife's uterus by mechanical means.	United States, 1884
Artificial Insemination: Donor	AID	Donor's semen is collected and deposited at the cervical os or in the woman's uterus by mechanical means.	United States, 1884
In Vitro Fertilization	IVF	After heavily medicating the woman with hormones to trigger ovulation, eggs are harvested and fertilized with father's sperm in a laboratory. Several of the resulting embryos are implanted in the mother's uterus.	England, 1978
Gamete Intrafallopian Transfer	GIFT	Eggs and sperm are inserted directly into the woman's fallopian tubes using a laparoscope. Embryos travel to the uterus for implantation.	United States, 1984
Zygote Intrafallopian Transfer	ZIFT	Eggs and sperm are combined in the laboratory. The resulting zygotes are then inserted into the woman's fallopian tubes and travel to the uterus for implantation.	Belgium, 1989
Preimplantation Genetic Diagnosis	PGD	Egg and sperm are united in the laboratory and the embryo is allowed to develop to 4–8 cells. One or two cells are removed and examined for harmful genes. Defective embryos are discarded; healthy ones are implanted in the woman's uterus.	United States, 1991
Immature Egg Harvest	IEH	Similar to IVF, the eggs are harvested from the ovaries while still immature, are cultured in the laboratory, fertilized, and transferred into the woman's uterus.	South Korea, 1991
Intracytoplasmic Sperm Injection	ICSI	In a laboratory setting, a single sperm cell is injected into an egg and then both are implanted in the woman's uterus.	Belgium, 1992

Are these embryos people, property, or their own entities worthy of respect? Like other adoptions, should a home study and background check be completed on the family receiving the fertilized ova? Some believe embryo donation is different, because most state laws presume that a woman who carries and gives birth to a child has earned the right to be a parent.

Other offshoots of IVF allow people who are carrying a severe genetic disease to be assured that their children will not be affected by the condition or carry the defective gene. Fertilized ova are examined for possible disease before being implanted in the uterus; those that are diseased are not implanted.

As wonderful as this may seem, concerns exist regarding what some would call the misuse of IVF. In Italy, a 62-year-old woman became pregnant using donated eggs and IVF before implantation in her uterus. She gave birth by cesarean section in 1994. A 59-year-old woman in England delivered twins by this method (Roan, 1997). A record was set for what is thought to be the oldest woman to give birth to a healthy infant, when a 67 year old Spanish native gave birth via cesarean section to two boys on December 29, 2006 in Spain. The unmarried woman is said to have told doctors in the U. S. fertility clinic where she sought care that she was 55, the clinic's cut off for treating single women ("Spanish Woman," 2006).

In some countries, legislation has been passed to prevent such situations. In January 1994, the French Senate opted to prohibit the use of reproductive options in certain cases (Capron, 1994). One can readily identify some of the difficulties in starting the mothering process at age 62 or 63, not the least of which would be living long enough to see the child reach adulthood. Quality-of-life issues also may be involved. If the mother is 62 when the child is born, she will be 67 or 68 when the child starts school and 75 when the child becomes a teenager.

In recent years another technological advance, **pre-implantation genetic diagnosis (PGD)**, has allowed physicians to pluck a single cell from an eight-celled embryo and determine whether that embryo has specific genetic alleles or the proper number of chromosomes. Using this technique, only healthy embryos can be selected for implantation; thus, some see this as the end of genetically inherited disease. Related to this is the concern that fertilized cells not implanted are usually destroyed—a procedure unacceptable to those who believe life begins when the sperm and ovum unite.

In one instance, parents with a child born with a lethal disease (Fanconi Anemia) wished to use this technique to select an embryo that would be immunocompatible with its older sibling. The cord blood from the newborn child could be harvested and used to treat the sister (Murray, 2003). Because no harm would occur to the child-to-be (only the cord blood would be recovered) and the older sibling would benefit, it was deemed morally permissible.

Other concerns focus on the fear that PGD will be used to make perfect babies (sometimes referred to as "designed babies") or to select embryos of one gender in preference to the other—a practice that is referred to as "family balancing," even when there is not a medical reason (such as hemophilia, Tay-Sachs, or sickle-cell anemia) for such action.

A study was conduced by the Genetics and Public Policy Center and reported in September 2006 of fertility clinics in which PGD was used. Of the 190 that responded to the on-line survey of 415 clinics, 42% reported providing the service for "non-medical sex selection purposes." Twenty-three percent reported initiating the procedure to produce a child who is an immunological match for a seriously ill sibling while ensuring that the baby also will be free of the genetic disease affecting the older sibling (Genetics and Public Policy Center, 2006). Ethicists find such practices troubling.

EXAMPLE

In Vitro Fertilization and Pre-Implantation Genetic Diagnosis

A Louisiana couple decided, after the death of their 3-year-old daughter from Tay-Sachs disease, not to risk having more children. They learned that they both carried one copy of the Tay-Sachs gene, which would result in a one-in-four chance of conceiving a child with the disease. Shortly thereafter, the couple were notified that a procedure had been developed through IVF and PGD, whereby technicians can remove one or two embryonic cells from those fertilized in vitro and test for the harmful gene. This allows only healthy embryos to be transferred back to the woman's uterus. This procedure resulted in the birth of a healthy child for this couple, and one who is not a carrier of Tay-Sachs disease.

Artificial Insemination

Other discussions revolve around the topic of **artificial insemination**, which is the planting of sperm in the woman's body to facilitate conception. Although we tend to think of this as a fairly new procedure, the first time artificial insemination is said to have been used was in Philadelphia in 1884. There are two kinds of artificial insemination: homologous (Artificial Insemination Homologous), in which the husband's sperm is used, and heterologous (Artificial Insemination Donor), in which a donor's sperm is used. Using the husband's sperm is by far the most common and creates the fewest problems legally, ethically, and morally. In some instances, the sperm from the husband and the sperm from a donor with similar physical characteristics are mixed together. As a result, if conception occurs, the couple could easily believe it was the husband's sperm that was accepted by the ovum.

Although some religious groups may have objections, few concerns arise when the husband's sperm is used. That is not true with donor sperm. If the woman is artificially inseminated with donor sperm without the knowledge and consent of her partner, the problems are multiplied. If conception occurs and the child is not biologically that of the husband, can one say that adultery has occurred? Others suggest that the husband should legally adopt the child. To some extent, this helps to clarify issues of inheritance, child support (if the couple should later divorce), and the legal status of the child.

A growing concern relates to the problem of the donor remaining anonymous and depriving children of knowledge of their parental and family background. For example, a child of an anonymous donor does not know whether there are familial disease tendencies or what their ethnic heritage might be. When an anonymous donor has been used for insemination many times in one community the potential exists for children with the same donor father to meet and marry.

Choosing Children Outside of Marriage

The National Center for Health Statistics identified that in 2004 more than 92,000 unmarried American women over the age of 35 gave birth (Hamilton, Ventura, Martin, & Sutton, 2005). Some of these women were in relationships with partners who fathered their children or they were partnered with a woman and used donor insemination. A large number of these women chose to have and raise children independently and saw artificial insemination as a logical solution to their desire to become pregnant.

While some argue against the artificial insemination of any unmarried woman on the basis that the traditional two-parent family composed of a man and woman is in the best interests of all children, others focus on the importance of having wanted children with parents who are thoughtful and committed to their well-being. This is an area in which people are choosing for themselves with little interference by society as a whole.

Recent years also have witnessed the adoption of children by those who are single or unmarried partners of both opposite sexes and the same sex. Such instances do not involve artificial insemination but, rather, a formal adoption process through the courts. Again, some of the same arguments are set forth against this process as against single women bearing children.

Surrogate Mothers

A **surrogate mother** is one who agrees to bear a child conceived through artificial insemination and to relinquish the baby at birth to others for rearing. This practice occurs with increasing frequency and in a variety of relationships and presents unique problems. The following represents one such situation.

Surrogate Mothering Within a Family

A 47-year-old woman agreed to serve as gestational surrogate for her own daughter, whose uterus had been removed because of disease. The daughter's eggs were inseminated with her husband's sperm and the embryos were then implanted in the mother, who gave birth to triplets when she was 48. Thus, this woman became the gestational mother and the genetic grandmother to triplets.

As you can see, these artificial means of reproduction have complicated even the language that we use. The term "biologic" is no longer adequate for making some critical conceptual distinctions. Macklin (1991, p. 6) states, "The techniques of egg retrieval, in vitro fertilization (IVF), and gamete intrafallopian transfer (GIFT), now make it possible for two different women to make a biological contribution to the creation of a new life." Macklin further believes that the woman who contributes her womb during gestation is also a biologic mother. We find terms such as "genetic mother" used to refer to the individual contributing the ovum, and "gestational mother" used to refer to the individual who provides the uterus in which the child develops. In some instances the surrogate mother is both.

Surrogate mothering within a family has caused fewer problems than have been seen when a stranger serves as the surrogate mother. Ethically, carrying a child for a family member out of love and concern and planning to remain in that child's life as part of the family reflect a commitment to the child and respect for the personhood of the child. The majority of serious conflicts have occurred in situations in which a woman has been paid to serve as a surrogate mother. A formal, contractual relationship is usually established. The couple who wishes to have the child agrees to pay all expenses associated with the pregnancy, and to pay the surrogate mother an agreed sum for her time and involvement. The contract must be carefully drawn up because it is illegal in all states to sell a child.

Many ethicists view parenting for pay as a gray ethical area that may fail to value the personhood of the child. This becomes apparent when things do not go as planned. What happens if the child is born with an anomaly, as occurred with a New York couple in 1982 who then refused to take the child? How are these dilemmas to be solved? What is to happen to the child? Who bears the responsibility?

Surrogate Mothering and a Child With an Anomaly

A man paid a woman to be artificially inseminated with his sperm and to carry his child. When the child was born with microcephaly (an unusually small brain), the man rejected the infant, stating that he could not be the father. The surrogate mother and her husband also did not want to accept the responsibility for parenting the child.

Recently, problems associated with surrogate mothering have centered on the surrogate mother's unwillingness to give up the child after birth (Fig. 10-1).

FIGURE 10-1 Complexities arise when surrogate mothers are unwilling to relinquish the infant after birth.

Surrogate Mothering and Custody

Baby M, as the court called her, was born to a surrogate mother who was impregnated with the sperm of a man for whom she agreed to bear the child. This man's wife, a pediatrician, chose not to bear a child because she had multiple sclerosis. Although signed agreements existed, the surrogate mother broke the contract within days of the baby's birth and asked for custody of the child.

Critical Thinking Activity

What safeguards would you recommend regarding IVF, artificial insemination, and surrogate mothers to ensure respect for the human condition? Be specific about how you believe these safeguards would be effective. Reflect on your proposals. Are there any you would change? Discuss your proposals with a classmate.

Sperm Banks

Another aspect of the artificial insemination issue is that of sperm banks. Sperm banks have been established in different parts of the United States for various reasons. Men who want to have a vasectomy may contribute to a sperm bank if there's a chance they may change their minds in the future. Men who will be exposed to high levels of radiation in their work, or during treatment of disease, may wish to have sperm stored because radiation may cause mutation of the genes or result in sterility. This allows them to father children at a later date without concern about the effect on the sperm.

In most cases, the medical community establishes sperm banks so that sperm is available for artificial inseminations. In California, a sperm bank exists that contains only sperm of outstanding and brilliant men. The idea was to create children with this sperm who will be genetically endowed with greater intelligence and creativity. Many find this unacceptable because it brings up the issue of creating a superior race. Concerns also have been raised regarding the possible number of offspring in a single community who might be genetically related without knowing it.

Are there ethical implications for the man who becomes a sperm donor and is the biologic father of a child, but assumes no ethical responsibility for who receives that sperm or for the resulting child and, in fact, has no knowledge regarding the use of his sperm? Some ask how a man can ethically father offspring and have no responsibility for their well-being.

Although there are strict safeguards for privacy of a sperm donor, the donor is known to the woman by a code number. In California, an organization called the Donor Sibling Registry, has been formed for individuals seeking half-siblings who share their donor father. Through identifying the sperm bank and the code number of the father, others with that same father can be identified. This organization (*DonorSiblingRegistry.com*) successfully links individuals who strongly believe that ties of family are strong and want to know these half-siblings. These donor-conceived children seek the same rights to know the identity of their biologic fathers as adoptive children have. This movement may create major changes in the area of donor insemination.

The Right to Genetic Information

All the issues of artificial insemination using donor sperm, surrogate mothering, single parenting, and sperm banks are further complicated by a recent trend toward providing individuals with information regarding their familial background, makeup, and history. You can readily anticipate the problems that would be created if donor sperm were used for insemination. In some instances, no record has been maintained regarding who donated the sperm.

As society emphasizes the importance of the role of fathers and the rights of children to know their family heritage, will anonymous sperm donation remain an option? How many individuals would be willing to donate sperm if it were to necessitate detailed background information? What might be the ultimate legal involvement? On the other hand, what are the rights of the child to know what genetic factors he or she carries? Whose rights should take precedence? Oregon has passed legislation opening birth records for adults adopted as infants to learn of their backgrounds, even though anonymity of the birth mother was guaranteed at the time of the adoption. Will tracking of sperm donors also become a concern in the future?

BIOETHICAL ISSUES CONCERNING DEATH

One of the most important areas of ethical debate revolves around the topic of death and dying. As mentioned earlier, the advent of life-saving procedures and mechanical devices has required redefinition of the term "death," caused us to examine the meaning of "quality of life," and created debates about "death with dignity."

Also associated with the issue of death are several companion concerns that did not exist before the technologic advances that occurred over the past 20 years. Some of these concerns relate to euthanasia, the right to refuse treatment, and the right to die. Other concerns relate to organs retrieved from the dying, because of the scarcity of these medical resources. Generally, the demand for donated organs far exceeds the number of organs available to meet the needs. Superimposed on all these issues is that of informed consent.

Death Defined

Until recently, the most widely accepted definition of death was from *Black's Law Dictionary*, which defines death as the irreversible cessation of the vital functions of respiration, circulation, and pulsation. This traditional view of death served us well until the development of ventilators, pacemakers, and other advances in medical science that made it possible to sustain these functions indefinitely. We also have learned that various parts of the body die at different times. The central nervous system is one of the most vulnerable areas, and brain cells can be irreversibly damaged if deprived of oxygen, while other parts of the body will continue to function.

Newer definitions of death have been built around the concept of human potential—meaning the potential of the human body to interact with the environment and with other people, to respond to stimuli, and to communicate. When these abilities are lacking, there is said to be no potential. Because this potential is directly related to brain function, the method most often used to assess capability is electroencephalography. Brain activity, with few exceptions, is said to be nonexistent when flat electroencephalographic tracings are obtained over a given period, often 48 hours. After this point, the person may be considered dead, although machines may be supporting the vital functions of respiration and circulation. Many institutions now accept this definition of cerebral death and use it as a basis for turning off respirators and stopping other treatments. It is also used as a basis for determining death when there is a desire to recover organs from the patient.

Planning for End-of-Life Issues

Increasing emphasis is being placed on prior planning for end-of-life issues. Identifying futile treatments is one aspect of this process. Another important consideration relates to patient self determination regarding these issues. Many hope that the use of such planning will decrease the ethical dilemmas in end-of-life situations.

Futile Treatments

Futile treatments are those that are evaluated by the health care team, the family, or both as being nonbeneficial or harmful to the patient (Moldow, Bartels, Brunnquell, & Cranford, 2004). For example, when an individual is dying of terminal cancer, treatment for a respiratory infection may be deemed futile because it will not alter the fact that the person is dying and will not restore a satisfactory quality of life. Identifying whether further treatment is futile may be extremely difficult. It is related to many assumptions about quality and quantity of life and, based on the best interests principle, places high demands on the individual responsible for decision making (Bailey, 2004). However, Schneiderman, Jecker, and Jonsen (1996) suggest that if, in the past 100 cases of the same nature, there was no change in the outcome based on the treatment, it can be considered futile. Others take a position that treatment never can be declared futile. In their thinking, the future cannot be predicted accurately, and if there cannot be absolute certainty about the outcome, then futility cannot be clearly identified.

Other problems may arise when futility is declared. To what extent should the patient be involved in the decision making? Does a patient have a right to treatment even if it has been identified as futile? What about cost considerations? Should insurance companies be required to pay for treatment that has been classified as futile? What about Medicare or Medicaid? Should there be differences in decisions based on age or quality of life?

Critical Thinking Activity

> Do you think that factors such as ability to pay, treatment of children or younger adults versus the elderly, the cost of the treatment, and the percentage of time the treatment is effective should be issues considered when deciding whether treatment is futile? Provide a rationale for each answer. What are your biases?

Ethical Issues Surrounding Advance Directives and Living Wills

End-of-life concerns often arise when the patient is unconscious or not able to participate in decision making. This raises the question of obtaining consent. A patient may have left advance directives such as a living will or durable power of attorney for health care, indicating preferences and identifying a substitutionary decision maker (see Chapter 8). If the patient has not done this, the law in each state specifies who may give consent when an individual is incapacitated. Would the ethical answer to this question be the same as the legal answer? Does everyone involved agree with the decision maker? Are there others who should be involved? Even the existence of advance directives does not eliminate the ethical concerns surrounding some of these situations.

In an attempt to gain greater control over the area of dying, many people now complete a variety of documents that have been titled advance directives. An **advance directive** is a legal document that indicates the wishes of an individual with regard to end-of-life issues.

In December 1991, the federal **Patient Self-Determination Act (PSDA)** went into effect. Passed by Congress in 1990, this legislation requires that all Medicare and Medicaid providers inform patients on admission of their right to refuse treatment. The intent of this legislation was to enhance an individual's control over medical treatment decisions by promoting the use of advance directives (see Chapter 8). The entire process has not been without its problems. The time of admission to a health care facility is often filled with anxiety, making it almost impossible to consider such matters. Most patients indicate that they prefer to discuss these matters with a doctor or nurse who is involved in their care, but in some settings, this task may be delegated to an admissions clerk.

In 1991, the American Nurses Association (ANA) issued *A Position Statement on Nursing and the Patient Self-Determination Act*. The ANA believes that nurses should play a primary role in implementation of PSDA, should facilitate informed decision making for patients, and should occupy a critical role in education, research, patient care, and advocacy (ANA, 1991).

A living will is a document that has been widely used as an advance directive (Fig. 10-2). In a **living will**, people identify what measures to include in care if they become terminally ill. The living will is often used to request that no extraordinary measures be implemented, although it can be used to indicate a preference that all possible actions should be taken. Although the

TO MY FAMILY, MY PHYSICIAN, MY CLERGYMAN, MY LAWYER

If the time comes when I can no longer take part in decisions for my own future, let this statement stand as the testament of my wishes:

If there is no reasonable expectation of my recovery from physical or mental disability, I, _____
request that I be allowed to die and not be kept alive by artificial means or heroic measures. Death is as much a reality as birth, growth, maturity and old age—it is the one certainty. I do not fear death as much as I fear the indignity of deterioration, dependence and hopeless pain. I ask that medication be mercifully administered to me for terminal suffering even if it hastens the moment of death.

This request is made after careful consideration. Although this document is not legally binding, you who care for me will, I hope, feel morally bound to follow its mandate. I recognize that it places a heavy burden of responsibility upon you, and it is with the intention of sharing that responsibility and of mitigating any feelings of guilt that this statement is made.

Signed _____

Date _____

Witnessed by:

_____

_____

FIGURE 10-2   The living will.

living will is not necessarily considered legal consent, it does reveal the desires of the person receiving care. It may help families to make decisions more confidently.

Another approach being used with increasing frequency is the signing of a **durable power of attorney for health care**. In this type of an agreement, an individual (referred to as the principal) may designate another person to have the power and authority to make health care decisions for the principal should the principal be unable to make those decisions. Durable power of attorney documents may simply name the decision maker, or may contain detailed preferences of the individual. The durable power of attorney goes into effect after the principal is no longer capable of making decisions, but not until this point is reached. These forms can be purchased in most office supply stores and become valid if signed before a notary public. However, it is best to consult an attorney before entering into such an arrangement (Fig. 10-3).

Euthanasia

Euthanasia, meaning "good death," may be classified as either negative or positive. The word, as it is generally applied, refers to the act or method of causing death painlessly so as to end suffering.

[PLEASE NOTE: This is a standardized legal document that may not be appropriate for a person in your particular situation. You should consult your attorney before signing this or any legal document.]

DURABLE POWER OF ATTORNEY FOR HEALTH CARE DECISIONS

I, _____ as principal, domiciled and residing in the State of Washington, hereby enter into a Durable Power of Attorney to provide informed consent for health care decisions pursuant to the laws of the State of Washington.

1. **Designation.** I designate _____ , if living, able and willing to serve, as my attorney-in-fact. If he or she is not living, able and willing to so serve, then I designate _____ , if living, able and willing to serve, as my attorney-in-fact.

2. **Powers.** The attorney-in-fact, as fiduciary, shall have all powers to provide informed consent for health care decisions on principal's behalf.

3. **Effectiveness.** This power of attorney shall become effective upon the disability or incompetence of the principal. Disability shall include the inability to make health care decisions effectively for reasons such as mental illness, mental deficiency, physical illness or disability, advanced age, chronic use of drugs, chronic intoxication, confinement, detention by a foreign power or disappearance. Disability may be evidenced by a written statement of a qualified physician regularly attending me. Incompetence may be established by a finding of a Court having jurisdiction over me.

4. **Duration.** This power of attorney shall remain in effect to the extent permitted by RCW 11.94 notwithstanding any uncertainty as to whether the principal is dead or alive.

5. **Revocation.** This power of attorney may be revoked in writing by notice mailed or delivered to my attorney-in-fact, and by recording the written instrument of revocation in the office of recorder or auditor of the county of my residence.

6. **Termination.**

   a. By Appointment of Guardian. The appointment of a guardian of the person of the principal terminates this power of attorney. The appointment of a guardian of the property only does not terminate this power of attorney.
   b. By Death of Principal. The death of the principal shall be deemed to revoke this power of attorney upon proof of death being received by the attorney-in-fact.

FIGURE 10-3   Durable power of attorney.

7. **Reliance.** The designated and acting attorney-in-fact and all persons dealing with the attorney-in-fact shall be entitled to rely upon this power of attorney so long as neither the attorney-in-fact nor person with whom they were dealing at the time of any act taken pursuant to this power of attorney had received actual knowledge or actual notice of the revocation or termination of the power of attorney by death or otherwise, and any action so taken, unless otherwise invalid or unenforceable, shall be binding on the heirs, devisees, legatees, or personal representatives of the principal.

8. **Indemnity.** The estate of the principal shall hold harmless and indemnify the attorney-in-fact from all liability for acts done in good faith and not in fraud on behalf of the principal.

9. **Applicable Law.** The laws of the State of Washington shall govern this power of attorney.

10. **Execution.** This power of attorney is signed on this _____ day of _____, 200 _____ , to become effective as provided in Paragraph 3.

Signature: _____
Print name: _____

STATE OF WASHINGTON)
) ss.
COUNTY OF KING   )

I certify that I know or have satisfactory evidence that _____ is the person who appeared before me, and said person acknowledged that _____he signed this instrument and acknowledged it to be h_____ free and voluntary act for the uses and purposes mentioned in the instrument.

FIGURE 10-3   (continued)

Negative Euthanasia

Negative, or passive, euthanasia refers to a situation in which no extraordinary or heroic measures are undertaken to sustain life. The concept of negative euthanasia has resulted in what are called "no codes" (also designated as DNR—do not resuscitate) in hospital environments. In these situations, hospital personnel do not attempt to revive or bring back to life persons whose vital processes have ceased to function on their own.

It is difficult to describe what constitutes extraordinary measures, and to determine on whom they should or should not be used. Is it one thing to defibrillate a 39-year-old man who is admitted to an emergency department suffering from an acute heart attack, and quite another to defibrillate a 95-year-old man whose body is riddled with terminal cancer and whose heart has stopped? Often, people who are involved in giving medical and emergency care develop an almost automatic response to life-saving procedures and have difficulty accepting dying as an inevitable part of the life process. This is particularly true when emergency personnel receive a 911 call and rush to the home of an individual who has requested that no extraordinary measures be taken to sustain life. Often cardiopulmonary resuscitation or other such efforts are started before the rescuers know of the request.

It is difficult to know when it is permissible to omit certain life-supporting efforts, or which efforts should be omitted. If the 95-year-old man who is dying of terminal cancer were also to develop pneumonia, should his physician prescribe antibiotics? This brings us to the distinction between stopping a particular life-supporting treatment or machine, and withdrawing treatment or not starting a procedure in the first place—that is, withholding treatment.

Some ethicists do not differentiate between withholding treatment in the first place and withdrawing treatment once it has been determined to be inappropriate or futile. They would see both as having the same position in terms of right and wrong. Those who support negative euthanasia support both withholding and stopping treatment. The general public often sees these as separate issues and may support withholding treatment, while not supporting the termination of treatment once it has begun. Increasingly, the legal system has supported withdrawing treatment that is determined to be futile. A landmark case in 2005 was that of Terri Schiavo, who was in a persistent vegetative state following a heart stoppage due to a chemical imbalance that occurred 5 years earlier. Her husband wanted her feeding tube removed, which would ultimately result in her death; her parents wanted the treatment continued. Finally the courts decided that the husband was the legal decision maker. He then had the feeding tube removed. Many ethicists supported this decision, arguing that Terri Schiavo's medical condition represented **fatal pathology**, pathology brought about by a disease process that can never be cured and is going to ultimately lead to the individual's death (Harvey, 2005). After her death, an autopsy did show that the areas of the brain that would have allowed any cognitive processes were destroyed.

Positive Euthanasia

Positive, or active, euthanasia occurs in a situation in which the physician prescribes, supplies, or administers an agent that results in death. On some occasions, a physician prescribes strong narcotics for a terminally ill patient and requests that the medication be given frequently enough to keep the patient comfortable. Nurses often are reluctant to administer a medication that they realize has a potentially fatal effect when given in that dosage. In such cases, the ethical intent of the action is often considered. Medications given for the comfort of the dying patient may be ethically justifiable even if they hasten death to some extent. This is based on the ethical concept of double effect, in which the acceptable effect (such as pain relief) is the purpose of the medication and the secondary effect (such as depressing respiration) is not the intended effect. This is not legally considered positive euthanasia. When nurses have difficulty with this issue, a patient conference with an oncology specialist or with a nurse skilled in the area of death and dying can help the staff to clarify values and deal with individual feelings.

Right-to-Die Issues

Right-to-die issues are gaining much more attention than in previous years. Kass (1993, p. 37) identifies four reasons for such a right to be asserted:

1. Fear of prolongation of dying due to medical interventions; hence, a right to refuse treatment or hospitalization, even if death occurs as a result
2. Fear of living too long, without fatal illness to carry one off; hence, a right to assisted suicide
3. Fear of the degradations of senility and dependence; hence, a right to death with dignity
4. Fear of loss of control; hence, a right to choose the time and manner of one's death

A great deal of controversy surrounds the issue of maintaining the lives of persons considered to be in a persistent vegetative state (PVS). Some of the issues that arise are the patient's rights, the family's wishes, and the cost to society. In most cases, the problems emerge when the life of a family member is being maintained through support measures that might be considered extraordinary.

In 1991, St. Francis-St. George Hospital in Cincinnati was sued in one of the first cases of its kind. The suit charged that the nurses should not have resuscitated an 82-year-old man when he suffered a heart attack. In so doing they disregarded the DNR status of the patient ("Hospital sued for 'wrongful life,'" 1991).

Withholding Treatment

Withholding treatment could be considered negative euthanasia. The following example is a historic case that occurred in 1963.

EXAMPLE

Withholding Treatment

A couple on the East Coast gave birth to a premature infant who was diagnosed as having Down syndrome, with the added complication of an intestinal blockage. The intestinal blockage could have been corrected by surgery with minimal risk; without surgery, the child could not be fed and would die. The Down syndrome, however, would have resulted in some degree of permanent mental retardation. The severity of the retardation could not be determined at birth, but would range from very low mentality to borderline subnormal intelligence. The parents, who had two normal children at home, believed that it would be unfair to those children to raise a child with Down syndrome and refused permission for the corrective operation on the intestinal blockage. Although it was an option, the hospital staff did not seek a court order to override the decision. The staff believed it was unlikely that a court would sustain an order to operate on the child against the parents' wishes, because the child had a known mental handicap and would be a burden to the parents financially and emotionally, and perhaps a burden to society. The child was put in a side room and was allowed to die, a process that took 11 days. When confronted with the possibility of giving medication to hasten the infant's death, both doctors and nurses were convinced that it was clearly illegal (Gustafson, 1973).

The situation above stimulates both ethical and legal questions. Would the approach have been the same if the infant had not been mentally retarded? Would the staff have been guilty of murder if the infant had been given medication to hasten death? If a court decision to proceed with the surgery had been requested and granted, who would have been responsible for the costs incurred? What are the rights of the child? Who advocates for those rights if the child is unable to do so?

Withdrawing Treatment

In some instances, a family may seek to have extraordinary life-support measures discontinued, (ie, **withdrawing treatment**). A landmark case is that of Karen Quinlan.

EXAMPLE

Withdrawing Treatment 1

Karen Quinlan was a young woman left in a vegetative state after suffering severe brain damage from chemical abuse that involved both drugs and alcohol. She was placed on a respirator, and her physicians believed that she would live only a short time if it were removed. Her parents requested that the respirator be discontinued, but because she continued to manifest a minor amount of brain activity, their request was refused. After previous petitions to the Supreme Court of New Jersey had been rejected, the courts ruled on March 31, 1976, that her parents could exercise her privacy right on her behalf, and the respirator was discontinued. Much to everyone's surprise, Karen continued to live after the respirator was stopped, although she never emerged from her comatose condition; she died in 1986 (Ascension Health, 2005).

This case represents a situation in which treatment was withdrawn even though the individual was not considered immediately terminal. Such cases represent difficult decisions for all involved and evoke legal, moral, and ethical questions in almost all instances. A similar case that attracted much attention was that of Nancy Cruzan.

EXAMPLE

Withdrawing Treatment 2

In March 1988, Joe and Joyce Cruzan requested through the Jasper County, Missouri, Probate Court that they be allowed to remove the gastrostomy tube that kept their daughter Nancy alive. Nancy had been in a PVS since an automobile accident in January 1983. Although the request was granted, Missouri's attorney general appealed the decision, asking for a clear precedent from a higher court. In June 1990, the U.S. Supreme Court effectively denied the request in asking for "clear and convincing" evidence of the patient's view. In reaching this point, a fine line was drawn between initially withholding medical treatment and later withdrawing it. In Missouri, once the family gives initial consent for treatment, they forfeit all power to undo that consent or to stop treatment. No other state has such a law (Colby, 1990). Treatment can be stopped in only two ways: if it can be demonstrated that it causes pain, or if the patient left behind clear and convincing evidence of his or her wishes prior to incompetency. The first was not an option because of Nancy Cruzan's PVS. Therefore, her parents presented a state court with testimony from her physician and three friends that Nancy would not have wished to continue existing with irreversible brain damage. The Circuit Court judge ruled that this met the test, and Nancy's feeding tube was removed on December 14, 1990. She died December 26th (Ascension Health, 2005).

Other cases have reached the headlines (such as the Terri Schiavo case mentioned earlier) as individuals and families have striven to have more voice in determining issues related to the right to die. In all cases, much conflict exists in the arguments put forth by those supporting the right-to-die and right-to-life movements. In 1990, Congress took a major step regarding this issue by passing the PSDA. Increasingly, states have supported the right of appropriate substitutionary decision makers to both refuse and withdraw medical treatment. Medical treatments include tube feeding, oxygen, medications, and intravenous fluids.

Of particular concern to nurses are their own feelings when a decision is reached to remove life-supporting measures, whether the measures are tube feedings or ventilators. Strong emotional attachments often form between the nurse and patient, even when the patient is in a vegetative state. Nurses who have worked to preserve the patient's dignity have great difficulty letting go. In some instances, patients are transferred to other facilities to die in an environment where the nurses are not so emotionally involved with the patient.

Positions on Withholding and Withdrawing Treatment

Several organizations and groups have issued guidelines for their members and others who would find them useful, with regard to the issue of withholding or withdrawing treatment. Key to all of these guidelines is whether the patient is legally competent (able to make decisions for him- or herself) or incompetent (in need of someone else to make those decisions). Table 10-3 outlines the date, organization, and major tenets of some of those positions.

Assisted Suicide

Assisted suicide involves helping another end his or her life. In June 1997, the U.S. Supreme Court rendered a decision on physician-assisted suicide (PAS). This decision took the position that there was no constitutionally protected right to PAS on behalf of terminally ill patients. In November 1997, the residents of Oregon supported PAS when they voted not to repeal the Death with Dignity citizen's initiative previously passed in 1994, despite the Supreme Court decision. Legal debate regarding its continuance is ongoing, with appeals, denials, and more appeals at increasingly higher court levels.

The Oregon Department of Human Services is required to monitor and collect data regarding the Death with Dignity Act. The seventh annual report indicates that in 2004, 40 physicians wrote a total of 60 prescriptions for lethal doses of medication, a decrease of eight from the previous year. Thirty-five of the 2004 prescription recipients died after ingesting the medication, 13 died from their illnesses, and 12 were alive on December 31, 2004. In addition, two patients receiving prescriptions during 2003 died in 2004 after ingesting their medication, thus giving a total of 37 deaths during 2004. Patients who used PAS in 2004 were similar to those in previous years, with the exception that they tended to be younger (median age 64, compared to 70). Males and females were equally likely to take advantage of PAS, with divorced and never-married individuals twice as likely to select this alternative. A higher education level was strongly associated with the use of PAS, with those with a baccalaureate or higher degree 8.3 times more likely to use PAS (Seventh Annual Report, 2005). Students wishing to further pursue information regarding this topic are encouraged to read the annual report at *http://oregon.gov/DHS/ph/pas/doc/year7.pdf*.

In April 2001, The Netherlands became the first nation to fully legalize euthanasia, a process that was 3 years in the making.

TABLE 10-3	POSITIONS ON WITHHOLDING AND WITHDRAWING TREATMENT	
	ORGANIZATION	**POSITION**
1983	President's Commission Report— *Deciding to Forego Life-sustaining Treatment*	Focused on the ethical, medical, and legal issues in treatment decisions. Distinguished between withholding (not starting) and withdrawing (stopping after it started) treatment without making a moral distinction between the two. Suggested that withholding may require more justification because the positive effects would not be known.
1986	American Medical Association— *Statement on Withholding or Withdrawing Life-prolonging Medical Treatment*	Stated that life-prolonging medical treatment and artificially or technologically maintained respiration, nutrition, and hydration, could be withheld from a patient in an irreversible coma even if death was not imminent (Fry, 1990).
1986	Office of Technology Assessment of the U.S. Congress—*Life-sustaining Technologies and the Elderly*	Issued the results of its study on the use of life-sustaining technologies on the elderly. Report noted that the most controversial of the technologies was that of nutritional support. Identified that the most troublesome aspect of nutritional support is whether it is intravenous feeding and hydration or a tube feeding (Fry, 1990).
1987	Hasting's Center—*Guidelines on the Termination of Life-sustaining Treatment*	Provided clear definitions of key terms and a general guideline for making decisions regarding treatment. Viewed nutrition and hydration as medical interventions, much as other life-sustaining measures. Placed emphasis on the patient's ability to make decisions and required case-by-case assessment (Fry, 1990).
1988	American Nurses Association— *Guidelines on Withdrawing or Withholding Food and Fluid*	Indicated that there were few instances under which it would be permissible for nurses to withdraw food or fluid from their patients. No distinction was made between withdrawing and withholding (ANA, 1988).
1992	American Nurses Association— *Position Statement on Foregoing Medically Provided Nutrition and Hydration*	Stated that the decision to withhold medically provided nutrition and hydration should be made by the patient or surrogate with the health care team. The nurse continues to provide expert and compassionate care to patients who are no longer receiving medically provided nutrition and hydration. Distinguished between medically provided nutrition and hydration and the provision of food and water (ANA, 1992).

The ANA has developed a position statement in which it states that the nurse should not participate in assisted suicide. Such an act is viewed as a violation of the Code for Nurses (see Chapter 9). It is the position of the ANA that the challenge for nurses should not be in legalizing assisted suicide. Rather, the role of the nurse should be directed toward reversing the despair and pain experienced in the last stages of life, and in fulfilling the obligation to provide competent, comprehensive, and compassionate end-of-life care (ANA, 1994).

The activities of a retired Michigan pathologist, Jack Kevorkian, who is alleged to have assisted patients in their suicide, received much media attention in the 1990's. Although eluding criminal charges for a number of years, in March 1999, Dr. Kevorkian was convicted of second-degree murder and the delivery of a controlled substance after CBS televised a video showing him administering lethal drugs. The first case in which he was charged but not convicted involved an Oregon woman with Alzheimer's disease. Dr. Kevorkian's release from prison in 2007 brought renewed attention to the issue of assisted suicide.

The Right to Refuse Treatment

The **right to refuse treatment** is an issue closely aligned with the right to die. However, it carries special implications that require separate consideration. Although we discussed some of the parameters of this issue in the previous section on the right to die, other aspects can create even bigger problems for the nurse. The moral, if not legal, precedent for refusing treatment occurred in 1971.

EXAMPLE

Refusing Treatment
Carmen Martinez was dying of hemolytic anemia, a disease that destroys the body's red blood cells. Her life could be maintained by transfusions, but her veins were such that a cut-down (a surgical opening made into the vein—the technology available at that time) was necessary to accomplish the transfusions. Finally, Martinez pleaded to have the cut-downs stopped and to be "tortured" no more. The physician, fearful of being charged with aiding in her suicide, asked for a court decision. The court ruled that Martinez was not competent to make such a decision and appointed her daughter as her guardian. When the daughter also asked that no more cut-downs be performed, the judge honored the daughter's request. He decided that although Martinez did not have the right to commit suicide, she did have the "right not to be tortured." She died the next day (Veatch, 1976).

People working in the health care field often are confronted with such dilemmas. Cases such as one in which a patient refuses to have a leg amputated, even though not having the surgery undoubtedly will result in death, often will make the news. The right to refuse treatment can take on additional implications when the patient, by refusing one type of treatment, is essentially demanding alternative medical management. Our support of the right to refuse treatment is based on a basic belief in and respect for the autonomy of the patient. When the refusal of medical intervention means that the individual is no longer a patient, it is known as a "negative right simpliciter" by bioethicists. In these cases, the patient's physician need only do nothing, as in cases in which patients discharge themselves from the hospital.

When the patient refuses treatment but does not withdraw from the role of being the patient, the matter becomes more complex. An example would be the patient who refuses to have a gangrenous toe surgically removed and demands to have it treated otherwise. These are referred to as positive rights. In the case of a patient with a gangrenous toe, one form of treatment may be more accepted than another, but both may be successful. A case illustrating this right occurred in 1993 in Chicago and attracted national attention.

EXAMPLE

Refusing a Form of Treatment 1
A Pentecostal Christian mother refused to have a cesarean section when physicians recommended the procedure because her fetus was being deprived of oxygen and would die if delivered vaginally. The courts upheld the patient's right to refuse the surgery. She later gave birth to an apparently healthy boy ("Baby born", December 31, 1993).

When children are involved, it is even more newsworthy, and again points out that there is as yet no consensus about when minors should be allowed to refuse treatment.

EXAMPLE

Refusing a Form of Treatment 2
In November 1994, 16-year-old Billy Best made national news when he ran away from home to avoid another 5 months of chemotherapy and radiation. Suffering from Hodgkin's disease, the high school junior was experiencing nausea, aching, and fatigue, as well as hair loss, from the treatment. He stated, ". . . I could not stand going to the hospital every week. I feel like the medicine is killing me instead of helping me." (Dorning, 1994).

Often in such cases, the parents refuse to have the treatment started, many times because of religious beliefs. The courts usually become involved in reaching a decision. The following 1952 case in Illinois is typical.

EXAMPLE

Refusing a Form of Treatment 3
Eight-day-old Cheryl suffered from erythroblastosis fetalis (Rh incompatibility). Her parents, who were Jehovah's Witnesses, refused to authorize the administration of blood necessary to save her life. The judge in the case ruled that Cheryl was a neglected dependent and overrode the parent's refusal. In such instances, the child is usually made a temporary ward of the court and legal documents are attached to the record authorizing the needed treatment. Such court decisions usually have been based on the premise that the right to freedom of religion does not give parents the right to risk the lives of their children or to make martyrs of them (Veatch, 1976).

When time is not a factor, the court may recommend that treatment be delayed until the child is 15 or 16 years old and can make a decision as an older minor. Other judges will rule just the opposite, deciding that it is cruel to place the burden of the decision on this older minor.

Situations like those that have been cited are always difficult for the people involved. Because nurses have the most contact with patients, they must examine their own feelings and attitudes. Nurses must recognize that patients also have the right to attitudes and beliefs. If a nurse decides that his or her feelings are so strong that they might interfere with the ability to give compassionate care, it would be wise to ask to be assigned to other patients (Fig. 10-4).

BIOETHICAL CONCERNS RELATED TO SUSTAINING QUALITY OF LIFE

With the increase in technology, bioethical concerns have expanded significantly to include issues related to maintaining or sustaining the quality of life through such procedures as organ transplantation, xenotransplantation, and stem cell research. We cannot discuss all of these in detail, but will provide an overview of the topics. We encourage those interested in this area to explore the topic further on the related Web sites listed at the end of the chapter.

FIGURE 10-4   People working in the health care field are frequently confronted with the dilemma of patients who may wish to refuse treatment.

Organ and Tissue Transplantation

Developments in the area of organ transplantation have created several issues deserving consideration. **Organ transplantation** is the process by which an entire organ is removed and replaced by a corresponding part. Tissue transplantation involves the use of tissues such as skin, bone, cartilage, and corneas. Developments in the area of organ and tissue transplantation have created several issues deserving consideration. Transplants can be done using tissue from one's own body; this is called an autograft. Transplantation using organs or tissue from a donor's body is known as homograft or allograft; it might involve organs such as the kidney, liver, pancreas, and heart, and tissues such as cornea, bone, or skin of another individual. Some organs (eg, the heart) must be transplanted immediately or the tissue will die. Others, such as the kidney can be stored for short periods. Many tissues, such as bone and skin, may be preserved for long periods of time. Organs require matching between the donor and the recipient, while most tissues do not. According to the United Network for Organ Sharing (UNOS), there are more than 90,500 individuals waiting for an organ transplant (UNOS, 2005).

Initially, the replacement for a diseased organ was obtained from a donor who had died. More recently, organs have been received from living donors. Between January and August 2005, UNOS listed 4,681 UNOS living donors, compared with 5,115 deceased donors. Transplants performed during this period numbered 18,995 (UNOS, 2005).

The supply of organs that can be used for transplantation has not been able to keep up with the demand. This concern resulted in the former Secretary of the Department of Health and Human Services (HHS), Tommy Thompson, announcing his "Gift of Life Donation Initiative" in April 2001. This initiative contained five major elements to encourage organ donation. Among these was a model donor card, which included provisions for designating whether all organs and tissues may be donated, as well as lines for signatures by two witnesses (Fig. 10-5).

FIGURE 10-5   Organ/tissue donor card.

This card may be downloaded from the Internet site *www.organdonor.gov/SecInitiative.htm.* Concomitantly, the number of bills in Congress that address the issue of organ transplant continues to grow.

Concerns About Procurement

Organ procurement refers to all the activities involved in obtaining donated organs. The idea of consent becomes important when we talk about organ transplantation and procurement. It is preferable to have the consent obtained from the donor. This has been facilitated in many states by the Uniform Anatomical Gift Act, which was drafted by a committee of the National Conference of the Commissions of Uniform State Laws in July 1968, and now by the Model Donor Card. People who are willing to donate parts of their bodies after death may indicate the desire to do so in a will or other written documents, or by carrying a donor's card. Many states also provide a space on the driver's license where individuals can authorize permission for organ donations.

The next-of-kin also must grant permission for the removal of organs and tissues after death. However, the time factor is crucial; the deaths are often accidental, and the relatives are often so emotionally distressed that the process of obtaining permission may be uncomfortable. Hospitals that receive Medicare funds are mandated to have required request policies in place. Typically, they have developed a procurement team that has received special preparation related to requesting organ donations. These are persons skilled in recognizing the stress being felt by the family and experienced in providing information that will be important to them. A growing number of hospitals are designating a nurse as transplantation coordinator to facilitate this process.

An interesting and controversial case related to obtaining necessary material for transplantation occurred in California in 1990.

EXAMPLE

Transplantation

An 18-year-old woman, an only child, was diagnosed as having chronic myelogenous leukemia. Although this form of leukemia responds favorably to bone marrow transplants, no compatible donor could be found after testing the girl's family and contacting the National Marrow Donor Program. In desperation, the parents decided to have another child with the hope that the new baby would have genetically matching tissue type. This required that the father have a vasectomy reversed and that the mother, age 43, go through another pregnancy, which resulted in a cesarean section. The baby proved a good match and was able to provide donor tissue for her sister (Kolata, 1991).

The case drew considerable attention, as medical ethicists voiced concern about creating one child to save another. Citing Immanuel Kant, a renown philosopher (see chapter 9), they argued that the baby was conceived, not as an end in itself, but for utilitarian purposes. Some medical ethicists argued in favor of the rights of the individuals involved, saying that it is not the concern of biomedical ethicists to intrude into matters affecting private citizens, especially when that intrusion approaches "intruding into a couple's bedroom." Still others say that striking cases must be brought before the public because an obligation to inform society exists.

Children and young people experience the most critical need for human organs. This has caused us to challenge previous decisions. A good example is that raised when considering organs removed from an anencephalic infant. An anencephalic infant is one born with only enough brain to support such vital functions as heartbeat and respiration. It has been estimated that about 60% of these infants are stillborn, and of those born alive, only about 5% will live longer than 3 days. Because anencephaly affects only the brain, other organs can be used for transplantation if the infant is kept alive on a respirator until an organ recipient is located. This challenges our definitions of death. How can current definitions of "brain" death be applied to a condition in which there is no brain as we normally recognize it?

Artificial Organs

Problems also arise regarding organ transplantations, especially because more people need organs than there are organs available. The skill of modern technology has resulted in the development and implantation of artificial organs such as the heart. Such technologic advances once were viewed as science fiction. As a result, historic cases such as the implantation of an artificial heart in Barney Clark in 1982 received a great deal of publicity. Over the years, the use of artificial organs has not proven effective for long-term use, but artificial organs have made it possible for individuals to live with the hope that a transplantable organ will become available. Over the past few years, a heart-assist has been developed and used to provide the patient's heart a rest and an opportunity to heal, in some instances reducing the need for heart transplantation. Work and research to develop better organs continues, and recipients are living longer, although the promise is far less than that with donated organs. The use of artificial joints, heart valves, and other prostheses continues to grow and to be successful.

Minority Groups and Organ Donation

Another issue that has emerged is that of minority differences regarding organ donation. Of the persons awaiting an organ for transplantation, approximately 50% represent minorities (Minority Organ and Tissue Transplant Education Program [MOTTEP], 2005). The risk of end-stage renal disease for African-Americans and Native Americans is three to four times higher than for the white population (Kasiske et al., 1991). Although minority groups donate in proportion to their population distribution, minority organ donations lag behind those from the white population, with more than 67% of cadaver donations coming from whites, 18% from African-Americans, 9.5% from Hispanics, and 3% from Asians (Organ Procurement and Transplantation Network, 2005). One of the reasons this presents a concern is that minorities form more than half of the kidney transplant waiting list. More minority donors are needed to increase the chances that a well-matched organ will be available to minorities awaiting transplants.

Several factors may affect reticence of minorities to donate organs. Some groups have identified religious beliefs and cultural customs as forbidding organ donation, although no major Western religion prohibits organ donation. Religious objection often stems from the high value attached to keeping the body intact ("Body and soul," 2002). African-Americans listed distrust of the medical community, fear of premature death, and racism as major barriers. Hispanics experienced language barriers and identified the importance of having the entire extended family involved in all decision making regarding donations. Puerto Ricans verbalized denial of death and fear of mutilation of the body as critical factors. Barriers to organ donation in Asian-American cultures included the belief that the body should remain intact to the grave and lack of respect during the handling of the body after death. Although Native Americans are theoretically supportive of organ donations, their rate of donation is low, probably due to lack of knowledge (Wheeler & Cheung, 1996). Although no single approach to organ donation fits all groups, efforts to decrease barriers to donation are being instituted.

MOTTEP has 15 sites across the country focused on educating the minority community in an effort to increase the number of minority donors and transplant recipients. MOTTEP represents African-American, Hispanic/Latino, Native American, Asian, Pacific Island, and Alaskan Native populations. It includes a health promotion and disease prevention component designed to reduce the incidence of conditions that can lead to organ failure. It can be reached at the Web site *www.nationalmottep.org.*

Critical Thinking Activity

Have you signed an organ donation card? If not, discuss the reasons why you have chosen not to do so. If you have, discuss the reasons why you have. Is there a possibility you will change your mind? Why or why not? What solutions can you suggest to help the nation deal with the shortage of organs needed for transplantation?

Concerns About Allocation

How will we determine who receives donated organs? Does elitism exist in their distribution—that is, does a rich individual have a better chance to receive an organ than someone who is poor? Medicaid and most insurance policies refuse to pay for the cost of many organ transplants, although Medicare usually covers the costs of corneal transplants and kidney transplants. Transplants are expensive procedures, often running into several hundreds of thousands of dollars. If money is required up-front, as it sometimes is, where can the needy person procure such funds? Other questions involve both donor and recipient. Should the donor or the donor's family have the right to say who will receive the organ? How does one get onto the list for an organ, and how can that need be made known? What about selling a healthy organ, such as a kidney? Current law makes it a crime to sell body parts.

Much has been written about the problem of selecting recipients for organ transplantation when the number of applicants exceeds the number of available organs. Many criteria have been suggested, and as one might anticipate, these criteria have arguments both pro and con; the criterion requiring medical acceptability is probably the only exception. Many transplants require that compatibility exist in the tissue and blood type of donor and recipient. In response to this problem, some centers transplant organs that are less well matched. This results in a higher rejection rate, but as immunosuppression improves, this is less marked than it was formerly. Other centers do not believe it appropriate to give a much-needed organ to a person whose body would have a high potential for rejection.

The criterion of the recipient's social worth is probably one of the hardest to defend, although it was used in the Pacific Northwest in the early 1960s to decide who should be allowed to live by kidney dialysis. Social worth, including past and future potential, was considered, and even such factors as church membership and participation in community endeavors were considered.

Some suggest a form of random selection, once the criterion of medical acceptability has been met. This could be either a natural random selection of the first-come, first-served variety, or an artificial selection process such as a lottery. A criticism of this method is that it removes rational decision making from the process.

We offer no suggestions to solve this problem but merely demonstrate the difficulty it presents. Even the issue of who should serve on the decision-making committee can be problematic. The potential for personal biases is a big concern.

In an effort to gather donations and disseminate information about individuals who need various organs, an Organ Procurement Program was started in Pittsburgh, Pennsylvania. This program was established to facilitate the matching of donor with recipient and to provide a central listing agency for those in need of transplants. Today, organ procurement agencies are located in all regions of the country. These groups carry out many activities related to organ procurement, including establishing groups for individuals who have received donated organs and their families, publishing newsletters, developing educational materials, increasing public awareness of the need for organs, and serving as a clearinghouse for organ procurement and matching. They are connected through the federally funded UNOS.

Concerns About Individual Property Rights

Concern for an individual's **property rights** regarding human tissues also has attracted attention. Developments in biotechnology allow profit-oriented companies to use human tissue to generate lucrative products, such as drugs, diagnostic tests, and other medically related materials. The modern legal system has consistently held that no property rights are attached to the human body (Swain & Marusyk, 1990).

Human Body Property Rights

In 1990, a Seattle man sued the University of California, two researchers, and two biotechnology and drug companies, because in 1976, he had sought treatment for hairy cell leukemia and subsequently had his spleen removed (which is the standard treatment). It was later discovered that the removed spleen contained unique blood cells that produced a rare blood protein, which then was used experimentally in the treatment of certain cancers and possibly AIDS. The patient was never told that his cells had great potential value, although he was brought from Seattle to Los Angeles frequently for blood and other tests. His cells were then developed into a self-perpetuating cell line to mass-produce the rare blood protein. The patient's suit claimed that the defendants wrongfully converted to their own use his personal property (ie, the blood cells) and that this was done without his consent (*Moore v. Regents of the University of California*, 1990).

Xenotransplantation

Xenotransplantation refers to the practice of using animal organs, cells, and tissues for transplantation into human beings. Some scientists believe that having a reliable supply of organs from pigs or other animals could solve the great shortage from human donors. It is in the stage of experimentation around the world.

Xenotransplantation usually involves organs or tissues from pigs and nonhuman primates. One case receiving national publicity was that of an AIDS patient in San Francisco who received the transplant of baboon bone marrow to bolster his weakening immune system. Since 1906, some 55 animal-to-human whole organ transplants have been attempted; none was successful (Fano, Cohen, Cramer, Greek, & Kaufman, 1999). Cases that received particular attention were the 1984 transplant of a baboon heart into Baby Fae (who died 20 days later) and the 1992 transplant of a baboon liver into a 35-year-old man (who also died).

In addition to the obvious problems associated with immune system rejection, of particular concern to some is the possibility of transmitting serious animal viruses and other microbes, so-called zoonotic diseases, to people. Fano and associates (1999) report more than 20 known, potentially lethal viruses that can be transmitted from nonhuman primates to humans. This has prompted pigs to become the donor of choice, and has led to attempts to alter pigs genetically so that tissues would be more adaptable to transplantation. In August 2002, a British biotechnology company announced the creation of the first so-called "double knock-out" pigs, genetically engineered to lack both copies of a gene that causes rejection (Cloning for xenotransplantation, 2005).

Concerns in England over the communicability of bovine spongiform encephalopathy through the ingestion of meat from ill animals has prompted the discussion of the potential for all animal organs to transmit diseases that would appear only years later. Even raising animals in a sterile environment has its limitations, because it is now being discovered that some diseases are transmitted from mother to fetus in utero. Some groups in England are urging that the xenotransplantation project be abandoned and that research into xenotransplantation be stopped because of the social cost and because of on-going suffering of animals inherent in such an approach.

In September 1996, the federal government proposed strict safeguards to provide protection. Representatives from the Food and Drug Administration (FDA), the Centers for Disease Control and Prevention, and the National Institutes of Health (NIH) developed the guidelines. The guidelines urged that patients and their families be fully informed of potential risks, and further required that any planned procedure be thoroughly screened and approved by a series of local institutional review boards, and by the FDA. The recommendations also require that transplants take place at a clinical center associated with an accredited biology and microbiology laboratory.

The Human Genome Project

A **genome** may be defined as the entire DNA in an organism, including the genes that carry information for making the proteins required by all organisms. These proteins determine such things as how the organism looks, how well its body metabolizes food and fights infection, and sometimes even how it behaves. Genomes have been studied for many reasons, including disease prevention, determination of the effects of radiation and chemicals on living species, and more recently, genetic therapy. DNA is made up of four similar chemicals called bases and abbreviated A, T, C, and G, and are repeated millions or billions of times throughout a genome. The order of As, Ts, Cs, and Gs is important because it underlies all of life's diversity, including whether an organism is human or of another species.

The **Human Genome Project (HGP)** was first proposed by Nobel prize-winning virologist Renato Dulbecco in 1986. Coordinated by the Department of Energy and the NIH, the project started in October 1990 and involved at least 18 countries in the international effort. The project was planned to last for 15 years; effective resource and technologic advances have accelerated the expected completion date to 2003. Several types of genome maps have already been completed, and a working draft of the entire human genome sequence was announced in June 2000 and the analysis was published in February 2001.

The goals of the project were to do the following:

- Identify all the approximate 30,000 genes in human DNA
- Determine the sequences of the 3 billion chemical base pairs that make up human DNA
- Store this information in databases
- Improve tools for data analysis
- Transfer related technologies to the private sector
- Address the ethical, legal, and social issues that may arise from the project (Human Genome Project Information, 2002).

An additional part of the HGP includes parallel studies being carried out on several nonhuman organisms, including the *Escherichia coli* bacterium, the fruit fly, and the laboratory mouse. Studying nonhuman organisms' sequences can lead to an understanding of their natural capabilities, which can be applied toward solving challenges in health care, energy sources, agriculture, and environmental cleanup.

Knowledge about the effects of DNA variations among individuals can lead to new ways to diagnose, treat, and someday prevent the thousands of disorders that affect us. This could unlock a plethora of bioethical concerns. Once this technology has been developed, where does it end? How is the information handled regarding issues of privacy and confidentiality? What is the impact if third-party payers gain access to the information? What might be the advantages and disadvantages of knowing the diseases to which you are susceptible? With whom should that information be shared? What would be the effects of manipulating stature, intelligence, or sex?

Does this project represent eugenics revisited? Who among health care providers will provide access to patients? Will the responsibility fall to the family practitioner, who will most likely be the first contact for those with a genetic disorder? How prepared are family practitioners for this type of care delivery?

More information regarding these issues can be obtained from the Web site, *www. ornl.gov/hgmis.*

Gene Therapy

An estimated 4,000 disease genes have been identified that reside with the genome. Identification and isolation of defective genes, and their replacement with functional genes (gene therapy), could result in the elimination of diseases that have plagued society for generations. Several significant conditions currently under study are cystic fibrosis, Huntington's disease, myotonic dystrophy, gout, and adult polycystic kidney disease.

In the genetic lexicon, the gene is a length of DNA that codes for a particular protein. The average human gene is a little more than 1,000 nucleotides long and, in many inherited disorders, only one or a few of these nucleotides is incorrect. For example, in sickle cell anemia, a single nucleotide causes the structural deformity that results in the characteristically distorted shape of the sickled red blood cell that prohibits the cell from adequately carrying oxygen to the body's organs and tissues. Seventy percent of the cases of cystic fibrosis may be due to the deletion of three nucleotides (Wine, 2006). Theoretically, **gene therapy** can take the form of somatic (body) or germ (egg and sperm) cells. Somatic gene therapy results in the recipient's genome being changed but the change is not passed down to the next generation. With germline gene therapy, not being actively investigated at the present time, the goal is to pass the change on to offspring. The genetic testing of eggs and the sex selection of embryos mentioned earlier in this chapter are a matter of selection; no cells are altered or changed.

Decisions on clinical applications of gene-therapy approaches are under the oversight of the federal government. The Office of Recombinant DNA Activities Advisory Committee evaluates protocols and makes suggestions for approval to the director of the NIH. Gene therapy policy conferences and gene therapy conferences designed to provide public information regarding research progress have been instituted.

To date, gene therapy is primarily experimental and has produced far more failures than successes. Positive results in mice do not necessarily promise positive outcomes for humans. Many of the basic problems with gene therapies have not been worked out. Finding a mechanism to insert the new gene into the body needs to be found. Scientists need a better understanding of how genes function. The problems associated with multigene disorders must be solved. Questions regarding the repair of genes versus the replacement of genes are yet to be answered. The high costs associated with this new technology present another concern. However, gene therapy offers a wide array of possibilities and undoubtedly will gain momentum in the near future.

Stem Cell Research

A **stem cell** is a special kind of cell that is able to renew itself and give rise to specialized cell types. These cells, unlike most other cells in the body, such as those of the heart or skin, are not committed to conduct a specific function. The cell remains uncommitted until it receives a signal to develop into a specialized cell. Scientists are now looking at a type of stem cell that is called "pluripotent," because those cells have the potential to develop almost all of the more than 200 different known cell types. These cells, which originate from early human embryos, may have the potential to generate replacement cells for a wide array of tissues and organs, including the heart, the pancreas, and the nervous system (DHHS, 2001). Thus, they offer hope for patients with diseases such as Parkinson's disease, diabetes, chronic heart disease, end-stage kidney disease, liver failure, cancer, multiple sclerosis, Alzheimer's disease and those with spinal cord injuries. Many of these conditions shorten lives, and no effective treatments have been found. In heart disease, for example, numerous heart cells are destroyed and the body cannot replace them. Doctors hope to inject patients with stem cells and then signal them to grow into new heart tissue thus engineering human organs (Weiss, 2005).

As progress was being made with tissue from early embryos, research was being conducted on adult stem cells, the only type to have been tested in humans. An adult stem cell is an undifferentiated cell that occurs in a differentiated tissue, renews itself, and becomes specialized. These adult stem cells are capable of making identical copies of themselves for the lifetime of the organisms. Sources of these cells include bone marrow, blood, the cornea and retina of the eye, the brain, skeletal muscle, dental pulp, the liver, skin, the lining of the gastrointestinal tract, and the pancreas. They are rare and often difficult to identify (DHHS, 2001). Because of this, the stem cells of human embryos are considered by some to be more desirable.

However, to retrieve the needed cells, the embryo is destroyed because the needed cells lie in the center of the blastocyst, a cluster of about 150 cells that has developed about 1 week after the ova is fertilized by a sperm. Thus, we find ourselves with the same ethical question raised earlier in this chapter: Do blastocysts equal human life? Many people, including antiabortionists, believe the answer is yes. Others find the benefits to be so great they tend to view the blastocysts as potentially human but not quite there yet.

Because research of this nature needs federal funding and approval to move forward, stem cell debate is a national issue. In August 2001, President Bush announced that federal funds could be used to study embryonic stem cells, but that taxpayer money could be used only to study the stem cells lines that met certain specific criteria in regard to "(1) the informed consent of the donors; (2) from excess embryos created solely for reproductive purposes; and (3) without any financial inducements to the donors." At the time of this decision, the White House announced that approximately 60 usable lines would be identified as available. But since that time, some of these lines have been found to lack the ability to continue to replicate, and fewer than two dozen appear to meet these requirements. Researchers wishing to work with other lines could do so only with private funding (Weiss, 2005). The concern is that the existing lines of embryonic stem cells are too limited to achieve the desired research objectives and that adult stem cells do not have the same potential. Those who want to see this research pushed forward want to use some of the thousands of leftover frozen embryos in storage at fertility clinics. The frozen embryos were created by couples who intended to use them for in-vitro fertilizations. The embryos can be left frozen for potential later use, donated to someone else who wants to have a child, or thrown out. Some privately funded research and research in other countries may continue with embryonic stem cells.

This is another issue to which there are no easy answers. However, as powerful and well-known individuals such as Nancy Reagan, Michael J. Fox, and Mary Tyler Moore push for legislation to support research, we can be assured of hearing more about the retrieval of embryonic stem cells for research.

Critical Thinking Activity

Given the arguments for and against stem cell research, what position would you take? Why do you hold this position? What are your biases? Discuss your position with someone who holds the opposite point of view. What are that person's strongest arguments?

OTHER BIOETHICAL ISSUES

Although our discussion cannot be exhaustive of the topic, certain events occur frequently enough in the health care delivery system that we would be remiss in not mentioning them.

Truth-Telling and Health Care Providers

The issue of whether to tell a patient something may not carry the emotional and bioethical impact that one experiences with concerns such as euthanasia, but it is often encountered in the health care environment. Although informed consent has forced a more straightforward approach between physician and client, the problem of having the patient fully understand the outcome of care still exists (see Chapter 9). Sometimes the question about telling the client the expected outcome of care results from a request made by a close relative, but most of the time it results from the persistence of past medical practices.

In such instances, the physician operates in a paternalistic role in relation to the client. Under this model of care, the locus of decision making is moved away from the client and resides with the physician. "Benefit and do no harm to the patient" is the dictum often cited as the ethical basis for this approach. It rationalizes that complete knowledge of his or her condition would place greater stress on the client. More recent discussions of medical ethics explore the rights of clients, particularly their right to make their own medical decisions. These discussions emphasize that in our pluralistic society, which also has fostered medical specialization to keep up with advances in knowledge and technology, physicians may be unable to perceive the best interests of their clients and to act accordingly.

Physicians do not agree on how much information should be provided to patients regarding their conditions. We usually experience a major controversy relating to this issue when a client has a terminal diagnosis such as cancer. Physicians may feel concerned that sharing bad news will result in unhappiness, anxiety, depression, and fear, and that the client suffering from a terminal illness will give up. In some cultures, such as Japan, this approach is widely considered appropriate, and both physicians and families strongly believe that those who are ill should be protected from bad news.

Physicians who argue the other side of the issue state that there exists a common moral obligation to tell the truth. They believe that the anxiety of not knowing the accurate diagnosis is at least as great as knowing the truth, especially if the truth is shared in a humane manner. These physicians also argue that one needs to have control over one's life and, if the news is bad, to have time to get personal affairs in order.

Regulations regarding informed consent and more aggressive treatment for all life-threatening conditions have minimized situations in which patients are not provided full knowledge of their condition. However, these situations still arise. Sometimes care providers are challenged as to the best ethical and legal approach when a family is from a different cultural background and strongly disagrees with giving full information to a patient.

Thus far, we have discussed situations in which information regarding a terminal illness may be shared with the client and family. At least one other circumstance that involves telling the truth is worth mentioning, although many examples could be included. One that we often see in the obstetric area of the hospital deals with sharing information with the parents of a newborn who is critically ill or who has a malformation. Sometimes physicians want to spare the mother unpleasant news until she is stronger. This occurs frequently enough for obstetric nurses to have labeled it "spare-the-mother syndrome." In some instances, the physician may want to delay giving information until suspicions can be validated. If the doctor is waiting for the return of laboratory tests to confirm suspicions of genetic abnormalities, several days may be required. If good communication exists between nurse and physician, so that the nurse is well informed, the nurse can provide emotional support and meet the client's need for information.

Another situation in which sharing the truth may be a concern occurs when a parent is diagnosed with a degenerative disease (such as Huntington's disease) for which there is no cure and that is an autosomal dominant trait (ie, there is a 50% chance that an offspring also will develop the disease). Should this information be shared with the offspring? Because there is also a 50% chance they will not develop the condition, is it wrong to compromise the individual's good life with bad news? What if the parent does not want the information shared and the physician believes it should be? Is ignorance bliss? What about the right to make informed choices and decisions (Taub, 2000)?

Although to tell or not to tell (or to delay telling) is a problem that exists between client and physician, nurses often become involved. Because the nurse is in contact with the client for a more extended time, he or she may be put on the spot by the client's questions. The nurse may feel that hedging on a response compromises the ethics of nursing practice. In such instances, a conference, whether formal or impromptu, that would involve the physician, nurses, and other appropriate members of the health team, may help everyone deal with the situation. The nurse who is a novice in the health care system should realize that anyone may initiate a client care conference, although appropriate channels of communication should be followed in organizing it.

The question of whether to tell has been applied to another issue in the health care delivery system in recent years. That controversy pits the rights to privacy of the individual who is HIV positive against society's right to be protected. Dr. Cary Savitch, who has treated AIDS patients since 1981, advocates universal testing. Dr. Savitch (1996, p. 140) states,

> Controlling the epidemic is the only means to limit needless suffering and death. Controlling the epidemic will not come at the hands of a vaccine or miracle drug. Controlling the epidemic requires prevention. Prevention requires knowing who is communicable. Knowing who is communicable requires universal testing.

Many express concerns about privacy and confidentiality. If universal testing for AIDS is mandated, what would be next? Others argue that if health care providers exercise proper precautions, little danger exists. Still others would find the cost of universal testing too great to make it realistic. There is no agreement among health care providers, activists, civil libertarians, and all concerned citizens regarding this issue, and the controversy is certain to continue.

Ethical Concerns and Behavior Control

Many people experience extreme discomfort when contemplating research into human behavior and **behavior control**. Although it may be one thing to work with atoms, molecules, and genes, it seems quite another to look at the science of human behavior.

Some of the problem seems to center around the fact that people define "acceptable behavior" in different and sometimes conflicting ways. When is behavior deviant? When is the client mentally ill? An excellent example is that of homosexuality, which the American Psychiatric Association at one time listed as a mental illness. Although many people may not approve of homosexuality, they would not classify all homosexuals as being mentally ill. Increasingly, society looks on sexual orientation as a personal matter.

The world has benefited from the work of many people whose behavior might not be looked upon as normal. Van Gogh cut off his ear; Tchaikovsky had terrible periods of depression; Beethoven was known for his uncontrollable rages. Some have suggested that Florence Nightingale's flights into fantasy could better be described as neurosis. Should this behavior have been changed? If so, by what methods?

We now can change behavior by several methods. Certainly one of the most common methods in which nurses will be involved is the administration of pharmacologic agents. Psychotropics are now one of the largest classifications of drugs in the United States. Many of these such as antianxiety agents and antidepressants are prescribed for people who wish to modify their feelings and behaviors. Other chemicals, such as alcohol, marijuana, cocaine, and lysergic acid diethylamide (commonly known as LSD), also change mood and/or behavior. Some of these are considered socially acceptable, whereas others are not. Some are socially acceptable to some people or to some cultures yet unacceptable to others.

Electroconvulsive therapy (ECT), known earlier as electric shock therapy (EST), has been used for years to treat severe depression. Although antidepressant drugs are more commonly used today, ECT is still used in many areas of the country for depression that does not respond to drugs. Opponents of this form of therapy, who see it as inhumane, are becoming an organized political force. Proponents point out that with the current safeguards, it can be an effective therapy.

Psychosurgery—for example, frontal lobotomy (portrayed in *One Flew Over the Cuckoo's Nest*)—was used in the 1930s. This is undoubtedly one of the most criticized treatment modalities because of its effect on the person. It is rarely used today, although another type of brain surgery is now being suggested for obsessive–compulsive disorder.

Psychotherapy can change other behaviors. Techniques include verbal and nonverbal communication between the client and the therapist. Although psychotherapy requires considerable time, it is widely used.

When are any of these methods justified? Who makes the decision? What behavior is beyond the realm of acceptability? Who determines this? How does behavior control mesh with our beliefs about the autonomy of the individual or with concepts of self respect and dignity? The issues of power and coercion pose a concern at this point. Problems related to involuntary commitment have moved this from the arena of ethics to that of legal determinants.

Halleck (1981, p. 268) has defined behavior control as treatment "imposed on or offered to the patient that, to a large extent, is designed to satisfy the wishes of others. Such treatment may lead to the patient's behaving in a manner which satisfies his community or his society." Certainly the need to control the behavior of others when such behavior is illegal or a threat to individuals or the community is not difficult to justify. But not all treatment is directed toward behavior that is illegal or threatens society—homelessness or depression might be examples. Halleck goes on to point out that the question of behavior control versus individual rights has become more critical because newer drugs and new behavior therapy (such as aversive therapy and desensitization) make it possible to change specific behavior more rapidly and effectively. Traditional psychotherapy, which works slowly, offers the patient time in which to contemplate the change and reject it if it is unacceptable.

Dworkin (1981, p. 278) has proposed a set of guidelines that preserve autonomy in behavior control, as briefly stated here. Although these guidelines are almost 20 years old, they continue to be recognized for the direction they provide.

- We should favor those methods of influencing behavior that support the self-respect and dignity of those who are being influenced.
- Methods of influence that destroy or decrease a person's ability to think rationally and in his or her own interest should not be used.
- Methods of influence that fundamentally affect the personal identity of the person should not be used.
- Methods of influence that deceive or keep relevant facts from the person should not be used.
- Modes of influence that are not physically intrusive are preferable to those that are (eg, drugs, psychosurgery, and electricity).
- A person should be able to resist the method of influence if he or she so desires, and changes of behavior that are reversible are preferable to those that are not.
- Methods that work through the cognitive and affective structure of a person are preferable to those that short-circuit his beliefs and desires and cause him to be passively receptive to the will of others.

Critical Thinking Activity

Review the guidelines for ethical treatment of psychiatric conditions. Which do you believe are the strongest, and why? Are there any that you question; if so, why? Are there any that you think should be added?

Rationing of Health Care

Perhaps no issue in health care will receive more attention in the next few decades than the **rationing of health care**. Technology has allowed people to live longer. New treatment modalities have become more expensive. Dollars do not exist within our current social system to make all forms of health care available to all who wish to receive it. What should be treated and what should not? Who should receive the treatment and who should not? Should age be a factor? Mental status? Ability to contribute to society?

Rationing is restricting the availability of some desired commodity to limited allotments. Most consider rationing to be a planned, thoughtful approach to a limited supply. Some would argue that we currently ration health care by restricting its availability to those with the financial means to pay, although none would argue that this is a carefully planned approach.

Some states have begun to address these issues. In 1989, the Oregon legislature passed several statutes that, among other things, created a process to establish health care priorities so that Medicaid and state-encouraged private coverage could provide the most cost effective and beneficial forms of care for the largest number of persons. Explicit in this legislation was the involvement of the public in the process of building consensus on the values to be used to guide health resource allocation decisions. Oregon has continued to lead the nation in health care reform, especially at the consumer involvement level.

In Vermont, a statewide public education and discussion project was initiated to explore public attitudes and values that underlie health care and the public's priorities in the allocation of health resources. The project focused on the need for individuals to make known their preferences with regard to personal treatment.

In New Jersey, a Citizens' Committee on Biomedical Ethics has taken the position that citizens have the right and responsibility to insist that their preferences and values influence the development of health care policies and the allocation of medical resources. They have launched a community health program to clarify the ethical and social issues surrounding the provision of health care in that state.

Other states are following these examples. Citizens are being asked to make informed decisions regarding health care. As a nurse, you have a vital role to play in the sharing of information regarding the delivery of health services. It is critical for you to anticipate some of the questions you may be asked and to analyze your own values (Fig. 10-6).

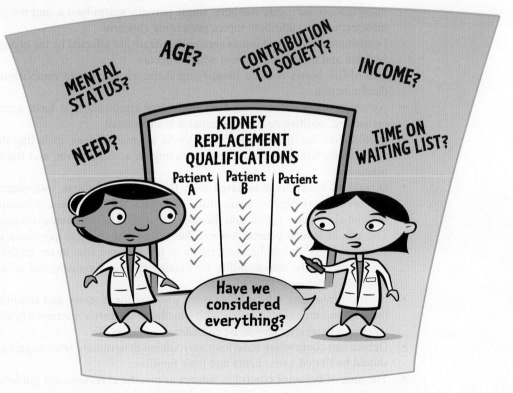

FIGURE 10-6 It is critical that you analyze your own values.

Critical Thinking Activity

What do you see as the major issues regarding the rationing of health care? Develop a list of the major health conditions for which you believe care should be funded. Identify those that should receive partial funding. List those that you believe should not be funded. Give a rationale for placing the various conditions on one of the three lists.

Key Concepts

- Bioethics is the study of ethical issues that result from technologic and scientific advances, especially in biology and medicine. The number of bioethical issues surrounding the delivery of health care is growing.
- Many bioethical issues can be divided into two major categories: those related to the beginning of life and those related to the end of life.
- Family planning (and the associated concern regarding age of consent) is one issue related to the beginning of life. Personal preferences and religious beliefs are critical determinants, and nurses should be prepared to meet the needs of all clients without imposing their personal values on clients.
- Abortion, amniocentesis, chorionic villus sampling, prenatal diagnosis, genetic screening, sterilization, the concept of eugenics, in vitro fertilization, artificial insemination, surrogate mothers, single parents, sperm banks, and the right to genetic information are additional topics presenting concerns.
- Fundamental bioethical issues concerning death are affected by the changing definition of death and the decision about when it occurs.
- End-of-life issues include identifying futile treatment and establishing patient self determination.
- Although many courts, based on individual circumstances, have accepted negative euthanasia, positive euthanasia remains controversial.
- Surrounding the discussion of right-to-die are many issues, including those related to withholding treatment, withdrawing treatment, assisted death, and the right to refuse treatment.
- Bioethical concerns associated with the process of organ transplantation include procurement of organs, availability of organs for minorities, allocation of organs, individual property rights, and the appropriateness of xenotransplantations.
- The area of human genetic research has raised many ethical questions, including how this knowledge should be used, rights to privacy, and who in the health care delivery system carries the responsibility for making testing, diagnosis, and cost-effective care available to patients.
- Stem cell research, which holds great promise for diseases and conditions for which there is no cure, is also laden with bioethical concerns, particularly those related to whether a blastocyst should be considered a human life.
- Debate and controversy have long surrounded determining what degree of information should be shared with clients and their families.
- The area of behavior control is subject to bioethical review, and guidelines have been established to preserve autonomy in behavior control.

- Rationing of health care commands major attention now. Many states have begun to establish citizen committees to respond to this concern.

Relevant Web Sites

American Journal of Bioethics, Bioethics Network: *www.bioethics.net*

Boston College, Nursing Ethics Network: *www.bc.edu/nursingethics*

Georgetown University, The Kennedy Institute of Ethics, National Reference Center for Bioethics Literature: *http://bioethics.georgetown.edu/nrc/index.htm*

International Society of Nurses in Genetics: *www.isong.org*

Johns Hopkins University, Bioethics Institute: *www.med.jhu.edu/bioethics_institute*

Medical College of Wisconsin, Center for the Study of Bioethics, Bioethics Online Service: *www.mcw.edu/bioethics*

Midwest Bioethics Center: *www.midbio.org*

National Catholic Bioethics Center: *www.ncbcenter.org*

National Coalition for Health Profession Education in Genetics: *www.nchpeg.org*

President's Council on Bioethics: *www.bioethics.gov*

Understanding Gene Testing: *www.accessexcellence.org/AE/AEPC/NIH*

United Network for Organ Sharing Transplantation Information Site: *www.unos.org*

University of British Columbia, W. Maurice Young Centre for Applied Ethics: *www.ethics.ubc.ca*

University of Southern California, Pacific Center for Health Policy and Ethics: *http://lawweb.usc.edu/Pacific_Center*

References

Alexander, S. (1962). They decide who lives, who dies. *Life. 53*, 102–125.

American Nurses Association. (1988). *Guidelines on withdrawing or withholding food and fluid*. Washington, DC: Author.

American Nurses Association. (1991). *Position statement on nursing and the Patient Self-Determination Act*. Washington, DC: Author.

American Nurses Association. (1992). *Position statement on foregoing medically provided nutrition and hydration*. Washington, DC: Author.

American Nurses Association. (1994). *Position statement on assisted suicide*. Washington, DC: Author.

Ascension Health. (2005). *Health care ethics: Cruzan, Nancy*. [On-line]. *www.ascensionhealth.org/ethics/public/cases/case 11.asp*. Accessed September 21, 2006.

Ascension Health. (2005). *Health care ethics: Quinlan, Karen Ann*. [On-line]. *www.ascensionhealth.org/ethics/public/cases/case21.asp*. Accessed September 17, 2006.

Bailey, S. (2004, January). The concept of futility in health care decision making. *Nursing Ethics, 11*(1), 77–83.

Bardia, A., Paul, E., Kapoor, S. K., & Anand, K. (2004 July–August). Declining sex ratio: Role of society, technology and government regulation in Faridabad district, Haryana. *National Medical Journal of India, 17*(4), 181–183.

Blackmun, H. (1981). Majority opinion in Roe vs Wade. In T. A. Mappes & J. S. Zembaty, *Biomedical ethics* (2nd ed.) (pp. 478–482). New York: McGraw-Hill.

Bush, G. W. (2001, August 9). Fact sheet: Embryonic stem cell research. [On-line]. *www.whitehouse.gov/news/releases/2001/08/20010809-1.html*. Accessed November 26, 2005.

Capron, A. M. (1994). Grandma? No, I'm the mother! *Hastings Center Report, 24*(2), 24–25.

Centers for Medicare & Medicaid Services. (2004). *National health care expenditures projections: 2002–2013*. [On-line]. *www.cms.hhs.gov/statistics/nhe/projections-2003/highlights.asp*. Accessed November 21, 2005.

Cloning for xenotransplantation. (2005). Bioethics.net. [On-line]. *http://bioethics.net/resources/index.php?sid=990418196&t=sub_pages&cat=16*. Accessed November 25, 2005.

Colby, W. H. (1990). Missouri stands alone. *Hastings Center Report, 20*(5), 5–6.

Congressional Kidney Caucus. (2002). *25 facts about organ donation and transplantation.* [On-line]. *www.house.gov/mcdermott/kidneycaucus/25facts.html.* Accessed September 24, 2006.

Department of Health and Human Services. (2001, June). *Stem cells: Scientific progress and future research directions, executive summary.* [On-line]. *www.nih.gov/new/stemcell/scireport.htm.* Accessed October 12, 2002.

Dorning, M. (1994, November 13). Teen-ager's refusal of treatment stirs debate. *San Diego Union Tribune*, p. A8.

Dworkin, G. (1981). Autonomy and behavior control. In T. A. Mappes & J. S. Zembaty, *Biomedical Ethics* (2nd ed.) (pp. 273–280). New York: McGraw-Hill.

Fano, A., Cohen, M. J., Cramer, M., Greek, R., & Kaufman, S. R. (1999). Of pigs, primates, and plagues: A layperson's guide to the problems with animal-to-human organ transplants. [On-line]. *www.mrmcmed.org/pigs.html.* Accessed December 22, 1999.

Fry, S. T. (1990). New ANA guidelines on withdrawing or withholding food and fluid from patients. In C. A. Lindeman & M. McAthie: *Readings: Nursing trends and issues* (pp. 499–507). Springhouse, PA: Springhouse.

Genetics and Public Policy Center. (2006). *Center study probes preimplantation genetic diagnosis.* [On-line]. *www.dnapolicy.org/news.release.php?action=detail&pressrelease_id=58.* Accessed September 21, 2006.

Gustafson, J. J. (1973, summer). Mongolism, parental desires, and the right to life. *Perspectives in Biology and Medicine*, p. 529.

Halleck, S. L. (1981). Legal and ethical aspects of behavior control. In T. A. Mappes & J. S. Zembaty, *Biomedical Ethics* (2nd ed.) (pp. 267–273). New York: McGraw-Hill.

Hamilton, B. E., Ventura, S. J., Martin, J. A., & Sutton, P. D. (2005, October 28). Preliminary births for 2004. Health E-stats. [On-line]. *www.cdc.gov/nchs/products/pubs/pubd/hestats/prelim_births/prelim_births04.htm.* Accessed December 3, 2005.

Harvey, J. C. (2005). Exploring the Terri Schiavo ethics meltdown. *Ethics Scoreboard.* [On-line]. *www.ethicsscoreboard.com/list/schiavo2.html.* Accessed March 29, 2005.

Hospital sued for 'wrongful life.' (1991). *American Journal of Nursing, 91*(5), 111.

Human Genome Project Information. About the Human Genome Project (2002). [On-line]. *www.ornl.gov/hgmis/project/about/html.* Accessed September 14, 2006.

Jacobson, J. (2005). AJN reports: When providing care is a moral issue. *American Journal of Nursing, 105*(10), 27–28.

Kasiske, B. L., Neylan, J. F., Riggio, R. R., Danovich, G. M., Kahana, L. Alexander, S., & White, M. G. (1991). The effect of race on access and outcome in transplantation. *New England Journal of Medicine, 324*, 302–307.

Kass, L. R. (1993). Is there a right to die? *Hastings Center Report, 23*(1), 34–43.

Killion, S. W., & Dempski, K. M. (2000). *Legal and ethical issues.* Thorofare, NJ: Slack, Inc.

Kolata, G. (1991, June 4). More babies being born to be donors of tissue. *The New York Times.* [On-line]. *http://query.nytimes.com/gst/fullpage.html?sec=health&res=9D0CE6d7163BF937A35755CDA967958260.* Accessed September 17, 2006.

Law, S. A. (1998). Sex discrimination and insurance for contraception. [On-line]. *www.crlp.org/pub_art_sylvialaw.html.* Accessed November 22, 2005.

Legal age of consent [table]. (2005). [On-line]. *www.ageofconsent.com.* Accessed November 21, 2005.

Lombardo, P. (2002). *Eugenics sterilization laws.* [On-line]. *www.eugenicsarchive.org/html/eugenics/essay_8.html.* Accessed September 14, 2006.

Macklin, R. (1991). Artificial means of reproduction and our understanding of the family. *Hastings Center Report, 21*(1), 5–11.

Miller, B. D. (2001). Female-selective abortion in Asia: patterns, policies, and debates. *American Anthropology, 103*(4), 1083–1095.

Minority Organ and Tissue Transplant Education Program. (2005). *Statistics: MOTTEP facts and figures.* [On-line]. *www.nationalmottep.org.ststs.html.* Accessed

Moldow, G., Bartels, D., Brunnquell, D., & Cranford, R. (2004). Why address medical futility now? *Minnesota Medicine.* [On-line]. *http://mmaonline.net/publications/MNMed2004/Moldow.html.* Accessed September 14, 2006.

Moore v. Regents of the University of California. (1990). 793P. 2d 479. 487–493

Murray, T. H. (2003, spring). New challenges in bioethics: Medicine, technology, and justice. *Phi Kappa Phi Forum, 63*(2), 39–43.

National Coalition on Health Care. (2005). *Health insurance cost: Facts on the cost of health care.* [On-line]. *www.nchc.org/facts/cost.shtml.* Accessed November 21, 2005.

Nuland, S. B. (1996). An epidemic of discovery. *Time Magazine Special Issue*, Fall, pp. 8–13.

Organ Procurement and Transplantation Network. (2005). *Transplants by donor types.* [On-line]. *www.optn.org/latestData/rptData.asp.* Accessed November 25, 2005.

Pellegrino, E. D. (2005). *The President's Council on Bioethics.* [On-line]. *www.bioethics.gov.* Accessed November 22, 2005.

Pilbeam, S. P. (1998). *Mechanical ventilation: Physiological and clinical applications* (3rd ed.). St. Louis, MO: Mosby.

Roan, S. (1997, April 24). Woman gives birth at 63: Ethical questions raised. *Los Angeles Times*, A1, A31.

Roberts, P. (1993, December 31). "Baby born into Path of Legal Storm". Chicago Tribune, p. 1.

Roe v. Wade, 410 U.S. 113 (1973).

Savitch, C. (1996). *The nutcracker is already dancing: The HIVs and the HIV-nots.* Ventura, CA: Teague House Press.

Schneiderman, L. F., Jecker, N., & Jonsen, A. (1996, October 15). Medical futility: Response to critiques. *Annals of Internal Medicine. Vol 125*(8), 669–674. [On-line].*www.annals.org/cgi/content/full/125/8/669.* Accessed September 14, 2006.

Seventh Annual Report on Oregon's Death with Dignity Act. (2005). Department of Health Services. [On-line]. *http://oregon.gov/DHS/ph/pas/docs/year7.pdf.* Accessed November 25, 2005.

Spanish Woman 67, becomes a mother with birth of twins. (2006, December 31). *Los Angeles Times*, A4.

Swain, M. S., & Marusyk, R. W. (1990). An alternative to property rights in human tissue. *Hastings Center Report, 20*(5), 12–15.

Taub, S. (2000). To tell or not to tell? *The American Journal of Bioethics.* [On-line]. *www.bioethics.net/printer.php?aid=135.* Accessed November 25, 2005.

United Network for Organ Sharing. (2005). U.S. Transplantation Data. [On-line]. *www.unos.org/data/default.asp?displayType=usData.* Accessed November 25, 2005.

Veatch, R. M. (1976). *Death, dying and the biological revolution.* New Haven, CT: Yale University Press.

Watanabe, M. "Body and soul." (2002, October 27). *Seattle Times*, p. A3.

Weiss, R. (2005). The power to divide. *National Geographic, 208*(1), 2–27.

Wheeler, M. S., & Cheung, A. (1996). Minority attitudes toward organ donation. *Critical Care Nurse, 16*(1), 30–34. [On-line]. *http://womenshistory.about.com/library/ency/blwh_comstock.htm.* Accessed October 16, 2002.

Wine, J. J. (2006). *Cystic fibrosis publications.* [On-line]. *www.stanford-edu/~wine/CF-pubs.html.* Accessed September 17, 2006.

Introduction to Leadership and Management Roles

The fourth unit in this textbook is devoted to topics that will assist you to move into the world of employment as a registered nurse (RN). The major focus is preparing you for the leadership role in nursing care that is expected of all RNs.

Chapter 11 provides the information on the basic structure underlying the health care environment including the mission and/or vision statement, organizational charts, chains of command, and approaches to governance. This chapter also discusses the forms of nursing care delivery, some major areas of nursing practice in which negotiation occurs including collective bargaining, and the purpose and expectations of a contract. The pros and cons of having a professional nursing association serve as the bargaining agent for nurses concludes the unit.

All RNs have responsibilities in regard to leading and managing others. The leadership and management roles of the nurse are highlighted in Chapter 12. You will find helpful information about how power is distributed and used in the health care system. The chapter concludes with a discussion of time-management issues.

As a leader in the health care system, nurses have specific responsibilities regarding delegation within the nursing team, and interacting with the interdisciplinary team. Leading requires the ability to build teams and to motivate others. These topics are explored in Chapter 13.

Skills related to leading change and managing conflict are also part of the professional role. Case studies and examples will help you gain an understanding of these activities. Additionally, nurses have responsibilities regarding the implementation of the medical plan of care, which necessitates the exploration of physician–nurse relationships, including both positive aspects and problem areas. Helping you to navigate these aspects of the system is the focus of Chapter 14.

11

Understanding the World of Health Care Employment

After completing this chapter, you should be able to:

1. Discuss the purpose of organizational mission and vision statements and statements of philosophy and describe how these are different.

2. Discuss the concept of organizational structure and analyze the relationships among organizational charts, chains of command, and channels of communication within the structure of organizations.

3. Delineate the characteristics of shared governance, analyzing the advantages of a shared governance approach.

4. Discuss the development of the Magnet Recognition Program for hospitals and list the characteristics required to achieve this status.

5. Describe various patterns of nursing care delivery, identifying the major characteristics of each and a situation in which each would be employed appropriately.

6. Discuss the history of collective bargaining as it applies to nursing.

7. Analyze the processes through which resolution is achieved in collective bargaining issues.

8. Identify at least four professional concerns that should be addressed in a contract for nurses.

9. Compare and contrast the characteristics of a grievance with those of a complaint.

10. Discuss the concerns nurses have regarding membership in a collective bargaining group and the reasons for each of these concerns.

11. Outline the advantages and disadvantages of having the state nurses' association serve as a bargaining agent for nurses.

Accountability
Agency shop
Arbitration/arbitrator
Authority
Authoritative mandate
Bargain in good faith

Binding arbitration
Bureaucracy
Case management
Case method
Centralized/decentralized/matrix
Chain of command

Channels of communication
Clinical ladders
Collective action division
Collective bargaining
Concession bargaining
Contract

Cross-training	Modular care	Protocols
Deadlocked	National Labor Relations Act	Ratified
Division of labor	National Labor Relations	Reinstatement privilege
Final offer	Board	Shared governance
Functional method	Negotiate/negotiation	Span of control—broad,
Government seizure	Organizations	narrow
Grievance/grievance process	Organizational chart	Standards of care
Impasse	Organizational hierarchy	Statements of philosophy
Informational picketing	Partnership models	Strike/strike-breaking
Injunction	Path of authority and	Structure
Interest-based bargaining	accountability	Team nursing
Job descriptions	Policy	Total patient care
Lockout	Primary care	Unfair labor practice
Mediation/mediator	Procedure	Union
Mission statement	Professional collectivism	Vision

As you seek employment as a professional nurse, you will most likely find that initial job in a health care organization. **Organizations**—formally constituted groups of people who have identified tasks and who work together to achieve a specific purpose defined by the organization—are the backbone of the American economy. We believe you will transition from student to staff nurse more easily and function more effectively in any organization if you have some understanding of the structure and makeup of organizations. By gaining an understanding of the makeup of organizations, you will be best equipped to participate effectively in the activities of the workplace. This also will help you anticipate some of the difficulties that may occur and, thus, handle them with greater ease and adeptness.

This chapter begins with a brief discussion of the structure of organizations and some of the most common conditions of employment, and then presents the most common avenues, including unions, through which employees participate in workplace decisions. Because we can only touch on these topics, you are encouraged to gain greater depth in this area by reading books devoted to this topic.

UNDERSTANDING ORGANIZATIONS

All organizations have structure and purpose. **Structure** refers to the way in which a group is formed, its chains of commands, lines of communication, and processes by which decisions are made. These comprise the formal working relationships and serve to identify who is accountable and responsible for the various jobs within the organization.

Mission Statement and Philosophy

All organizations have a purpose, or a reason for existing. The purpose of an organization is expressed in its **mission statement**, which outlines what the organization plans to accomplish, including its goals and function. Sometimes mission statements incorporate **statements of**

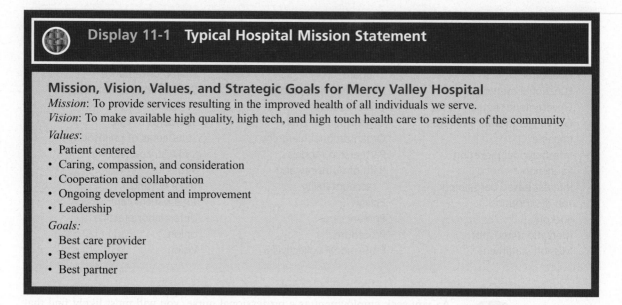

Display 11-1   Typical Hospital Mission Statement

Mission, Vision, Values, and Strategic Goals for Mercy Valley Hospital

Mission: To provide services resulting in the improved health of all individuals we serve.

Vision: To make available high quality, high tech, and high touch health care to residents of the community

Values:
- Patient centered
- Caring, compassion, and consideration
- Cooperation and collaboration
- Ongoing development and improvement
- Leadership

Goals:
- Best care provider
- Best employer
- Best partner

philosophy (beliefs), purpose, and goals or objectives into a single statement; other times, the philosophy, purposes, and goals are addressed in a statement separate from the mission statement. The mission of an organization may be combined with a **vision**, which is a broad conceptual view of what the organization desires to be and do. Welch & Welch (2005) states that the development of a mission statement is the responsibility of top management and cannot be delegated to anyone. Although input can be gathered from many sources, it must ultimately be created by those held accountable for it. Display 11-1 provides examples of mission and vision statements.

Mission and vision statements serve as a standard against which an organization's performance can be evaluated. A large research hospital might incorporate into its mission statement obligations for research, teaching, and the care of clients with complex problems. A smaller community hospital may reflect a goal of meeting the health care needs of citizens of the community in its mission statement. The hospital's ability to meet these goals would be reviewed as part of the overall evaluation of the organization.

Critical Thinking Activity

Based on your perception of the needs of the community in which you live, write a mission statement for a hospital. How did you arrive at the decision to offer the services you outlined? What facts support this decision? What services did you not include? Examine your response for personal biases.

Organizational Structure

To continue operation, any organization must make enough money to meet expenses and to improve and develop; some also seek to provide a profit return to investors. This is as true in health care as it is in retail businesses. A central goal of most organizations is to seek an organizational structure that is efficient while providing maximum cost effectiveness. As the values and priorities of our society change and as new technology becomes available, health care organizations also must make adaptations. Thus, today we encounter a health care system experiencing tremendous transformation (see Chapter 1).

The structure of an organization outlines the formal working relationships and identifies who is accountable and responsible for the various jobs required within the organization, Thus, it refers to the way it is put together to accomplish its goals. Breaking work into pieces or tasks, which are assigned to various individuals or groups, is known as **division of labor**. Size, age, services, technical components, and environment influence the structure of an organization. The concept of organizational structure is credited to a German social scientist, Max Weber, who is known as the father of organizational theory. He highly valued **bureaucracy**—the administration of institutions through departments or subdivisions managed by sets of officials who followed an inflexible routine. Historically, hospitals have functioned in the bureaucratic mode.

Types of Structure

The power to make decisions is a key factor in the structure and function of any organization. With regard to the decision-making process, organizations may be described as having a centralized (or tall) or a decentralized (or flat) structure. An organization is depicted as **centralized** when the authority to make decisions is vested in a few individuals. For example, in the patient services area of a hospital, major decisions may be made by the vice president of patient care and two or three associates (Fig. 11-1).

Conversely, when the decision making involves a number of individuals and individual employees are responsible for making decisions in areas in which they have expertise, the organization is said to operate in a **decentralized** fashion. Major decisions may be made by the individual closest to the action, and a head nurse or unit manager may be responsible for more than one patient care unit. Currently, many organizations are going through a process of restructuring to embrace a transformational approach to decision making that places the responsibility for finding solutions to problems at the site where the activity occurs. Later in this chapter, we discuss the concept of shared governance, which embraces a decentralized structure and function (Fig. 11-2).

Another type of organizational structure, the **matrix** structure, may be either flat or tall. The unique characteristic of the matrix structure is that a second structure overlies the first, creating two directions for lines of authority, accountability, and communication. An organization will have an underlying structure (either tall or flat) that is the functional structure over which is imposed a project structure. In short, the individuals in the functional structure perform the duties of operating and maintaining the organization, and the individuals in the project structure oversee the application of various projects or special responsibilities. The relationship that exists among individuals in the project structure is outside the regular chain of command of the underlying structure. We typically see the matrix structure in large, multifaceted organizations. Individuals with special expertise or authority in an area serve as resource persons for several departments, all of which can benefit from the knowledge. For example, in Figure 11-3, three types of expertise (financial services, planning and marketing, and quality assurance) cross all aspects of this large hospital corporation, which includes acute care, long-term care, and home care. Another example of a matrix-type relationship could be illustrated when a nurse with expertise in gerontologic nursing provides assistance, advice, and information to employees in each branch of this hospital organization.

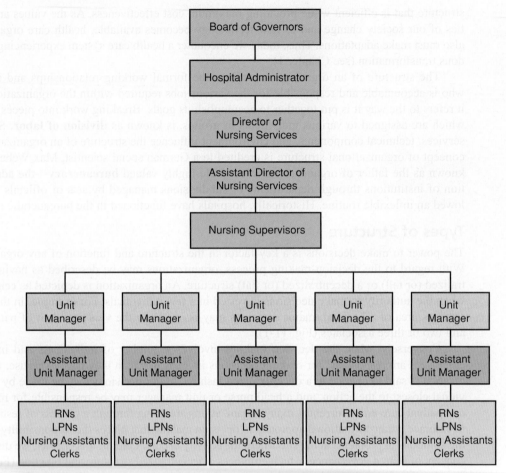

FIGURE 11-1   Centralized (tall) organizational structure of nursing service.

ORGANIZATIONAL RELATIONSHIPS

When examining organizational function, it is important that you identify relationships among people and departments and realize where the authority and accountability are placed within that organization. When one has **authority**, it means that the individual has the power or the right to take action, give directions or commands, and to make final decisions. **Accountability** refers to being obliged to answer for one's actions and sometimes, as when certain tasks are delegated, for the actions of others. A synonym for accountability is responsibility. We will discuss both authority and accountability in more detail in the section on shared governance.

Most organizations have several ways of expressing and defining the relationship of one worker to another. Organizational charts, chains of command, channels of communication, job descriptions, and policies and procedures provide different views of organizational relationships.

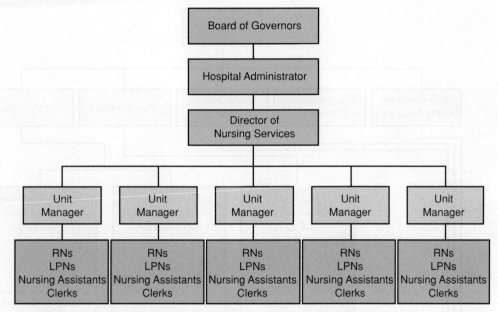

FIGURE 11-2   Decentralized (flat) organizational structure of nursing service.

Organizational Chart

The structure of any large group comprises both a formal and an informal organization. The formal organization can be seen on an organizational chart. The **organizational chart** is a graphic, pictorial means of portraying roles and patterns of interaction among parts of a system. It identifies formal chains of command, communication channels, and the authority for decision making.

The organizational chart typically is represented on the page by boxes stacked in a pyramid formation. The greatest authority exists at the top of the chart (often a single box), and authority declines as you move toward the base (many boxes). Persons occupying jobs at the top of the organizational chart are considered administrators, executives, or management, and individuals with jobs closer to the base are considered employees or staff members. Located between these two levels is an area known as middle management, comprising those who coordinate and control activities of specified groups of workers.

The organizational chart may take one of several forms, reflecting the type of administration operating within that organization. One term used to describe these forms is **span of control**, which refers to the number of employees supervised by a manager. A **narrow** span of control exists when a manager has responsibility for only three to five subordinates. If, however, the organization operates with a **broad** span of control, it places authority and responsibility for decision making in the hands of fewer individuals, with each manager supervising a large number of employees. The larger the number of individuals to be supervised, the more difficult it is to control each worker through direct observation. If two organizations of equal size were to exist—one with a narrow span of control and the other with a broad span

FIGURE 11-3   Matrix organizational structure of nursing service.

of control—the organization choosing to implement a narrow span of control would have more managers.

Organizational charts have limitations. One limitation of the organizational chart is the difficulty in keeping it current. Positions and people change frequently, and each change requires updating the chart. However, the primary limitation of the organizational chart is the fact that it does not depict the informal structure of the organization. In most groups, we find an informal organization, sometimes called the "grapevine," that represents informal or social relationships. The informal organization is not depicted on an organizational chart or formally acknowledged in any specific manner, but it can often have a profound effect on how an organization functions.

This informal structure has its own leaders and communication channels. It is responsible for much of the socialization that occurs among employees of the organization and creates a sense of belonging. There also may be unwritten and informal rules and expectations regarding performance, dress, communications, and other factors that affect group operation.

Chain of Command

All organizations have a chain of command. The **chain of command** represents the **path of authority and accountability** from individuals at the top of the organization to those at the base of the organization. It is often referred to as the **organizational hierarchy**. Thus, in hospitals we typically find that the nursing administrator gives directions to and evaluates the performance of the assistant administrator, who, in turn, gives directions to and evaluates the performance of the nursing unit manager, and so forth. When we look at this process from the base of the organization to the top, we often use the language "reports to"—indicating that the unit manager is accountable to the assistant administrator, and the assistant administrator is accountable to the nursing administrator. Similarly, we find the registered nurse (RN) giving direction to and overseeing the activities of the practical (vocational) nurse and the nursing assistant. The length of the chain of command varies depending on the size of the organization.

Some individuals are represented as having accountability to those above them but also hold some accountability to other departments. These represent collaborative rather than authoritarian relationships. For example, a clinical nurse specialist in wound care might hold some accountability to nurses on all units but she has no authority to compel them to consult with her or follow her suggestions.

Almost without exception, the salaries commanded by persons at the top of the organizational hierarchy are greater than those of persons close to the base. Accordingly, the experience, educational requirements, hours worked, and responsibilities are greater for persons with positions near the top of the organizational chart.

Channels of Communication

Channels of communication are, as the name implies, the patterns through which messages are delivered within an organization. The channels of communication usually reflect the chain of command; they run up and down the organizational chart, moving from one level of responsibility and authority to the next. Thus, the nurse manager communicates concerns and information to the assistant administrator, who either has the authority and responsibility to deal with the problem or relays the concern to the nursing administrator. The nursing assistant reports her concerns to the staff nurse, who either has the authority to deal with the issue or reports it to the head nurse or clinical manager. Some types of communication move along to individuals in parallel positions.

For nurse managers to report a concern directly to administrators rather than to assistant administrators to whom they report is referred to as "looping" the system; it is generally considered improper and inappropriate to skip or bypass any level in the communication system. For example, if a staff nurse disagrees with a pharmacy technician who delivers medications to the unit, and takes this problem directly to the nursing supervisor without first discussing it with the unit manager, this individual is looping the system. You can see how this would put the unit manager at a distinct disadvantage, should the supervisor ask about the incident.

■■ COMMUNICATION IN *ACTION*
■■

Missing Supplies

Mary Allioto had been working on a medical unit of a community hospital for four months. Over that period of time she noted that one of the nursing assistants, Jane, often left with towels, wash cloths, and other unit supplies in her backpack. Mary approached Jane as they were leaving one afternoon and said, "I've noticed that you often carry home towels and other unit supplies." Jane quickly replied, "Oh, these ones are becoming ragged and should not be used anymore." Further conversation suggested that Jane would continue to remove unit items. Mary decided she needed to report this to her unit manager. Talking with the manager in private, Mary explained, "On several occasions within the past 3 months I have noticed Jane leaving the hospital with unit supplies in her backpack. I asked her about it 2 weeks ago and she stated that the supplies were worn and should not be used with clients. I thought you should know about this." The unit manager thanked Jane and said, "I'll look into it."

Not all communications follow the formal pathways. New approaches to leadership and management have encouraged communication outside those lines if the result is accomplishing a desired action more efficiently. The informal structure of the organization mentioned earlier also functions outside the formal pathways, often communicating messages much more rapidly than within the formal structure.

EXAMPLE

Informal Communication Networks

Betsy Archer had been working on a medical unit of a community hospital for about 4 months. During lunch, a colleague said, "I hear that our unit will be the first to start on the new computerized charting system." Betsy replied, "How do you know that? The newsletter said that the hospital has not even decided on a vendor for computerized charting. I thought we were going to get to evaluate systems before the final choice." Her colleague replied, "Oh, they didn't mean that people at our level would get to evaluate the systems. That is all done. My friend in technology says the decision is made, and they are making plans for implementation right now and we are first! Jenny [the unit manager] will find that out at that manager's meeting she is going to today."

Job Descriptions

Job descriptions form another important aspect of any organization. **Job descriptions** are written statements, usually found in policy manuals, that stipulate the duties and functions of the various jobs within the organization, and the scope of authority, responsibility, and accountability involved in each position. Job descriptions should explain the role of each individual working for the company or organization, from the chief executive officer to the janitor.

Sometimes job descriptions are very specific; other times they are more broadly stated. If broadly stated, policy and procedure manuals may help to specify a task or responsibility. Job descriptions provide the foundation for performance standards for each position and should provide the basis for evaluation. Job descriptions also may include competencies expected of employees and can provide the basis for competency-based orientation. As the RN delegates more care to those with lesser educational preparation, it is critical that job descriptions provide sufficient description of the competencies of various workers, so that the document can be used to guide delegation activities (see Chapter 13 for more information on delegation).

Job descriptions also are important when cross-training is used in the organization. **Cross-training** involves teaching one member of the health care team to perform functions usually associated with another position. For example, a respiratory therapist might learn to perform basic patient care skills and, when not needed for respiratory therapy treatments, be available to answer lights and respond to patient needs. Cross-training is viewed by some administrators as a method by which costs can be reduced through the efficiency of having an individual able to do more than one set of tasks within the organization. The effectiveness of cross-training between different disciplines has not been well documented. Certainly issues related to scope of practice, liability, and patient safety must be considered. Patients may express concerns if care providers wearing an identification badge stating they are a radiological technician are functioning as a phlebotomist.

Cross-training of nurses between differing specialties has become common, and many nurses welcome the employment flexibility this provides. It also allows nurses to move with greater comfort from one area of the hospital to another when patient census surges or drops in an area. As you enter into your first nursing position, check with your state board of nursing to learn what position your practice act has taken regarding cross-training.

Job descriptions also may describe **clinical ladders**. A clinical ladder differentiates and defines the skills and performance expected of nurses in terms of advancing levels. Typically, three or four levels of performance are defined, with each higher level having greater responsibility and authority than the previous one. A new graduate usually enters the system as a clinical nurse one (or similar title), moves to clinical nurse two, and then to clinical nurse three as that individual becomes more proficient. Salary increases typically accompany movement from one level to another, and the responsibility the individual is expected to assume also increases.

Sometimes additional formal education or continuing education is required for advancement. Through this process, the nurse is supported and encouraged to develop greater clinical expertise. The clinical ladder also serves as a mechanism for recognizing and rewarding nurses who wish to remain in direct care positions rather than seek administrative positions.

Policies, Protocols, Procedures, and Standards of Care

A **policy** may be defined as a designated plan or course of action to be taken in a specific situation. In organizations, the governing board holds the responsibility and authority for ensuring that appropriate policies are adopted. The governing board usually delegates the development of policies to the chief administrative officer. The administrator usually delegates the responsibility for development of policies for a specific department to individuals or groups in the department that will be most affected by the policy. Once their work is completed, the policy is returned to the governing board for review, possible revision, and adoption. The management within the organization is responsible for ensuring that the policies are followed and that more specific policies are developed if necessary.

Written copies of all policies usually are placed in a policy manual that is available in each department, or a current copy may be available on-line in the institution's computer network. On-line policy manuals ensure that all departments refer to the most current policy and that the information is always available. Depending on the area in which you are employed, you will find varying needs for referring to the policy manual in your role as a new employee. As you might anticipate, the need for special policies related to occurrences in an emergency department, delivery room, or a critical care unit is greater than in a general medical or surgical unit in a hospital. When you are confronted with a new nonclinical problem to solve, always check your policy manual to see if it offers guidance.

Special unit policies are sometimes termed **protocols**. A protocol is a detailed standard plan for patient care. For example, the protocol for dealing with a patient seen in the emergency department suffering from a dog bite determines the wound assessment instrument to be used, a reference to the procedure to be used for wound care, when tetanus immunization would be included in care, discharge criteria, and teaching needed (Ellis & Hartley, 2005). Protocols may be available on-line so that any unit confronted by an unusual situation has access to the protocol even when it is not commonly used. For example, nurses on a surgical unit might need protocols for postpartum care for a woman who recently delivered and is suddenly hospitalized after an automobile accident.

Procedure manuals contain the written instructions describing the accepted method for satisfactorily performing a particular nursing activity (**procedure**), often describing it in a number of steps. Each unit or department should have a procedure manual. In the manual, you might find a procedure for changing the dressing on a central intravenous line, administering chemotherapy agents, and doing many other procedures, such as catheterizations. Procedures may also be available on-line.

Institutions are giving nurses more responsibility for developing institutional policies and procedures, and serving as representatives to various committees that monitor, review, and update policies and procedures. As hospitals move to broader spans of control and to greater involvement of all employees in decision making, grassroots participation in policy formation is becoming more common. The nature of a policy and the breadth of its scope will determine whether it needs further review within the organization.

Standards of care are authoritative statements that describe a common or acceptable level of client care or performance. Thus, standards of care define professional practice. In 1991, the American Nurses Association (ANA) formulated general standards and guidelines for nursing practice; now in their second edition, they reflect a general standard of practice. Additionally, standards for more than 20 areas of specialty practice have been developed. (The individual standards can be purchased from the ANA, or all may be purchased as a package.) They apply across the nation, are broad and general in nature, and have the purpose of establishing the best practice and eliminating as much variation as possible. Similarly, state practice acts contain language describing the standard of practice that applies to all nurses licensed in that state.

Each agency also may develop standards of care for patients with selected health care problems. These more detailed and specific standards may take the form of standard nursing care plans. Some standards are being incorporated into documents termed "care pathways," "critical pathways," or "clinical pathways." These are intended to serve as guides to direct the health care team in daily care. The individual standard organizes and sequences the care and describes the care required for a patient at specific times in the treatment. It involves a multidisciplinary approach and identifies both the care activities and the outcomes for each 24-hour period of hospitalization. These specific standards of care become the basis for evaluation of care, quality improvement within the organization, and cost analysis.

⊕ SHARED GOVERNANCE

Few industries have felt the impact of technology as much as health care. Ranging from new systems of information and communication to different administrative structures to changing approaches to systems of evaluation to highly technical equipment, the health care delivery system has seen a radical acceleration in all forms of technology. In the realm of administrative structure, one of the more important changes has been the recent move to a pattern of shared governance within health care agencies. Governance establishes how the power and authority for decision making is structured within an organization.

The Shared Governance Model

Shared governance is a professional practice model in which the nursing staff and the nursing management are both involved in decision making, as opposed to the administrative decision area being controlled by management. As described by Porter-O'Grady (2003, p. 251), it is "a structural model through which nurses can express and manage their practice with a higher level of professional autonomy." Hinshaw (2002, p. 92) further describes shared governance as a system in which nurses have organizational autonomy as reflected in control over their practice, and have input into "the broader unit and decision-making processes pertaining to patient care." Fundamental to the successful implementation of shared governance is the belief that staff nurses at every level within the organization should govern their practice and be involved in decisions that affect that practice; it enables staff nurses to assume greater levels of autonomy and control over their practice. It involves the concepts of equalitarianism, collegiality, and shared professional accountability. Thus, shared governance is more than a structure—it is also a philosophy (Caramanica, 2004).

Shared governance originated during the mid-1980s, when concepts of participative management and decentralization were popular in organizational literature. It gained further status and recognition as an alternative to bureaucratic management during the 1990s. This structure allows nursing staff to make major decisions within the organization and attempts to get the decision-making process as close to where the action occurs as possible, typically through the development of internal councils. It manifested itself in the health care delivery environment somewhat in response to the work of organizational theorists such as McGregor (1960) and Herzberg (1966), who supported the concept that the employee is an organization's most valuable resource and, as such, should be encouraged to grow and contribute to organizational goals. Often, this pattern of organization is paired with the concept of total quality improvement, which has as its hallmark emphasis on the customer (Alexander et al., 1994).

There is no single model for shared governance and its structures, and processes can be different in every organization (Hess, 2004). Early descriptions of the shared governance format stated that it may take a councilor model, in which committees and councils have defined authority and functions; a congressional model that involves an elected representative system; or an administrative model consisting of committees or forums in which people communicate and share ideas (Porter-O'Grady, 1987). The committees or councils result in staff actively participating in management, and, as a consequence, gaining autonomy, control over the work environment, and greater job satisfaction. Often, councils report to a nursing executive board that serves as a coordinating and approval body. Within this framework, the nurse is held to greater accountability within the context of peer-defined and peer-operated parameters (Porter-O'Grady, 1990).

The Effect of Shared Governance on the Role of the Manager and Staff Nurse

In a shared governance model, the traditional role of the supervisor as one who hires, evaluates, promotes, and fires becomes a thing of the past. The nurse manager's role becomes one of facilitator, integrator, and coordinator of the processes that support the work of the staff nurse who has been empowered to control his or her own practice (Caramanica, 2004). It requires that managers learn to share authority over key areas such as scheduling. In some instances, it has required that they give up seats on various hospital committees to staff nurses. Managers are required to understand their own change style, decision-making style, and leadership style (Brooks, 2004). The inability of managers to make these changes has been a major impediment to the success of shared governance. Many managers find their new and changing role difficult to accept.

The implementation of a shared governance structure requires that staff nurses understand that it is their right and professional obligation to participate in how decisions are made about nursing practice (Brooks, 2004). They need to participate in professional development sessions that increase nurses' understanding of the decision-making process, team building, group dynamics, leadership and budgeting, and how to participate in and conduct meetings.

The Pros and Cons of a Shared Governance Model

The shared governance model has waxed and waned in hospitals over the past 25 years. Strong advocates for the empowerment, autonomy, and professional development of staff nurses encourage the implementation of shared governance. Because shared governance models were introduced to improve nurses' work environments, satisfaction, and retention (Anthony, 2004), some argue that its structure will help lessen the impact of the nurse shortage.

Nurses engaged in evidence-based practice (see Chapter 6) argue that this practice requires inquisitive professionals to have solid decision-making skills, including the ability to ask relevant questions, critique research studies, and examine research findings in the context of clinical practice. They believe the environment that most facilitates and nurtures critical thinking and autonomous decision making is that of shared governance in which engagement and participation are encouraged (Zuzelo et al., 2003).

Nurses involved in Work Place Advocacy, which endeavors to strengthen nursing's voice and ensure nurse involvement in workplace decisions, also see shared governance as an avenue by which to accomplish their goals. Some of characteristics shared in common include accountability, empowerment, conflict resolution, and patient advocacy. Both approaches are seen as improving the status of nurses in the workplace as well as improving the quality of nursing care delivered (Green & Jordan, 2004).

Others have questioned the continuance of shared governance models in today's health care system. The re-engineering and restructuring of the health care delivery system, which has resulted in multi-hospital systems, consolidations, mergers, and the use of nurses as primary care providers and case managers, also may result in the demise of shared governance, or in its assuming a different format. The time involved in shared governance is costly to an organization, and the cost-effectiveness of shared governance in terms of patient outcomes is being questioned.

In all instances, a system for evaluating the effectiveness of shared governance needs to be put into place. Evidence that sorts actual costs of the various shared governance models is needed. Information that examines the returns on the investment in terms of what is attained, and in relationship to retention rates, nurse satisfaction, and vacancy needs to be gathered and analyzed (Herrin, 2004).

Critical Thinking Activity

Interview nurses who work in a shared governance environment. Identify what they find satisfying about shared governance. How would they like to see it changed? If shared governance is not used in your area, interview nurses about the concept of shared governance and how they believe it would improve patient care. Contact your state nurses association and learn what information it has regarding shared governance.

MAGNET HOSPITALS

Along with the concept of shared governance, within the past 20 years the hospital workplace has witnessed the development of the Magnet hospital concept. The Magnet Award is a nursing award for excellent patient care. In the early 1980s, the American Academy of Nursing recognized that acute care facilities, in particular, were having difficulty attracting and retaining RNs. They appointed a task force on hospital nursing practice to examine the situation. The task force determined that it was necessary to research the various factors involved in creating environments that would attract and retain professional nursing staff (McClure, 2005). Nurse researchers, sponsored by the ANA, conducted "reputational" studies to identify successful hospitals and a body of literature developed from these studies.

Initially 41 hospitals were selected as Magnet Hospitals. Gold Standards were then identified. In 1991, the American Nurses Credentialing Center (ANCC) established a program through which hospitals could apply to be designated Magnet Hospitals (Kramer & Schmalenberg, 2005). Table 11-1 outlines the phases of development of quality hospital recognition and the focus of each phase.

As the study of hospitals continued, characteristics emerged that resulted in the hospital being considered a good place to work. In the initial study conducted by Kramer and Schmalenberg (2005), 14 Forces of Magnetism were identified. Over time, some of these became outdated; for others the operational definition changed. These forces were narrowed to 10 items staff nurses identified as important to enabling them to give quality patient care, and eventually down to 8 (see Display 11-2). Note that many of the Forces of Magnetism relate to characteristics of hospitals discussed earlier in this chapter (ie, flat, decentralized organizational structures; shared governance; and nurse autonomy). Other concepts are tied to processes such as team building and participative leadership, which are discussed in Chapters 12 and 13. The various Forces of Magnetism can be used by the individual nurse to assess a potential employment setting in relationship to its support for professional practice.

Although the initial impetus for Magnet Recognition was initiated by nurses and is carried out through the ANCC, it should be emphasized that the Magnet effort involves all departments and disciplines within the institution. Excellent patient care is an interdisciplinary process. Hospitals seeking this designation tend to view it as a journey with participants in the process experiencing feelings of pride, satisfaction, and enthusiasm (Ellis & Gates, 2005).

TABLE 11-1	PHASES OF QUALITY HOSPITAL RECOGNITION	
TYPE	**TIME PERIOD**	**FOCUS AND ACTIVITY**
Original Magnet Hospitals	1983–1989	Study focused on the structure—outcome relationship. Outcomes were based on hospitals that were considered a good place to work, resulting in attraction and retention. Nursing Work Index developed to measure nurse job satisfaction and productivity of quality patient care. Forty-one hospitals initially were identified.
Gold Standard of Magnetism	1989–1993	Focused on the structure, process, outcome relationship. Culture of the hospital assessed and caregiver and IPR processes identified.
ANCC Magnet Recognition Program	1991–present	Focused on simultaneous evaluation of structure and outcomes based on foundational structural elements of the Scope and Standard for Nurse Administrators. "Forces of Magnetism" criteria added, which looked at hospital characteristics and attributes—14 forces were identified.
Quality Nursing Care Processes	1993–present	Focused on process and eight structural features were identified by staff nurses as "Essentials of Magnetism."

Compiled from Kramer & Schmalenberg, 2005; Goode, Krugman, & Diaz, 2005.

PATTERNS OF NURSING CARE DELIVERY

The nursing department of any health care institution carries major responsibility for the quality of nursing care delivered. Throughout the years, the structure of the delivery of care has taken many forms. The particular pattern of care that is in common use has changed about every 20 years. Among the factors influencing the delivery pattern selected in each era were the types of patients served, the type of care provided, the cost of the care, the structure of the hospital, and the number and education level of potential employees. Perhaps a wider variety of patterns of care is being used today than at any other time in nursing's history. In the following section, we

Display 11-2   Eight Essentials of Magnetism

- Support for education
- Clinically competent coworkers
- Autonomous nursing practice
- Positive RN–MD relationships
- Supportive nurse manager
- Control over nursing practice
- Adequate staffing
- Culture that values concern for the patient as paramount

Compiled from Kramer & Schmalenberg, 2005.

describe the typical implementation of several patterns of care delivery. However, remember that you might find a particular pattern of care practiced a little differently in different settings.

Case Method

The **case method** was the first system used for the delivery of nursing care in the United States (around the beginning of the 20th century) and should not be confused with the term **case management** practiced today (more discussion occurs later in this chapter). With the case method, the nurse worked with one patient (or case) only and was expected to meet all of that patient's needs. The nurse often lived in the patient's home and was expected to assume other household duties, such as cooking for the patient and family and light housekeeping, when not busy with the patient. Nurses worked long hours and were poorly paid. Advancing technology and increasing costs made this type of care delivery impractical, but vestiges of its structure can be seen in today's home health nursing. However, the role of the RN in home health care is typically one of assessment, planning, skilled intervention, supervision of care provided by a home health aide, and evaluation of the client's progress.

Functional Method

The **functional method** of care delivery emerged during the Great Depression of the 1930s. This method allowed for the care of greater numbers of patients in hospitals and for use of advancing technology. At this time, the industrial model of narrowly defined and frequently repeated tasks revolutionized manufacturing. The idea that this would transfer into all types of work environments was widely accepted.

Typically, the head nurse assigned nursing tasks to the various persons employed on the unit, according to the level of skills required for performance. One nurse might take all temperatures, another would do all dressings, while yet another administered all medications, charted them, and provided a list of replacement needs to the head nurse. Assignments varied depending on the size of the unit, the number of personnel available, and the skill level of the personnel. The head nurse gave a report to the next shift.

Although economical and efficient, this system of care delivery had the disadvantage of fragmenting care—no single individual was responsible for the planning of the care. Patients were confused about who was caring for them, and communication among caregivers was lacking. Individual nurse–patient relationships were limited. Nursing care came to be viewed as a list of procedures and tasks. This pattern of care still may be used in long-term care facilities or subacute units, largely because of the educational preparation of the care providers. Some nurses are concerned that the economic push in today's health care institutions may see many hospitals returning to functional approaches to care.

Team Nursing

The concept of **team nursing** was introduced in the early 1950s, with the promise that it would result in more patient-centered care. It also was responsive to the nursing shortage that followed World War II (see Chapter 4) and the involvement of nurse aides and licensed practical (vocational) nurses (LPNs) in patient care. This approach to care is based on the premise that each unit will have two or more teams composed of variously educated care providers. For example, a team might be composed of two nurse aides, an orderly, an LPN, and an RN. A more experienced RN would be the team leader. Team members work together, each performing those tasks for which they best prepared. The

FIGURE 11-4   Team conference, planning, and communication are critical elements of team nursing.

team leader makes assignments, has overall responsibility for the care of patients on the unit, might administer all medications, and gives a report to the team that follows on the next shift. An important part of this form of nursing is the team conference, during which members of the team meet to communicate about the needs of their patients and to plan for care. Without the conference and the communication, team nursing might be little different from functional nursing. Today, as we see more health care facilities decreasing the number of RNs and adding more unlicensed assistive personnel, team nursing has again become a prevalent method of care delivery (Fig. 11-4).

Total Patient Care

During the late 1970s and early 1980s, many hospitals returned to a **total patient care** type of assignment, in which an RN or LPN is assigned for all care needs. A nurse is assigned to the care of a group of four to six patients, depending on patient needs and how acutely ill each patient is. This returns a greater sense of control to nurses, gives them a greater sense of autonomy, and fosters a greater sense of involvement in the whole spectrum of care and patient outcomes. This type of care focuses on the total person (from which its name is derived), rather than on a collection of tasks or procedures.

Some have suggested that this approach to care is too costly because an individual with less training could satisfactorily complete many of the tasks performed by the RN and at a lesser cost. Additionally, the continuity of care may be at risk as nurses, who have the right to change care plans, replace one another on shifts and alter the original plan of care. However, recent studies demonstrating the relationship between nurse–staffing levels and quality of care in hospitals would question this conclusion. Needleman and colleagues (2002), in examining the outcomes of more than 6 million medical surgical patients in 799 hospitals in 11 states across the country, determined that hospitals with the higher proportion of care delivered by RNs and the greater number of hours of care per day by RNs resulted in better care for hospitalized patients. When the proportion of care given by RNs was greater, complications such as pneumonia, bleeding, blood clots, urinary tract infections, and cardiac arrest were fewer. These data would indicate that decreased complication rates, shorter lengths of stay, and decreased readmission rates for patients, plus the employment of fewer assistive personnel who have greater turnover rates, offset the additional direct care costs. This is consistent with other studies that have resulted in similar findings (Brown, 2001; Domrose, 2002).

Primary Care Nursing

In a pattern of **primary care**, which came into popular application in the 1980s, one nurse is assigned the responsibility for the care of each patient from the time the patient is admitted to the hospital until that patient's discharge. The primary nurse is responsible for initiating and updating the nursing care plan, patient teaching, and discharge planning. An associate nurse works with this same patient on other shifts and on the primary nurse's day off, carrying out the plan of care developed by the primary nurse.

Obvious benefits of this method include the continuity of care for the patient and job satisfaction for the nurses because they have more autonomy and control. Whether this method is more expensive has been the subject of debate. Health care administrators argue that the salary costs for RNs make this a more costly approach to care.

Under this system, every nurse is a primary nurse for a few patients and an associate nurse for others. Sometimes the nurse functioning in an associate role has difficulty following the plan of the primary nurse or may disagree with the established plan of care. The patient's condition also may change rapidly, requiring the plan to be changed without consulting the primary nurse. Another concern is the level of expertise and commitment required of all nurses, and the fact that nurses who work autonomously with patients soon forget how to delegate responsibilities.

Modular Care

Modular care gained popularity in the mid-1980s. Patient care units were divided into modules, and the same team of care providers consistently was assigned to a particular module. An RN served as team leader of each module, with LPNs and nursing assistants making up the team. In this sense, modular nursing looked a lot like team nursing. Each module was stocked with its own linens, medications, and supplies.

This form of care delivery has the advantage of offering continuity of care, because the same team cares for the same group of patients each day. It also has the advantage of involving the RN in planning and coordinating care and results in more efficient communication because of the geographic closeness of the unit. The disadvantages center on the increased costs of stocking each unit, and the fact that many hospitals, with long corridors and halls, do not lend themselves architecturally to a modular design (Komplin, 1995).

Partnership Models

In some areas of the country, there currently exists a trend toward **partnership models**, in which patient care is provided to a group of patients by an RN and either an LPN or an unlicensed nursing assistant. If an unlicensed care provider is involved, this individual does non-nursing tasks and the RN provides the professional care. When an LPN is employed, the patient care is shared, with the RN responsible for planning and directing the care. This form of care delivery may also be referred to as "care pairs."

Case Management

Case management, although not a system of care delivery in the sense that we have mentioned earlier, involves nurses in the role of managing patient care and bears mention here. Case management refers to a system in which the health care services are controlled and monitored carefully to ensure that policies are followed, that neither too much nor too little care is provided, and that costs are minimized. A key to case management is the identification of a critical pathway for care and treatment that includes specific timelines and protocols. The case manager typically follows the patient from the diagnostic phase through hospitalization, rehabilitation, and back to home care, ensuring that plans are made in advance and that the patient receives care that will achieve the most positive outcomes. The case manager may not provide direct care but is responsible for managing the patient's interaction with the entire health care system. For a more detailed discussion of case management, please refer to Chapter 1.

RNs are the health care professionals who most often act as case managers. In some settings, social workers also act as case managers. Case managers may be employed by third-party payers (such as insurance companies) or by health care agencies (such as hospitals or long-term care facilities). Case managers employed by a particular institution also might be involved in wellness programs (eg, blood pressure management, stress management, smoking cessation programs, and exercise classes).

Some objections to this form of care delivery come from physicians, who see the role of the case manager as an infringement on their historic rights of autonomy in decision making. Providers may also believe that the case manager is more concerned with cost factors than with what is best for the individual, arguing that quality is sacrificed to cost containment.

Critical Thinking Activity

Compare the various patterns of nursing care delivery with the pattern being used in a facility where you currently receive clinical experience. Analyze the pattern in current use and evaluate whether another pattern of care delivery would be more or less effective. Provide a rationale for your answer.

WORKPLACE ACTIVITIES THAT INVOLVE NEGOTIATION

Negotiation involves the exchange of ideas and values for the purpose of reaching a mutual decision regarding a particular situation. While it occurs on a day-to-day basis as we work with others, it often is also a part of the mediation process. The following section of this chapter discusses some of the major activities in health care environments when negotiation occurs.

The Grievance Process

A **grievance** is a circumstance or action believed to be in violation of a contract (or of policies of an institution if a contract is not in place). The **grievance process** represents an established and orderly method to be used in the adjustment of grievances between parties. In this sense, it represents a problem-solving mechanism.

If a contract exists, the steps to be used in mediating grievances are usually included in that document. If there is no formal contract, internal policies exist that outline grievance procedures. Perhaps you are aware of grievance processes from your student handbook, where the processes in place in an educational program are shared with students.

Grievances usually are related to interpretations of a contract or to policies and procedures. They may occur as a result of a misunderstanding or difference of opinion about the contract or its language, or as a result of direct violations of policies or of the contract. Although either the management or an employee can file grievances, in most instances, it is an employee who initiates the case.

The grievance process spells out in writing a series of steps to be taken to resolve the area of dissension and a timeline for accomplishing those steps. Initially, the employee and the immediate supervisor attempt to resolve the disagreement through an informal talk. If no resolution occurs, the discussion moves to the steps of the grievance process, involving others within the organization. The steps include providing notifications and responses in writing, adhering to strict time lines for action, and eventually involving people at higher levels within the organization (eg, representatives from the bargaining unit, a grievance chairperson, the personnel director, and administrative representatives). Perhaps the services of an arbitrator will be needed toward the end of the dispute. Failure of either side to comply with the timelines that are in effect regarding its own actions or responses ends the process. If an arbitrator is involved, that person's decision is usually binding.

It is important to differentiate between complaints and grievances (Fig. 11-5). Employees may have complaints that are not violations of the contract. For example, Nurse No. 1 may object that she was required to float from the postpartum unit to the nursery; she had been oriented to the nursery but preferred to work in the postpartum unit. Nurse No. 2 was required to float from a medical unit to a surgical unit to which she had not been oriented. If the contract in this hospital stipulates that no one would be floated to a unit to which he or she had not been oriented, Nurse No. 1 had a complaint, whereas Nurse No. 2 had a grievance.

At one time, the absence of grievances was thought to be an indication of an effective, well-managed organization; however, that may not be the best indicator of the organization's health. It is entirely possible that problems are not being addressed. By the same token, a high number of grievances may indicate problems within the organization. These problems also may relate to the language of the contract or the education of the employee regarding the conditions of employment. Another barometer of the health of an organization is the level at which the grievances are resolved. It is most desirable to settle most grievances at the informal level, without the involvement of an arbitrator.

The grievance procedure may sound like many steps that take a great deal of time, and indeed this is true. Although most grievances are settled short of arbitration, they are still time and energy consuming. Grievances can best be avoided if everyone has a good understanding of the terms of employment and if sound personnel policies are developed and applied consistently and equitably. A part of the orientation of new employees to an organization should be spent reviewing and explaining these features. Open discussions between the employees and management to review mutual concerns and share information help reduce the number of grievances. Mutual respect is a critical element in any organization.

FIGURE 11-5 It is important to discriminate between complaints and grievances.

Critical Thinking Activity

What are the reasons that grievance processes need to be spelled out? How would you determine whether an issue is a grievance or a complaint? What resources are available to you as you search for the answer?

Collective Bargaining

Collective bargaining consists of a set of procedures by which employee representatives and employer representatives negotiate to obtain a signed agreement (contract) that spells out wages, hours, and conditions of employment that are acceptable to both. A key word in this definition is **negotiate**. The goal of negotiations is to obtain a signed agreement, which is a legal contract that spells out in writing the decisions that are reached. Colosi and Berkeley (1994, p. 3) define negotiation as "a process which affords the disputants an opportunity to exchange promises and make binding commitments in an effort to resolve their differences."

Because of nursing's long history as a profession of dedication, altruism, and service, collective bargaining initially was a controversial issue within nursing. Some saw this process as detracting from the professional role of the nurse and ethically improper.

Today, however, nurses are vitally concerned about contracts, services, third-party payers, comparable worth, patients' rights, shared governance, staffing ratios, and a host of issues that can be discussed at the bargaining table. Nurses believe that people who choose nursing as a career should have the opportunity to have some voice in patient care assignments, length of the work day and week, fringe benefits, and wages, without losing face with the public at large, members of the medical profession, or other colleagues. Additionally, at a time when nurses are campaigning for a safer practice environment free of mandatory overtime and other work issues, collective bargaining takes on a new countenance—an avenue by which to address these and other work concerns and gain control over practice. If you plan to work in a health care facility in which nurses bargain collectively, study the following section carefully.

History of Collective Bargaining

As early as the 1850s, Horace Greeley, a reformer, publisher, and politician, was generating interest in and giving impetus to collective bargaining issues in his editorial columns in the *New York Tribune*. During the early part of the 20th century, efforts by workers to organize were met with opposition from employers, government officials, and some members of the public. After the Great Depression, which immobilized the United States in the late 1920s and early 1930s, several laws were enacted to help improve workers' conditions. Franklin D. Roosevelt was elected president in 1932, and his New Deal administration saw the passage of the National Industrial Recovery Act. One result of this act was the creation of the National Recovery Administration, whose purpose was to administer codes of fair practice within given industries. The nation was called on to accept an interim blanket code that established a 35- to 40-hour workweek for workers, minimum pay of 30 to 40 cents an hour, and prohibition of child labor—all issues that had long been advocated by nurses. Students wishing to learn more about this act are encouraged to type "National Recovery Administration" into their browser and follow the many leads provided.

Passage of the National Labor Relations Act. On July 5, 1935, the **National Labor Relations Act (NLRA)** became the national labor policy of the United States. Also known as the Wagner Act, for Senator Robert F. Wagner (who introduced the legislation), the NLRA gave workers federal protection in their efforts to form unions and organize for better working conditions. It listed as unfair practice any actions on the part of employers that would interfere with this process. Senator Wagner wanted management and labor to resolve their mutual problems through a system of self-government. This act also created the **National Labor Relations Board (NLRB)**, a quasi-judicial body that was to ensure proper enforcement of the conditions of the legislation.

The NLRB has the responsibility for administering the NLRA. In addition, it has two primary functions: to conduct secret-ballot elections that will determine that the majority of employees of a unit desire the representation of a given union in collective bargaining procedures, and to prevent and rectify unfair labor practices committed by employers or unions. It also has the responsibility for determining to which of the eight bargaining units established for health care workers various employees will be assigned. This is important to nurses because it enables them to have a separate unit and, therefore, to deal with issues important to their role in health care delivery.

The original NLRA used the term "labor organization," which was defined in language that could be interpreted to exclude nursing and several other professions, such as teaching and medicine that were organized through professional organizations. These early labor unions often were viewed negatively by the public—an image that was reinforced in movies, in newspapers, and on radio. Often portrayed as rowdy, aggressive, and hostile, unions did not seem to fit well in nursing.

In 1947, the original NLRA was amended through the Taft-Hartley Act (also known as the Labor Management Relations Act). Because of heavy lobbying by hospital management, the act was written in such a way as to specifically exclude nonprofit hospitals from the legal obligation of bargaining with their employees. Although the administrations of some hospitals chose to negotiate salaries and working conditions with their employees, many did not, and no legal action could be taken to force the process (Kalisch & Kalisch, 2004).

Further Federal Legislation. On August 25, 1974, the Taft-Hartley Act was amended to provide economic security programs for those employed in nonprofit hospitals, and brought health care facilities and their employees under the jurisdiction of the NLRB. Nonprofit hospitals were legally required to bargain with nurses for better wages, hours, staffing conditions, and patient–nurse ratios, and for a voice in hospital governance. To ensure that the public would be protected from strikes or work stoppage, several amendments were attached to the NLRA passed in 1974, including the requirement of longer notification periods and provisions mandating participation in mediation.

Federal legislation passed in 1962 enabled employees of federal health care institutions to participate in collective bargaining. In 1967, investor-owned hospitals and nursing homes also were included, and the ANA was identified as the bargaining agent for the nurses of the Veterans Administration hospitals. Legislation passed in 1970 included nonprofit nursing homes in the collective bargaining process. Concurrently, the Service Employees International Union (SEIU) and other labor-related organizations were also bargaining for nurses.

Activity of the American Nurses Association. Although nurses were not permitted to engage in collective bargaining activities until 1974, by 1931, the ANA was publicly recognizing its obligation regarding the general welfare of its members, and developed within its organization a legislative policy addressing this concern. Some suggest that this effort was spurred by the fact that other groups, particularly the SEIU, an affiliate of the American Federation of Labor/Congress of Industrial Organizations (AFL/CIO), were actively working to organize health care workers. Other factors also were important. Before 1930, most nurses were employed in public health, visiting nurse, or private duty positions. Students, aides, and orderlies, under the direction of a head nurse, delivered much of the care in hospitals. As more care was delivered in the hospital setting, the number of nurses employed by these facilities grew. The existing working conditions affected more people.

In 1946 the ANA's House of Delegates approved a resolution that called upon the state nurses associations to work actively to secure the general and economic welfare of its members. The ANA has worked constantly since those early years to provide leadership and support to nurses as they negotiate salaries, working conditions, benefits, and governance opportunity. In 1966, they adopted the Resolution on National Salary Goal, which established a salary goal of not less than $6,500 per year for entry-level RNs. Lacking the right to bargain collectively for salaries, nurses sometimes used mass resignations as a method to change employment conditions.

The United American Nurses (UAN) was established in 1999 and exists as an affiliate of both the ANA and the AFL-CIO. It is composed of members of the ANA's constituent states' (constituent nurses associations) local bargaining units. The UAN assists the state nurses associations to organize work hours, staffing levels, health and safety, and wage benefits and issues.

TABLE 11-2	ANA ACTIVITIES RELATED TO COLLECTIVE BARGAINING AND WORKPLACE ADVOCACY
YEAR	**ACTIVITY**
1931	Developed within its organization a legislative policy addressing general welfare concerns of its members.
1945	Appointed a committee to study employment conditions.
1946	Established the ANA Economic Security Program as an outcome of the 1945 study. State nurses associations encouraged to act as exclusive bargaining agents for their memberships.
1947	Collective bargaining between nurses and hospital administrations implemented in several states with negotiated contracts in effect.
1949	ANA is certified as a labor organization.
1950	No-strike policy adopted officially by ANA due to concern for the image of nursing.
1967	ANA identified as the bargaining agent for nurses in Veterans Administration hospitals.
1968	No-strike policy rescinded.
1991	ANA embarked on a Workplace Advocacy Initiative to improve the work environment of nurses.
1999	UAN established as an autonomous arm of ANA to carry out collective bargaining for nurses at the national level and to coordinate the work of state collective bargaining units.
2000	Commission on Workplace Advocacy established to address the needs of individual nurses in the workplace not represented by collective bargaining.
2003	The Center for American Nurses established as an outgrowth of the Commission on Workplace Advocacy. Created a new membership category for Associate Organization Members and addresses challenges and opportunities individual non-union nurses face in their practice environments.

In 2000, the Commission on Workplace Advocacy was established by the ANA House of Delegates. Its purpose was to work through policy and legislative activities that affect nurses in all work environments, both those who participate in collective bargaining and those who do not.

Following on the heels of the establishment of the Commission, a new membership category for Associate Organizational Members was created in 2003. The Center for American Nurses was established to deal with issues of workplace advocacy. The Center offers tools, services, and strategies designed to make nurses their own best advocates in their practice environments. Although the Center is independent of the ANA, the organizations are linked through an Affiliation Agreement in effect through 2008. Under this agreement, the Center coordinates with, purchases administrative services from, and is co-located with the ANA.

Table 11-2 summarizes the activities of ANA in relationship to collective bargaining and workplace advocacy.

Understanding the Basic Concepts of Collective Bargaining

Intelligent and effective bargaining begins with an awareness of the process itself. The information that follows is designed to provide a better understanding of the terms and processes involved in bargaining collectively to achieve an agreed-upon contract.

Bargaining and Negotiating. To **negotiate** means to bargain or confer with another party or parties to reach an agreement. It implies that there will be discussion of the terms of the agreement and suggests that there will be give and take—that neither party will obtain all items asked for in the contract. Ideally, negotiations would proceed in a somewhat philosophic vein, moving toward reasonable compromises that would allow each side to achieve many of the conditions it requested, but this does not always occur.

A typical bargaining session has three phases. The early sessions include a formal exchange of proposals, during which each side may ask for more than it knows it can expect to receive and emphasize its commitment to certain issues. The second phase gives the most attention to secondary issues. The third phase occurs as the deadline approaches and primary issues are discussed realistically. Throughout all phases, each side presents "solid arguments," explaining its position and developing a "we vs. they" approach (Budd, Warion, & Patton, 2004).

Several forms of bargaining have evolved. **Interest-based bargaining** represents a non-traditional style of bargaining that attempts to problem solve differences between labor and industry (Williams, 2004). It is intended to allow parties to jointly problem solve ways to meet each side's interest or what each side wants, rather than taking a bottom line approach. Brainstorming and information sharing are techniques used to develop ideas and options (Budd, Warino & Patton, 2004). After establishing shared values and goals, the two parties then begin to work out their differences regarding specific policies and conditions. Interest-based bargaining is gaining attention as a less adversarial process, which may preserve effective working relationships and lessen feelings of alienation between supervisory personnel and employees involved in the union.

Another variation sometimes seen is concession bargaining. **Concession bargaining** is a process in which there is an explicit exchange of reduced labor costs for improvements in job security. This occurs with increasing frequency. An example would be a shift in emphasis from one that asks for increases in salary to one that focuses on eliminating the practice of calling nurses and telling them not to report for work because the census has dropped (on such days, the nurses do not receive salary). These are issues that seriously concern nurses today.

Unions and Collective Action. A **union** is a legally authorized organization that has been empowered by its members to negotiate and enforce a contract. Therefore, in order to engage in collective bargaining, employees must choose a union that will represent them. This usually is done through an election. The major areas in which a union may bargain are the wages, hours, and working conditions of its members.

When a branch or part of a professional association assumes the role and responsibility of a union, as often occurs in nursing, the negotiating group may be known as a **collective action division**, although it is legally considered a union. A professional organization works under the same legal constraints as any other union. It provides legal counsel and representatives to assist with negotiations, may lobby on behalf of issues, or may participate in other activities that would further the economic welfare of nurses. It oversees the development of the contract, monitors adherence to the contract, and represents employees in any grievance process.

Contracts. The conclusion of the bargaining process should result in a signed contract that converts to writing the agreements that have been reached. A **contract** is "an agreement between two or more parties, especially one that is written and enforceable by law" (*www.freedictionary.com*). This signed contract is enforceable under law and cannot be changed by either party acting unilaterally.

Some would suggest that the contract is the most important product of the collective bargaining process because it is a legal agreement on all issues that have been discussed. It provides the foundation for further activities. Unlike the policies of an agency, which can be changed by management alone, the agreement of both management and employees is required for any change to be made in a contract. The contract remains in effect until breached or terminated. Most negotiated contracts define the period of time—usually 2 or 3 years—during which the established conditions are effective.

Before being put into effect, a contract must be **ratified**. This means that the members of the bargaining group must accept the terms of the contract. This is usually done by a vote of the membership. Factors to be considered in a contract will be discussed later in this chapter.

Rules Governing Labor Relations. When two parties agree to begin the negotiation process, it is understood that both will **bargain in good faith**. Bargaining in good faith is a poorly understood concept, but generally it means that the parties will meet at regular times to discuss (with the intent to resolve) any differences over wages, hours, and other employment conditions. Failure to carry out these activities could lead to an unfair labor practice.

An **unfair labor practice** is any action that interferes with the rights of employees or employers as described in the amended NLRA. It is not possible to discuss all of these in detail; however, some examples follow. An employer must not interfere with the employee's right to form a union or other organized bargaining group, join the group, or participate in the group's activities. The employer may not attempt to control a group, once organized, or to discriminate against its members regarding hiring or tenure. Most important, the employer must bargain collectively and in good faith with representatives of the employees.

Likewise, labor organizations have constraints placed on their activities. They, too, must bargain in good faith. They must not restrain or coerce employees in selecting a bargaining group to bargain collectively. They may not pressure an employer to discriminate against employees who do not belong to the labor organization.

One of the issues brought up in negotiations that usually results in a dispute is that of **agency shop**. When an agency shop clause is in effect, all employees are required to pay dues for membership. There are several variations in provisions related to an agency shop. If, because of religious or philosophic beliefs, employees are unwilling to pay dues to the bargaining group, provisions may be made to pay the same sum to a nonprofit group, such as a church or foundation. In some instances, those who are already members of the union are required to remain members for the life of the contract, although no one is required to become a member. In some states, laws referred to as "right to work laws" forbid the establishment of an agency shop.

The obvious advantage of an agency shop, from the workers' point of view, is encouraging membership in the union. The union is required to represent all employees, both members and nonmembers. Negotiating a contract, monitoring compliance with its provisions, and facilitating the grievance process may be costly. The union, therefore, desires to have a greater percentage of paying members to support these activities. Additionally, the union will be stronger when negotiating when more of the employees are members. Those who oppose agency shops may not agree with the actions or positions of the union and therefore not wish to support it financially. Another group are those without philosophical differences with the union but who would rather not pay the cost.

Settling Labor Disputes

When labor disputes arise, several actions can be taken to help resolve the differences. Initially, of course, the parties continue to negotiate, and may agree to extend the negotiation period if progress in settling differences is being made. When the two parties doing the negotiating cannot come to agreement on an issue, they are considered to be at **impasse** or **deadlocked** on the issue.

Mediation and Arbitration. Perhaps the most commonly used method of seeking agreement between parties when negotiating has not been successful is through **mediation** and **arbitration**. A **mediator** is a third person who may join the bargainers to assist the parties in reconciling differences and arriving at a peaceful agreement. Although the mediator may join the parties at any point in the negotiations, due to the cost of mediation, most negotiations proceed until things are at an impasse. Mediation involves finding compromises, and the mediator assists with this. He or she must gain the respect of both parties and must remain neutral to the issues presented.

An **arbitrator** is technically defined as a person chosen by agreement of both parties to decide a dispute between them. The primary difference between a mediator and an arbitrator is that the mediator assists the parties in reaching their own decision, whereas the arbitrator has the authority to actually make the decision for the parties if necessary. However, the terms mediator and arbitrator and mediation and arbitration often are used interchangeably; in fact, a mediator may also serve as an arbitrator (Fig. 11-6).

Arbitration may take several forms. It may be mediation-arbitration, in which a third person joins the parties in the negotiation process before any serious disputes arise. This person's role is to act as a mediator, who attempts to keep the parties talking, suggests compromises, and helps establish priorities. If an agreement is not reached by a specified date, or if it appears that the issue is deadlocked, with neither party willing to compromise, the mediator then assumes the role of an arbitrator and makes a decision based on the information gained in the role of mediator.

Another form of arbitration is called **binding arbitration**. This means that both parties are obligated to abide by the decision of the arbitrator. Some people see this as the least desirable alternative in settling disputes because it may result in a decision that is not satisfactory to either side, but one by which both must abide. It has been suggested, in instances in which binding arbitration is used, that the parties spell out exactly which of the issues are to be decided by the arbitrator. Binding arbitration has the advantage of resolving deadlocked issues without a strike. It also encourages both parties, knowing that the arbitrator's decision may not please either side, to reach a compromise on their own.

One type of binding arbitration uses a **final offer** approach. Employer and employee bargaining representatives reach agreement on as many issues as possible. The deadlocked issues and a final position (final offer) from each side are then presented to the arbitrator, who is obligated to select only the most reasonable package. The arbitrator may not develop a third alternative, which would split the difference. The final offer approach encourages both sides to come up with a realistic package and serves to close the gap on issues, as each side seeks to maintain some control over the outcome of the deliberations.

One criticism of any type of arbitration is the expense involved. Arbitrators must be paid for their services. Arbitration is also criticized because it undermines voluntary collective bargaining

FIGURE 11-6   The arbitrator's decision may not really please either side.

and allows parties to avoid unpleasant confrontation with their own difficulties by shifting that responsibility to a public authority. However, it is useful in preventing the disruption of services.

Arbitration may be requested from the American Arbitration Association or from available state, public, and private mediation and conciliation services. The American Arbitration Association is a nonprofit, nonpartisan organization that, for a nominal fee, can provide a list of qualified arbitrators. Most states have available groups, such as the Public Employees Relations Commission, that also can provide a list of mediators and arbitrators.

Strikes and Lockouts. When the negotiation process breaks down, lockouts and strikes are likely to occur. A **lockout** occurs when an employer refuses to allow the employees to work. It is done to force employees to agree to the terms offered by the employer. The employer may close a place of business, or the employer may choose to remain open, discharge the workers, and use replacement workers. One readily can see how undesirable this would be in the health care system, but it has occurred in rare instances.

A **strike** occurs when workers refuse to continue to work until certain demands are met, thus imposing economic hardship and pressure on the employer. When the negotiation process breaks down, employees may use the strike to emphasize the need to improve their working conditions, salaries, and benefits. The most recent strikes by nurses, however, have been over issues related to patient care rather than those related to the economic status of the nurses. Striking places a serious economic hardship on employees and therefore is not undertaken lightly. Sometimes a strike is used to gain public attention to the labor dispute and to create public pressure for a settlement. This is only successful if the public agrees with the position of the striking workers.

At one time, nursing strikes were viewed by some as unprofessional and detrimental to the health of the community and, as indicated in Table 11-2, were forbidden by ANA policy until 1968. When strikes occurred, they drew major media attention and it was feared that they would damage the image of nurses and nursing.

Some nurses view with great concern the issue of whether nurses should participate in strikes if negotiations break down. These nurses believe that the withholding of services from patients is unethical and unprofessional, and therefore, personally unacceptable. Others view the strike as a final method for bringing attention to the needs of the nurse as a citizen. Fortunately, as bargaining groups representing nurses become more knowledgeable and skilled in the process, strikes occur less frequently. Disagreements at the bargaining table are more commonly resolved through mediation and arbitration, much to the relief of many professionals.

Strikes in nursing are undertaken only with advance notice, to enable patients to be transferred to another facility and to make other plans for care of individuals in the community. Typically, arrangements are made with another hospital to admit patients during the strike, and all elective procedures are canceled. The striking nurses may also agree to provide staffing to critical care, labor and delivery, and emergency departments of the facility in which the strike occurs. Often the notification that nurses intend to strike on a certain date is sufficient incentive to move negotiations to the point of settlement.

In spite of efforts to avoid them, strikes do occur in nursing. When this happens, it is often an unpleasant experience for all. Those who choose to cross picket lines may be subjected to harassment and verbal abuse by their colleagues. Those striking for better working conditions and patient safety may feel betrayed by nurses who make the strike less effective. Nurses may feel pitted against one another as well as against the management (Williams, 2004).

Reinstatement Privilege. A **reinstatement privilege** is a guarantee offered to striking employees that they will be rehired after the strike as positions become available, provided that they have not engaged in any unfair labor practices during the strike, and provided that the strike itself is lawful. The hospital may replace a striking nurse during the strike. If strikers agree unconditionally to return to work, the employer is not required to rehire a striking nurse at that time. However, recall lists are developed, and if the nurse cannot find regular and equivalent employment, he or she is privileged to recall and preference on jobs before new employees may be given employment. Nurses may lose their reinstatement privileges because of misconduct during a lawful strike. For example, strikers may not physically block other nurses and person-nel from entering or leaving a hospital during a strike. Strikers may not threaten nonstriking employees and may not attack management representatives. These types of activities usually do not occur during strikes conducted by nurses, but are not outside the realm of possibility.

Other Methods of Influencing Settlement. There are a wide variety of methods by which solutions can be reached in the negotiating process. The following discussion briefly addresses the more formal and far-reaching of these activities.

One method of reaching solution is to employ an **authoritative mandate**, in which a pres-ident, secretary of labor, or other high-ranking or influential person encourages a peaceful set-tlement. This is usually employed when the situation becomes critical and when continuance of a strike would cause problems for a great number of people.

Another technique is **informational picketing**, which involves employees carrying infor-mational signs outside of the institution. Informational picketing is not designed to stop work, but rather to inform the public of the concerns under dispute and to create public pressure on behalf of the union and the employees; it happens frequently. Other methods of obtaining community support also may be employed. These include newspaper editorials, letters to the editor, and even paid advertisements. Rallies and marches may be used to draw public attention to the issues.

In some instances, an **injunction** may be requested. This results in a court order that requires the party or parties involved to take a specific action or, more commonly, to refrain from taking a specific action. Employers may use this measure to forestall or end a strike. Unions may use this measure to stop a lockout.

In still other instances, an institution or company may be subjected to **government seizure** and operation. Government employees are then used to run the plant, firm, or industry in ques-tion. This is seldom seen in the health care industry, for obvious reasons. However, this option was used in Montana in 1991, when state employees decided to strike. The National Guard was called in to replace striking state patrolmen.

What to Look for in a Contract

The negotiation process should ultimately conclude in the development of a written contract that is signed by both union and management representatives.

A contract must meet certain specified criteria to be legally binding. It must result from mutually agreed-upon items arrived at through a "meeting of minds." Something of value must be given for a reciprocal promise, that is, professional duties for an agreed-upon sum. Contracts can be enforceable whether written or oral, but are easier to work with when written. Written contracts are also considered formal contracts (Killion & Dempski, 2000).

Although each agreement will differ, most contracts have a fairly general format. Display 11-3 includes items included in that format.

Issues Negotiated in Contracts

Many have come to believe that the collective action of nurses provides one of the best avenues for achieving professional goals and exercising control over nursing practice. Provision 6 of the ANA Code (2001) states, "The nurse participates in establishing, maintaining, and improving health care environments, and conditions of employment conducive to the provision of quality

Display 11-3   Items Typically Included in Contracts

- A preamble stating the objectives of each party
- A statement recognizing the official bargaining groups
- A section dealing with financial remuneration, including wages and salaries, overtime rates, holiday pay, and shift differentials
- A section dealing with nonfinancial rewards, that is, fringe benefits such as retirement programs, types of insurance available, free parking, and other services provided by the employer
- A section dealing with seniority in respect to promotions, transfers, work schedules, and layoffs
- A section establishing guidelines for disciplinary problems
- A section describing grievance procedures
- A section that may explicitly state codes of conduct or professional standards

health care and consistent with the values of the profession, through individual and collective action." As nurses are called on to assume greater responsibility for complicated decisions and control over practice, collective bargaining through a professional organization may provide the means to implement the concept of collective action. Today, the terms and conditions of employment have taken on a prominence over wages and hours in contract negotiations. Common issues to be negotiated include the following:

- Provisions for shared governance
- Mandatory and voluntary overtime
- Acuity-based staffing systems
- Use of temporary nurses
- Protections from reassignments and other issues related to assignment of duties
- Provisions for orientation to the work environment and continuing education
- Whistleblower protection
- Health and safety provisions such as free vaccines and needle safety
- "Just cause" language provision for discipline and/or termination
- Provisions for nursing and interdisciplinary practice committees (Budd, Warino, & Patton, 2004)

The manner in which the bargaining is conducted greatly influences how it will be perceived. Nurses as a group need to develop the skills necessary to communicate to the public the importance of their role in health care delivery. They must be able to handle conflicts and work toward resolution while maintaining integrity and dignity. Nurses need to become enlightened and informed, and they need more than a superficial understanding of the process of collective bargaining.

It is important that, as a new graduate, you know whether there is a contract in effect in the institution in which you seek employment or in the community in which you plan to work. You should also be knowledgeable about the terms of the existing contract so that you might best fulfill your obligations, and recognize and benefit from the provisions to which you are entitled. The organization to which you are applying for employment can provide you with a copy of the current contract. Contact state nurses associations for information regarding the organization that represents nurses in a particular hospital or facility. They can also provide a copy of any contracts that have been negotiated for which they represented the nurses.

Critical Thinking Activity

As a new employee in a hospital, how will you explore the matter of learning whether there is a contract? Whom will you ask? How will you obtain a copy of the contract? What will you do if the contract includes language that you do not understand? What would you do if you were in total disagreement with some of the stipulations of the contract?

Issues Related to Collective Bargaining and Nursing

Four major issues of collective bargaining affect the nursing profession. The first of these relates to the fact that some nurses see collective bargaining as unprofessional. The second is the issue of which bargaining group will represent nursing when nurses participate in collective bargaining. The third issue is an individual one and relates to the question of whether to join a union when one exists; and the fourth deals with the role of the supervisor.

These issues may take on greater or lesser importance depending on the area of the country involved, the length of time the nurses in that area have been participating in collective bargaining, and the group chosen to represent the nurses at the bargaining table. As a staff nurse, you may, at some time, have to make a decision regarding whether to strike. In making this decision, you want to be well grounded in the issues at hand, and knowledgeable about the arrangements that have been made for continuance of services in emergency situations and in special hospital areas, such as labor and delivery.

Collective Action and Professionalism. The argument against unionism has its roots in the history of nursing itself. Nursing was perceived by many, including nurses, as a selfless, all-serving, altruistic calling. The act of caring for others, even if that meant subordinating the individual to the goals of that care, was to be compensation enough for the services rendered. The strong religious influences that pervaded the early development of nursing added to this concept of the profession (see Chapter 4). Early leaders in nursing espoused this dedication to its arts.

Another factor that has hampered the strong development of unionization in nursing is the socialization of women and the fact that nursing is primarily a woman's profession. Although more men now enter nursing, currently fewer than 10% of the RNs in the United States are male. Early social beliefs that a woman's role should be submissive, supportive, and obedient were extremely compatible with the expectations that our society placed on nurses. The paternalism that has existed in the health care delivery system has also made the process of collective bargaining for nurses a slow one (see Chapter 4). The combination of the role of women and the role of the nurse under earlier paternalistic practices had the nurse caring for the "hospital family," looking out for the needs of all (from patient to physician) and being responsible for keeping everyone happy (Ashley, 1976). The tendency to see the physician as the father figure in the health care system, the nurse as the corresponding mother figure, and the patients as the children has done little to promote the autonomy of nursing as a profession. A quote by Campbell (1980, p. 1286) illustrates this historical use of the family concept in health care: "If we are to keep unions out of the profession we, as nurses, must make every effort to build loyalty and a family feeling among our fellow nurses."

Today we see nurses involved in collective bargaining in greater numbers than ever before. Several factors are responsible for this change. Wilson and colleagues (1990) have identified these as the following:

- The focus on the continued high cost of health care and the need to examine this rise; the scrutiny that has been placed on employees' salaries as part of this process
- The fact that nurses constitute the largest number of employees in hospitals (nearly half)
- Changes in the NLRA allowing nurses to bargain collectively.

Representations for Nurses. As collective bargaining has become accepted for those in the nursing profession, the number of groups that seek to represent nurses at the bargaining table has constantly increased, with many groups now bargaining for nurses. Representation is determined by elections that are supervised by the NLRB. To become the certified collective bargaining representative of a group of employees, the organization in question must receive 50% of the votes cast, plus one.

When nurses first began to organize, the ANA, through the state nurses associations, was the sole bargaining representative; this group still represents more nurses than all other organizations combined. However, some would contend that it is not realistic for one group to work with the professionalism aspect of nursing as well as with the issues of wages, benefits, and working conditions. This has encouraged other organizations to vie for the representative position.

A large number of nurses are also represented by the American Federation of Teachers, the Teamsters Union, the National Union of Hospital and Health Care Employees, The Federation of Nurses and Health Professionals, United Food and Commercial Workers, or the SEIU. In some instances, as with the SEIU, the organization represents other workers employed in the organization. The SEIU organizes what are called "wall-to-wall" unions, in which all employees of all categories from housekeeping and maintenance to nurses and pharmacists belong to one bargaining unit. This may be favored by hospital administration, which often expresses frustration with the number of groups with whom they must carry out negotiations. However, when the SEIU is bargaining for all employees, it has the distinct disadvantage of diluting the ability of nurses to include professional issues in the negotiation process.

Nurses face a difficult decision when choosing which group can represent them best. In past years, this decision has occupied perhaps more time and effort on the part of nurses than has the actual bargaining. Those who have strong allegiance to the ANA contend that only RNs should bargain for RNs. One of the reasons given for this position is that in collective bargaining, nurses face different issues than other workers. Many believe that only nurses can effectively negotiate such items. These people contend that hospital administrations, fearing the power of labor unions, will bargain more constructively and positively with nurses themselves. They also believe that the ANA will be a stronger, more united organization if it serves as both the professional association and the bargaining agent.

The state nurses association serves as a collective bargaining agent in most states. To do this, they must organize in such as way that the collective bargaining is separated in terms of finances and control from the other activities of the organization. Those who are members but not part of a collective bargaining unit pay lesser dues than those who are part of a collective bargaining unit. Only those who are part of bargaining units have a vote regarding collective bargaining issues. At the national level, the UAN is formed by the state association collective bargaining units and has been kept separate from the other activities of the ANA. In addition to helping the state organizations work together, the UAN can also act as a collective bargaining agent for multi-state healthcare organizations and for states that do not have a collective bargaining arm. Thus, the ANA and its constituent state organizations have tried to address the concerns of those who believe one organization cannot fulfill both roles.

Some nurses prefer two organizations—one to represent issues related to professionalism and another to negotiate salaries. This results in cost factors, because both organizations would collect dues. Many consider the cost of belonging to the ANA and to the state association to be very high, with dues of approximately $350.00 per year. Additional, equally expensive membership dues in another organization might be prohibitive. Second, many believe that the union would become the dominant force between the two groups, because money and working environment issues both speak strongly.

There are no easy answers to this question, and it will certainly be one of the biggest issues facing nurses in the future.

Critical Thinking Activity

If the collective bargaining agent in the hospital in which you worked was other than the state nurses association, would you belong to both organizations? What factors would you use to support your decision? Why are these factors important to you?

The Decision to Join or Not to Join. Once nurses have gained an understanding of collective bargaining and have developed a personal philosophy about the professional role of the nurse, they are ready to make a decision regarding membership in the bargaining unit.

In working with students who are soon to embark on professional careers, we find that it is easier for them to decide whether to bargain collectively than it is to decide to part with the money that is required for membership. Many nurses want better working conditions and higher salaries, but are all too willing to let someone else fund these endeavors and work to achieve them.

It is in response to these concerns that many agency shop clauses have been added to contracts. Those who are members and are active in the negotiation process believe it is inappropriate for some to benefit from the labors of the bargaining process without having contributed, at least financially, to the effort. The presence of agency shop clauses may serve as either an asset or a deterrent to recruitment, depending on the applicant's viewpoint.

COMMUNICATION IN *ACTION*

Seeking Information Regarding a Union

Will Jones had just begun working at the medical center. He was given a copy of the contract for RNs during his orientation. He was also given the name of a union representative on his unit. During his first week there, he approached the representative and said, "Hi Carol, I was told you are the union representative for our unit. Do you have some time to talk with me at lunch? I would like to understand more about the process here." She replied, "Sure—let's plan to go down to the cafeteria at 11:30—first lunch. Does that work for you?" He said, "That is when I was scheduled for lunch too. Just so you know, I don't really know anything about the union, what its goals are, the issues here, or anything. I hope you can help me get that kind of information." Will had set the stage to become a knowledgeable participant in the bargaining process.

Critical Thinking Activity

Do you support the concept of nurses becoming members of a union? If so, should all employees of an organization be required to pay membership fees? Analyze your response to this question and provide the rationale to support your views.

Collective Bargaining and the Role of Supervisor. In 1994, a nursing home argued before the Supreme Court that the LPNs in its employ were supervisors (because of their role in directing nursing assistants in patient care) and, therefore, were not protected by the NLRA. The Supreme Court, in a 5 to 4 decision, ruled in favor of the nursing home. Nursing organizations engaged in collective bargaining have expressed serious concern about the implications of this ruling for all nurses. Labor groups expect to lobby for legislation that would alter this interpretation of the NLRB ("Striking at bargaining . . . ," 1994).

This issue was again addressed in February 1996, when the NLRB ended nearly 2 years of deliberation by ruling that charge nurses at Alaska's Providence Medical Center could not be called supervisors simply because the role requires some direction of other workers. The board stated that the essence of the nurse's role was judgment, and went on to explain that authority that arises from professional knowledge is distinct from the authority of a front-line manager ("NLRB to the Supreme Court," 1996). The issue continues to occur with surprising frequency.

Changes in the Number of Bargaining Units. Within hospitals, there are many different positions and job titles, ranging from professional staff through office staff to those responsible for hospital maintenance. In nursing alone, there are groups of RNs, LPNs, and nursing assistants. As these groups have been granted authority to organize into bargaining units, concern has been expressed about the number of unions with which any hospital administration must bargain at any given time. Some fairly elaborate estimates have been made regarding the amount of time demanded by the collective bargaining process.

When the NLRA was first passed in 1974, the NLRB specified that seven employee bargaining units would exist within the health care industry (Wilson et al., 1990, p. 37). The seven groups were RNs, physicians, other professional employees, technical employees, business office employees, clerical employees, and skilled maintenance employees. In 1984, the NLRB determined that bargaining units would be decided on a case-by-case basis. This resulted in reducing the number of bargaining units to three: all professionals, all nonprofessionals, and guards.

In 1989, the NLRB proposed a new rule that resulted in the establishment of eight collective bargaining units. At this time, it was also determined that the rule would apply to hospitals of all sizes. In response, the American Hospital Association (AHA) sought and obtained a permanent injunction against the rule. Subsequently, all-RN units were legally approved. The latest activity regarding this issue occurred in April 1991. The U.S. Supreme Court upheld the NLRB in its authority to define bargaining units for health care workers in acute care hospitals, and allowed for all-RN bargaining units ("Supreme Court okays . . . ," 1991). As might be expected, the AHA and the ANA occupied opposite points of view regarding this issue.

Changing Trends With Regard to Collective Bargaining

At one time, economic concerns and working conditions may have been the principal motivators for collective action. However, by the mid-1980s, subtle, and at times not so subtle, changes occurred throughout the United States regarding collective bargaining, unionism, and labor-management relations.

Some working in the area of contract management have reported a shift from the adversarial relationship that historically had existed between the employee and the employer (which focused on salaries, work hours, and the like) to one that placed greater emphasis on the quality of work life.

The Thrust of Collective Bargaining in Nursing. The focus of collective bargaining issues changed during the 1990s. As nurses have become more comfortable and knowledgeable about the bargaining process, their energies have been directed toward many issues. Originally focusing on wages and benefits, today the major concerns of nurses also include staffing patterns, involvement in decisions affecting patient care, cross-training, the use of unlicensed assistive personnel, workplace safety and the rights of employees to know the hazards with a work environment, comparable worth, and discriminatory practices against employees (both male and female). This shift in emphasis reflects the general acceptance of the process of collective bargaining by nurses and the fact that significant headway has been made through this process regarding basic issues. This change of thinking is borne out by a vote of the House of Delegates of the American Medical Association to develop an affiliated national labor organization, under the NLRA, that would support the development and operation of local negotiating units to represent employed physicians. Self-employed physicians were barred from joining collective bargaining units by antitrust laws ("Docs vote . . . ," 1999).

Elimination of Unions and Strike Breaking. A trend seen in health care institutions during the 1980s, and persisting in some areas today, is an effort toward eliminating unions. Although technically illegal when referring to methods used to eliminate an existing union, the movement has been expanded to include a wide range of legal activities that slow down collective bargaining or prevent a union from forming or functioning effectively. Pressured by rapidly escalating health care costs, and influenced by the changing attitudes toward work, hospital administrators have hired consultants and law firms to assist and advise in discouraging and impeding organizational activities.

Another closely related approach involves mutual cooperation between management and the union without undermining the legitimate roles and rights of either. The union encourages wholehearted employee participation by its members while exercising flexibility on issues. With this approach, the union should have input into the managerial decision-making process through representation on committees at every level of the organization. Unions should be expected to be cooperative with management but not be co-opted. Management must be fair with the union, neither seeking to destroy the union nor meekly acquiescing to every union demand (Colosi & Berkeley, 1994).

Strike breaking refers to efforts directed at causing employees on strike to cease the strike without having reached an agreement. In an effort to break a strike, employers hire temporary nurses at very high wages plus living stipends to entice them to come to work. One temporary agency specializes in providing nurses as strike breakers. In Portland, Oregon, the temporary nurses were housed in a hotel and transported to and from the hospital in a bus with blacked-out windows. Their salaries (without the cost of transportation and stipends) were significantly higher than the maximum requested by the striking nurses (Oregon nurses strike, 2002). That strike was finally settled by the intervention of the governor of the state as a mediator, and a contract agreement was finally reached.

The Impact of Shared Governance on Collective Bargaining. Although the greater involvement of staff nurses in health care agency decision making may have a significant impact on the collective bargaining process, the number of nurses represented by collective bargaining is increasing. When both collective bargaining and shared governance are present, there is a separation of those issues that are the purview of the union and those issues that can be decided within the shared governance structure. If there is a union, it has the responsibility and authority to negotiate those things that fall under wages, benefits, and working conditions, such as the use of agency nurses, work load, and policies regarding floating from one unit to another. The shared governance committees work with clinical standards. Each nurse has greater accountability for participation in decision making outside of the bargaining process and for implementing decisions that have been made.

Looking to the Future

As with many of the issues with which nursing wrestles, there are no easy answers to the matter of collective bargaining. Some view it as an absolute necessity; others find it unethical. And there are many who would prefer to play ostrich with regard to the entire concern, hoping it will not be necessary. Williams (2004) makes the following four recommendations regarding collective bargaining, all of which demonstrate opportunities for nursing leadership grounded in ethics:

- Because nurses are creative and powerful problem solvers, they should recognize the power that they have to observe, identify, and improve processes within the health care system.
- Nurses must recognize health care and hospital administrators as health professionals and be familiar and respectful of their ethical and professional obligations.
- Nursing curricula should provide graduates with a working understanding of all aspects of the ANA Code, especially provision six, which addresses collective action and advocacy.
- When selecting leaders and spokespersons for their groups, care should be taken to choose those who are able to listen, understand, and communicate the interests and problems identified by the other parties at the negotiating table. Powerful and creative leadership requires understanding both sides.

Key Concepts

- Mission statements provide information about critical elements of the organization. They explicitly outline the purpose of the organization and may also contain the philosophy and goals of the group. These statements serve as a benchmark against which an organization's performance may be evaluated.

- Organizations may be structured a number of ways. Some are tall and centralized, where the authority to make decisions is vested in a few individuals. Others are flat and decentralized, with a number of individuals involved in decision making.

- All organizations have chains of command, channels of communication, and spans of control that describe lines of authority and accountability. These can be depicted in organizational charts, which represent the formal organization and are a pictorial means of portraying roles and patterns of interaction among parts of a system.

- Written job descriptions outline the roles and responsibilities for all employees and are a necessary and vital part of any organization.

- Policies and protocols guide the activities of the employees as they carry out their responsibilities.

- Shared governance, a form of practice model that involves decision making in which both nursing staff and management participate, results in a decentralized organization and often results in greater job satisfaction for nurses because they have more control over practice.

- In the late 1980s, studies were conducted to determine what factors resulted in hospitals attracting and retaining RNs. Characteristics of these hospitals were identified and the awarding of Magnet status to hospitals that achieve these goals has resulted. The process is carried out under the auspices of the ANCC.

- Patterns of nursing care delivery have varied over the years and include the case method, the functional method, team nursing, total patient care, modular care, and primary nursing.

- Case management provides an approach to delivery of all patient care services (not just nursing) over an entire hospital stay or even throughout an entire health care concern. Nurses are involved in case management and may serve as case managers.

- Many workplace issues require negotiation. Major among these are grievances, collective bargaining contracts, and workplace safety issues.

- A grievance is an alleged violation of the provisions of the contract or institutional policies. Should a grievance arise, all steps must be followed as outlined in order for the grievance to be addressed effectively. Nurses need to distinguish between issues that are grievances and those that are simply complaints.

- Since 1974, nurses have bargained collectively for salaries, working conditions, and benefits. Collective bargaining may also negotiate for nurses' participation in committees focused on improving patient care and patient care standards and other issues of concern to nurses including staffing patterns, mandatory overtime, use of temporary nurses, workplace safety, and discriminatory practices.

- Approaches to collective bargaining vary and include the historic adversarial approach, interest-based bargaining, and concession bargaining.

- Interest-based bargaining attempts to problem solve differences between labor and industry. Nurses can play a powerful leadership role in the process.

- The collective bargaining process culminates in a contract that places in writing the decisions reached at the bargaining table. Key aspects of a contract are the wages and benefits, issues of seniority and layoffs, grievance procedures, termination procedures, and working conditions (including professional involvement).
- One of the issues surrounding nurses and collective bargaining is related to which group should do the bargaining for nurses. Many believe this process is best conducted by a professional nursing organization; others believe they are served best by an organization that has collective bargaining as its only focus.
- Trends regarding the collective bargaining process include constructive adversarialism, union busting, strike breaking, and changes in the number of bargaining units.

Relevant Web Sites

Magnet Status:
http://nursecredentialing.org/magnet
http://nursingworld.org/ancc/magnet/index.html

Shared Governance:
www.sharedgovernance.org

Unions:
AFL-CIO: *www.nursefriendly.com/unions*
American Nurses Association: *http://nursingworld.org.* (click on "United American Nurses")

Support:
www.Nursinghands.com

References

Alexander, M. K., Bourgeois, A., & Goodman, L. R. (1994). Total quality improvement: Bridging the gap between education and service. In O. L. Strickland & D. J. Fishman, *Nursing issues in the 1990s* (pp. 280–289). Albany, NY: Delmar Publishers.

American Nurses Association. (2001). *Code of ethics for nurses with interpretive statements*. Washington, DC: American Nurses Publishing.

Anthony, M. K. (2004). Shared governance models: The theory, practice, and evidence. *Online Journal of Issues in Nursing, 9*(1), Manuscript 4. [On-line]. *http://nursingworld.org/ojin/topic23/tpc23_4.htm.* Accessed January 13, 2006.

Ashley, J. A. (1976). *Hospitals, paternalism and the role of the nurse*. New York: Teachers' College Press.

Brooks, B. A. (2004). Measuring the impact of shared governance. *Online Journal of Issues in Nursing, 9*(1), Manuscript 1a. [On-line]. *http://nursingworld.org/ojin/topic23/tpc23_la.htm.* Accessed January 13, 2006.

Brown, S. J. (2001). Research evidence linking staffing and patient outcomes. *Orthopedic Nursing, 20*(1), 67–68.

Budd, K., Warino, L., & Patton, M. (2004, January 31). Traditional and non-traditional collective bargaining: Strategies to improve the patient care environment. *Online Journal of Nursing 9*(1), [On-line]. *http://nursingworld.org/ojin/topic23/tpc23_5.htm.* Accessed January 13, 2006.

Campbell, G. J. (1980). In opinions: Is bargaining unprofessional for nurses? *AORN Journal 31*(6), 1289.

Caramanica, L. (2004). Shared governance: Hartford Hospital's experience. *Online Journal of Issues in Nursing, 9*(1), Manuscript 2. [On-line]. *http://nursingworld.org/oijn/topic23/tpc_2.htm.* Accessed January 13, 2006.

Colosi, T. R., & Berkeley, A. E. (1994). *Collective bargaining: How it works and why*. New York: American Arbitration Association.

Domrose, C. (2002, August 12). Changing tides. *NurseWeek (Mountain West Ed.), 3*(11), 17–19.

Ellis, B. & Gates, J. (2005). Achieving magnet status. *Nurse Administration, 29*(3), 241–244.

Ellis, J. R. & Hartley, C. L. (2005). *Managing and coordinating nursing care*, 4th ed. Philadelphia: Lippincott Williams & Wilkins.

Fuller-Jonap, F. (1994). Collective bargaining in nursing: Benefits, issues, and problems. In O. L. Strickland & D. J. Fishman, *Nursing issues in the 1990s* (pp. 33–45). Albany, NY: Delmar Publishers.

Goode, C. J., Krugman, M. E., & Diaz, J. (2005). The pull of magnetism: A look at the standards and the experience of a western academic medical center hospital in achieving and sustaining Magnet status. *Nursing Administration, 29*(3), 202–213.

Green A., & Jordan, C. (2004). Common denominators: Shared governance and work place advocacy—Strategies for nurses to gain control over their practice. *Online Journal of Issues in Nursing, 9*(1), Manuscript 6. [On-line]. *http://nursingworld.org/ojin/topic23/tpc23_6.htm*. Accessed January 13, 2006.

Herzberg, F. (1966). *Work and the nature of man.* New York: World Publishing Company.

Hess, R. G. (2004). From bedside to boardroom—Nursing shared governance. *Online Journal of Issues in Nursing, 9*(1), Manuscript 1. [On-line]. *http://nursingworld.org/ojin/topic23/tpc23_1.htm*. Accessed January 13, 2006.

Herrin, D. M. (2004) Shared governance: A nurse executive response. *Online Journal of Issues in Nursing, 9*(1), Manuscript 1b. [On-line]. *http://nursingworld.org/ojin/topic23/tpc23_1b.htm*. Accessed January 13, 2006.

Hinshaw, A. S. (2002). Building magnetism into health organizations. In: M. L. McClure & A. S. Hinsaw (Eds.), *Magnet hospitals revisited: Attraction and retention of professional nurses.* Washington, DC: American Nurses Publishing.

Kalisch, P. A. & Kalisch, B. T. (2004). American Nursing: A History, 4th ed. Philadelphia: Lippincott Williams & Wilkins.

Killion, S. W., & Dempski, K. M. (2000). *Legal and ethical issues.* Thorofare, NJ: Slack, Inc.

Komplin, J. (1995). Care delivery systems. In P. S. Yoder Wise, *Leading and managing in nursing,* (pp. 411–435) St. Louis, MO: Mosby.

Kramer, M., & Schmalenberg, C. E. (2005). Best quality patient care: A historical perspective on Magnet hospitals. *Nursing Administration, 29*(3), 275–287.

McClure, M. L. (2005). Magnet hospitals: Insights and issues. *Nursing Administration, 29*(3), 198–201.

McGregor, D. (1960). *The human side of enterprise.* New York: McGraw-Hill.

Needleman, J., Buerhaus, P., Mattke, S., Stewart, M., & Zelevinsky, K. (2002, May 30). Nurse-staffing levels and the quality of care in hospitals. *New England Journal of Medicine, 346*(22), 1757–1766.

"NLRB to the Supreme Court: Labor law protects nurses." (1996). *American Journal of Nursing, 96*(4), 67, 72.

"Oregon nurses strike for pay, health care." (2002). *The American Nurse.* [On-line]. *http://nursingworld.org/tan/janfeb02/inbrief.htm*. Accessed January 23, 2006.

Porter-O'Grady, T. (1990). Nursing governance in a transitional era. In N. L. Chaska, *The nursing profession: Turning points,* (pp. 432–439). St. Louis, MO: CV Mosby.

Porter-O-Grady, T. (2003). Researching shared governance: A futility focus. *Journal of Nursing Administration, 33*(4), 251–252.

Porter-O'Grady, T. (1987). Shared governance and new organizational models. *Nursing Economics, 5*(6), 281–286.

"Striking at bargaining rights, court says RNs are supervisors." (1994). *American Journal of Nursing, 94*(7), 67, 70–71.

"Supreme Court okays all-RN unit." (1991, June). *American Nurse 33*(3), 1.

The Free Online Dictionary by Farlex Inc. (2005). [On-line]. *www.thefreedictionary.com/contract*. Accessed April 24, 2005.

Welch, J., & Welch, S. (2005). *Winning.* New York: HarperCollins Publishers, Inc.

Williams, K. O. (2004). Ethics and collective bargaining: Calls to action. *Online Journal of Issues in Nursing.* [On-line]. *http://nursingworld.org/ojin/ethicol/ethics_15.htm*. Accessed January 13, 2006.

Wilson, C. N., Hamilton, C. L., & Murphy, E. (1990). Union dynamics in nursing. *Journal of Nursing Administration, 20*(2), 35–39.

Zuzelo, P. R., Seminara, P., McGoldrick, T., & Karbach, H. (2003, July). Facilitating evidence-based practice in a shared governance nursing organization. A description of a symposium conducted at a preconference on International Evidence-Based Practice sponsored by Sigma Theta Tau International, July 9, 2003. [On-line]. *http://stti.confex.com/stti/preinrc14/techprogram/session_1636.htm*. Accessed January 13, 2006.

12

Initiating the Leadership and Management Role

LEARNING OUTCOMES

After completing this chapter, you should be able to:

1. Compare and contrast the skills involved in leadership and management.
2. Differentiate between the terms "authority" and "accountability."
3. Discuss the major theories regarding leadership.
4. Compare and contrast the three prevailing leadership styles.
5. Analyze the factors that have resulted in the development of transformational leadership.
6. Describe the relationship of power and empowerment and identify ways by which one individual can empower another.
7. Explain emotional intelligence and why it is an important quality of a leader.
8. Analyze methods by which the development of leadership style can be enhanced.
9. Describe the basic characteristics of effective communication.
10. Analyze the communication strategies that are essential for effective leadership, identifying the critical role of each.
11. Describe the elements of an effective performance-appraisal system, including the conduct of the interview.
12. Analyze the importance of time management and evaluate methods that will help overcome major time wasters and procrastination.

KEY TERMS

Accountability
Authority
Autocratic/authoritarian leadership style
Charisma
Coercive power
Communication
Connection power

Democratic/participative leadership style
Empowerment
Emotional intelligence
Expert power
Informational power
Job descriptions

Laissez-faire/permissive leadership style
Leadership
Leadership/management style
Legitimate power
Management
Mentor

Mindfulness	Procrastination	Reward power
Motivational power	Professional standards	Theories of leadership
Multicratic leadership	Referent power	Time management
Performance appraisal	Responsibility	

The novice in the area of health care administration can easily be dazzled by the many terms populating the literature devoted to the topics of leadership and management. Words such as authority, responsibility, accountability, team building, empowerment, coaching, mentoring, motivating, and collective power are but a few of those incorporated into articles, monographs, and books addressing the topic of successful leadership and management. What do these terms mean to you as you begin reading this chapter? What will they mean to you when you finish this course? In what ways will the meanings gain greater significance as you begin your career as a staff nurse? What will the terms mean as you begin to assume a leadership role in patient care?

UNDERSTANDING LEADERSHIP AND MANAGEMENT

Although the terms "leadership" and "management" are often used interchangeably, differences exist in how each is practiced in the work situation. At some point in your nursing career, you likely will fill both roles: leader and manager. Understanding the uniqueness of each will help you be effective in either position. Let us explore the differences and how they are applied in the work situation.

Leadership refers to the ability to guide, motivate, and inspire, and to instill vision and purpose. As you read this, you probably can think of individuals you know who possess strong leadership abilities—your class president or the person who arranges and guides your study sessions, for example. To provide leadership, you must be able to influence the beliefs, opinions, or behaviors of others and to persuade others to follow your direction. This can be accomplished in a number of ways, referred to as leadership styles, which we will discuss later.

Management refers to activities such as planning, organizing, directing, and controlling with the purpose of accomplishing specific goals and objectives within an organization. Essentially, management involves coordination and integration of resources to accomplish specific tasks. Often management positions are roles to which one is appointed or hired after a competitive job application and interview. This appointment grants the manager the power to direct others and the responsibility for ensuring that certain tasks within the organization are completed effectively and efficiently. In other words, the authority to act is gained by virtue of the position one holds within the organization.

The very best managers also are leaders, although this may not always happen. Conversely, not all leaders are officially managers in the sense we have defined it. A foremost authority on leadership and organizational management, Warren Bennis (2003), has stated that managers are people who do things right, while leaders are people who do the right thing. Individuals may become leaders because of the way in which they inspire others to follow them. Can you think of a situation in which an individual was a leader but did not have the role of manager? Similarly, can you think of any situations in which the manager lacked the ability to lead a group of people? Can you recall situations in which the manager also was a leader?

UNDERSTANDING ACCOUNTABILITY AND AUTHORITY

Three terms are frequently associated with leadership and management roles: accountability, responsibility, and authority. Are you clear about the definitions of each of these terms?

Accountability and **responsibility** are terms with similar meanings. They refer to the obligation to answer for one's actions and to accomplish what you have agreed to do. For example, the team leader assigns you the care of four patients and you agree to that assignment; therefore, the patients' care is your responsibility. You have an obligation to provide timely care to that group of patients and to achieve the desired outcome regarding that care.

By virtue of the state Nurse Practice Acts, nurses are held responsible or accountable for their actions. This means they must provide the necessary care competently and in compliance with accepted standards, using sound judgment, thinking critically, and delegating wisely. Failure to perform in a responsible manner could result in legal action being taken against the nurse if harm occurs to the patient.

Nurses have always been accountable for the care they give from both a personal and a professional standpoint. However, as we have witnessed the rapid technologic, fiscal, and operational changes occurring within the health care system, the term now carries stronger legal implications. Nurses face greater legal vulnerability because of consumer rights, the public availability of records, and increased patient involvement in health care decision making. This intensifies the need for nurses to be aware of the legal aspects of nursing and of the laws that protect the client. Legal aspects of care are discussed in greater detail in Chapter 8.

Individuals are accountable for their own actions and also for some of the actions of those they supervise. Thus, we see that tasks can be delegated, but accountability cannot. Nurses who delegate tasks to assistive personnel continue to be accountable for that care (see Chapter 13). For example, if you ask the nursing assistant to check the vital signs of four of your patients, you are asking the assistant to act in your place. You are still accountable for that activity (ie, that the vital signs are accurately measured, reported, and documented). This accountability has become a sensitive issue for nurses as, in an effort to contain costs, more unlicensed assistive personnel are hired to replace licensed staff.

Authority can be defined as the power to influence, give directions, command, take action, and make decisions. Traditionally, we have considered it the manager's job to command or make decisions. In this sense, the manager authored all critical decisions. As you read further, you will note that in today's work environment, authority is more often shared. Accompanying this shared authority and decision making is a mutual responsibility for outcomes. We will discuss this concept in greater detail after we have talked about leadership.

In the ideal work situation, workers are given the amount of authority needed to carry out the responsibilities expected of them. However, many nurses experience frustration because they must be accountable for activities without the authority to affect the situation or create change. For example, a nurse has the responsibility of ensuring that all patients receive competent care, but the nurse may have no input into the performance appraisal of nursing assistants working on that shift. Therefore, the nursing assistants may not be as responsive to the nurse's instructions as they should be. Or perhaps a nurse has the responsibility for seeing that there are adequate supplies on a unit but has no opportunity to affect the unit's budget.

EXAMPLE

Accountability Without Authority

John Jones, a registered nurse (RN), works on the night shift. He works with two nursing assistants. All nursing assistants are taught the skills expected in their job description by the staff development department. During his orientation to the hospital, John was informed that all nursing assistants were taught basic care skills and how to measure vital signs. They also were cross-trained as phlebotomists. The nursing assistants were expected to draw the blood for morning lab work. However, John quickly discovered that one of the nursing assistants on his shift was not able to draw blood successfully. When he spoke with the other RN on his unit about this, she said, "You will find that lots of them really don't have that skill. You will just have to draw the blood yourself. Nobody really says anything to them if they don't do it and it makes their job easier if they don't draw blood. Some are even afraid to draw blood because they are afraid of the potential for contracting HIV." John replied, "But that really increases my work load at a busy time. Isn't there any way that I can require them to go back and get the skills they need?" The other RN replied, "Nope, you just have to make sure everything gets done on time." John discovered that he was accountable for the care by the nursing assistants but had no authority over their practice.

Critical Thinking Activity

Think for a moment of behaviors you noted in your clinical experiences this past week. What behavior did you observe that was a clear demonstration of authority? What were the characteristics that made it so? Can you recall a situation in which an RN accepted responsibility for an action that had been taken? How was this done?

THEORIES OF LEADERSHIP

Let's talk briefly about the various **theories of leadership** (Table 12-1). Just as knowledge of theories of nursing can help us to understand nursing (see Chapter 4), leadership theories help us to describe and understand the processes of leadership. As a society, we have studied leadership theory since about the mid-20th century, and a number of theories have been set forth, far too many to discuss in detail in this text. The theories of leadership listed in Table 12-1 are those most frequently cited as helpful in understanding specific situations.

As a student preparing for graduation from your nursing program, you may wonder how all the information on leadership theories relates to you. Health care represents one of the largest businesses in the United States. Historically, the administrative structure in hospitals has been predominately bureaucratic, with a few decision makers and many followers. That situation is changing as more hospitals adopt a pattern of transformational leadership. But that will not be true in all organizations, nor will it reflect the attitudes of some of the individuals with whom you will work. Having basic knowledge of the various approaches to leadership will help you understand the environments in which you work and will help you determine the leadership approach you wish to develop.

Current emphasis in most management literature is placed on transformational leadership. Today's health care work environment relies on teamwork and shared decision making. Many believe that in this environment, the goals of the organization are most likely to be met

TABLE 12-1	MAJOR THEORIES OF LEADERSHIP
GENERAL CLASSIFICATION, THEORY, AND THEORIST	**ESSENTIAL CHARACTERISTICS AND COMMENTS**
Trait	Focuses on certain characteristics of the leader.
Great Man theory	Promotes the concept that certain people were born to be leaders because they inherited a set of special characteristics qualifying them for such responsibilities. Because leaders are "born," this theory suggests that leadership cannot be developed.
Attribution theory	Suggests that leadership relates to personal attributes people tend to characterize leaders as having, such as height, social background, creativity, assertiveness, initiative, integrity, ability, intelligence, etc.
Charismatic theory	Often listed as a quality of other theories, this theory relates to a special charm or allure possessed by the leader that inspires others to follow and give allegiance. Sometimes this type of leadership is said to emerge in times of crisis and change.
Attitudinal	Theorizes that attitudes of the leader result in the leader's behavior.
Ohio State Leadership Studies	Describes leadership behavior as related to initiating structure and consideration of employees.
Michigan Leadership Studies	Describes leader behavior as employee oriented or production oriented.
Managerial grid (R. R. Blake & J. S. Mouton, 1964)	Identifies five management styles best described on a grid, in which each style combines elements of concern for production and concern for people.
Situational	Suggests basis of leadership is the situation or environment and the behaviors of leaders in response to the situation.
Contingency theory (Fred Fiedler, 1967)	Examines factors in the situation, particularly the skills of the leader and that individual's position of power in the organization, as determinants of leader effectiveness.
Path–Goal theory (Robert J. House, 1971)	Relates effective leadership to leader's ability to minimize obstructions to goals, identify outcomes that workers want to achieve, and reward the followers for high performance and achievement, thereby increasing worker satisfaction and productivity.
Transactional leadership (sometimes referred to as *Exchange leadership*) (J. M. Burns, 1978)	Examines leadership in terms of striking a bargain in which there is a mutual exchange between leaders and followers of benefits for work. Leader diagnoses problems in the organization, work group, or situation and is a caretaker who facilitates workers' motivation, satisfaction, and performance.
Contemporary Theories	Includes theories most commonly in use at the present time.
Transformational leadership (Heinrich von Pierer, 1994)	Places emphasis on the collective purpose and mutual growth of both the leader and the follower and de-emphasizes differences in the roles of the leader and followers. Leader activities include creating a vision, building relationships, developing trust, and building self-esteem. Leader makes subordinates aware of how important their jobs are, helps them build skills, and motivates them to work for the good of the organization.
(Peter Senge et al., 1994)	Identifies the role of the leader as that of a strategic visionary; promotes "learning" organizations in which the leader is the teacher who builds a shared vision.

if transformational leadership is employed. As you study the attributes of transformation leadership in Table 12-1, you will note that the differences in the role of the leader and the followers are de-emphasized. When effectively implemented, transformational leadership can result in agreements about priorities, shared values, perceived common goals, and meaningful purposes (Bass, 2001). You can see how this would be desirable in a health care environment.

Leadership/Management Styles

Lewin (1951) described three prevailing styles of behavior observed in leaders/managers that we refer to as **leadership** or **management styles** (Display 12-1). Sometimes these styles also are listed among the behavioral theories of leadership. The focus of these three styles is on the amount of control the manager assumes over the actions of the workers and the beliefs of the leader/manager about the nature of workers (which is why they may be referred to as behavioral theories). Note that the extremes extend from situations in which the manager makes all the decisions to situations in which virtually no direction is given to workers. In addition to the individual characteristics of the leader, several other variables will determine the type of manager a nurse might be. The type of organizational structure will influence leadership styles. How authority is centralized or dispersed throughout the organization also affects leadership styles. The

---

 Display 12-1   Leadership/Management Styles

Autocratic/Authoritative
Majority of decisions determined by the manager
Dictates work to be done and who will do it
Provides little opportunity for input or suggestions from followers
Gives little feedback or recognition for accomplishments
Communication flows downward, with emphasis on completing the task
Works well in emergency situations where time is of the essence
May be preferred style when working with unskilled or uneducated employees

Democratic/Participative
Input to decision-making encouraged among workers
Leaders see themselves as coworkers
Communication, consensus, and teamwork stressed
Leader leads by providing information, suggesting direction, supporting coworkers
Communication flows both up and down
Human relationships important
Considered the preferred style in the majority of work situations

Laissez-faire/Permissive
Little or no direction or guidance provided
Coworkers develop their own goals, make their own decisions, and take responsibility
Decision-making dispersed throughout the group
Provides maximum freedom for individuals and motivates workers to perform at high levels
If used inappropriately, a leadership vacuum may occur, in which an informal leader may arise

Multicratic
Combines the positive features of authoritative, participative leadership styles
Leader provides a maximum of structure when the situation requires it
Leader provides maximum group participation when needed
Support and encouragement provided to subordinates at all times

communication patterns, which are directly tied to organizational structure, also will influence leadership styles. Equally important is the situation at hand.

Autocratic or **authoritarian leadership**, in which the leader/manager makes the majority of the decisions, may be essential in emergency situations that call for immediate action. When faced with life-threatening conditions, as we frequently see in emergency departments, the leader may be in the best position to make judgments and decisions. Little time exists to contemplate and build consensus regarding the best approach or to allow discussion for alternative actions.

Laissez-faire or **permissive leadership**, in which little or no direction or guidance is provided, is at the other extreme and provides the least structure and control. It is highly effective for situations in which coworkers can develop their own goals, make their own decisions, and take responsibility for their own actions. An example might be seen in an inpatient psychiatric unit where a certain amount of autonomy and self-direction are an important part of the unit's operation.

Democratic or **participative leadership**, in which input to decision making is encouraged among workers, represents the middle ground. The democratic leader focuses on involving subordinates in decision making. There are various methods to accomplish this, such as asking for input, developing a consensus, voting, or delegating decisions to others. It is most effective when the decision or task at hand does not require urgent action and when subordinates have the ability to make meaningful contributions.

A fourth leadership style, not identified by Lewin, is probably the one that is most frequently used in health care. **Multicratic leadership** combines the most favorable aspects of all styles as mediated by the circumstances at hand. A multicratic leader provides maximum structure and direction when the situation calls for it and provides for maximum group input into decision making when conditions are conducive to such an approach. Support, encouragement, and recognition of subordinates and their contributions are always present. Learning when to use each of the various approaches is something that a new graduate will need to study and to practice, just as with other nursing skills.

Critical Thinking Activity

In addition to the examples provided in the text, identify a health care–related situation in which each of the leadership styles would be appropriately employed. Provide the rationale for choosing that particular leadership style in the situation. What are the advantages of that leadership style? What are its limitations?

Changes in Approaches to Leadership

Nothing operates in isolation or in a vacuum; approaches to leadership are no exception. As you may surmise from the information in Table 12-1 and Display 12-1, the leadership systems have changed as societal values and norms changed.

As a society, we have experienced tremendous growth in information systems and technology. As a result, individuals at all levels within an organization have access to data. Access to information is no longer reserved for a few selected individuals at the top of an organizational chart but is now available to many. Employees at all levels within an organization are knowledgeable about goals, operations, rewards, and critical areas. The information explosion also has brought a more intelligent and informed customer to the health care arena, the impact of which can be seen in the changing language by which this person is referred—once patient, then client, now more frequently consumer or customer.

Today, more informed workers are developing into self-directed teams. This has resulted in managers spending time developing the abilities of others rather than directing them. Approaches to leadership have moved from authoritarian styles to a more collaborative leadership style, with the individuals closest to the problem helping to find solutions to it. This concept is demonstrated in a statement attributed to General Colin Powell: "The people in the field are closest to the problem. Therefore, that is where the real wisdom is" (Harari, 2002).

The strategies used for developing human resources have undergone significant changes. Many organizations, health care facilities included, are encouraging employees to be involved in decision making. The leadership required for this type of organization must be much different from that seen in the 1950s, when the manager instructed and directed and the worker acted and followed. Business leaders today would suggest that leadership needs to be visionary, ethical, supportive, facilitative, motivational, and open to new ideas. It also needs to provide for shared decision making and be responsive to the needs of those it serves. The effective leader must be able to communicate clearly and effectively, build consensus and inspire people to do their best, deal well with ambiguity, and maintain diplomatic and productive relationships.

THE CONCEPT OF POWER

Power, as we refer to it in a leadership sense, is the ability to do, act, or produce; the ability to control others. In other words, power refers to the ability an individual has to get things done. The concept of power forms a basis for action in transformational leadership.

Types of Power

French and Raven (1959) identified five types of power based on the source of that power (Display 12-2). You can find all of these types of power at work in nursing. The most obvious of these forms can be seen in such positions as clinical director of nursing or director of coordinated care management. Individuals carrying out these responsibilities enjoy **legitimate power**—that which occurs by virtue of the position held in the institution.

Referent power is gained by an individual because others like and admire that person or what the person symbolizes. This can be observed when one selects a mentor or an individual after whom he or she wants to model behavior. The mentor has referent power that translates into the ability to change the behavior of those being mentored. Mentoring has gained much popularity in the past few years, and new graduates are encouraged to find a mentor when they begin their careers. We will discuss mentors in more detail later in this chapter. Referent power is often associated with **charisma**. Charisma is a combination of characteristics that makes a person appealing and that attracts others. Charisma includes the way the leader acts, talks, walks, and relates to others. It is sometimes listed separately as a theory of leadership (Howell, 1997) and also is included often in the list of traits in the trait theory.

Reward power can be seen anytime one individual rewards another with positive statements, compliments, or other ego-boosting comments. It is also seen in promotions, salary increases, and awards. Even beginning nurses will find reward power available to them if they focus on giving recognition to others' strengths and accomplishments.

Display 12-2   Types of Power

Legitimate power	Power based on an official position within the organization. Often referred to as authority, in which manager has the right to direct others and workers are obligated to respond. Activities typically include making decisions on behalf of the organization and acquiring or controlling human and material resources.
Referent power	Power an individual has because others identify with the leader or what that leader symbolizes or represents. It also exists because others see the leader as powerful, as in the case of political figures.
Reward power	Power achieved by having the ability to grant favors or give rewards to others. Rewards might be in the form of praise, commendation, respect, or support.
Coercive power	Power that occurs because of the ability to place sanctions on another individual in the form of verbal threats, withholding pay increases, undesired assignment, or warnings. The opposite of reward power, it is based on the fear of punishment.
Expert power	Power gained through the possession of special knowledge, skills, or abilities that are respected by others.
Informational power	Power that is gained by having information or data that is important to others.
Connection power	Power that represents the cumulative effect of more than one person working toward a goal; for example, people working together to bring about a change or influence legislation.
Motivational power	The ability of the leader to stimulate the interest, enthusiasm, or participation of others with regard to a common goal.

▪▪ COMMUNICATION IN *ACTION*
▪▪

Using Reward Power

Jessica Brown was a new RN on the surgical unit. She worked with a charge nurse who had worked at the hospital for many years. After the end of the shift, Jessica stopped to talk with the charge nurse. "I just wanted to take a couple of minutes to thank you for the great job you did as charge this evening. I cannot believe how many details you kept straight and how you were still able to take the time to help me with that difficult IV start. It has really made a difference for me that you are willing to help me learn. Thanks a lot!"

Although Jessica was the newest person on the shift, she found that she could use reward power. Because Jessica was a willing learner and expressed her appreciation for learning opportunities, the charge nurse was very willing to help and felt rewarded for her efforts.

Coercive power involves using threats of punishment to enforce desired behaviors. Coercive power also has its place in nursing. If you fail to practice safe, competent nursing after you are licensed, the board of nursing has the power to compel you to change behavior by the threat of revoking your license to practice (see Chapter 7). For example, if unsafe practice is the result of chemical abuse, an employer can force an employee to enter treatment for chemical dependency, with the threat of job loss for failure to do so.

Expert power involves having specialized skills and abilities that serve to accomplish desired goals or influence others to follow one's leadership. Expert power is observed every day on hospital units. As nursing becomes more specialized, the individual with particular skills, knowledge, and ability will have power in the area where these skills are important.

Two other forms of power have been added to those originally identified by French and Raven. **Informational power** (Heineken & McCloskey, 1985) exists when an individual possesses information that others need or want to accomplish a goal. An individual who has access to information about the unit's budget or one who is more informed about policies that guide behavior of others is an example of someone with informational power.

Connection power is the cumulative effect of more than one individual working toward a goal. Connection power is responsible for the effectiveness seen in networking. Nurses who work collaboratively develop connection power. Connection power also can occur by working with persons who command power, respect, or access to desired positions or places. You will observe nurses using connection power as they work with other professionals in the health care system. You will also see nurses who are politically involved exercising connection power.

Motivational power is a new term. It refers to one's ability to arouse in others an excitement and enthusiasm for what they are doing. Because of its inherent or internal nature, motivation must be generated by the individual as opposed to being provided from outside. Motivational power, therefore, refers to the ability of the leader to stimulate the interest, enthusiasm, or participation of others with regard to a common goal. It involves recognizing the elements that drive individuals or creates satisfaction for them. McGregor's (1966) Theory X and Theory Y, Ouchi's (1981) Theory Z, Herzberg's (Herzberg, Mausner, & Snyderman, 1959; Herzberg, 1966) Satisfiers and Dissatisfiers, and Maslow's (1954) Hierarchy of Needs are all examples of approaches to motivation (see Chapter 13). In transformational leadership, motivational power is seen when the leader shares information, involves others in decision making, recognizes accomplishments, and rewards behavior (Fig. 12-1).

EXAMPLE

Considering Attributes When Selecting Team Members
The nursing administrative group at Columbia Community Hospital was anticipating a major change in the system of patient care delivery. As they discussed plans for implementing this change, it was decided that a small team to pilot the program would be a sound approach. They then wanted to select individuals to work in the pilot program. Melissa Worth had worked at the hospital for four years. A skilled decision maker full of enthusiasm and energy, she was welcomed by all nursing groups. Her positive attitude and ability to relate to others made her a favorite among the staff. When it was suggested that she lead the group to pilot the new program, everyone was in agreement.

Melissa possessed motivational power in that she was able to instill enthusiasm in others as well as herself. In order for a change to take place, those in the administrative group knew that motivation for change would be a key ingredient.

Thus, we see that power is derived from a variety of sources and is used in a number of different situations. It is important for all nurses to realize that they have a power base and to seek positive ways to use it to bring about improvements in the health care system that will benefit patients and society as a whole.

FIGURE 12-1 Motivational power is seen when the leader recognizes the accomplishments of others.

Empowerment

The concept of empowerment has received a great deal of discussion in the past decade. **Empowerment** refers to the process by which one individual who has power is able to share it with another. It involves making others partners in the decision-making process by providing them with necessary knowledge and reinforcement. Perhaps you have already learned about empowering your patients. Transformational leaders seek to empower their followers and thus transform the work environment. Blanchard, Carlos, and Randolph (1999) state, "The real essence of empowerment comes from releasing the knowledge, experience, and motivational power that is already in people but is being severely underutilized."

Transformational leaders openly share information with workers so that everyone is aware of problems and the need for action. The leader provides a vision of what is to be accomplished and helps workers to understand that they are an integral part of the group. Workers are delegated authority for decision making and for helping to find solutions to problems. Transformational leaders work at developing the skills of workers, who then develop a strong sense of self and are motivated toward achievement. Empowered workers have a greater sense of satisfaction derived from goal achievement. None of this could occur if workers were not empowered initially.

Empowerment is not easily achieved. Some organizations do not support empowerment of employees. Supervisors themselves may not be empowered within the organization. Some supervisors lack the self confidence necessary to empower others and fear loss of control if workers assume greater responsibility in decision making. In other instances, the supervisors may have moved into their roles while working in hierarchical organizations and may find it difficult to shift their approach to management in a new setting. Some employees do not want the accountability and responsibility that are required of the empowered individual.

Organizational Characteristics That Support Empowerment

Senge, Kleiner, Roberts, Ross, and Smith (1994, p. 51) refer to organizations that support empowerment as "learning organizations" and identify a number of characteristics of the learning organization. They include the following among these characteristics:

- People feel they are doing something that matters and that all individuals are growing and enhancing their capacity to create. Values and visions are shared.
- The belief exists that people are more intelligent as a group than they are individually and that visions of the organization emerge from all levels.
- The knowledge in the hearts and minds of employees is one of the organization's greatest resources.
- Employees are encouraged to learn what is going on at every level within the organization.
- People feel free to inquire about another's values and assumptions, and mutual respect and trust exist among individuals, thus freeing people to take risks and openly assess results.

Empowering Others

Nurses are expected to practice according to professional standards. However, nurses function within the constraints of their employment settings, and this affects their ability to engage in true professional practice. As we indicated earlier, if the organization does not support the empowerment of people, it is much more difficult to accomplish. If you want to work in an organization that empowers its employees, you will want to set this as one of your goals when seeking employment following graduation (see Chapter 15). An organization that is involved in transformational leadership styles also will support (and require) the empowerment of employees. The two are intricately interwoven. Manojlivich (2005) found that unit level leaders who empowered staff nurses enhanced the professional practice behaviors of those nurses. Other employees are also affected by nursing leaders who empower others. When nursing aides in long-term care are empowered by inclusion in decision making, outcomes for residents improve (Barry, Brannon, & Mohr, 2005.)

As you move into positions of responsibility, what are the behaviors and characteristics that you must possess to empower others? How can you motivate others to assume more responsibility and accountability for their actions? Display 12-3 provides a list of personal characteristics that are critical to being able to empower others and identifies some behaviors that help to create those characteristics. How many of those characteristics do you currently possess? Which ones will you need to develop?

Empowering others can be accomplished through a variety of strategies. These are appropriate for any situation in which the goal is to give others power and control over a situation.

For a person to gain more control over a situation, that individual must be knowledgeable. So a first step in empowering is often the open sharing of information. Everyone must be aware of the underlying situation, the nature of the problems, and why change is needed. Sharing information with others also is an important aspect of gaining the trust of your followers. Without information, others cannot act responsibly. They need to know how the organization works and the factors that impinge upon a situation.

Once individuals are aware of the problems and situations being faced, they can be involved in setting the goal or developing a vision of what is to be accomplished. Through this process,

Display 12-3   Personal Attributes That Support Empowering Others

Trustworthiness
- Honest in relationships with others
- Honors commitments, follows through on promises
- Can be relied upon
- Is predictable with regard to responses to others

Integrity
- Accepts responsibility for own actions
- Gives credit to others for things done well
- Is fair and just in relationships with others
- Is sincere
- Possesses sound moral values

Self-Confidence
- Knows one's abilities and limitations
- Models the values and behaviors desired of others
- Maintains a confident body language
- Is able to control one's own feelings and behavior
- Is not arrogant, conceited, or boastful

Sensitivity
- Is kind and thoughtful in interactions with others
- Actively listens to others
- Recognizes things that are important to others
- Is free of cultural and racial biases

Intelligence
- Is reasonable in decision-making
- Learns from experience
- Able to respond quickly and successfully to new situations
- Maintains keen approach to problem solving
- Seeks new information regularly

Skill in Communicating
- Communicates clearly and concisely
- Listens to others
- Knows when not to talk
- Maintains positive body language
- Is sensitive to nonverbal cues
- Does not interrupt others when they are speaking

the employee becomes more vested in achieving the desired outcome and buys in to the excellence expected and the productivity needed to accomplish it. Along with this, team members need to know the ranges or boundaries within which they can act (Blanchard et al., 1999).

Another characteristic of empowering others is involving them in finding solutions to the problems once they are aware of the problems being encountered. This is where the collective intelligence of the group is useful. Rather than support the belief that only the leader can propose workable solutions, empowered employees are respected for their contributions and first-hand knowledge of a situation. Ideally, employees will become involved in the development of strategies to accomplish the goal or vision.

Reaching this point in any organization requires that the leader has been able to help workers develop their skills. It involves teaching, team building, and coaching abilities on the part of the leader (see Chapter 13). Workers must gain confidence in their ability to make correct decisions and take appropriate action. Employees need to be able to see themselves as members of influential teams, with the ability to discover new resources. Recognizing the accomplishments of others, sharing credit, valuing honesty and openness, and rewarding behavior are important aspects of this development. As a result of feeling empowered, employees understand the valuable contribution they make.

Like many other endeavors, empowering others has no straight line to success; some days are good, others not so good. Do not expect too much success early on. Being successful requires that you maintain an optimistic attitude, persevere in your goals and activities, and remain steadfast in your commitment to them. Continual assessment of yourself and the situation is essential. Be honest with yourself, and at the same time avoid being overly critical of your own behavior. Remember that the art of empowering others, like other skills you have mastered, can be learned.

Critical Thinking Activity

Think of a situation you have experienced or observed in which an individual was empowered. What were the factors that resulted in the individual being empowered? How did that individual respond? What additional actions might have made the empowerment even greater? Which of the behaviors that helped empower the person would you want to use? Which ones would you not use? Why did you choose these behaviors?

ENHANCING YOUR EMOTIONAL INTELLIGENCE

With increasing frequency, we hear the term "emotional intelligence," which is sometimes referred to as emotional quotient. **Emotional intelligence (EI)** refers to the essential quality of understanding how emotions function within oneself and others and the ability to use emotions effectively. It is considered by some to be as critical to high performance as is basic intelligence. As a result, a number of large businesses are now assessing an individual's EI before hiring that person into an important position in the organization or before making promotions.

Emmerling and Goleman (2003) list five components of EI: self awareness, self regulation, motivation, empathy, and social skill. These five components are interdependent, each affects the others, and they create the "whole" that is EI.

Self Awareness

Self awareness involves recognizing and understanding your own moods and feelings. It also includes appreciating how your emotional behaviors affect others. When this skill is well developed, individuals typically see themselves realistically and are able to act confidently. Developing self awareness requires an ongoing commitment to examining your own feelings and behavior and noting their effects on yourself and on others. It may be likened to holding up a mirror to yourself and inspecting yourself very critically.

EXAMPLE

A Targeted Self Assessment

Jodie Ellington was an RN working in a long-term care facility. She found that she dreaded going to work in the morning. One day, she sat down after work and thought to herself, "What is going on here? I always loved working with the elderly, and now I don't even want to go to work. The nursing assistants have been asking me what is wrong because I am so critical of everything." As she began reviewing what was happening at work, her responses to what was happening, and her dreams for a career in nursing, she became aware that she had always thought in terms of working directly with the elderly, helping them to be more independent, helping them to find joy in the later years. Her job was one of managing documentation, supervising nursing assistants, and organizing the delivery of services. Her unhappiness with a job that had so little resident contact had spilled over into the way she was treating the nursing assistants. She realized that she still loved working with the elderly and that she needed to consider a career change into a different role in gerontologic nursing. Meanwhile, she was going to change how she treated those with whom she worked. They really worked very hard and needed to be appreciated for that.

Self Regulation

Self regulation refers to the ability to control inappropriate impulses and to think before acting (Habel, 2005). Research on mindfulness training indicates it is a positive strategy for managing emotionally charged situations (Kabat-Zinn, 2005). **Mindfulness** is a process of being aware of the present while keeping distressful thoughts away. Persons who have developed skill in this area continue to respond to human emotions such as anxiety, anger, and sadness, but they do not overreact to them and are able to direct them in positive ways. Lack of self regulation is seen in the person who has emotional outbursts and the one who breaks down and cries and is unable to function if criticized. While tears of sadness can be appropriate, an inability to manage responses in order to function seriously inhibits one's effectiveness.

To increase your ability to self regulate, try to develop the ability to not take things personally. Managing your own emotions may be the biggest and most difficult to control. You might begin by using stress-management techniques. Deep-breathing exercises, stress relief through physical exercise, and meditation may all help. Using such techniques as deep breathing when faced with an emotional situation may give you time to decide how to react rather than simply reacting from immediate feelings. However, you may still find yourself in a situation where you cannot control your emotions. In such cases, you need to exit the situation.

Simply saying, "Please give me a few minutes," may be adequate. Think before you leap. Self-help books and practiced meditation can assist in this process (Habel, 2005). Another important point is that you should not put into writing anything that you would not want to say before a large group of people. This includes writing in e-mail or on personal blogs. These are not private and may be shared widely, thereby creating many other problems for you in the work environment.

Motivation

Motivation relates to the desire to achieve or get things done. The motivated individual is optimistic and works in self-directed ways toward positive goals (see Chapter 13 for more discussion of motivation). The motivation discussed here is self motivation, the ability to set goals, standards, and expectations for yourself and meet them. As a new graduate, seeking new learning experiences is an example of self motivation. Volunteering to serve on committees or accepting a challenging assignment are other activities that demonstrate self motivation.

Empathy

You are well acquainted with the meaning of empathy from your other nursing courses. Empathy involves the ability to read accurately and respond appropriately to the emotions of others. Expressing empathy for others is important to effective functioning in groups or teams. Individuals who have developed this skill listen carefully to what others say and react in effective ways to this information. You have used this skill in working with patients and their families. You can use it when working with others also. When responsible for directing the activities of others, do not control unpleasant situations by talking. Listen carefully to what is being said. Recognizing others' distress with words such as, "I know we are working short-handed this morning, but if we all pull together, we can do it." Maintain eye contact when listening to others; it helps assure them that they have your attention.

Social Skills

Social skills, also referred to as people skills, center on being able to relate to many different types of people and groups. Goleman (1998) calls this "friendliness with a purpose." Greeting people when you meet them, remembering and using preferred names, listening with interest, and using the common courtesies of "please" and "thank-you" are all a part of social skills. Individuals who possess people skills initiate conversations with others, look for opportunities to interact, and respond positively to the communications of others. Being a pleasant and courteous member of the health care team demonstrates social skills.

Developing Your Own Emotional Intelligence

Although EI may be learned from life experience, it does not improve greatly without sustained effort and attention. A number of techniques have been suggested to enhance one's EI. As we frequently have suggested in this book, EI begins with a thorough self assessment. Table 12-2 contains statements that will assist you in this exercise.

How did you do on the self assessment? Did you have many areas where you answered "seldom"? Were most of your responses "usually"? What would you like to improve? Which techniques will help? Improving your ability to identify your own emotions and how they are perceived by others is critical.

TABLE 12-2	SELF-ASSESSMENT OF EMOTIONAL INTELLIGENCE			
ITEM	ALWAYS	USUALLY	SELDOM	NEVER
I am able to recognize my emotions and I know what they are.				
I consistently think before I act and do not act rashly.				
I am aware of my own behavior and can describe how it affects others.				
I am able to manage my own feelings in a wide variety of situations.				
I consistently express my negative emotions in an acceptable manner.				
I am able to remain calm and collected when interacting with people who are angry or verbally abusive.				
I am self-motivating and do not require someone else to get me going.				
I find it easy to empathize with others and they frequently share feelings with me.				
I can identify when emotions can be used effectively and when not.				
Others would describe me as an optimistic person.				

EXAMPLE

Dealing with a Stressful Day

Dennis Damon is the unit manager on a busy medical unit. Today he met with other unit managers and representatives from hospital administration to discuss budget requests for next year. Each unit manager had prepared an information sheet identifying needs for the coming year with rationale and anticipated cost for each. Dennis was not surprised that it was a stressful meeting and that tempers occasionally flared. Nonetheless, he left the meeting feeling tense and on edge. On his way home, he dropped by the health club and played a fast-paced game of racketball. When he left the club, he was relaxed and felt more able to think constructively about the concerns of the day.

DEVELOPING YOUR LEADERSHIP STYLE

In today's health care environment, all professional nurses will find themselves involved in working conditions that require some leadership skills. Both acute and long-term care facilities use assistive personnel who have less educational preparation and who require direction from RNs. This trend will increase as long as the shortage of RNs continues. As you move into the world of employment, think about your own leadership style. What approach will you use when directing others? How will you develop those skills? The following suggestions may help to enhance this process:

- *Continue to learn and to grow.* You will be expected to demonstrate competence and knowledge. These attributes can be developed and maintained only when you continue to seek and find answers to problems you encounter, many of which you may not have studied in your nursing program. Subscribe to a nursing journal that focuses on content related to your area of practice so that your clinical knowledge continues to grow. Attend meetings and participate in committees so that you learn more about the organization in which you work.

- *Seek out a role model or a mentor.* A **mentor** is a more experienced individual who is willing to support and guide an individual who is new to a work environment and who systematically develops a subordinate's abilities through tutoring, coaching, and guidance. In selecting a mentor, look for someone whose abilities and career accomplishments you admire and who is willing to make the extra effort required to assist in your growth. The mentor will help you navigate the system until you are capable of doing so on your own. The mentor can provide counsel and guidance regarding issues that concern you. This person can also suggest committees or groups in the workplace that create opportunities for you to learn and excel. The mentor can coach you to perfect your performance and can provide a sounding board when needed. This person can protect you by helping you deal with negative feedback and teaching you about rules that are not written in any policy manual. The mentor helps you seek solutions, provides inspirational motivation, and provides individualized consideration. It is a fortunate novice who has a good mentor (see additional content on mentors in Chapters 3 and 13).

- *Maintain your personal physical resources.* One of the significant criticisms directed at today's health care environment by those who are employed in it is the high level of stress encountered daily. This stress can best be managed when a person is physically and mentally fit. Everyone needs time to unwind, to relax and rest, and to find the time and energy to reflect on work activities. It is important to maintain outside interests and relationships that help to round out life and provide diversion from the stresses of work. As you move into the world of employment, be certain that your lifestyle includes a healthful diet, exercise, rest, and relaxation.

- *Retain an open mind and develop flexibility.* Individuals who are open to new ideas and who can cope with unpredictable circumstances have an advantage in the workplace. Remember that there is often more than one way to approach a problem. Locking into only one way of viewing things or one method of dealing with a situation limits one's growth, can create tension in the workplace, and may result in using the wrong approach to solve a problem. Learn as much about the organization in which you are employed as you can. Developing a broad view of how the organization functions will help you to see where you and your unit fit in. Be willing to compromise and to negotiate; these skills are critical to any good team player. Ask questions when you are not sure.

- *Demonstrate respect and consideration for others.* All individuals bring unique perspectives and contributions to the workplace that should be valued. Sometimes encouraging others to do their best requires patience and understanding. Help others to grow just as you want others to assist you. Observe the basic behaviors considered to be social skills. Practice common courtesies and etiquette. Address people by the name by which they wish to be addressed. Be polite and considerate to others, and generally you will find they will return this behavior. Be sensitive to things that may be distressful to those with whom you work. Trust people and share information—it helps others to know you believe in them.

- *Believe in yourself.* Develop your own self confidence. Give yourself credit for the things you know you do well. Identify the things that you need to learn more about and do so. Develop a body language that inspires confidence in others; walk tall. Maintain good grooming and dress. Become articulate in your communication patterns and remember the importance of being a good listener. Review the language you use in reference to yourself. Don't discount your own skills and abilities or minimize your accomplishments. In others words, develop a professional demeanor.

COMMUNICATING EFFECTIVELY

After reading the above material, you have an appreciation for how important effective communication is to your ability to provide leadership. The concept of communication is not new to you. In previous studies, you learned that **communication** involves the sending and receiving of a message from one person to another. Let's list some of the other things that you know about the communication process:

- Communication occurs in four settings: intrapersonal, interpersonal, group, and societal. Intrapersonal occurs when you talk to yourself. Interpersonal occurs between two or more individuals. Group communication takes place when a number of persons are involved. Societal communication relates to an entire society or culture.
- Communication takes several forms, notably, verbal, nonverbal, and written. Verbal communication occurs in the use of words. Nonverbal involves one's body language and dress and includes facial expressions, body positions, eye contact, boundaries, and body movements. Written communication is that which is recorded, as in charts, memos, letters, and the like.
- Verbal and nonverbal communication systems interrelate, and may either complement each other or contradict each other. For example, if you say, "It doesn't matter to me" and at the same time shrug your shoulders, the messages complement each other. However, if you say, "Please tell me more" but look away, you have given two different messages. Looking away can suggest you don't really care.
- Certain skills can facilitate the communication process and result in therapeutic communication or communications that are goal directed. Therapeutic communication has a purpose and direction and employs processes to achieve established objectives. It focuses on the needs of the other person and involves active listening and observation.
- The words we use when communicating can mean different things to different individuals. Chief concerns include the use of figures of speech, jargon, slang, and idioms with which not everyone is familiar, such as "She heard it straight from the horse's mouth" (meaning from a reliable source) or "Up a creek without a paddle" (meaning in a difficult situation without a means of exiting). Another example is abstract messages that use vague terms, such as asking a patient in an urgent care center, "What brings you here?" when inquiring about symptoms and receiving the reply, "A car."

- Communication involves feedback that allows us to know which messages were received and understood as intended and which messages need correction. Feedback performs a regulatory function and helps us to evaluate the communication process.
- Communication is influenced by a variety of factors, including a person's perceptions and values. Words represent generalized symbols that may vary from individual to individual. Your perceptions can be altered by crises and anxiety-producing situations.
- Blocks to communication occur when unhelpful responses are made, such as generalizing, labeling feelings, making judgmental statements, or changing the subject. Blocks to communication can involve such things as telling the individual how to do something that he or she has already learned. Belittling others' feelings, disagreeing, disapproving, refusing to admit that a problem exists, or being defensive are other examples of blocking communication.
- Communication is culturally sensitive and culture-bound as a result of impressions formed at an early age about how the world is structured. This applies to both verbal and nonverbal behavior. For example, not all cultures maintain eye contact during communication in the manner of those in the Western culture. In some cultures, such as Native American, Appalachian, Indochinese, Asian-American, some Mexican-American, and some African-American, it is not acceptable to make eye contact when talking because it is a sign of disrespect (Videbeck, 2006). Touch, which is a nonverbal form of communication, may be viewed differently by different cultures. Although it may be comforting to some, others may see it as an invasion of personal space.

In the past few decades, electronic devices have significantly affected our communication systems. The computer, e-mail, faxes, the Internet, cell phones, and personal digital assistants (such as the Palm Pilot®) have greatly increased the ease and speed with which we can communicate with one another. At the same time, it has resulted in ethical concerns about the sharing of information, how it is stored, and who has access to it. Increasingly, the care provided to clients is recorded electronically.

USING COMMUNICATION SKILLS IN THE LEADERSHIP ROLE

The importance of being able to use communication skills effectively in a leadership role cannot be overemphasized. Swansburg and Swansburg (2002) state that 80% of a higher-level manager's time is spent on communication, with 9% of the time spent writing, 16% of the time spent reading, 30% speaking, and 45% listening. Ustun (2006) points out that communication skills are an essential element of professionalism and are necessary for being able to affect others. To be an effective leader, one must possess an adequate understanding and application of communication techniques. The following are some basic guidelines for skillful communications:

- *Communications should be clear.* A message being given to others should be free of ambiguities, and the person receiving the message should have no difficulty interpreting what is meant. If messages are not understood, the individual being addressed should ask for clarification. However, in the health care environment, we often work with nursing assistants who come from other cultures. They may have difficulty questioning a superior, partially because they may not want to offend someone in a position of authority. Sometimes they do not want to acknowledge that they do not understand because they fear it will cost them their job. Instead, they may nod, smile, or give other nonverbal cues that suggest understanding.

▪▪ COMMUNICATION IN *ACTION*

Determining Understanding

Alice McAdams worked as the evening charge nurse in a local long-term care facility. Her nursing team was composed mostly of nursing assistants from an Asian culture. Hard working and eager to please, they struggled with English as a second language. During care planning time, Alice said to two of them, "I would like you to do range of motion exercise on Mrs. Howard and then get her up in a chair for 30 minutes." Both assistants smiled and looked at one another, but Alice was not sure her instructions were clearly understood. She then said, "Now, can either of you tell me how you are going to do that? How will you know it is okay to get Mrs. Howard up?" The assistants rather shyly smiled and one volunteered, "We move her joints and then put Mrs. Howard into chair." "That is correct," said Alice. "And how will you know if it is okay to get her up?" "If she says she no, we don't get her up," replied the other. "Well, it is important that she get out of her bed, so if that happens, please come get me so that I can talk with her and explain. But if she says she is dizzy or not feeling well, check with me before getting her up. I will check with you later to see how things are going."

In this situation, Alice clarified that the nursing assistants knew what they were to do and also that they understood the importance of getting the resident out of bed. She also offered her help should it be needed.

- *Communications should be concise.* This applies to both verbal and written messages. We should work at stating the necessary information as briefly as possible while still providing enough data to be clear. The longer messages become, the more extraneous information is included, and the longer it takes for someone to receive the communication. Learning to communicate in a concise and clear manner is another learned skill that will improve as we become more proficient.

- *Communications should maintain a positive approach or perspective.* When problems arise, individuals respond better to communications that give positive direction, are not fault finding or accusatory, and that focus on finding a solution rather than on the problem itself. When people become defensive, their energy is diverted to self protection rather than to problem resolution, and they become stressed. This detracts from accomplishing the goals.

▪▪ COMMUNICATION IN *ACTION*

A Slippery Floor

John Brice worked in a busy urgent care center. After a hectic afternoon of seeing an unusually large number of clients, John noticed a puddle of water on the floor as he was walking down the hall to greet yet one more patient. In the next room, two licensed practical nurses who helped staff the clinic were relaxing over a cup of coffee. Both would have had to go past the puddle of water to get to the room. John walked into the room and said, "I notice there is a puddle of water in the hall. We don't like to leave things like that because falls and injuries can result. I need to get to the patient in Room C, but could one of you please see that the water is cleaned up? It is important to maintain a safe environment." Both got up to get a rag to clean up the spill.

In this instance, John did not focus on the fact that the spill had been overlooked in favor of a coffee break, nor did he overlook the hazard because he did not have time to address it personally. He was courteous in his request and explained why it was important.

- *Communication should recognize and accommodate diversity.* Any work environment presents a variety of personalities, cultures, educational experience and capabilities, and gender differences. Maintaining an open mind and being willing to listen to others will help in difficult situations. While being sensitive to cultural values, it is equally important not to stereotype. Recognizing and acknowledging that differences often occur in the communication patterns of men and women is also important. For example, men tend to communicate with a purpose to achieve a particular goal and as a tool to deliver information. Women, on the other hand, more often value the role communication plays in relationships (Cherry & Jacob, 2002).
- *Communicating effectively involves active listening.* Active listening tells others that you value both what they have to say and their membership in the team. Active listening involves hearing the facts in the verbal message but also listening for feelings, values, and opinions and observing the nonverbal cues. A busy work situation may not lend itself to this type of communicating. You may need to assess the situation as to its urgency. If it is not urgent, you can arrange to meet later to discuss the concern. When time is available, remember to use the communication skills you have learned earlier: accepting, focusing, reflecting, clarifying, questioning, paraphrasing or restating, and summarizing. Listen for vocal cues such as pressured speech or slow, hesitant responses. This will assist you to understand the context of the situation. A major deterrent to active listening is the fact that we often begin to formulate a response to the individual with whom we are communicating before that person has finished talking. This prevents us from listening to all the cues in an individual's message to us.

It is difficult to think of any time in nursing when one would not use communication skills, but certainly some of the situations calling for the effective use of communication skills include conflict management, negotiations, delegation, assessment, discharge teaching, documentation, and any situation involving interviews. In addition to the interview that is part of data collection from clients and the interviews commonly used in employment activities (see Chapter 15), the interview plays a significant role in performance appraisals.

PERFORMANCE APPRAISAL

Performance appraisal represents a formal process by which an individual's performance is reviewed and evaluated against established standards, most commonly a job description. It might also be appropriately referred to as performance evaluation, performance review, or performance assessment. At all times, the focus should be on the performance and not on personality characteristics of the individual being evaluated. Accreditation standards established by various private, federal, and state agencies that review health care organizations require regular performance appraisal as part of the approval process.

The primary objectives of performance appraisal are to maintain or improve employee performance and to enhance the development of employees. As a result of the performance appraisal, the employee should know how he or she has been performing and what he or she can expect in the coming months. Performance appraisals also can be a part of identifying individuals for special assignments or for advancement within the organization. Properly conducted, they can also provide the institution with information regarding the effectiveness of its recruiting and hiring processes.

Guidelines exist for conducting good performance appraisals. All performance appraisals should be based on standards. The standards used to evaluate the performance must be clear, objective, and known in advance by the employees being evaluated. Additionally, the individual being evaluated should know who will be doing the evaluation. This is especially true if it is someone other than the immediate supervisor. The performance appraiser needs to be schooled in the process. Often the guidelines for conducting a performance appraisal are spelled out in the collective bargaining agreement that governs working conditions. The process should be consistently applied and the rewards and disciplinary actions understood by all involved. It should occur at regularly scheduled intervals. The individual being evaluated should know what will be done with the evaluation once it is completed and after it has been shared with the employee (Display 12-4).

Often those responsible for conducting the performance appraisal as well as those being evaluated have an aversion to the process. Some of the reasons managers dislike the process relate to the amount of time it consumes, the fact that unpleasant messages may have to be transmitted (many persons are hesitant to criticize others), and fear of legal repercussions. Persons being evaluated may dislike the process because it feels much like receiving a report card or because the process is intimidating. As a new graduate, you should find the process very similar to the end-of-the-term clinical evaluation conference you experienced with your clinical instructors.

Display 12-4   Characteristics of an Effective Performance Appraisal System

- The appraisal system has administrative support
- Evaluation is based on standards such as job description or other well-defined criteria
- Clear criteria exist for the evaluation used
- Employees know who will be evaluating them
- Evaluation procedures are consistently applied
- Evaluations are conducted in a timely fashion
- Evaluators are well trained in the use of the appraisal system
- The appraisal interview is a two-way communication
- All individuals know the related rewards or disciplinary action
- The final disposition of the evaluation is known to the employee

Hopefully, they helped you to grow and improve your performance, just as performance appraisals in the work situation should help you grow professionally.

Criteria for Evaluation

All performance evaluations, whether formal or informal, should be based on appropriate standards of performance. Standards of performance include job descriptions, policies and procedures, and professional standards of practice. To ensure that the daily worklives of employees are linked to the mission, vision, and values of the organization, these also must be integrated into the standards of performance at all levels (Ingersoll, Witzel, & Smith, 2005).

Job descriptions contain statements that describe the duties for which the employee is responsible. These usually include reporting relationships and accountability. To be useful for evaluation they should be up-to-date and clearly written to avoid ambiguous interpretation.

Policies and procedures should be taught as part of the employee orientation processes and relate to patient care activities, as well as to timeliness, absenteeism, and participation in agency committees. More institutions are including customer relationship skills in their policies. By this, they usually are referring to the aforementioned people skills. They may even have an entire program for employee actions. For example, in one facility the customer relationship procedures include that when meeting a person who looks lost or confused, any employee must stop, ask if there is a concern, offer assistance, and even escort the person to the correct place if that is necessary. This is required of everyone from the custodian to the vice presidents and is being strictly monitored and included in employee evaluations. The goal is that the institution will become known as friendly and helpful and a place where one would like to receive health care.

Professional standards are "authoritative statements that describe a level of care or performance common to the profession of nursing by which the quality of nursing practice can be judged" and that reflect the values of the profession. (Dochterman & Grace, 2001, p. 235). Standards of practice reflect expectations for the behaviors of professionals in relationship to specific areas of practice and may be developed by professional organizations such as the American Nurses Association. Standards of care, which reflect expected processes and outcomes that should occur for individual patients, may be developed by health care agencies or by regulatory groups.

The mission, vision, and values of organizations were discussed in Chapter 11. They cannot be achieved if all employees of the organization do not support them. If the mission of an organization is to serve an underserved population, then employees who are developing new programs and services should be expected to include underserved populations in their planning. If the values of the organization reflect a particular religious viewpoint and the employee does not support that view, then the organization is undermined in adhering to its values.

Instruments Used in Performance Appraisal

Instruments are the forms and tools used in the performance appraisal process. They should be designed around the pre-determined standards described above. A number of different instruments can be used for the performance appraisal. Table 12-3 identifies some of the more commonly used approaches. In nursing, a rating scale is frequently employed. It has the advantage of being easy to use and does not require a great deal of time to complete. The most critical aspect is that the assessment methods and the instruments used should focus on what the person actually does as opposed to personal characteristics of the individual.

TABLE 12-3	COMMONLY USED PERFORMANCE-APPRAISAL SYSTEMS
SYSTEM	**DESCRIPTION**
Rating scales	Comprises a list of behaviors or characteristics to be evaluated and a rating scale to indicate the degree to which the criterion is met. Rating scales may be numeric (1–5), lettered (A–E), graphic (always, frequently, seldom, never), or descriptive. Rating scales are a widely used type of evaluation instrument in nursing.
Checklist	Describes the standard of performance; the evaluator puts a checkmark in a column (usually yes or no) as to whether the employee demonstrates the behavior. Behaviors can be weighted based on importance.
Essay or narrative	Calls for evaluator to write several paragraphs outlining the employee's strengths, weaknesses, and potential. The evaluator may be provided with a guide for development of the narrative.
Critical incident	Requires that the evaluator observe, collect, and record specific instances of the employee carrying out responsibilities critical to the job. Incidents must be recorded regularly.
Group appraisal methods	May take one of two forms. The first involves using multiple judges. Several people form an appraisal team, typically the immediate supervisor and three or four other supervisors who have knowledge of the work being evaluated. Each person does an independent evaluation and then the results are combined. The second form may be used as a supplement to a supervisor's evaluation. Members of a team evaluate one another and team members' evaluations are included in the final evaluation. All persons use exactly the same job-based criteria for their evaluations.

In addition to knowing the basis of the performance appraisal, the person being evaluated should know who is going to be doing that assessment and when it will occur. In some organizations, the appraisal process may also include a self evaluation. In such instances, the employee and the manager would use the same instrument to guide the evaluative process and would compare ratings during the appraisal interview.

The Appraisal Interview

As pointed out above, the primary objective of performance appraisal from the organization's perspective is to maintain or improve performance. However, the manner in which it is accomplished can make a significant difference.

The interview associated with the performance evaluation should occur in a timely fashion, be held in a setting that provides for privacy, and have a constructive focus. The dialogue may include both positive and negative feedback. Positive feedback is information that communicates to others what they have done correctly. Negative feedback is more difficult because it identifies areas of unsatisfactory performance. Giving negative feedback takes skill and experience and is a significant part of the coaching role mentioned earlier in this chapter. Negative feedback is best provided at the time the incident occurs and should be objective and accurate. For example, if you see a nursing assistant moving from client to client without washing her hands in between contacts, do not wait until the formal evaluation conference to correct the behavior. Employees usually want frequent and continuous informal appraisal or feedback on their performance and it should not be left until the formal interview.

As a new graduate working in a health care facility, you are more likely to be the one being evaluated as opposed to being the one doing the evaluation. (However, hopefully the institution provides some means by which you can evaluate your superior.) There are some steps you can take to assist with the interview aspects of this performance appraisal session.

Effective performance appraisal is a two-way street. Before the interview, prepare three or four questions that you can ask during the interview session. These might be as simple as "How do you think I am doing given the time I have been here?" or "Are there ways that you think I might organize my work more efficiently?" Both of these questions would indicate that you are eager to try to improve your performance and meet the demands of the job. Should your manager have a tendency to fill the time with friendly chit-chat, the questions will help to focus the interview.

If you believe that some of the statements made by your manager are not accurate or are broad generalizations, challenge the statements. Of course, you will want to do so in a polite and constructive manner. Ask your manager to talk about the specifics of your behavior and performance. For example, if the manager says, "You seem to have difficulty completing tasks on time," ask for an example of a particular task that should have been done more efficiently. This will bring the conversation back to specifics rather than dealing in generalities. Be prepared for the fact that this could result in more negative feedback than might have otherwise occurred. If you receive negative feedback, it should be accompanied with some constructive suggestions for improvement. If the suggestions are not provided, ask for guidance, such as, "Okay, what can I do to work more effectively?" Then set a time frame with your manager for the improvement. If you receive ratings that you believe are inaccurate, negotiate with the manager about the rating. If you can convince the manager that factors were overlooked, he or she may be willing to change the score. It is difficult to predict how the manager will react to this response, but if you truly believe the rating is not accurate, you have nothing to lose. However, you must accept those statements that are a true reflection of your performance, even though they may be negative. These behaviors will be ones you will want to work at improving. Display 12-5 identifies some of the aspects of a performance interview that we all desire. Be certain that you consider these when you are being evaluated or if you are responsible for evaluating others.

 Display 12-5   Employee Expectations of the Appraisal Interview*

- A feeling that they were dealt with fairly
- An appreciation for their contribution to the organization and its goals
- Recognition of special accomplishments, efforts, or endeavors
- Some indication of how their performance can be improved, with specific recommendations on how it can be achieved
- An honest appraisal of future potential or prospects
- A sense of being fairly rewarded financially relative to others who are in the same position
- A sense that they have been allowed to contribute to the appraisal session and discussion, and that the evaluator actively listened to the comments.

*Adapted from McConnell, C. R. (1993).

■■ COMMUNICATION IN *ACTION*
■■

Providing Negative Feedback

Patricia Black, unit manager, was not looking forward to the performance interview she had to conduct with Richard Wilson, a new graduate who has just completed his first 3 months of employment. Although obviously trying hard, Richard was consistently late to work and his tardiness upset the operation of the entire unit. When Richard arrived at her office, she offered him a beverage and invited him to sit down at the table across from her. Using the standard evaluation form developed by a nursing committee in the hospital, Patricia reviewed Richard's strengths as a new employee. He seemed pleased that his efforts have been recognized. Then she discussed his habitual lateness. She said, "However, I do have a concern, Richard. You arrive on the unit 20 to 30 minutes late on an average of 2 days a week. For example, this week you were 25 minutes late on Monday and 20 minutes late on Thursday. This disrupts the start of the day for the unit because we count on everyone being here at the start of the shift. Can you explain to me why you believe it occurs?" Richard took a sip of his beverage. "Well," he said, "I know it is a problem. You see, I never was an early riser. Most of my jobs in the past have started in the afternoon. As a student, I always tried to get into the afternoon clinicals. Perhaps I am not cut out for a 7:00 AM shift."

"That may be true," agreed Patricia. "Nonetheless, the hospital has a policy that all new graduates spend a 6-month orientation on the day shift so that they best can learn the policies and procedures of the hospital. When you have completed that period, we could think about rotating you to the later shift. For now you need to develop some strategies for correcting your tardiness. Do you have any ideas?"

"Well," replied Richard, "I guess I could begin by setting my alarm clock 30 minutes earlier."

This manager recognized the strengths of the employee but did not neglect discussing areas of concern. While acknowledging Richard's statement of the problem, the nurse manager placed the responsibility for solving it on Richard and did not try to solve the problem for him. The employee, when directly asked to develop a plan, responded with a concrete proposal.

Behaviors to Avoid in the Interview

McConnell (1993, p. 81) identifies four simple "do nots" for the appraisal interview. As you become responsible for evaluating others and then sharing this information with others, you will want to consider these "do nots":

- Do not argue with the employee. It is counterproductive and destroys communication.
- Do not scold or reprimand the employee. Behavior needing a reprimand should have been dealt with when it occurred.
- Do not dispense personally referenced advice. Providing constructive instructions is part of the evaluation and is often considered advice from the supervisor. It should not be confused with advice that has a personal reference rather than advice of a professional nature. Making statements such as "If I were you, I would . . ." possess a personal reference and should not be a part of the appraisal process (Fig. 12-2).
- Do not wield your authority by making statements designed to coerce, intimidate, or demonstrate your power. The employee already understands your role, and wielding authority in this way will destroy the two-way nature of the process.

FIGURE 12-2 Personally referenced advice should not be a part of a performance appraisal interview.

Common Problems With Performance Appraisal

In the best of circumstances, performance appraisal probably falls somewhat short of accomplishing the goals for which it is intended. McConnell (1993) has identified five areas in which problems can occur. The area that creates the greatest difficulty is motivational weaknesses and shortcomings on the part of managers who are responsible for the evaluations. Good evaluation systems require the total support of top management. All persons involved must believe in the process and its value.

The second concern cited relates to confusion as to what is being evaluated. We have already stressed the importance of evaluating performance, but all too often the focus strays to personality. In fact, 15 or 20 years ago it was not uncommon for statements on evaluations to include "cheerful," "smart," "likeable," and "attractive." Perhaps you once had a job that included such statements in your evaluation.

System administration barriers also can cause the evaluation process to fail. We have already stated that all persons must believe in and support the appraisal system. Often, managers find the process to be unpleasant and time-consuming. Evaluations will be done late, hurriedly, or not at all. Systems work best when someone or some department has the responsibility for ensuring that all the steps in the evaluation process are completed in a timely and appropriate manner. This includes training for those persons who will be doing the evaluations. Training in the use of the evaluation instruments and the process helps to decrease variations in rating from manager to manager and will reduce inconsistencies in application of the process.

The discomfort sometimes felt by the evaluators may also present a problem to the appraisal system. Many people dislike giving feedback to others when it is aimed at correcting shortcomings or weaknesses. We shy away from criticizing others, especially when it is discussed face to face. As a result, one of two things may happen. The manager may tend to gloss over the areas that need improvement, or the manager may come down too heavily on the negative concerns. Neither approach is appropriate. Criticism, when given, needs to be assertive, constructive, and specific and relate to a particular behavior required in the job.

The last problem area relates to fear of legal repercussions. As employee organizations have gained strength and recognition, managers have concerns that actions may be taken against them either in a legal form or in the nature of complaints, grievances, or appeals. Apprehensions of this nature are less common when all aspects of an appraisal can be supported by specific examples. When assessments are completed using specific criteria and definable measures, unsupportable judgments are less likely to occur. Maintaining consistency is as important as avoiding surprises. Evaluations should focus on what an employee does, not who the employee is.

Critical Thinking Activity

Think back to the last time you were evaluated. What were the positive aspects of that evaluation interview? Were there any negative aspects? How did you feel throughout the interview? How could the interview have been made more productive?

Evaluating Your Manager

Most organizations supportive of personnel evaluation will provide an opportunity for you to evaluate your supervisor. Be certain to adhere to all the principles that you would want observed in your own evaluation. Work from clearly stated job expectations, a job description, or other document outlining the standards to be observed. Deal with aspects of the position, not the personality. Word any negative comments as positively as possible. Try to form the comments into constructive criticism. Avoid the use of words like "always" and "never." Rarely are statements that include these words completely true. If you can think of some corrective action or constructive suggestion that would make the situation better, include it. Do not attempt to address areas about which you have no knowledge—just indicate that you cannot respond to those criteria. Be fair, kind, and honest.

TIME MANAGEMENT

As a new graduate, one of the biggest challenges you may face in your first position is organizing and using your time efficiently—a process known as **time management**. As a student, the number of patients assigned to your care was typically fewer than those you are assigned as a regular employee. In addition, you have not had time to become efficient in many of the technical procedures required in your job. Because time is finite, time management skills become essential. Like many other areas you have already mastered, time management can be learned.

Principles of Time Management

As you work at learning to manage time more effectively, some general principles will be of assistance to you. The following principles can be applied in every setting and will facilitate your work in any role:

- *Understand yourself.* Learning to manage your time begins as many other behavior-related concerns: with a thorough assessment of yourself. This includes giving attention to your basic physical needs and identifying things that restore and enhance your level of energy, as well as examining individual patterns of behavior. Adequate nutrition, sufficient rest, appropriate exercise, and relaxation are all part of appearing in the work environment in the best possible condition to perform. Analyze your body rhythms and determine when your energy is at its peak. Plan activities requiring the greatest energy output and concentration to coincide with these peaks whenever possible. Are there things that boost your energy, such as a cup of tea, a break, or a snack? Generally, it is considered unwise to skip breaks or lunch to capture more time. Your efficiency, and perhaps your disposition, will suffer. What things create the greatest stress for you? How can they be mitigated or avoided? What activities help you best deal with stress?

- *Take control of your own time.* Responding to the requests of others results in one of the greatest expenditures of time. These requests may be for assistance or simply directed toward socialization. In either case, they can rob you of needed minutes and hours.

We recognize that it is difficult to say no, especially when a colleague asks for assistance. However, there are clear-cut situations in which it is easier. The first of these occurs when you are asked to assist with something for which you lack the necessary skill. You need to honestly recognize these instances and decline involvement when they occur. For example, if a seasoned nurse on the unit asks you, as a new graduate, to watch a critical patient while she takes a break, and you lack the needed knowledge to safely evaluate that patient, it is essential that you refuse. You do not want to jeopardize the patient's safety.

There are times when honoring a request, although you are capable of performing the necessary actions, will make it impossible for you to complete your own assignment in a timely fashion. In such instances, be honest and say, "I'm sorry, I simply cannot take the time right now." Although this is difficult, particularly at first, it is preferable to trying to do too much.

Interruptions also rob us of valuable time. In addition to stopping an action in process, we often have to restart or reorient ourselves to the task at hand before starting again—all lengthening the time it takes for completion. You may need to be assertive with those who have a tendency to interrupt you frequently; explain as kindly as possible that you cannot be interrupted.

Some activities, such as developing a patient's plan of care, require thoughtful attention. Seeking a quiet place where you are least likely to be disturbed will increase your efficiency in completing the plan. Some hospitals now structure units with a room located away from the major area of activity where such tasks can be carried out.

Perhaps the greatest time waster is social chit-chat. Nurses typically are a gregarious group, and while no one intends to waste time, it just happens. Although it is fun and interesting to learn what other team members are doing, it is easy to lose 15 to 30 minutes in such an exchange. If you find yourself frequently involved in such conversation, excuse yourself by saying, "I need to check my patient now, but can we discuss it during break time or over lunch?" If your message is communicated in a kind and genuine manner, feelings will not be hurt and people will not feel put off (Fig. 12-3).

- *Develop a time schedule.* Developing a time schedule or a plan for how you use your time helps you to stay focused and to avoid interruptions. It also requires that you set priorities. You can do this for long-term activities as well as for those to be completed in a shorter period. Once you have established a basic plan, develop a to-do list and determine which activities must be done first, which second, and so on. Look at your

FIGURE 12-3. Perhaps the greatest time waster is social chit-chat.

to-do list and determine whether there are any items on it that can be deleted, or whether some items can be delegated to someone else; remember, however, that you retain responsibility for professional care that is delegated. To-do lists will help you to avoid forgetting to do something that is important. They also serve as reinforcement to many individuals who are amazed at how many items they have completed in a given period.

Dealing With Procrastination and Time Wasters

Two final behaviors that help manage time are related to avoiding time wasters and managing the tendency to procrastinate.

We all experience time wasters. Certain occurrences in our day-to-day existence are sure to rob us of valuable time. Mackenzie (1997) has identified a list of 20 common time wasters that include telephone interruptions, drop-in visitors, ineffective delegation, personal disorganization, socializing, attempting to do too much, poor communication, and lack of self discipline. To some extent, time wasters are unique to each individual. One individual spends too much time on the telephone, another makes too many trips to the water fountain, while another only manages by crisis. When you complete your personal analysis suggested earlier, look at ways in which you spend your time and decide which of those activities represent time wasters. Once identified, make plans for eliminating or decreasing the time spent in such activity.

Some individuals are more inclined to procrastinate than others. If procrastination has been a big part of your life, avoiding it may be the most difficult of the tasks we have outlined. **Procrastination** is defined as a chronic delay in carrying out actions that are necessary to accomplish important tasks (Ellis & Hartley, 2005). Delaying a task can result in it seeming to be much larger, more time-consuming, or more difficult than it actually is. Perhaps you have experienced these feelings in the past when you have put off writing a paper due for class or postponed starting an important assignment. Researchers include fear of failure, lack of interest, and feelings of anger or hostility among the many explanations for procrastination. Regardless of the basis of the behavior, an important step in correcting it lies in making a personal commitment to complete tasks on time. This involves establishing realistic deadlines and adhering to them.

Kanarek (1996) provides five suggestions for dealing with procrastination. First, she suggests that you start working on a project for 10 minutes and quit if tired or bored. Often, at least half an hour will pass and you will have made progress. Second, she suggests that you save the best for the last, a form of reward. Third, make a game out of things: Challenge yourself to handle one task in less than half an hour and make a game of seeing how quickly you can complete tasks you have been putting off. Fourth, break tasks into smaller, more manageable units, and, fifth, tell others of your plans, thus putting pressure on yourself to do what you have indicated you are going to do.

Determine the time of day when you are most productive. Some of us work best in the morning, others find mid-afternoon to be their industrious time; still others function most efficiently in the evening. When you have determined what works best for you, use this time to initiate projects. This will make the task seem less overwhelming.

Barriers to Effective Time Management

The modern health care environment poses many barriers to the individual's ability to manage time effectively. These barriers may be either within the system or within the individual.

One of these barriers is a system in which more is expected of the individual that can be accomplished in the work day. For many nurses, patient care loads have increased both in numbers of patients and in terms of the acuity of patients. In a study by Kalisch (2006), nurses were surveyed in regard to care that was omitted because of time pressures. Routine omissions included basic care measures such as ambulation, turning, feeding, and hygiene, as well as the more professional behaviors of patient teaching and surveillance. For system-wide problems with load and demand, answers must be found in the system. Nurses may influence the system through shared governance or collective bargaining. Examining the work environment before accepting a position may help you guard against this problem.

Another system barrier lies in whether the nurse truly has any control over the personal practice. Those who do not perceive that they have control often give up on planning because they feel it does not change the situation (Claessens, Van Eerde, Rutte, & Roe, 2004). Thus, the system problem underlies the failure to use planning as a time management strategy.

Personal issues that may interfere with time management include both physical and mental health problems. For those with physical health problems, it may not be possible to move at the consistent speed required in many direct care nursing positions. The nurses facing physical health problems may need to consult with the human resources department or with a career counselor to identify positions that mesh with their health status. Mental health problems such as depression cause serious deficits in the individual's ability to initiate and complete tasks (Adler, McLaughlin, Rogers, et al., 2006). When a nurse finds that he or she cannot complete work, a self appraisal in terms of mental health and possible discussion with a counselor may be needed. Successful treatment of mental health problems will enable the person to function effectively.

Critical Thinking Activity

Identify one activity about which you procrastinated. Using the material discussed above, determine why you delayed completing the task. Does this occur frequently? What steps can you take in the future to avoid such behavior? In what ways will you benefit from avoiding procrastination?

Key Concepts

- Differences exist in how leadership and management are practiced. Leadership refers to the ability to persuade others to follow your direction, to motivate, to inspire, and to instill vision and purpose, while management refers to activities such as planning, organizing, directing, and controlling resources.
- Accountability and responsibility often are used synonymously and refer to the obligation to answer for one's actions and to do what is promised. Authority can be defined as the power or right to give directions, take action, and make decisions.
- A number of theories exist regarding leadership. The theories can generally be classified as trait theories, attitudinal theories, situational theories, and contemporary theories.
- Three major leadership styles prevail: autocratic or authoritarian leadership, laissez-faire or permissive leadership, and democratic or participative leadership. Each is appropriate in a particular situation or setting.
- A multicratic leadership style that combines the most favorable aspects of all styles is probably most frequently used in health care.
- Theories of leadership evolve with social cultures. Currently, a leadership approach referred to as transformational leadership is advocated by many theorists. A transformational leader shares information and decision making with all employees.
- Power refers to the ability an individual has to get things done. Empowerment refers to the process by which one individual who has power is able to share it with another. Both are essential components of effective leadership.
- For individuals to realize their full potential, they must be empowered. Empowerment occurs when information is shared; individuals are involved in goal setting and finding solutions to problems and decision making, and when efforts are recognized.
- Emotional intelligence refers to the ability to use emotions effectively. This involves recognizing one's emotions and how they affect others. Emotional intelligence is a critical quality in high-performance areas.
- Emotional intelligence has five components: self awareness, self regulation, motivation, empathy, and social skill.
- Leadership is a skill that can be developed. You can enhance the development of your leadership skill by continuing to learn and grow, seeking a role model or a mentor, maintaining your personal physical resources, retaining an open mind and developing flexibility, demonstrating respect and consideration for others, and believing in yourself.
- Communication is a critical part of everything we do. It occurs in intrapersonal, interpersonal, and group settings, and is experienced in verbal, nonverbal, and written forms that may complement or contradict one another. Therapeutic communication has purpose and direction, focuses on the needs of others, and involves active listening. Words mean different things to different individuals, and feedback allows us to know which messages are received and how they are understood. Communication is influenced by a variety of factors, and blocks to communication occur when unhelpful responses are made. Communication is culturally sensitive and culture-bound.
- In the leadership role, communications should be clear and concise, should maintain a positive approach or perspective, should recognize and accommodate diversity, and should involve active listening.

- Performance appraisal represents a formal process by which an individual's performance is evaluated. Employees know who will be conducting the evaluation and where the records will be placed. Good performance evaluation systems are based on appropriate standards of performance, have top management support, are conducted in a timely fashion, involve a two-way communication, and assist the employee to grow in his or her position. Evaluators have training for this responsibility.
- Effective performance appraisal interviews are a two-way communication system that recognizes an employee's accomplishments and provides direction and motivation for further growth. The interviews are conducted in a setting where privacy can be ensured.
- Time management involves learning to use your time more effectively and efficiently. To accomplish this, you must understand yourself, take control of your own time, develop a time schedule, avoid procrastinating, and avoid time wasters.
- You can avoid time wasters by examining the ways in which you spend your time and then deciding which of those activities were time wasters. Once identified, they can be decreased or eliminated. Making a game of tasks that you want to delay doing can help prevent procrastination. Breaking tasks into smaller, more manageable units can also help.
- When inability to complete required job components is due to system problems, a system change is required. If physical or mental health inhibits individual functioning, that must be addressed in order to manage time effectively.

Relevant Web Sites

Electronic Resource Center/Management Sciences for Health: *http://erc.msh.org*
National Council of state Boards of Nursing: *www.ncsbn.org*
National Library of Medicine: *http://nlm.nih.gov*
NursingNet: *www.nursingnet.org*
Nursing World: *http://nursingworld.org*

References

Adler, D. A., McLaughlin, T. J., Rogers, W. H., Chang, H., Lapitsky, L., & Lerner, D. (2006). Job performance deficits due to depression. *The American Journal of Psychiatry, 163*(9), 1569–1575.

Barry, T., Brannon, D., & Mohr, V. (2005, June). Nurse aide empowerment: Strategies and staff stability: Effects on nursing home resident outcomes. *The Gerontologist, 45*, 3.

Bass, B. M. (2001). The ethics of transformational leadership. KLSP: Transformational Leadership Working Papers. Academy of Leadership Press. [On-line]. *www.academy.umd.edu/publications/klspdocs/bbass_pl.htm*. Accessed March 7, 2006.

Bennis, W. (2003). *On becoming a leader: The leadership classic—Updated and expanded*. Cambridge, MA: Perseus Books Group.

Blake, R. R., & Mouton, J. S. (1964). *The managerial grid*. Houston: Gulf Publishing.

Blanchard, K., Carlos, J. P., & Randolph, A. (1999). *The 3 keys to empowerment*. San Francisco: Berrett-Koehler Publishers.

Burns, J. M. (1978). *Leadership*. New York: Harper & Row.

Cherry, B., & Jacob, S. R. (2002). *Contemporary nursing: Issues, trends, & management* (3rd ed.) St. Louis, MO: Mosby–Year Book.

Claessens, B. J. C., Van Eerde, W., Rutte, C. G., & Roe, R. A. (2004). Planning behavior and perceived control of time. *Journal of Organizational Behavior, 25*, 937–950.

Dochterman, J. M., & Grace, H. K. (2001). *Current issues in nursing* (6th ed.). St. Louis, MO: Mosby.

Ellis, J. R., & Hartley, C. L. (2005). *Managing and coordinating nursing care* (4th ed.). Philadelphia: Lippincott Williams & Wilkins.

Emmerling, R. J., & Goleman, D. (2003) *Emotional intelligence: Issues and common misunderstandings.* Consortium for Research on Emotional Intelligence in Organizations. [On-line]. *www.eiconsortium.org/research.* Accessed March 9, 2006.

Fiedler, F. E. (1967). *A theory of leadership effectiveness.* New York: McGraw-Hill.

French, J., & Raven, B. (1951). The basis of social power. In Cartwright, D. & Lander, A. (Eds.), *Studies in social power* (pp. 150–167). Ann Arbor, MI: University of Michigan: Institute for Social Research.

Goleman, D. (1998). What makes a leader? *Harvard Business Review. 76*(6), 93–102.

Habel, M. (2005). Emotional intelligence helps RNs work smart. *NurseWeek: Mountain Edition, 6*(16), 13–14.

Harari, O. (2002). Behind open doors: Colin Powell's seven laws of power. *Modern Maturity, 45*(1), 48–50.

Heineken, J., & McCloskey, J. (1985). Teaching power concepts. *Journal of Nursing Education, 24*(1), 40–42.

Herzberg, F. (1966). *Works and the nature of man.* New York: World Publishing.

Herzberg, F., Mausner, B., & Snyderman, B. B. (1959). *The motivation to work.* New York: John Wiley.

House, R. J. (1971). A path-goal theory of leadership effectiveness. *Administrative Science Quarterly, 16*, 321–338.

Howell, J. M. (1997). *Organization contexts, charismatic and exchange leadership.* Academy of Leadership Press. [On-line]. *www.academy.umd.edu/publications/klspdocs/howell.html.* Accessed March 7, 2006.

Ingersoll, G, L., Witzel, P. A., & Smith. T. C. (2005). Using organizational mission, vision, and values to guide professional practice model development and measurement of nurse performance. *Journal of Nursing Administration, 35*(2), 86–93.

Kabat-Zinn, J. (2005). *Wherever you go, There you are: Mindfulness meditation in everyday life.* New York: Hyperion.

Kalisch, B. (2006, October/December). Missed nursing care: A qualitative study. *Journal of Nursing Care Quality.* [On-line]. *www.nursingcenter.com/library/JournalArticle.asp?Article_ID=668515.* Accessed October 14, 2006.

Kanarek, L. (1996). *Everything's organized.* Franklin Lakes, NJ: Career Press.

Lewin, K. (1951). *Field theory in social sciences.* New York: Harper & Row.

Mackenzie, A. (1997). *The time trap.* (3rd ed.). New York: American Management Association.

Manojlovich, M. (2005). The effect of nursing leadership on hospital nurses' professional practice behaviors. *Journal of Nursing Administration. 35*(7/8), 366–371.

Maslow, A. (1954). *Motivation and personality.* New York: Harper & Row.

McConnell, C. R. (1993). *The health care manager's guide to performance appraisal.* Gaithersburg, MD: Aspen Publishers, Inc.

McGregor, D. (1966). *Leadership and motivation.* Cambridge, MA: MIT Press.

Ouchi, W. G. (1981). *Theory Z: How American business can meet the Japanese challenge.* Reading, MA: Addison-Wesley.

Senge, P. M., Kleiner, A., Roberts, C., Ross, R. B., & Smith, B. J. (1994). *The fifth discipline fieldbook: Strategies and tools for building a learning organization.* New York: Doubleday, a division of Bantam Doubleday Dell Publishing Group, Inc.

Swansburg, R. C., & Swansburg, R. J. (2002). *Introduction to management and leadership for nurse managers* (3rd ed.). Sudbury, MA: Jones & Bartlett Publishers.

Ustun, B. (2006). Communication skills training as part of a problem-based learning Curriculum. *Journal of Nursing Education, 45*(10), 421–424.

Videbeck, S. L. (2006). *Psychiatric mental health nursing.* (3rd ed.). Philadelphia: Lippincott Williams & Wilkins.

von Pierer, H. (1994). Informatik und informationstehnik als basis industrieller innovation. *Informatik Spektrum, 17*(2), 77–78.

13

Working With Others for Patient Care

LEARNING OUTCOMES

After completing this chapter, you should be able to:

1. Discuss why teams are essential in health care settings and identify key factors in effective team function.
2. Analyze the differences between multidisciplinary and interdisciplinary health care teams.
3. Discuss the various roles the nurse may assume on a health care team.
4. Discuss the relationship of physicians and nurses within the health care team, and identify actions nurses can take to facilitate positive interactions.
5. Describe the team-building process and identify behaviors that will strengthen a team.
6. Discuss the role of a coach in the health care environment.
7. Discuss the concept of motivation and give examples of intrinsic and extrinsic motivational factors.
8. Describe steps that can be taken to motivate others.
9. Explain the process of delegation and why it is necessary in today's health care environment.
10. Outline the steps to be followed for effective delegation.
11. Identify factors to be considered when care should not be delegated.

KEY TERMS

Accountable	Interdisciplinary health care	Synergy
Assignments	Motivation/motives	Team
Coaching	Multidisciplinary health care	Team building
Credibility	Nursing teams	Unlicensed assistive personnel
Delegation	Satisfiers/motivators	(UAP)
Dissatisfiers/hygiene factors	Scope of practice	

In all health care settings, many different health care workers provide differing skills to meet patient needs. In Chapter 1, we discussed the various health care occupations; in Chapter 11 we described patterns of nursing care practiced in different health care settings. Here we will discuss the importance of teams and some of the strategies for effectively building teams and motivating the diverse group of individuals involved in delivering health care. The importance of effective delegation also will be addressed. Strategies for leading change and managing conflict will follow in Chapter 14.

TEAMS AND HEALTH CARE

In general, a **team** is a group of people working together for a common goal. The very nature of health care requires the development of health care teams and collaboration among all the variously prepared individuals caring for a particular patient or within a given setting. In today's health care environment, individuals who represent a wide variety of disciplines combine to form a patient care team. This team could include a nurse, a physician, a pharmacist, a nutritionist, a social worker, clergy, a physical therapist, a speech therapist, a respiratory therapist, and housekeeping staff members, just to name a few. Sometimes their roles overlap. For example, both the social worker and the registered nurse (RN) may see discharge planning as an important part of their work.

At this point, you may think, "So what has that got to do with me? Health care teams have been there forever, and when I go to work I will not have much effect on the functioning of a team." But nothing could be further from the truth. The health care environment literally abounds with teams. An ad hoc committee that comes together to work on refining a policy or protocol could be viewed as a team. A group of nurses and assistants that works a particular shift or in a particular area could be viewed as a team. An assembly of variously prepared health care workers that plans a particular client's care is also a team.

What makes a team different from any other group of people who come together for a purpose? A team is a special kind of group. Teams enable us to capture the skills, abilities, and creativity of all persons that work with the group, a factor that is critical in today's health care environment. The strength of teams can be found in the various skills, abilities, values, and personalities of its members. Teams make things happen and create solutions to problems. What one person may not think of, another person very well might. When a team functions as it should, it generates a kind of synergy that makes the work of all members greater than the sum of the contributions of the individuals comprising the group. Teams are often led by facilitators or coaches rather than leaders, may set their own goals as opposed to having them set by the organization, have communication patterns that flow both up and down, and have members who share responsibility for decisions and outcomes (Baguley, 2002). Thus, we can expand our definition to say that a team is a group of people working toward a shared goal in ways that maximize the individual skills of each member and for which they all share responsibility.

Multidisciplinary and Interdisciplinary Teams

When the knowledge and skills of many disciplines are used to meet the total needs of the patient, we refer to it as a **multidisciplinary health care** team. Each team member has special skills brought from a particular health care discipline and is able to focus on different problems as he or she applies the expertise of that specialty to the same patient. The term **interdisciplinary health care** team adds the concept of coordination and collaboration between disciplines that usually are considered distinct. In interdisciplinary teams, the work of the members, while focused on their individual specialties, is coordinated with effective communication occurring among the various members of the team. The terms multidisciplinary and interdisciplinary are often used interchangeably, although, theoretically, greater coordination occurs in the interdisciplinary team approach.

Nurses are in a pivotal position to affect how the team functions because they contact all the various individuals who are involved in the team. The nurse, with input from other disciplines, develops the patient's plan of care. The nurse can help move the team from a multidisciplinary approach to a more interdisciplinary approach. This role requires finely tuned interpersonal and coordinating skills as well as excellent communication proficiency.

Critical Thinking Activity

Review the number and background of caregivers in the clinical area to which you are currently assigned. How many health careers are represented? What are the primary responsibilities of each area? If responsibilities overlap, what are they? Who is responsible for bringing the individuals together as a team? Who is responsible for coordinating all the various patient care activities, such as x-rays, lab work, treatments, and the like?

Communication Within the Health Care Team

To be successful in this team environment, recognize the importance and contribution of each person and the necessity for teamwork. Respect should be the hallmark of all relationships within health care. Although their education differs significantly, the nursing assistant should receive the same respect as a team member as does the physician or the pharmacist. The same characteristics that demonstrate respect toward a patient may demonstrate respect toward coworkers. From using their preferred name when you address individuals, to avoiding intrusion upon privacy, to using language that reflects courtesy and consideration (such as saying "please" when making a request), you have many opportunities to demonstrate respect for others.

Trust in the integrity and purpose of all individuals on the team creates the foundation for successful interaction and problem solving, as well as for team building. Others must be able to trust that you will fulfill your obligations and carry through on responsibilities, regardless of the role you play on the team. They need to be able to predict your response to various situations. Conversely, you must be able to trust that they will fulfill their responsibilities. When you find yourself unable to meet commitments, you maintain trust when you are honest with others and address the issue in a straightforward manner. Letting others know that a situation has changed or that you will be unable to complete something promised is the only ethical way to handle the circumstances.

Sharing information is central to building trust and responsibility among team members. When we share information, there is an implied element of trust that the information will be handled appropriately. There is also the indirect message to the person to whom the message is communicated that they are valued and are important enough in the scheme of things to have the information.

Building Trust Through the Sharing of Information

On 4-North, the schedule of work hours was always posted two weeks in advance of the first work day of that schedule. However, the unit manager, Janie Bright, had been unable to complete the schedule because of heavy demands on her time regarding budget issues being addressed by nursing administration. Knowing that this was an important issue with the staff, Janie shared information regarding the delayed posting at the change of each shift, explaining the reason for the delay and giving a date by which the schedule would be available. She also apologized for any problems this might create for her team members.

Relationships Within the Health Care Team

In health care settings, there has been a pervasive tendency for individuals to align relationships into a hierarchical system. Thus, some people see themselves as being of higher status or more important than others and develop an expectation of having more power within the system. This occurs within disciplines as well as among disciplines. Those in lesser-paid jobs frequently are assigned lower status and typically have less power. Often, they accept this as the expected way the system will operate. Some are even content with this because they do not want the added responsibility that often accompanies a higher-level position.

The approach to working with teams has changed significantly over the past century, with the quality improvement movement having a major effect. Three early Americans laid the foundation for quality-improvement initiatives: W. Edwards Deming (Demings's 14 Points), Joseph M. Juran (Quality Planning Road Map), and Armand V. Feigenbaum (Total Quality Control) all worked in Japan in the early 1950s at the invitation of that country. Their work was adapted and expanded in the latter half of the 20th century by a new wave of thinkers, including Philip B. Crosby, Tom Peters, and Claus Moller, all of whom pushed for quality improvement. Along with Kaoru Ishikawa, Genichi Taguchi, and Shigeo Shingo, all from Japan, this group of men is often referred to as the Quality Gurus (wise teachers) ("The Quality Gurus," 2007) because of their interest in improving quality. Their work led to many changes in approaches to management, especially with regard to respect for everyone in the system and trust among various members of the team. Trust and respect, as mentioned earlier, are considered vital factors in creating a work environment that will result in quality products, including quality health care.

Nursing Teams

Nursing teams focus on the provision of nursing care. RNs, licensed practical nurses (LPNs) (known as licensed vocational nurses, or LVNs, in Texas and California), nursing assistants (with various titles), as well as nursing students, may all be part of a nursing team. In most situations, it is anticipated that the RN will lead the nursing team. However, in some long-term care facilities, LPNs lead nursing teams because there are so few RNs. In that situation, however, an RN must be available for oversight of the nursing care. There are a wide variety of nursing teams in different settings. Some nursing teams are small, composed of two or three persons; other teams may be quite large.

FIGURE 13-1 Many times the nurse wears more than one "hat" and performs several roles simultaneously.

The Many Roles of the Nurse

Traditionally, the public and even some nurses have thought of the nursing role as being one of providing care. That certainly remains true in today's health care environment. Providing care is the heart of nursing. However, the role of the nurse has expanded to include many other responsibilities and obligations. Nurses often find themselves simultaneously carrying out several responsibilities, each of which might be viewed as "wearing a different hat" (Fig. 13-1).

The Nurse as Educator

An important role filled by the nurse is that of educator. As a patient educator, the nurse is responsible for ensuring that patients and their families have a clear understanding of post-hospital care. They must be sure the patient and family know when to take medications, what side effects need to be reported, and a host of information related to recuperation. As a leader of the nursing team, the RN plays a key role in the ongoing education of team members with lesser educational preparation. RNs improve patient care through **coaching** and teaching staff on an ongoing basis. As a member of the community, the nurse is an informal educator who can provide important information related to health issues for friends and others within the community. In an era when health promotion and health maintenance are emphasized, this role is more important than ever.

EXAMPLE

Assisting a Client to Understand and Comply with Medication Orders
Jane Allard, an 87-year-old female, was being seen as an outpatient in a large health maintenance organization. After a routine physical with blood work, the physician placed Jane on 3 mg of warfarin daily, told her to discontinue taking the 325 mg of aspirin she took each day, and asked her to return for more blood work in two weeks. He then hurried on to the next waiting patient. Mary Beth, the nurse in the clinic, talked with Jane following her examination. She learned that Jane had taken aspirin for many years and was convinced

that the cause of her blood being "too thick" was related to the fact that she ate too much raw spinach in salads because she liked it so much. Mary Beth realized that Jane planned to adjust the dosage of the warfarin on her own and without the knowledge of the physician. Jane also stated she really did not want to quit taking her aspirin daily. She planned to treat her condition by not eating any more spinach. Mary Beth sat down with Jane and explained that it was very important that she take the medications exactly as ordered. She encouraged Jane to use a soft tooth brush, to watch for any signs of bruising, and to be sure to return to have the blood work in two weeks. She further explained that if Jane adjusted the dosage of the medication, then it would influence the results of the blood work and the doctor would not be able to assess whether the dosage prescribed was appropriate for Jane. She was able to get Jane to promise to take the medication exactly as prescribed and discontinue the aspirin for the next two weeks. Later in the day, Mary Beth made a special point to seek out Jane's physician and discuss Jane's resistance to taking the medication as ordered so that he might review the situation with Jane during her next appointment.

The Nurse as Patient Advocate

The nurse also fills the role of patient advocate. The health care system has become so complex (see Chapter 1) that clients may need assistance in moving through it. It is often the nurse who is keenly concerned with ensuring that patient rights are not violated, that care is of high quality, and that service is provided in a timely manner.

When serving in an advocacy role, the nurse can assist the patient to be involved in informed decisions that affect that individual's health care. Since 1991, advocacy has been included in the ethical standards of clinical practice prepared by the American Nurses Association (ANA). Because nurses spend more time with patients than do other health care workers, they are in a prime position to fill this role, may have a keener understanding of the patient's desires and values, and have an established trust relationship.

The need for advocacy can originate from a number of causes, including patients' lack of knowledge and understanding of the health problem, confusion about the way the health care system operates because of the complexity of the system, ethical and legal concerns, frailty or disabling conditions that will not allow patients to speak for themselves, or perhaps inadequate care.

The Nurse as Counselor/Coach

Tied closely to the role of advocate is that of counselor or coach. In their educational programs, nurses are provided with interpersonal knowledge and skills that allow them to assist others to express their concerns, seek alternative approaches and second opinions, and ask questions. Through such activities, the nurse is able to empower the client and family. Assisting those with less experience to move into effective roles within the organization is an important aspect of the responsibility of more senior individuals (see Chapter 16 on mentoring).

The Nurse as Manager and Leader of Teams

Nurses also occupy roles as managers and leaders of health care teams. Often this involves serving as a change agent within the health care environment. Leadership and management were discussed in Chapter 12, and we will discuss the change process in Chapter 14.

The Nurse in Nursing Informatics and Research

The RN can fill a wide variety of other roles in health care. Two roles that we see more frequently relate to nursing informatics and nursing research (see Chapter 6). The need for information management in health care has never been greater, and nurses are in a unique position to take a key role in data management for decision making. Similarly, as the profession stretches to enlarge to a body of knowledge that is uniquely nursing, the demand for nurses who will participate in research increases.

Critical Thinking Activity

You have just moved into a new position in the long-term care facility where you have been employed for 6 months. The position requires that you do more teaching and counseling of staff than you have done in the past. What resources will you tap to gain information to increase your skill in these areas? Which persons might you contact? How will you assess your new competencies? How can you be alert to personal biases?

Nurse–Physician Relationships

Nurses work more closely with physicians in the acute care or long-term care setting than any other group. The relationships of nurses with physicians may be very positive, but they also result in some of the most stressful encounters for nurses. Because this stress plays a key role in job satisfaction, studies have been done focusing on nurse–physician relationships. When these relationships lack respect and trust, the result is a difficult working environment and potential for ineffective patient care. Interpersonal relationships always are the result of actions by both parties, and both are responsible for their success. Here we will look at strategies the nurse can use to positively influence nurse-physician relationships. Sirota (2007) suggests two: improving communications with physicians and empowering nurses.

Treating the physician with respect and expecting respect in return is no different than relationships you might have with other individuals with whom you have worked and interacted. It requires that we are considerate, are sensitive to factors in the environment, and respond in a manner similar to that which would be pleasing to us. Expecting to be treated with respect is the first step to receiving it. Social skills that include basic courtesies such as using appropriate names and titles, saying please and thank you when appropriate, and creating a pleasant environment while working are all examples of steps that can be initiated to set the tone in a relationship that will engender respect.

Nurses must be mindful that they work and communicate within the **scope of practice** of nursing. Nurses can jeopardize their license and endanger the relationship with physicians by stepping over the boundary of nursing practice and into medical practice. Although a collaborative role allows for all team members to contribute ideas regarding patient welfare, it is important that nurses remain in the realm of nursing practice when initiating suggestions for care.

Ensuring competence and possessing excellent nursing skills fosters positive nurse–physician relationships. If procedures are not carried out correctly, if medication errors occur, or if the nurse appears inept in a particular situation, it can be anticipated that the physician will be critical of the behavior. Nurses are empowered when they feel secure in their knowledge and expertise.

A study that looked at nurse–physician relationships and how they affected nurse satisfaction and retention (Rosenstein, 2002) identified five key circumstances or events that resulted in disruptive physician behavior. These occurred at the following times:

- After placing calls to physicians
- After questioning or seeking to clarify physicians' orders
- When physicians were concerned that their orders were not being carried out correctly or in a timely manner
- After perceived delays in the delivery of care
- After sudden changes in patient status

Rosenstein (2002, p. 27) defined disruptive behavior as "any inappropriate behavior, confrontation, or conflict ranging from verbal abuse to physical and sexual harassment." Nurses can help reduce the occurrence of this disruptive behavior in several ways. When placing calls to physicians, be certain that you have all necessary information available before placing a telephone call. Be certain that assessments are complete and that you have all needed vital signs and other information. This is doubly important if that call is made in the middle of the night. None of us appreciates being wakened from a sound sleep, especially if we know we have a busy day ahead. A physician might be distressed if the call were made without adequate assessment data to allow a decision to be made.

■■ COMMUNICATION IN *ACTION*
■■

The Patient With a Changing Condition

Patricia White worked the 11 PM to 7 AM shift in a small community hospital. She cared for a patient admitted to the unit during the evening shift who had been involved in a serious motorcycle accident resulting in multiple injuries. Although morphine sulfate 1 mg had been administered intravenously (IV) every hour, the patient continued to complain of pain, particularly in the abdomen. Patricia knew Dr. Whittle, the patient's physician did not like to be disturbed during the night; however, she was concerned that the medication had not helped relieve the pain. She called Dr. Whittle and said, "This is Patricia White on 3-South at Mercy Hospital. I am calling about your patient Jim Short who was admitted this evening following a motorcycle accident. Despite the fact that I have given him morphine sulfate 1 mg IV every hour, he continues to complain of pain, particularly in his abdomen rating it as an 8 on a scale of 1 to 10. His vital signs show some change with a slight drop in blood pressure from 130/80 to 122/72 in the past 3 hours. His pulse is slightly increased from 80 to 88 over that same time period. His neuro signs remain normal. He is alert and complaining." Dr. Whittle replied, "Make him as comfortable as you can, and I will be there in 30 minutes. There may be more injury than we first believed. Please, tell him I am on my way and prefer that he not have more medication until I see him."

In the communication example above, the nurse carried out the responsibility of alerting the physician to the needs of the patient. Recognizing that the phone call would awaken the physician, she gave detail about the patient to assist with orientation to the situation. She provided the physician with assessment data to help understand the patient's condition. She did not suggest treatment or medications, as that would have been outside her scope of practice.

It is important that nurses follow through on their own responsibilities. When it is necessary to question an order, the nurse is obligated to discuss that order with the prescriber (who is most often the physician). However, it should be done politely and in a considerate manner. Often it is not what is said, but the manner in which it is said, that will result in a positive or negative exchange. Provide information such as assessment data to help substantiate your concern. Because nurses are held legally **accountable** if incorrect doses of a medication are administered, learn to question orders in a pleasant and polite manner.

Recognize and allow for situations in which the emergency nature of what occurs with the client may require haste in getting things done, and that what appears as domineering or demanding behavior on the part of the physician is part of ensuring that care is rendered quickly and efficiently. A difference exists between meeting the demands of the situation and being disruptive or rude.

Fortunately, the number of physicians who display inappropriate behavior is small. Sometimes a physician's angry and rude response to nursing inquiries makes nurses reluctant to contact the physician when the patient needs medical care. If you are sure that you have fulfilled your nursing responsibility through appropriate assessment and communication, continue to seek the care the patient needs. Part of your own legal and ethical responsibility is to continue the quest for care and not be intimidated. This also is the hallmark of patient advocacy. If the physician refuses to respond, berates you instead of clarifying the medication order, or displays other such behavior, contact the appropriate person in the organization. This may be the nursing supervisor, but in some instances, the head of the medical staff for the unit should be contacted. If an emergency exists, communicate that clearly and you may need to contact an emergency department physician or some other hospital resource.

If the situation is not urgent for the patient, you may confer with your manager and determine the best course of action. You have a right to expect that the health care agency will support an employee in situations of abusive behavior. Many health care facilities have policies, procedures, or protocols in place for dealing with such issues. Check to determine whether the institution in which you are employed has such guidelines; if so, follow them in dealing with the situation. If those in the expected chain of command neither follow through nor provide support, you may want to look for other methods to remedy the problem. You might have a union that will support a grievance, or you may find support in the human resources department, where individuals are more familiar with employment laws and standards.

Critical Thinking Activity

It is 2:00 AM on a busy surgical unit. A new surgery patient, who had abdominal surgery late the previous afternoon, is experiencing a great deal of pain. You have administered all the medication for which orders were left. You are going to call the attending surgeon but you know that she has surgery early the next morning. What should you consider before calling? What information should you have? Are there other persons with whom you should discuss this before making the call?

TEAM BUILDING

Having looked at nursing teams and relationships among team members, let us focus our attention on activities of the nursing leader or manager on enhancing the strength and functioning of the team members. In the late 1980s and 1990s, the concept of team building began to receive a great deal of attention in business environments as well as in health care. This can be attributed in part to the changes occurring in management strategies, as managers responded to guidelines that had evolved from recommendations designed to improve quality. In implementing a quality-improvement process, managers need to have a concern for the satisfaction of staff and must demonstrate respect for staff and their abilities. Without these attributes, team building will not be successful.

Team building itself sometimes seems rather nebulous. People aren't quite sure what it is. For purposes of our discussion, we will refer to our earlier definition of a team: a group of people working together toward a shared goal in ways that maximize the individual skills of each member and for which they all share responsibility. The goal of team building is to create a type of **synergy**, in which the effect of everyone working together toward the shared goal results in a greater total effect than could be achieved by the sum of the efforts of everyone working individually. Synergy is a concept that ties closely to interdisciplinary health care models.

Teams and team building are not new. The most obvious forms of it that exist in today's world can be found in the sports arena, where teams and team functions are integral to the activities that take place. Much of the literature about team building comes from the area of athletics. As we look at the idea of team building, we will draw some analogies between the concepts we are presenting and their implementation in athletics.

Team building begins with involving all members of the team in identifying the goal and establishing the steps to be taken to achieve that goal. If it is a sports team, the goal is to win the game; that is, the team wants to score more points than its opponent. In health care, the goal is to provide the highest quality health care and patient satisfaction, measured in a wide variety of ways in today's health care environment (see Chapter 1). Through the process of goal setting, members of the team recognize the importance of their role in and contribution to the work of the team. All members of the team have an ownership in the process and the product.

Teams are composed of a diverse membership, with a variety of skills and abilities represented, each with a special role to play on the team. On a football team, for example, some block, some pass, some carry the ball, and others kick, all using the skills that they bring to the game. In health care, some have special knowledge of pharmacy, some of medicine, some of respiratory therapy, some of nursing, with each member contributing to the patient's recovery. There are informal roles as well the formal roles. The formal role relates to an individual's contribution to the team goal or purpose and relates to the individual's job preparation (eg, physician, therapist, nurse, or pharmacist). The informal roles are defined by natural skills and talents. For example, some have natural abilities to smooth over potentially volatile situations, some individuals are good at detail, others have a bent for creative ideas, and some are able to energize a team. Teams need to recognize both the formal and informal roles of their members.

Many of our life experiences have not encouraged team behaviors. Our early schooling may have emphasized individual achievement, recognizing those who excelled over others. Many of our work experiences may have occurred in environments where decisions were made by a few and passed down to others who were expected to follow though without questioning. Work was accomplished by a group directed by a supervisor (Blanchard, Randolph, & Grazier, 2005). Thus, as we move into a work environment that requires greater team work, we need to make mental shifts that place more value on working together and less on personal triumphs. Perhaps your nursing program has provided opportunities for you to practice these skills.

Central to building effective teams is the belief that those who are closest to problems may best be able to provide the sound solutions to address the concern. All share in the problems that occur; all share in the success that is achieved. In bringing together members of the team, the manager needs to establish a working environment that recognizes and values the contribution of each individual on the team. Abilities are acknowledged. This serves another purpose as well. It helps each team member to feel necessary and included in the team and that the member's contribution is important. They become engaged, feel valued, and take pride in the activities of the team.

Another part of team building relates to celebrating successes. Think of the soccer team that rejoices when a goal is scored. The efforts of the individual who scored the goal and the person who assisted are recognized, and all team members share in the accomplishment. As we look at building health care teams, we need to look for opportunities to celebrate the good things that happen. This will help members appreciate one another and the effort that has been made as a group.

Leaders focus on how problems can be corrected rather than on how they occurred. Again, making a comparison with the field of athletics, if a basketball team consistently breaks through the defense and scores baskets, the opposing team comes together, revises its plays, and tries another approach. Similarly, in health care, if one approach to treatment does not provide the outcome desired, a conference is held and other strategies are discussed and decided upon. The focus centers on how things can be made better rather than on what was not working right.

Team building works to eliminate individual faultfinding. On the volleyball court, if a team member allows a point to be scored, that member is not made to feel at fault. Rather, the team looks for ways to tighten the defense to prevent giving up more points. In a good team-building situation, this would be the desired approach. Instead of spending valuable time discussing with a nursing assistant why the dinner trays were not promptly delivered for the evening meal, helping that individual develop an organized approach to tray distribution would have more long-lasting and better results. The role of the manager often becomes more one of coach than that of boss.

Critical Thinking Activity

As a new graduate, you have accepted a position on the medical unit of a community hospital. After working for 1 month, you have determined that the morale among the nurses and nursing assistants on the unit is low, that they do not function as a team, and that they don't have much team spirit. What can you do about this situation? Where would you begin? What are your limitations?

BECOMING A GOOD TEAM MEMBER

Although you eventually may carry major responsibility for leading a nursing team, when you initially move into a staff nurse position, you will likely be a member of a team rather than its leader. How can you best fulfill that role? What questions do you need to ask yourself? What behaviors do you need to enhance? Which ones should you try to eliminate? How do you know?

Once again, we suggest a self assessment. How well do you listen? Communication is very important among team members. But sometimes we forget that listening is just as important, sometimes more important, than talking. People who are a good listeners learn things that others may miss. Good listeners communicate a message to others that they are interested in what is being said and value the individual who is speaking.

Do you communicate your ideas clearly? It is important to team effort that you contribute ideas and concerns when appropriate. Contributions should be constructive and should be expressed in positive language that does not imply a lack of respect for previous ideas or approaches.

Can you accept criticism? Part of growing and improving involves having one's actions evaluated. Evaluation should involve feedback and it may not always be glowing. Maintaining a positive approach in such a situation is a mark of emotional maturity. Pouting, clamming up, withdrawing, or having an emotional outburst are not appropriate responses. Feedback and recommendations can be steps toward professional growth. Analyze your performance honestly and make changes where needed. As Joe Montana (2005) states in his book *The Winning Spirit*, fail fast and move on.

Do you support others? Just as you want support in the role you play in a group, others need support also. When someone does a task well, let him or her know you noticed. Give credit where credit is due. Statements such as, "I think Warren has a good idea" or "I'd like to try Wendy's approach" are supportive in nature. And when things are going poorly for another, be helpful and encouraging. Offer your assistance if it is appropriate to do so.

Do you ask good questions and contribute? One of the reasons why teams succeed is because they use the collective intelligence of all members. If you fail to share your ideas or ask pertinent questions that will lead to new approaches or prevent poor ones, you are letting down other members of your team.

Are you a team player? Are you willing to give a little to accomplish the goals of the team? This means making team goals your goals and, in some cases, giving up a little of the spotlight. There may be more than one effective path to the goal. Team players are willing to take the path that someone else prefers rather than insisting on their own preference.

Can you deal with conflict? Conflict is a natural part of our lives. When we are unable to deal with conflict, we may become frustrated, jealous, or angry or may withdraw from the situation. Conflict must be dealt with in ways that are constructive and positive rather than negative (see Chapter 14).

Are you self motivating? Being able to set your own time lines and commitments and meet them are indications of self motivation. Demonstrating ability and confidence to manage what you do are important behaviors to nurture. Display 13-1 summarizes these questions you can use to assess your competence as a team member.

THE COACHING ROLE

Much is written in nursing literature today about the coaching role. The activities of the team leader often involve one of coaching less experienced members of the team as we strive to involve all team members in decision making and team effort. Whitworth and colleagues (1998) describe coaching as a collaborative process that is focused on actions that will move the individual forward through the process of learning and result in helping people achieve goals. The

Display 13-1   Questions to Assess Your Competence as a Team Member

- Are you a good listener?
- Do you communicate ideas clearly?
- Can you accept criticism?
- Do you support others?

- Do you ask good questions and contribute?
- Are you a team player?
- Can you deal with conflict?
- Are you self motivating?

learning may be associated with job skills, understanding the operation of the organization, meeting new challenges, increasing efficiency and productivity, or other issues specific to the organization. The goal is to help the individuals who are being coached to fulfill their potential. Coaching replaces the old style of leadership in which the leader told staff members what to do with a style in which the leader assists the members to learn to handle situations on their own, thus building a stronger team.

In a coaching role, a more senior nurse supports and nurtures the learner, providing positive reinforcement as well as information. Rather than telling less experienced nurses what to do, the coach might ask how they plan to approach a problem and then help refine the plan so that success will be realized. It involves asking reflective questions and providing feedback. Coaching may be consultative, educational, motivational, or a combination of all three.

An individual who accepts the coaching role must possess certain qualities. This individual must be competent and emotionally stable. He or she must be willing to take risks, be honest and credible, communicate clearly, and possess energy and enthusiasm.

In some ways, the coaching role is as much a style of management as a unique approach in and of itself. The unit manager who can coach teams to efficient and effective performance will have a much happier and more motivated group of workers than the manager who tells them what to do.

MOTIVATING OTHERS

Team building and motivating are closely related. What team building is to a group, motivating is to an individual. Motivating others to perform at their best for the benefit of the organization is a huge task. It requires strong people skills, leadership, clear personal goals, and participatory supervision.

Understanding Motivation

Motivation encompasses the sum of all those individual factors that cause or impel an individual to do something. Individual factors, called **motives**, are generally referred to as extrinsic or intrinsic.

Extrinsic motives include things such as salary, the work environment, and recognition by others, in other words, factors outside the individual. As far back as we can remember, society has relied on a combination of threat and reward to get people to do what it wants them to do. These

FIGURE 13-2   Rewards provided by the manager are external motivators.

threats and rewards are considered external motivators. Much of our early history saw a predominance of the threat or punishment as a motivator. Persons were threatened with punishment if they did not perform well. As time went on, rewards were introduced and those who performed well were rewarded for their action. Today, the use punishment or threat is considered less effective in motivating individuals than are rewards for work well done. However, there are times when the organization cannot afford to continue to increase rewards that are financially costly to the organization. Managers and leaders must then find other types of rewards to motivate workers.

Intrinsic motives are more difficult to work with than extrinsic motives because they arise from within the individual. Some would argue that all motives are intrinsic and that the most we can do is try to foster within the individual the desire to act in a certain way, to perform certain activities, or to strive for certain goals, because the motivation to do so originates from within the person who will be doing the acting. Those who adhere to that approach state that when we talk about motivating others, it is limited to those acts of persuasion that will fire the inner desire within another individual to take the desired action (Fig. 13-2).

When it comes to grades, why do some individuals strive for As, while others are satisfied with Cs? Why do some seek leadership roles within organizations, while others prefer positions that may capture a lower salary but be less stressful? Why do some people seek doctorate degrees, while others believe a high school diploma will provide them with all the education they need? A lot of study and a number of theories have been set forth to explain why people make the choices they do from among a variety of possible behaviors.

You may already have learned about human needs as motivation and that needs appear in a hierarchy, with unmet needs creating motivation. People engage in actions that help them to meet their needs (Maslow, 1954). Abraham Maslow, an American psychologist whose work has been popular since the 1950s, established the highest level of functioning as self actualization. The needs for food, shelter, belonging, esteem, and self-esteem (in approximately that order) provide motivation for behavior. Self actualization, the highest level, occurs when esteem needs are met and the individual is no longer driven by the need to prove him- or herself.

Herzberg and colleagues (1959) and Herzberg (1966) discussed **dissatisfiers** or **hygiene factors** and **satisfiers** or **motivators**, which were essentially independent of one another in his Motivation-Hygiene theory. His theory stated that people focused on the environment in which they were working when dissatisfied with the job. His hygiene factors related to conditions under which the job is performed and include such things as organizational policies, working conditions, salaries, status, and job security. When satisfied with working conditions, they focused on the job. Satisfiers referred to feelings regarding the work itself and included such items as achievement, professional growth, recognition, responsibility, and advancement. When workers are satisfied, work performance increases.

Another approach to motivation suggests that some people are motivated by a desire affiliation, the desire for power, or the desire for achievement (McClelland, 1953, 1961). Affiliation referred to the desire for friendly, close social relationships—to be liked. Power referred to the need to be in control—to manage things. Achievement related to the desire to excel, advance, succeed, and grow. Much of today's focus on motivating behavior in others centers on people's desire to achieve.

McGregor (1966) suggested that some managers operate as if people are motivated only by fear of the manager's displeasure or the potential for a concrete reward, such as pay. These would be considered extrinsic factors. Labeled Theory X, it supported the concept that most people would rather be directed than assume responsibility for creative problem solving. They found work distasteful, were motivated primarily by physical and security needs, and needed to be managed through close supervision. McGregor recommended another approach to managing people that started from the viewpoint that most people want to do well and that tapping into this basic tendency was the way to motivate people. It assumes that people welcome opportunities to make contributions and can be self directed and creative. McGregor labeled this Theory Y.

A central concept for you as a beginning nurse is that different factors motivate different people and that one individual might be motivated by one factor at one point in life but by another factor at a different time. Keeping a broad view of what might motivate others will enable you to work more effectively to motivate nursing staff. Table 13-1 summarizes the theories mentioned above and describes how they may be used to motivate people.

Developing Your Ability to Motivate Others

As a team leader, how will you motivate others? What behaviors on your part will encourage others to perform at their best? What people skills can you develop that will assist you in working with others? A key aspect of being successful in this area relates to your ability to develop the kind and quality of relationships with others that will positively influence the way they perform. It is important to get to know the people with whom you work. As previously discussed, different things motivate different people. Personal praise may result in outstanding performance in one individual; another may respond best when given new responsibilities or challenging **assignments**. You will want to know your team members well enough to know what things you can do that will bring out the best in them. The behaviors discussed below are summarized in Display 13-2.

TABLE 13-1	APPLICATION OF THEORIES OF MOTIVATION	
THEORIST & THEORY	**DESCRIPTION**	**APPLICATION**
Maslow Hierarchy of Needs	Established a pyramid of human needs ordered from simple to complex. The needs at the base of the pyramid are physiological (food, shelter), then self-preservation, affiliation (love, belonging), esteem (confidence, recognition), and self-actualization (maximum achievement).	Facilitate opportunities for workers to meet as many basic needs as possible in the workplace, thus attracting more workers.
Herzberg Motivation-hygiene	Dissatisfiers/hygiene factors prevent job satisfaction and result in workers focusing on work conditions. Satisfiers/motivators promote work performance and work achievement.	Provide enriching opportunities for workers in the work environment Recognize performance.

McClelland
  Affiliation, power,
  achievement
	Major motivators are the need to belong, the need to control, and the need to succeed.	Foster opportunities within the work environment for gratification of needs.

McGregor
  Theory X
  Theory Y
	Theory X: Workers are dissatisfied and are motivated by fear of the manager's displeasure. Need to be supervised.
	Theory Y: Workers are satisfied, self-directed and creative, enjoy work.
		Broaden employees' responsibility, involve them in decision making.
		Recognize achievements.

Inspire Trust and Confidence

As you examine the personal behaviors that will help you motivate others, give serious consideration to the things that people do to inspire trust and confidence in others. What helps build **credibility** – the assurance that people can count on you to do what you say you are going to do when you say you will do it? Behaviors that lend credibility to actions include exercising good judgment, and being knowledgeable about procedures, policies, and protocols. Performing in a timely fashion is also critical. You will want to be even-tempered and patient, even in stressful situations. As a result of developing these qualities, others will view you as a person from whom they can seek answers and directions.

Role Model Behaviors

You will want to model the behaviors you want to see in others. In doing so, you set the pace for your team. When you are energized, others also will be energized. When you respond to

---

Display 13-2   Personal Behaviors that Motivate Others

- Inspire trust and confidence from others
- Role model the behaviors you want to see in others
- Treat others respectfully
- Give recognition for things done well
- Maintain a positive attitude

others in a positive way, it becomes contagious and others respond positively. Avoid any behaviors that would undermine a team member's motivation, such as being arrogant, showing favoritism, telling jokes that put down others, making racist statements, or issuing threats.

Treat Others Respectfully

Foster all opportunities to take pride in the accomplishments of the team and share ideas for improvement. Find ways to let your team members know you care about them as individuals. Show a genuine interest in things that are important to them. Be sensitive to problems they may encounter away from the workplace as well as within. Learn what their personal goals and aspirations are and encourage activities that will help them to reach those goals. Avoid gossip or humor that makes someone else the object of the joke. Do not talk about one person with another. When you need to speak to someone about a problem, do so privately.

 COMMUNICATION IN *ACTION*

Avoiding Gossip

One evening at dinner, Sarah, a new graduate, ate with an LPN and a nursing assistant from her unit. The nursing assistant said, "I get so tired of Jennie [another LPN] always showing how smart she is!" The LPN replied, "I know just what you mean—you would think she was the nurse manager or something. Sarah, haven't you noticed how bossy and controlling Jennie is?" Sarah replied, "I feel really uncomfortable discussing Jennie behind her back. It seems unfair. I guess if it is a problem for you, maybe you should try to talk to Jennie about it." She then introduced a new topic of conversation. Sarah has not labeled the others but has indicated the behavior of gossip is not one in which she will participate. She laid the framework for others to expect that she will not gossip about them.

Recognize Achievements

Receiving recognition for things done well helps motivate many people. Even those who answer shyly, "It was nothing" appreciate having their efforts acknowledged. Giving praise for accomplishments also means that you will be working closely with individuals, so that you know when they have done something well. Praise and recognition, even in the form of a thank you, serve as great reinforcers and encourage people to keep trying. Most individuals seek to please others by their performance and need to know when that has been achieved. If you can offer this praise in public, it will reap even greater rewards. You have heard before that we praise publicly and correct privately. This is certainly true when trying to motivate others to do their best.

Another aspect of encouraging individuals to perform at their best focuses on having them know that their opinion is wanted and valued. This means involving them in decision making. We talked earlier in this chapter and in Chapter 12 about involving those closest to the action in the decision-making process. People perform better when they believe they are important and contributing to the team effort—that they are valued. You can provide the opportunity for others to have input into decisions and to articulate their thoughts and opinions. When you initially try this, you may run into resistance. When encouraging others to participate in decision making, you may get the response, "That's what they pay you for." If this occurs, continue to offer opportunities for input. If this is a new experience for the team member, that individual may doubt your sincerity. Developing a genuine approach when working with others creates the basis of trust and respect as mentioned at the beginning of this chapter.

Maintain a Positive Attitude

When working with others, maintaining a positive attitude will help both you and those with whom you work. If you avoid becoming upset and angry, you can respond to problems or errors more effectively. This may require using your sense of humor when things go awry. The discomfort of many situations can be decreased by being able to laugh at things that fail to meet our expectations. In contrast, becoming upset or angry if something is done incorrectly will only cause your team members to avoid you. They will consider you unapproachable, and communication will decrease. The opportunity to build the strength of the team will be missed.

A final word should be said about redirecting the efforts of others. Especially when working with unlicensed assistive personnel, you may identify techniques that are incorrect or approaches to client care that need improvement. When this occurs, always focus your comments on the observed behavior you believe needs to be changed, not on the individual's personal characteristics. You will find it useful to ask personnel for their own commitment to make the needed change in behavior or performance. This places the responsibility for correct performance on the individual. Then, when you observe the corrected behavior, be certain to positively comment about it. More discussion related to supervising the actions of others follows later in this chapter.

■■ COMMUNICATION IN *ACTION*
■■

Lost Privacy

John Wilson was making rounds of the patients in a long-term care facility when he noticed a nursing assistant with an elderly resident. The assistant was preparing to move the resident onto a commode, but the curtain was not pulled. John moved to the bedside and simply said, "Here, let me get that curtain pulled for you," and pulled the curtain around to protect the resident's privacy. When the nursing assistant was finished, John approached her privately and said, "I am concerned that you did not pull the curtain when you were assisting the resident to the commode. Our residents have to be provided modesty and privacy. You must always remember to pull the curtain before providing care. Can I get your assurance that you will work on that?" He avoided making general statements such as, "You are inconsiderate and careless of the modesty of our residents," but was specific about the incorrect behavior and the rationale for the correct behavior. Also, John asked the nursing assistant to make a commitment to changing her own behavior.

🌐 DELEGATING

When you first began your clinical experience, you may have felt that you and your classmates were the only people who needed to be directed in what to do. As you progressed, you may have become aware that staff nurses were directing the actions of all the individuals on the nursing team. In today's health care environment, all RNs have the responsibility for supervising the activities of those who have lesser educational preparation than they. It is possible that you have already had to provide direction to a nursing assistant or an LPN.

Delegation is the process by which one individual is able to accomplish necessary tasks with and through others. It is an important management process and allows organizations to function effectively and efficiently. The ANA (1997) defined delegation as "the transfer of responsibility for the performance of an activity from one individual to another while retaining accountability for the outcome." An example would be an RN asking that a nursing assistant help a client ambulate in the hall. The nursing assistant assists the client to walk, the RN is still responsible for seeing that the client ambulates, and that it is completed safely and documented in the client's record.

In today's health care environment, which uses variously prepared caregivers, the importance of being able to effectively delegate responsibilities is critical. Nurses would not be able to complete their duties, tasks, and responsibilities without the ability to delegate some nursing activities. Delegating effectively requires that you have skill in the ability to guide, teach, and direct others. And like other skills you have mastered, it can be learned.

The ANA (1997) also has made a distinction between the delegation and assignment of tasks. They have defined assignment as "the downward or lateral transfer of both the responsibility and accountability of an activity from one individual to another." It is intended that the assignment would be made to an individual of skill, knowledge, and judgment. The two critical elements of this distinction are the accountability for actions when delegating to another and the skill, knowledge, and judgment of the person to whom tasks are assigned. Assignments given to assistive personnel may involve making beds, passing water, answering lights, and taking specimens to the lab. In the clinical environment, tasks for which the nursing assistant is accountable and tasks that are delegated both may be referred to as "assignments." This causes some confusion in discussions. For practical purposes, keep in mind that the nursing assistant can be accountable for some routine tasks, but that accountability for outcomes for patient care remains with the RN who is supervising the nursing assistant.

Reasons to Delegate

There are a number of reasons that we delegate certain tasks to others. Primary among these is the current trend in health care facilities to allow the RN more time for critical aspects of care by hiring **unlicensed assistive personnel (UAP)** to perform those tasks that they can perform safely. This also results in cost cuts, as a UAP commands a much lower salary than does an RN. At one time in nursing, a primary care model of care delivery was popular in which the RN performed all nursing care activities for a group of patients (see Chapter 11). Although this was a desirable approach from a patient care standpoint, it was very costly. In an effort to contain costs, hospitals restructured and redesigned staffing patterns to change the skill mix of employees who provided care. In other words, staffing patterns decreased the number of RNs and included caregivers with lesser educational preparation to provide certain aspects of care. This change was predicated on the assumption that many tasks occurring on a nursing unit do not require the skills of an RN. Individuals with lesser educational preparation can carry out certain aspects of care such as taking vital signs, ambulating, transporting clients, and performing basic procedures. This allows the RN to focus on activities such as client assessment, care coordination, and teaching. In this way, delegating provides for effective time management.

Another reason to delegate relates to the positive effect it can have on building team spirit. As team members to whom work is delegated are able to effectively perform the tasks assigned to them, a sense of satisfaction is created and self-esteem is increased. Thus, teams function more effectively.

Critical Aspects of Effective Delegation

For delegation to be effective and to ensure that the quality of patient care remains high, a number of factors must be considered. Review these factors before you begin delegating tasks to others.

It is critical to remember that although you have asked someone else to carry out a nursing task, you are still accountable for the care that is given (see the discussion of accountability in Chapter 12). You need to be able to ensure that the task will be completed in compliance with accepted standards, in a timely fashion, and that the activity, along with the patient's response, if appropriate, is adequately documented.

Knowing When Not to Delegate

Are there tasks that should not be delegated? When should I not delegate a task? What are the situations in which I should retain responsibility for doing the task? How will I know the difference? These are questions frequently asked by the nurse who is just moving into the role of managing the activities of others.

Certain tasks cannot be delegated. The most obvious of these are activities that are not within the scope of practice of the individual to whom you might delegate the task. Any activity that requires knowledge and judgment that is unique to the function of an RN cannot be delegated to others. Thus, you would not ask or expect a UAP to do assessments or evaluations or make decisions that require nursing judgment.

You may not delegate responsibilities that call for professional judgment, skill, or decision-making ability. An RN must complete all assessments of the client and client needs. Information from the assessment that is important to the client's care then needs to be communicated to any person to whom care is delegated. The ability to do a thorough assessment and to not overlook some critical need is part of the nursing judgment acquired through your education. Someone with lesser preparation might overlook that need. For example, if you admit to your unit a patient with head trauma, the assessment of that patient cannot be delegated.

You may not delegate roles that are limited to licensed individuals under the nursing licensure laws. For example, giving medications cannot be delegated, because medication administration involves assessment, understanding of appropriate procedural safeguards, knowledge of pharmacology, and the ability to evaluate the effectiveness of the medication. Because of this, the law limits who may administer medications. Display 13-3 summarizes information on what should not be delegated.

Identifying to Whom to Delegate

You can delegate only to a person who is competent to perform the task delegated. The nurse who is delegating tasks must know and understand the level of care that can be performed by the person to whom the task is being delegated. In other words, you need to understand staff members' competency level or, if they are licensed, their scope of practice—what activities a person with a particular license may legally perform. The scope of practice for RNs and for LPNs is outlined in state practice acts and may vary from state to state (see Chapter 7). You will want to be familiar with the practice acts of the state in which you are employed. When working with someone

Display 13-3   Situations in Which Delegation Is Inappropriate

- When the activities to be delegated fall outside the scope of practice of the person to whom they would be delegated. You cannot delegate something the individual is not allowed to do.
- When the activities to be delegated require independent, specialized nursing knowledge and judgment. This protects the safety of the client.
- When the activities to be delegated fall within job description and role of the registered nurse and delegating it would erode that role. This would apply to situations in which the nurse is responsible for evaluating the performance of others.
- When the work situation will not allow time for adequate supervision of those to whom tasks are delegated. Delegated tasks must be supported and supervised at all times.

who is not licensed, you will want to be knowledgeable about job descriptions, specific competencies, and agency policies and protocols.

Determining What to Delegate

The tasks delegated to assistive personnel should not require nursing judgment while being carried out. This implies that the tasks should be routine in nature, ones that can be performed according to certain exact standards, and that the client's condition be relatively stable. We have said it before, but it bears repeating—activities that require specialized nursing skill, knowledge, or experience cannot be delegated. It is the use of this specialized nursing judgment that constitutes the heart of professional nursing.

The anticipated outcome of the care that is being delegated should be reasonably predictable. For example, if the responsibility for checking the vital signs of a patient is assigned to an LPN, the result will be the accurate assessment and recording of the patient's vital signs.

Tasks associated with any situation requiring ongoing assessment, complex observations, additional instructions, or critical decisions should not be delegated. Again, these activities require the use of nursing judgment and, therefore, should be completed by the RN. This would apply to any situation in which a client's condition is unstable, changing, or whose acuity level is high.

Supervising Delegated Tasks

The supervision of delegated activities is essential. The ANA (1997) defines supervision as "the active process of directing, guiding and influencing the outcome of an individual's performance of an activity." This means that an individual with greater skill and education is available, usually in person, but occasionally through alternate means, such as written or verbal communications, to give directions and ensure that activities are carried out properly. For delegation to be successful, there must be sufficient personnel and adequate time to provide the needed supervision and follow up. If either of these is missing, problems may result.

Matching the Task to the Person to Whom it Is Delegated

When delegating, you have the responsibility for ensuring that a match exists between what care the client needs to have performed and the level of competence and understanding of the person being asked to provide that care. In this way, you are assured that the tasks that are delegated are not beyond the ability of the individual asked to do them. This requires that you know members of your team and their abilities. It also requires that you understand the legal scope of practice of the various members of your team. This can be an important consideration in situations in which an RN is floated into a special care unit to assist during especially busy times. Aspects of care in that unit that are specialized should not be delegated to someone who has not had the necessary additional training and education required to render safe care, even if that person has the RN license. Rather, the floated nurse should be asked to perform those aspects of care with which he or she is familiar.

The Five Rights of Successful Delegation

If you have followed all these guidelines when delegating responsibilities to others, in all likelihood you will have also followed the five rights of successful delegation. The National Council of State Boards of Nursing (NCSBN) issued these five rights in 1995, when changes in delivery of patient care first included use of UAP and similar care providers (NCSBN, 1995). (Typically, this includes positions with job titles such as nurse aides, certified nurse assistants, nurse technicians, patient care technicians, personal care attendant, or unit assistants.) The five rights as identified by the NCSBN are found in Display 13-4.

Suggestions for Successful Delegation

A number of elements can result in delegation either enhancing or compromising patient care. Following the steps in the nursing process will help ensure the best outcomes.

Assess the Situation

Before you decide which aspects of care you can ask others to do and which you should complete yourself, be certain that a complete assessment of the client has been done. You will want to know what that individual's needs involve, what priorities have been set, the goals of care, the time you have to accomplish the care, and other factors that impinge on the situation.

If you are to make a good match between the skills of the person to whom you delegate responsibilities and the complexity of the task, you must know the abilities of the person to whom you will delegate tasks. This can sometimes be determined through hospital protocols that establish the competencies of various levels of caregivers or via job descriptions that define what an individual in a certain job category is capable of performing. If the individual is licensed, you can be guided by what that category of worker can legally do. The length of time they have worked in that position or on that unit can also give some guidance. The best way to understand

Display 13-4   The NCSBN'S Five Rights of Delegation

- Right Task
- Right Circumstances
- Right Person
- Right Direction/Communication
- Right Supervision/Evaluation

what individuals can and cannot do is to have worked with them for a sufficient period of time. If you are unfamiliar with the skills of a particular worker, you will need to provide greater supervision as you begin working with that person.

Initially, you will want to delegate only those tasks that have the highest level of predictive outcome, that is, those that are routine and standard. In so doing, you are also considering the potential for harm to the client and how difficult a particular task is to perform. You will note that your process of assessment has broadened to include the patient, members of your team, and the work situation.

Plan Your Actions

At this point, you will need to compare in your mind the information you have about the skill level of your team and the nursing care activities to be accomplished. Using the information you have gleaned in your assessment, you will then identify the specific persons to whom you may delegate the various tasks. Plan the time to give them their assignments to ensure that you have adequate opportunity to clearly communicate your expectations. Also plan time for them to ask any questions they may have regarding the assignment.

Think about the situations that may require you to provide teaching and guidance to your team members. You will want to create an environment in which those you direct feel comfortable asking for assistance or instruction regarding procedures and skills with which they are less familiar. This could include the actual skill itself, but do not forget areas such as communication, priority setting, and critical thinking.

Implement Your Plan

As you begin to direct the activities of others, your instructions should be complete, easily understood, and able to be followed correctly. What activities need to be completed immediately? Which ones can be done later in the shift? Whose should time be organized? What are the expected outcomes? If you are working with an individual whose primary language is not English, this may take more time (see "Communicating Effectively" in Chapter 12). Be certain that the assistants know what to report back to you and when you want to receive that information. What information can be left until the end of the shift? What data should be shared immediately (Fig. 13-3)? Listening carefully to their response to your instructions will help you to know that they have understood what you want accomplished. Watch for both verbal and nonverbal cues to their comprehension of your expectations. Ask them to repeat back to you what they plan to do and when. Ask whether they have any questions before beginning their work. Tell them where you will be if they need assistance.

Supervising care constitutes an essential part of delegation. Supervising care means that you know what is occurring with the patients and the staff, what has been accomplished, what remains to be done, and what problems may have occurred in the process. This requires that you check with individuals throughout the day to determine how they are progressing, what problems they may be having, or what assistance or instruction they may need. Asking questions such as, "How are you progressing with your task?" or "Are you having any difficulties with care?" or "Is there anything with which you need help?" will provide opportunity for feedback. If you find that a team member is behind in the tasks you have delegated, plan adjustments that will allow completion of the care. You many need to help the individual set new priorities, or you may need to find another person to assist with the completion of care if you are unable to do so yourself.

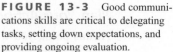

FIGURE 13-3   Good communications skills are critical to delegating tasks, setting down expectations, and providing ongoing evaluation.

Sometimes the individual who is a novice in the supervising role finds it difficult to know when to step in and assist and when to step back. Initially, you may be so concerned about doing a good job that you micromanage the situation. When you delegate responsibilities, provide an appropriate amount of autonomy for the person to decide how to accomplish the work. Generally speaking, once you delegate a task you should not take it back. This is a good opportunity you use your skills as a coach. Ask questions that will help people to whom tasks are delegated find the answer for themselves. Cueing questions such as, "What did you do the last time you had this to do?" or "What do you think will work best?" stimulate individuals to begin to solve problems for themselves, elevates their self-confidence and builds stronger teams. If your assistance is required, provide just that—assistance—rather than taking over the situation. You want to develop team members who have confidence in their own abilities and who feel they are valued members of the team.

Evaluate the Results

When you are responsible for the activities of others, evaluating the outcomes of care is more important than ever. Remember, the fact that you have delegated part of it to another person does not absolve you of the responsibility of seeing that it is completed according to established standards and in a timely manner. You will want to evaluate all patients in your care and determine that their needs have been met to the highest degree possible. Be certain that all documentation is complete and done according to standards. Talk with members of your team to obtain needed information about the care they gave and any observations they made in the process of providing that care. Asking questions such as, "Did any problems arise while care was being given?" or "How did Mr. Drummer respond to the range of motion you performed?" or "Did Mrs. Winston

Display 13-5   Suggestions for Effective Delegation

- Know what your team members are able to do, including their scope of practice and educational preparation.
- Plan ahead to avoid problems, decide what tasks to delegate.
- Match the task to be accomplished with the abilities of the individual to whom you are assigning the task.
- Communicate clearly the task you are delegating and your expected outcomes.
- Provide the necessary authority and responsibility to accomplish the task to the individual to whom you are delegating.
- Monitor and assess the performance of the task.
- Provide positive feedback as is appropriate; take corrective action when necessary.

seem comfortable when you finished?" or "How much apple juice did Julie drink?" will help elicit responses.

If, in your evaluation, you believe there is some aspect of care that has been done well, comment on it. We all like to know our efforts are appreciated and to receive recognition for a job well done. Positive feedback is a powerful motivator. A pat on the back along with a few positive words lets people know their work is appreciated. On the other hand, if corrections need to be made in the care, be certain that such conversations occur in a private, supportive manner. Display 13-5 summarizes suggestions for delegating successfully.

EXAMPLE

Appropriate Delegation of Tasks

Annett Jordon, RN, is employed in the labor room of a busy metropolitan hospital. The staff members are experiencing a particularly busy morning, with all birthing rooms full and many mothers expected to deliver within the next hour. Nursing administration has sent another RN, Belinda, to the area to assist with care. Annett quickly interviews the floated RN about her experience in the birthing area and determines that it is minimal and occurred 2 years ago when Belinda was a student. She determines that Belinda has had recent experience in recovery room. She decides to assign Belinda to the care of two mothers who have just delivered. She asks that Belinda check their blood pressure every 15 minutes, take their pulse, watch until IVs have been completed and then discontinue them, assess for full bladders, and check lochia. She assures Belinda she will return to check the height and condition of the fundus. In this situation, Annett carefully assessed the situation and the person who had been sent to assist on the unit. By her careful attention to the principles of delegation, she ensured that all the patients had appropriate professional nursing care.

Blocks to Effective Delegation

Situations exist in today's health care environment that result in blocks or barriers to effective delegation. If these blocks can be eliminated or reduced, delegation will be more satisfying to all who are involved.

Lack of Job Descriptions

The first serious block to good delegation is the lack of current and complete job descriptions for all employees within the institution. As mentioned earlier, the RN must know the abilities and competency of members of the nursing team. These are most commonly found in the job descriptions of the institution. As new positions are created, management should form and distribute clear job descriptions. Communicating the content of the job descriptions is just as important as developing the documents. This will help ensure that the individual responsible for delegating tasks has access to the information and can use it for decision making. Similar to this problem is that of job descriptions that are not kept current. Jobs may be changed and tasks redistributed, but job descriptions reflecting these changes may not be completed. Thus, those needing the information find themselves having to make decisions without being fully informed.

Time Required to Delegate and Supervise

A second concern rests with the time required to effectively delegate and supervise. Many nurses believe they do not have enough time to spend with their patients. Time that is taken to plan, implement, supervise, teach, coach, and evaluate activities delegated to others may be viewed as taking even more time away from that spent at the bedside. This is especially true when working with inexperienced UAPs, who may require a lot of teaching and support. The high rate of turnover in UAP positions heightens the frustration. There are no simple answers to this problem. To some extent, these are system problems that need to be addressed at a level higher than the individual nursing unit. The best action you can take in such situations may be to let your supervisor know that the problem exists. Perhaps longer periods of orientation can be planned for the assistants or better screening in the hiring process.

Inadequate Training

A final block to effective delegation rests with inadequate training both for those who will be involved in patient care and for those who are moving into management positions. Formal orientations to the facility and to on-the-job-type skills for the position the employee will fill help ease new employees into their roles. This is also true for those who will be responsible for supervising the new employees or who are new to the management role. It is one thing to know how to provide quality care to a small group of patients and quite another to oversee the activities of a team that is caring for a large group of patients. As with other situations in nursing, you will develop greater skill with experience.

Key Concepts

- A team is a group of people working together for a common goal. Because of the diverse disciplines that are now involved in health care, the effective functioning of the health care team is critical to the provision of quality health care. Trust and respect of others are key ingredients in team function.
- Health care teams have moved from being multidisciplinary to interdisciplinary in which the skills of a variety of health care professionals come together on behalf of the patient. The nurse has a key role in coordinating the efforts of the team.

- Nurses have a number of roles other than that of provider of care. They may serve as an educator, a patient advocate, a counselor/coach, or a manager and leader for the nursing team. They might also work in nursing informatics or in nursing research.
- Nurses and physicians fill key positions on the health care team. The relationship between these two care providers must be symbolized by mutual respect and consideration. Nurses can take positive actions to help assure that this occurs.
- Many leaders in health care are using team-building techniques to strengthen the functioning of their teams. Team building involves setting common goals, recognizing the contribution each person makes to the team, involving others in decision making, focusing on problems rather than individuals associated with the problem, and sharing in accomplishments.
- As important as leading a team is being a good team members. Most new graduates begin in the role of team member. You need to be able to assess your abilities as a team member.
- The coaching role is being seen more frequently in health care. Rather than telling a younger nurse what to do, an individual serving as a coach helps them search for answers providing necessary support, encouragement, and information.
- Motivation encompasses the sum of all the factors that cause an individual to do something. To motivate individuals, the leader must understand personal behaviors and role model those that are desired in others.
- Delegation is the process by which one individual is able to accomplish necessary tasks with and through others. It is an important management process and allows the health care system to function efficiently. Nurses remain accountable for all nursing care that is provided. It is important to follow the guidelines for effective delegation and know which aspects of care can never be delegated.
- The five rights of successful delegation include the right task, the right circumstances, the right person, the right direction and communication, and the right supervision and evaluation.
- Nurses cannot delegate aspects of care that require nursing judgment, including such activities as patient assessment.

References

American Nurses Association. (1997). *Attachment I: Definitions related to ANA 1992 position statements on unlicensed assistive personnel*. Kansas City, MO: Author.

Baguley, P. (2002). *Teams and team-working*. London: Hodder Headline Plc.

Blanchard, K., Randolph, A., & Grazier, P. (2005). *Go team! Take your team to the next level*. San Francisco: Berrett-Koehler Publishers, Inc.

Herzberg, F. (1966). *Works and the nature of man*. New York: World Publishing Co.

Herzberg, F., Mausner, B., & Snyderman, B. B. (1959). *The motivation to work*. New York: John Wiley.

Maslow, A. (1954). *Motivation and personality*. New York: Harper & Row.

McClelland, D. (1953). *The achievement motive*. Norwalk, CT: Appleton-Century-Crofts.

McClelland, D. (1961). *The achieving society*. Princeton, NJ: Van Nostrand.

McGregor, D. (1966). *Leadership and motivation*. Cambridge, MA: MIT Press.

Montana, J., & Mitchell, T. (2005). *The Winning Spirit*. New York: Random House.

National Council of State Boards of Nursing. (1995). *Delegation: Concepts and decision-making process*. Chicago: Author.

"Quality Gurus." (2007). [On-line] Available http://*www.qualitygurus*.com/gurus/ Accessed June 2, 2007.

Rosenstein, A. H. (2002). Nurse–physician relationships: Impact on nurse satisfaction and retention. *American Journal of Nursing, 102*(6), 26–34.

Sirota, T. (2007) Nurse/physician relationships: Improving or not. *Nursing* 2007, 37(1) 52–56.

Whitworth, L., Kimsey-House, H., & Sandahl, P. (1998). *Coactive coaching: New skills for coaching people toward success in work and life*. Palo Alto, CA: Davis Black Publishing.

14

Leading Change and Managing Conflict

LEARNING OUTCOMES

After completing this chapter, you should be able to:

1. Discuss situations in the health care environment that create a need for change.
2. Describe two models of change that can be used to facilitate the change process and reduce resistance to it.
3. Identify three strategies for change and explain how each can be effective.
4. Discuss actions that can be taken to facilitate change.
5. Describe the role of the change agent.
6. Explore your personal response to change and how you might more successfully adapt to changes in your work environment.
7. List the various sources of conflict in a health care setting.
8. Discuss the way in which conflict can have positive outcomes.
9. Describe win-lose, lose-lose, and win-win outcomes and give an example of each.
10. Describe the types of conflict that exist explaining the differences among them and citing an example of each.
11. Explain five strategies for managing conflict and give examples of appropriate situations for the use of each.
12. Discuss the techniques you will want to employ to be prepared for conflict.

KEY TERMS

Champion
Change
Change agent
Conflict
Conflict management
Conflict resolution
Driving forces
Empirical–rational strategy
Intergroup conflict

Interpersonal conflict
Intrapersonal conflict
Lose-lose outcome
Movement stage
Normative–reeducative
  approach
Organizational conflicts
Power–coercive strategy
Reactive change

Refreezing stage
Restraining forces
Role ambiguity
Role conflict
Stakeholders
Unfreezing stage
Win-lose outcome
Win-win outcome

With few exceptions, people like those things that are familiar and comfortable. We often become dismayed when our favorite store closes or a brand of merchandise we have used for a period of time is discontinued. Our zone of comfort operates best when things are predictable and when life is not full of surprises that require us to make adjustments in the way things are done. But change is to be anticipated. One of the most constant features of today's health care environment is the inevitability of change. It will occur whether we want it to or not. How we are able to manage change may be a key factor in determining how successful we are.

Just as change is inevitable, so is conflict. Conflict has existed since man inhabited the earth. From squabbles you had with your siblings or friends as a child, to irritations you experience in the adult world, conflict exists in your life. And, again, how you are able to handle conflict may affect your professional success.

This chapter is devoted to explaining the processes of change and conflict. It offers suggestions for managing each.

LEADING CHANGE

Change has been defined as "a significant disruption in established patterns of behavior and/or expectations" (Carr, Hard, & Trahant, 1996, p. 67). As an individual who will have the responsibility for managing others, you need to know how to deal with change yourself and how to help others deal with the change process.

Origins of Change

Typically, change occurs because of either internal or external forces that are brought to bear on the individual or the organization. Internal forces come from within the individual or the individual organization. External forces originate outside the entity experiencing the change. In Lewin's theory of change (described in the next section), both of these are termed **driving forces**, those that push the system toward change.

In the health care environment, many forces for change may exist. Internal changes within health care organizations can result from new ideas about the system of nursing care delivery, changes in the way pharmacy will dispense medications, the opening of new units, or the implementation of a new computerized system for charting. All of these might be initiated because of the goal of improving the quality of patient care and/or patient satisfaction. Change might also be required to reduce costs due to economic constraints. Or it could be initiated to improve the work environment, thus creating greater employee satisfaction (eg, the introduction of a shared governance structure).

Internal forces that create the need for change may include the desire to advance oneself, to retire, to marry, to find a more challenging job, and so forth. Other internal factors, such as a desire for more efficiency, greater competence, and additional education that would give individuals greater knowledge, also create change.

External forces abound in the health care environment. One external factor that creates the need for change in the health care field is technology. For example, long ago the electronic thermometer replaced the glass mercury thermometer, and even the electronic thermometer has undergone changes since first being introduced. Computerization, automatic monitoring devices, and mechanical lifts are additional types of technology requiring changes in practice.

Additional external forces creating the need for change might include new legislation, new standards, and changing population demographics of the people served. Examples of these include legislation requiring staffing levels or limiting overtime, accreditation standards that are revised, and an increase in the number of uninsured individuals in the community. The Americans with Disabilities Act was responsible for many changes, not only in health care facilities but also in many other places that serve the public. The Patient Self-Determination Act, also known as the Danforth amendment required significant changes, particularly in long-term care facilities. Health care agencies currently are experiencing changes mandated by the Health Insurance Portability and Accountability Act related to patient's privacy. Other situations that create the need for change include insurance company requirements for different documentation procedures and the closure of companies that have provided services.

Regardless of the reason for the change, you can anticipate that things will not remain the same. And whether the change is internal or external, whether it is within the individual or the organization, you will want to be able to work with the change and, if in the position of providing leadership, be able to assist others in the process.

Planned and Unplanned Change

Planned change has been defined as "the deliberate design and implementation of a structural innovation, a new policy or goal, or an overt change in operating philosophy, climate, and style" (Thomas & Bennis, 1972, p. 289). Thus, planned change has a definite design and structure established to facilitate the process, including time lines, identification of stake holders, goals, plans for implementation, and processes for evaluation. Thoughtful planning often results in more effective and efficient change processes and is essential for projects that are complex or large in scope and that require greater time, resources, or skills.

Change also may be unplanned and occur as a reaction to another issue. This is referred to as **reactive change**. Reactive change occurs when some problem or event arose to require a different way of doing things.

EXAMPLE

A Case of Wrong Medication Setting the Stage for Change

A nurse on a medical unit of a community hospital became concerned when she noticed that the Toprol-XL, a medication to treat hypertension, sent from the pharmacy looked different from the medication she had administered to a patient for the previous dose. She placed a call to the pharmacy, and a pharmacist came to the unit to double check the medication. The medication order had been filled with Topamax, an antidepressant used in the treatment of seizures. A team was quickly put in place to recommend actions to prevent such incidents from occurring. The final result of this team process was a requirement that prescribers include both the trade and generic names of a drug and that the indication for ordering be written on all medication orders. Additionally, nurses were required to confirm that the drug ordered was appropriate to the patient's condition.

Lewin's Theory of Change

A noted authority on the subject of change is Kurt Lewin (1951), whose theory of change is one of the most widely accepted and remains in current use today. His change theory identified that change has three stages: the unfreezing stage, the moving stage, and the refreezing stage.

The Unfreezing Stage

According to Lewin, the **unfreezing stage** occurs when an individual is motivated by the need to create a change. This person becomes a **change agent**, the person who is responsible for facilitating the change process with others. Having gathered data, identified the problem, and decided that change is needed, the change agent sets about making others aware of the need for change. The change agent attempts to "unfreeze" or lessen the resistance to change or selects someone else who can help to unfreeze the current position. Those who will be affected by the situation requiring change are notified about why the change is needed and they also become discontented with the current situation. The problem is then diagnosed and the best solution selected. Thus, those who will be involved begin to see the need for the change. For change to be successful, people must believe that it is necessary. It avoids having individuals blindsided (taken unaware) by proposed changes that will affect their way of operating. It instead enlists their cooperation.

The Movement Stage

The second phase of Lewin's theory is called the movement stage. During the **movement stage**, the person initiating the change identifies strategies that will facilitate the change and then plans and implements them. The person leading the change needs to be knowledgeable, be respected, and have sufficient power within the organization for others to accept direction from this individual. The process of facilitating change is described below.

The Refreezing Stage

In the final phase, the **refreezing stage**, the changes are integrated and stabilized and become part of the value system of the organization. The change agent helps to stabilize the change that has been made in the organization so that it becomes part of everyday operation. This step is necessary to prevent the system from reverting to old patterns of behavior. Refreezing occurs when the new behaviors have occurred frequently enough that people are comfortable with them and feel rewarded because of them. Most changes need between 3 and 6 months before being totally accepted. During this time, the change agent supports those affected by the change and helps them adapt to it.

Driving and Restraining Forces

Lewin (1951) also described driving and restraining forces that affect change. As described previously, driving forces are those that push a system toward change. The external, system-related, and internal factors that result in the initiation of change that were discussed previously are driving forces.

Restraining forces, on the other hand, pull the system away from change. These may include economic factors that make the change too expensive. It might be the lack of staff who have the knowledge and skills to make the change. In some instances, it may be that the change dramatically affects one group more than others and the group strongly resists the change. If the change is mandated by external forces, many individuals resist what they feel to be a loss of control or choice. Perhaps the group has experienced too many changes recently to add another to the work environment, for example. And if people are not prepared for change, or if they are threatened by it, they will not support it.

Systems may maintain equilibrium through the interaction of the two forces. For change to occur, the balance between the driving forces and restraining forces must be altered so that the driving forces outweigh the restraining forces.

Other Theories of Change

A number of other individuals have set forth theories related to change. Each of these theories explores a different aspect of change or addresses change from a different framework. Every theory may have value depending on the situation.

Lippitt, Watson, and Westley (1958) built on the work of Lewin. Their theory begins by recognizing and diagnosing the problem, determining the ability to change, selecting the change, planning, implementing and evaluating the change, and then stabilizing afterward. This presents a logical method of approaching change and may sound very much like the problem-solving methods with which you are already familiar.

Rogers and Shoemaker (1971) identified five factors that determined successful planned change: relative advantage, compatibility, complexity, divisibility, and communicability. Relative advantage refers to the change being thought of as better than the status quo. Compatibility refers to the change possessing values that are similar or compatible with the existing values held by the individual or group. Complexity suggests that simple techniques are more readily adopted than more complex ones. Divisibility states that changes attempted on a trial basis will have a greater chance of succeeding. Communicability implies that the easier the change is to describe, the more likely it will grow. The proper balance of all factors would result in achieving the desired change.

Asprec (1975) described four behaviors that help one to recognize resistance to change:

1. Active resistance through frustration and aggression
2. Organized passive resistance or resisting change as a group
3. Indifference by ignoring or attempting to divert attention elsewhere
4. Acceptance on the surface or by not openly opposing change.

This writer emphasized the importance of decreasing the resistance in order to reach the goal set forth in the change process.

In 1990, Perlman and Takacs, focusing on the emotions change evokes and using death and dying literature as a base, listed 10 emotional stages or phases that are experienced throughout the change process. These phases include the following:

- Equilibrium—there is a sense of peace or balance before the change occurs
- Denial—the reality of a change is denied, thus draining energy from the process
- Anger—energy is used to prevent the change from occurring
- Bargaining—effort and energy go into attempting to eliminate the change
- Chaos—energy is diffused with an accompanying loss of identity and direction
- Depression—no energy remains to produce results
- Resignation—energy is used to passively accept the change
- Openness—renewed energy becomes available
- Readiness—energy is used to explore new events
- Reemergence—energy is rechanneled, resulting in feelings of empowerment

This theory focuses on the strong feelings most people have about the change process. As you work with change, explore some of the ideas described by these authors more fully.

Much of the more recent thoughts about facilitating change focus on assisting those affected by the change to make adjustments in their attitudes, work habits, and lives (Quinn, Spreitzer, & Brown, 2000).

Developing Strategies for Implementing Change

Along with the theories that have been developed to explain and facilitate the change process, strategies for implementing change have also been identified. We will discuss some of the most commonly recognized strategies for change.

Empirical–Rational Strategy

The **empirical–rational strategy** suggests that individuals will follow their rational self-interest once it is revealed to them (Benne, Bennis, & Chin, 1976). This means that people will accept change when they see it as desirable and when it fits with their personal interests. This strategy is based on reason and knowledge and is often used to implement technologic changes. This strategy might be useful in helping to shift from paper documentation of care at the nurses station to one using a computer at the bedside. When individuals understand how much easier and more accurate computer charting will be, they will be more eager to learn how to use it and will learn the process more quickly.

For this strategy to be effective, it is important that every initiative for change have a clear purpose and goal. Those involved in the change process need to know why the change is necessary and what will be gained by completing it. Sometimes this is not easily accomplished, because there may not be adequate information regarding all details involved. Make efforts to collect and share as many facts and figures as is possible.

Power–Coercive Strategy

A **power–coercive strategy** is in use when a leader orders change and those with less power or position comply (Benne et al., 1976). The use of this strategy requires that the change agent have official authority to mandate the change. The compliance of those affected rests in their desire to please or with their fear of the sanctions that might accompany noncompliance—things such as loss of employment, rewards, advancement, or other benefits. We may see this strategy used when new laws are enforced, such as occurred when the minimum data set was mandated for use in long-term care.

Normative–Reeducative Strategy

The **normative–reeducative approach** to change states that change will take place only after changes have occurred in values, attitudes, skills, and significant relationships (Benne et al., 1976). To accomplish this, those who will be involved in the change must necessarily be included in working out the plans for the change. Mutual trust and collaboration are hallmarks of the process. If conflict occurs, the process of change must be delayed until the conflict is resolved. Table 14-1 summarizes these three strategies for change.

Selecting the Change Agent

Once the decision has been made to implement a change, some person or group must be responsible for leading that change. This may be an individual within the organization who is particularly

TABLE 14-1	STRATEGIES FOR CHANGE
Empirical–rational	Individuals will accept change when they see it as desirable and fitting with their personal interests.
Power–coercive	A leader orders change and those with less power must comply.
Normative–Reeducative	Change will take place only after there have been adjustments in values, attitudes, skills, and significant relationships.

From Benne, K. D., Bennis, G., & Chin, R. (1976). Planned change in America. In W. G. Bennis, K. D. Benne, R. Chin, & K. E. Corey (Eds.), *The planning of change*. New York: Holt, Rinehart and Winston.

knowledgeable about theories of change and skilled in assisting people in the process of change, or it may be someone hired from outside the organization who has the skills needed to bring about the process. On occasion, teams are established to bring about a change. In all instances, the change agents engage "in the exercise of power, politics, and interpersonal influence" (Buchanan & Badham, 1999, p. 615). In organizations that have adopted continuous quality improvement, the change agent is often referred to as the **champion**. Within that system, anyone could have an idea for improvement of the organization.

Facilitating Change

As with many other management and leadership skills, facilitating change can be learned. One of the first aspects that must be recognized and dealt with relates to overcoming the resistance to the change.

Understanding Resistance to Change

Because making a change will require that we alter the way we have been doing things, most people are initially resistant to change. In 1990, Senge stated resistance to change "arises from threats to traditional norms and ways of doing things (p. 88). Carr and colleagues (1996) reiterated this concept: "Resistance to change is mainly an effort to maintain the status quo" (p. 73). We become comfortable with the way that things have been done and may be apprehensive of new approaches that require us to change established patterns of behavior. The new approaches may take additional time to learn or may be threatening to us if they involve skills with which we are not entirely familiar. Resistance to change may be the basis of sayings such as, "If it's not broken, don't fix it." In some instances, resistance to change occurs because of fear for job security. People may be concerned that the change will eliminate their position or that they will not be able to handle the demands required by the change. A major role of the change agent is to overcome resistance to change.

Most authorities on change agree that change is most easily implemented when it is the result of a collaborative process (the normative–reeducative approach). This means involving everyone who is going to be affected by the change or those referred to as **stakeholders**. All persons involved need a good understanding of the change, why it is necessary, how it is to be accomplished, and what will be the benefits. Suggestions from those affected by the change need to be built into the change model whenever possible. Mutual trust and respect must exist among all persons working with the change.

Display 14-1   Communication Skills for Facilitating Change

- Communicate openly, frequently, and honestly
- Provide as much information as possible
- Allow for questions and suggestions
- Accept feedback constructively
- Address rumors quickly
- Supply facts when perceptions are incorrect
- Listen actively to people's concerns, feelings, and objections
- Remain matter-of-fact and avoid being argumentative or defensive

The Importance of Communication

One of the most valuable tools for facilitating change and overcoming resistance to it is communication. Communication should remain open throughout the entire process. The whys and hows of the change need to be communicated frequently, and regular feedback should be provided. When questions arise, answer them in an honest and straightforward manner. Often during the change process, rumors will begin to circulate. Address these rumors as quickly as possible and supply facts where perceptions are incorrect. Listen to and address the concerns of those affected by the change to the best of your ability. People need the opportunity to express their fears and possible losses they believe will occur when the situation is changed. They need time to grieve those losses. Their feelings need to be accepted, not disputed. Provide opportunity for input and suggestions and implement these when possible. Display 14-1 identifies some of the communication skills to be used in facilitating change.

▪▪ COMMUNICATION IN *ACTION*
▪▪

Resistance to Developing New Processes

Janet Chasey, a unit manager on the medical floor, announced, "Hi folks, thanks for taking the time to come to this staff meeting. I'll be very brief because I know you all have things to do and places to go. The only agenda item is to inform you that a committee is being formed by nursing administration to develop and implement a standardized approach to communication between caregivers when patients are moved from one department to another within the hospital." One nurse responded, "It really isn't fair to ask us to take on a committee when we are already overworked." Another said, "It just sounds like more paperwork to me! We don't need that!" A third spoke up, "I think the forms and taped messages we currently use are more than adequate. Why change what isn't broken?" Janet patiently explained, "There is a new standard set by The Joint Commission. It requires that we have a standardized process to ensure that all information about the patient's condition is shared, including allergies, potential problems, medications, and stability of vital signs." She further explained, "The whole purpose of this is to make patient handoff safer, and I know that is your concern too. Maybe one or two of you might like to be involved in developing the process and help shape the direction it takes." Elsa, who had graduated from her nursing program the previous year spoke up, "I have never been involved in setting up a policy or procedure. It would probably be a good thing to learn. You can put me down for that committee." By respecting their concerns, explaining carefully, and pointing out shared goals, Janet was able to achieve her objective of having a unit member participate.

Assessing the Setting

Before beginning the change process, it is important to have a good understanding of the existing power structure within the setting where the change is to occur. Who within that area gets things done and makes things happen? Where is support typically found? Where—or with whom—can obstacles be anticipated? Are there values one must be sensitive to? Are there factors present that could prevent the change from taking place?

If you are in a position to decide whether to make a change, or when to make that change, consider when the last change occurred in the area. Because change is stressful to individuals, there needs to be downtime between changes. Abrahamson (2004) identifies a condition he calls repetitive-change syndrome, of which change-related chaos is a part. Change-related chaos refers to the continuous state of upheaval that happens when too many changes are trying to be instituted. People lose track of who's doing what and why and may become anxious, cynical, frustrated, and/or burned out. If it is possible, delay making a change if those affected by it have recently experienced other changes.

Thinking and Planning

Successful change is well thought out and planned. A process similar to that which you have used in the application of the nursing process provides good guidance. First of all, once a problem that might benefit from change has been identified, data need to be gathered that will assist with the diagnosis of the problem. Is it a problem? Why is it a problem? Who does it affect? How are they affected? Might there be a better way to approach the situation? What would the costs be in terms of time? What would be the personal cost to those affected? What would be the effects of not addressing the problem? Should we move forward with the change or look for other solutions?

Once a reasonable amount of data have been gathered, begin to plan. Who needs to be involved? Who should be the key players? How might the change best be implemented? When would be the best timing? What resources will be needed? What needs to be done to help those affected to unfreeze? What needs to be built into the plan that will help to ensure that the changes remain in place? What additional training and education will be necessary? Display 14-2 highlights these questions.

Early in this process, those who are going to be affected by the change need to be included. They need to be informed of intentions to make changes and be brought into the collaborative process for planning. Mutual objective setting will help motivate others toward change. Smith (1996) includes, as one of his management principles related to change, ensuring that each person always knows why his or her performance and any change matter to the purpose and results of the whole organization. Providing maximum information is important, as is calming concerns about the personal effects of the change. Those who will be affected need to realize how they can benefit from the change. Positive relationships must be built between the change agent and those experiencing the change.

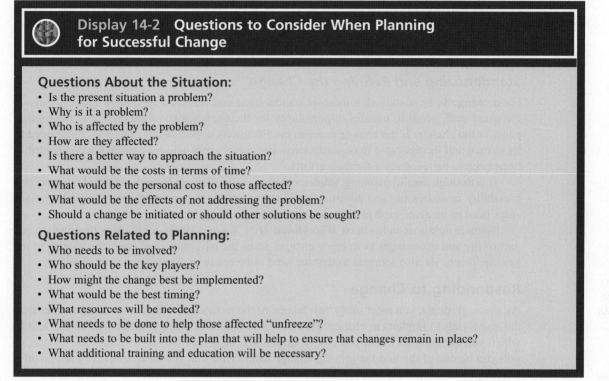

Display 14-2   Questions to Consider When Planning for Successful Change

Questions About the Situation:
- Is the present situation a problem?
- Why is it a problem?
- Who is affected by the problem?
- How are they affected?
- Is there a better way to approach the situation?
- What would be the costs in terms of time?
- What would be the personal cost to those affected?
- What would be the effects of not addressing the problem?
- Should a change be initiated or should other solutions be sought?

Questions Related to Planning:
- Who needs to be involved?
- Who should be the key players?
- How might the change best be implemented?
- What would be the best timing?
- What resources will be needed?
- What needs to be done to help those affected "unfreeze"?
- What needs to be built into the plan that will help to ensure that changes remain in place?
- What additional training and education will be necessary?

Implementing the Change

Once plans are well formulated and people who will be affected have full information as well as a role in the process, the change needs to be implemented. Establishing a timetable is often useful.

Generally it is wise to implement change as quickly as possible. The slower the change process, the greater the opportunity for individuals affected by it to ruminate on how things were, to build up anger, and to develop fears and resentment. Once dates have been announced, it is unwise to change them or to postpone actions, because people will become suspicious and/or critical of the process. If delays are necessary, share the full explanation of the reason(s) for the delay. This is a continuation of the open communication process. Recognize and praise positive efforts toward making a change. Celebrating milestones of accomplishment throughout the entire process can generate team spirit. It helps create feelings of well-being about the change and builds a bond among those who are involved in it.

Evaluating the Change Process

Monitor the change process throughout its implementation and evaluate it after it is completed. This will provide the information that will indicate whether the change is accomplishing the desired outcome. Evaluation provides information about how people are adjusting to the change and how satisfied they are with it—data that are crucial to sustaining the change. When implementing and evaluating change, remember that change does not occur instantly but rather over a period of time. Additionally, the pace of change is not regular. It tends to have periods when it slows down and other periods when there are spurts. The slower periods can be viewed as reflective time, when the individuals involved in the change have the opportunity to assimilate new facts, approaches, values, and other items involved in the change.

Standardizing and Refining the Change

For a change to be sustained, it must be standardized and refined. The change agent, if outside the usual staff, needs to transfer responsibility for the continuance of the project to the participants in the change. If the change requires modifications in policies or protocols, those need to be written and incorporated in organizational manuals. People who have made notable contributions need to be recognized for their efforts.

It is through careful planning, implementation, and follow-up that successful change occurs. Flexibility in addressing and adjusting problems that arise is important. Interpersonal relationships need to be given high priority during this time.

Spencer Johnson, in his book *Who Moved My Cheese?* (1998), reminds us that change is a part of life and encourages us to enjoy change, savor the adventure, and enjoy the aspects of the new approach. He also reminds us that we need to be ready to change again and enjoy it.

Responding to Change

As a new graduate, you most likely will be one of the individuals affected by change rather than the one trying to implement change. How will you react if a change must occur on the unit to which you are assigned? Will you drag your feet and be one of the last to accept the change, or will you be one of the first the join the change team? How can you be an effective participant?

Learn About the Change

Take all available opportunities to learn about any anticipated changes. Attend scheduled meetings and read all announcements that are circulated. If there are matters that seem unclear to you, ask questions at the appropriate time. Learn what the benefits will be for you and for others. Discuss your thoughts and findings with others and share any suggestions you have. Validate any information about which you may not be certain. Rumors often run rampant during the process of change. Be sure you are dealing with facts rather than rumors.

EXAMPLE

Concern for a Job During Restructure

The nurses on 4-South knew that their unit was in serious need of remodeling and updating. Yet, when it was announced that patients would be transferred and the unit would be closed, many became concerned about their positions. Small groups of nurses would gather in corners and ask questions of one another. Nurses discussed it during their coffee breaks. Soon a rumor was circulating that they would all be laid off during the remodel. Several decided to submit their resignations and look for work elsewhere. After receiving three resignations from the same unit within 1 week, the head of the human resources department made an appointment to talk with the surgical supervisor about the resignations. Afterward, the supervisor immediately scheduled a meeting with the unit staff. He explained the plans for the remodel, the time lines, and assured the unit staff that during the remodel process they would all be assigned to other units. He further explained that individual appointments would be made with each employee to determine that person's work preferences.

Express Your Concerns

As you learn about the anticipated changes, you may develop concerns about various aspects. If you have concerns, express them. If you are anxious, there are probably others who share your feelings. The person or persons responsible for leading the change cannot read your mind, so it is critical that you share your apprehensions. Remember that most often those who are closest to a situation are the individuals who understand it best. When setting forth your concerns, think a minute before you speak. Organize your thoughts. Be clear, concise, and unemotional. Speak clearly in a well modulated voice.

Actively Listen

We often are encouraged to actively listen when working with others. Active listening involves focusing entirely on what the other person is saying and refraining from other mental activities (Fig. 14-1). This works well in many situations, including conflict, which we will discuss later in this chapter.

FIGURE 14-1   Active listening means focusing entirely on what the other person is saying and avoiding other mental activities.

The following behaviors are usually included in active listening:

- Always be respectful and courteous
- Use constructive language, both in verbal and nonverbal (eg, body language) communication
- Remain calm and unemotional
- Maintain eye contact
- Do not interrupt
- Be serious but cheerful
- Use nondirective techniques to encourage the person to share concerns
- Ask for clarification as needed to facilitate your understanding

Listen carefully to the responses that are given to your concerns. If you are not clear about what has just been said, ask the other individual to please repeat it. You need to truly listen to the other person's responses, however. Too often people are so busy thinking about what they will say next that they do not hear the explanations that are being provided.

You will find that if you actively participate in the change, it will be much easier to move into the new behaviors it may require. Change can be energizing for some individuals. It often opens the door for new opportunities. It can provide empowerment and enjoyment if managed correctly.

Critical Thinking Activity

You have just learned that a new form of charting is being initiated on your unit. As a new employee, you have just become comfortable with the current system, which was quite different from anything you used as a student. You are dismayed that you will now need to learn a new system. What steps can you take to participate effectively in this change? How can you develop a more positive attitude toward this change? What will facilitate the process for you? What role do you see for yourself in the change process? If you become really frustrated during the change process, to whom will you speak?

MANAGING CONFLICT

We have talked about collaboration and collaborative relationships throughout this textbook. Some would propose that the opposite of collaboration is conflict. Let's now look at how one might deal with conflict.

Certainly conflict is not a new topic to you. You have dealt with it from the time you were a child. It is a part of everyday living. The very nature of conflict is what keeps attorneys, marriage counselors, mediators, and arbitrators in business. Our ability to work positively with conflict may determine our success in today's world. Conflict also occurs in the work environment. The many groups that must function as a whole in health care delivery leave that setting primed for conflict. It is critical that you learn to deal with conflict, because progress stops if it is left unresolved.

Conflict and Nursing

Conflict, broadly defined, results when people with differing values, interests, goals, needs, or approaches come together to address a common concern. Because people view things from different perspectives and bring different values to the situation, incompatible ideas, approaches, or resolutions can occur. The settling of a conflict is known as **conflict resolution**. The process through which the conflict is recognized and resolved is called **conflict management**. The critical element is not that conflicts come about—but how we deal with them.

In Chapter 13, we discussed the conflict that can occur between physicians and nurses. As nurses command a more independent role in patient care, become involved in evidence-based practice, and accept responsibility and accountability for their actions, they may feel devalued if their suggestions for care are not acted upon, thus leading to anger and a breakdown of communications.

In Chapter 11, we discussed collective bargaining, a major area in which there can be discord. This can occur nurse to nurse and nurse to administration. Unfortunately, conflicts at the bargaining table may spill over into conflicts in the workplace.

As nurses exercise professional judgment, differences of opinion may arise regarding the best approach to treatment for a client. There may be disagreements about staffing patterns, particularly during the holidays. Overlapping roles can result in conflict, and not having sufficient resources, either monetary or physical, can cause discord. Often the utilization of space in the health care environment leads to conflict.

These represent just a few of the many situations in nursing in which disagreements can happen. Conflict leads to stress and the disruption of professional relationships. As you will see in Chapter 15, the consequence of all this can be burnout.

Phyllis Kritek (2001), author of *Negotiating at an Uneven Table*, reflects on nurses and conflict, noting that conflict is pervasive in nursing, endemic and integral to the role. She questions why this is so and asks whether it is because most "nurses are women, or because they are socialized to be conflict-aversive, or essentially conservative, or primarily healers, or inherently nurturant" (p. 474). Regardless of the answer, all nurses must be skillful in dealing with conflict (Fig. 14-2).

The Positive Side of Conflict

Note that conflict can have positive aspects; not all conflict is serious, ominous, or intimidating. Conflict can result in personal growth and development. We learn by contrasting our values and beliefs with those of others. As we learn about others, we learn about ourselves.

Conflict can provide the impetus for change. It can contribute to innovation and creativity. When conflict is a major part of any operation, reasons for its presence must be sought and alternatives set forth. Thus, new approaches are tried. For example, conflict over the use of completing morning baths during busy and rushed morning hours could result in a more flexible bathing routine for patients that schedules some baths for the evening.

Conflict also helps employees of an organization to have a better understanding of one another's jobs and responsibilities. As health care becomes more specialized, differences become greater and give rise to conflict. Conflict may result in people from different areas sitting down and talking to resolve the problem (Fig. 14-3). As talk continues, a greater appreciation for others can develop, thus creating unification within the organization.

Conflict can also open new channels of communication. As efforts are made to eliminate sources of conflict, new approaches and avenues may evolve. Similarly, conflict can be a positive source of energy and creativity (Fig. 14-4). It may serve to invigorate people. A good disagreement has the potential to sharpen people's awareness, to get them thinking, and to put new spark into their work.

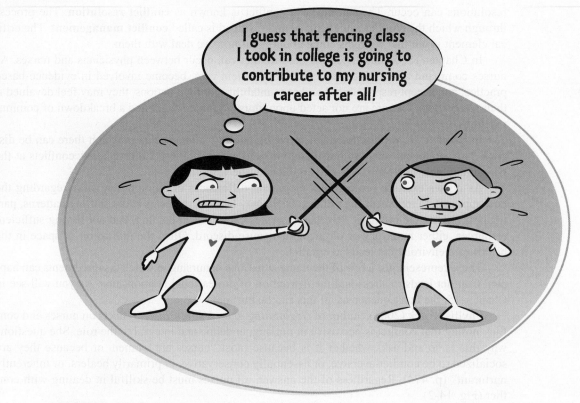

FIGURE 14-2   All nurses should be skillful in dealing with conflict.

Types of Conflict

Conflict can be looked at from a number of perspectives and broken into several categories. Your approach to dealing with the conflict may vary depending on the type of conflict that exists.

Intrapersonal, Interpersonal, and Intergroup Conflict

Intrapersonal conflict occurs within one's self in circumstances in which a choice must be made between two alternatives. Choosing one alternative means that you cannot have the other. An example would be a situation in which the nurse must decide whether to participate in a committee on nursing practice that will take time away from direct patient care or decline the opportunity in order to spend more time with patients. Either choice carries benefits and drawbacks. The conflict that occurs is within the nurse who must decide, which is more important personally.

Interpersonal conflict occurs between or among individuals. This is where differences in values, ideas, perceptions, and goals play an important role. If one nurse believes that the most important aspect of care is that every patient has a complete bath every day, and another nurse believes that having all patients ambulate is more critical and there is not time for both, an interpersonal conflict results. The basis of the conflict is the difference in what each perceives as the first priority in nursing care. Ethical issues such as abortion, gene therapy, stem cell research, do-not-resuscitate orders, and decisions to withdraw or withhold treatment can result in conflict

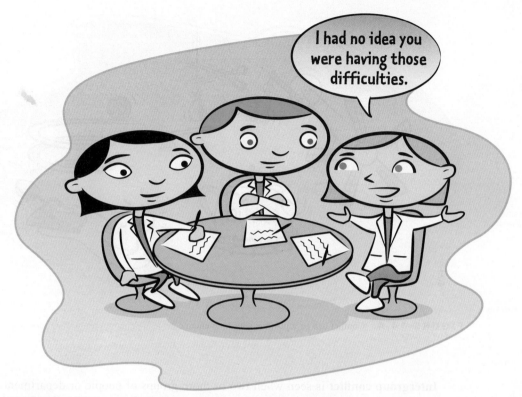

FIGURE 14-3 When people from different areas sit down to talk to resolve a problem, they often gain a greater appreciation for one another.

among those responsible for delivery of care. Different leadership styles and organizational climates can also result in interpersonal conflict.

EXAMPLE

Too Many Managers
The unit manager on 5-South decided to accept a higher position in the organization. He was replaced by an interim manager. Within a month, a permanent new manager was hired to provide leadership to the staff on the unit. However, within a short period of time, nursing staff members on the unit had worked with three different managers, each with a different management style and different expectations. This resulted in unrest and increased conflict among members of the staff. These confrontations, disagreements, and episodes of anger gave evidence of the stress created by the changes.

Critical Thinking Activity

Think of an interpersonal conflict that you recently observed or in which you were involved. What was the basis of the disagreement? How did the individuals conduct themselves during the heat of the conflict? How were the issues resolved? How might the conflict have been avoided?

FIGURE 14-4   Conflict can be a positive source of energy.

Intergroup conflict is seen when two or more groups of people or departments struggle for power, authority, territory, or resources. Each group tends to perceive the situation only as it affects that group. Each group acknowledges only its own value and positive aspects, attributing negative aspects to the other group. Negative stereotypes form, hostility develops, and communication deteriorates. This can be especially true if the group includes racial minorities who feel discriminated against. Intergroup conflicts can occur between those who work on different shifts of a nursing unit—the evening shift personnel critical of the day shift and the day shift people believing that their job is harder than that of the evening shift. Intergroup conflicts might also occur between the nursing staff and the housekeeping staff over setting priorities for cleaning rooms and preparing them for new admissions. The housekeeping staff members may have a set of priorities based on how personnel are distributed, while the nursing staff members may want the priorities to change and flex based on their perceptions of patient needs. Intergroup conflicts can increase in both number and perception when those in one group spend time recounting to others within their group all the perceived inadequacies of the other group. As they do this, they may gather additional anecdotes to support their own perceptions. Thus, the conflict is maintained and spread.

Organizational Conflict

Some conflicts originate within the structure and function of an organization. Typically, the policies, procedures, channels of communication, and style of management, and similar factors related to organizational operations generate them. These are termed **organizational conflicts**. In organizational conflict, the leader's role and behavior are particularly important to both the origin of the conflict and to the resolution of issues.

Role ambiguity and role conflict are major causes of organizational conflict. **Role ambiguity** refers to a situation in which the role is not clearly defined. **Role conflict** occurs when two or more individuals have role descriptions that overlap. This frequently occurs because of the lack of good job descriptions and clear communications regarding what is expected. An example of role conflict could be seen in the provision of discharge planning. Both the registered nurse and the social worker clearly may view this as an important aspect of their professional responsibilities, and the job descriptions of both may include this aspect of patient care.

The structure of the organization may also lead to conflict. The term "turf" refers to the territory that one or one's group controls. Turf battles are not uncommon in organizations, with various individuals within the system attempting to protect, expand, or advance the area for which they are responsible. Again, good job descriptions, organizational charts, chains of command, channels of communication, and the like will minimize the advent of this type of problem (see Chapter 11).

Conflict within an organization also can arise when a scarcity of resources exists. Dove (1998) refers to this as conflict of interest. Scarcity of resources refers not only to money but also to supplies, equipment, space, personnel, and similar necessities. When the budget for the organization is developed, not all requests are likely to be funded. Competition occurs as various departments vie for the resources that are available. As nursing moves into one of the greatest shortages experienced in recent years, conflicts related to securing and retaining adequate nurse staffing can be anticipated.

Conflict Outcomes

Filley (1975) identified three positions or outcomes of conflict that have become so well known that they are often included in our everyday language.

One type of outcome addressed by Filley (1975) is the **lose-lose outcome**, in which there are no winners. The resolution of the conflict is such that it is unsatisfactory to both parties. An example can be seen in collective bargaining relationships that stalemate and go to arbitration. The arbitrator in the case may make decisions that neither side finds totally acceptable (see Chapter 11 for more discussion of collective bargaining).

A second type of outcome is referred to as **win-lose outcomes**, in which one person obtains desired goals in the situation and the other individual fails to receive what is desired. Certainly the most obvious example of this would be elections for public office, in which decisions are made by majority rule with only one winner possible. An example in a hospital environment might be one unit receiving all the money available for new equipment, while the other areas receive none. Although this may have been the most prudent approach if the budget for new equipment was very small and dividing it would have meant that no department actually could get what it really needed, it remains an example of a win-lose situation.

The last and most desirable type of outcome is the **win-win outcome**. In such situations, both parties walk away from the conflict feeling they have achieved most of the things that were important to them. For example, if we are working on a project and everyone feels good about it when it is done and each individual reaps some rewards, it is a win-win situation for all.

Strategies for Coping with Conflict

The approach that you use to deal with conflict will depend on a number of factors. The investment you have in the situation will be one major consideration—there is an old adage that advises us to pick our battles carefully. This suggests that not all differences or conflicts are worth the effort of resolving them. The nature of the conflict, the individuals that are involved, your ability to influence the outcome, and the possibility of retribution are all elements that will affect the situation. Thus, a wide variety of approaches to the management of conflict exist. They tend to fall into one of five categories.

Withdrawing From or Avoiding Conflict

You employ the strategy of avoiding or withdrawing from the conflict when you choose not to address the issue at hand. Some would also refer to this as denying the existence of the conflict, sometimes with the hope that if it is ignored it will go away. There are many times when this approach is appropriate. This includes situations in which the conflict clearly is not your problem, when there is little or nothing that you can do about it, when there is more to lose than to be gained by becoming involved, when you lack sufficient information about the conflict and its cause, or when the problem will straighten itself out if given time. It is also a good approach to use if the situation is volatile and individuals need some time to regain composure. For example, one of two staff nurses who are becoming distressed about an issue might say, "You may be right, let's find a time to talk about it later." The issue may never be discussed later, or the parties involved in the disagreement may gain new understandings that change their perspectives.

Although appropriate at times, avoiding conflict is often preferred by people who are very uncomfortable with conflict situations, and it may not be the best approach. In a competitive society, individuals who will back away from a conflict can be taken advantage of. It is important to learn to advocate for yourself as well as for your clients. An example might be a situation in which both you and another nurse want to be off-duty Halloween evening so that you can participate in your children's trick-or-treat activities. Although the other nurse enjoyed that evening off last year, you again concede to her request because you do not want to deal with her comments and criticisms if you are awarded the evening off.

Smoothing or Accommodating

Smoothing or accommodating conflict involves trying to relieve feelings associated with conflict without solving the underlying problem. It may involve apologizing for something that is not one's fault, stating agreement with a position with which one does not truly agree, or taking action that one does not really support to stop the feelings of conflict from occurring. Similar to avoidance of the issue, smoothing or accommodating may also be referred to as surrendering to the conflict. In such situations, it is easier not to address the issue and to deal with feelings of anger than it is to deal with the conflict.

We see this approach used by individuals with a strong need to be liked, or those who are overly concerned with the welfare of others. They tend to take the martyr or self-sacrificing approach that will result in a peaceful environment. An individual who wishes to preserve harmony or build up social credits may employ this technique.

There are times when smoothing or accommodating is appropriate. It may be the best approach if the conflict and anger that accompanies it disrupts the work situation or interferes with the immediate needs of the patients. In such situations, harmony and constancy are important. If the outcome does not matter to you, or if you obviously are wrong, this is a good approach. If you have little chance to win, or if this represents a situation in which you can lose the battle but win the war, it is appropriate.

Forcing the Issue or Competing

Competing or forcing the issue in a conflict situation means you are working exclusively for your own solution to the problem. You may have taken this approach because you believe you know more about the issues involved than others or when your values will allow no other compromise. Typically individuals who use this approach are accustomed to being the winner and often fail to consider the needs and opinions of others. Thus, it can prevent good problem solving and innovative approaches. This would be considered a win-lose outcome—one person wins, others lose. It is an aggressive approach that could result in retaliation at another time. However, it might be the best approach if you observe a violation of ethical or legal standards.

Negotiating and Compromising

Compromising and negotiating involve give and take; one factor is balanced against another. It is the approach to the conflict seen in collective bargaining—one factor in the situation is balanced against another. It serves to minimize the losses for all parties while allowing each to realize some gains. It may be the approach of choice if the opposing goals are so incompatible that no resolution can be reached and discussion has stalled. It also would be appropriate if an immediate settlement to the issue were needed because of time constraints or other factors.

Problem Solving and Collaborating

Although problem solving or collaborating to achieve a mutually agreed-upon plan of action may be the most difficult to achieve, many believe this to be the best approach to conflict. It encourages participants in the conflict to work toward common goals and to work toward consensus. The process can be time-consuming and requires that all persons involved come to the table willing to examine and discuss issues openly and honestly. If effective in resolving the conflict, it is viewed as a win-win situation for everyone.

Personal Preparation for Conflict

If you find yourself in a conflict situation, try to be as prepared as possible to deal with the conditions at hand. This is often hard to do at the time the conflict occurs.

One of the best techniques is to practice for the situation. Rehearse what you will say. Think about the tone of your voice, the speed with which to talk, and your body language. Think positively about yourself. Be confident. Visualize what a successful interaction would be like.

When engaged in the confrontation, do not interrupt others. Give them an opportunity to express their position. When they talk, practice the good listening skills discussed earlier in this chapter. Insist that you are given the same courtesy of uninterrupted explanation. Politely saying, "Please let me finish" usually ensures that you can continue presenting your position.

Be clear and concise in presenting your point of view. Long, complicated presentations lose everyone's interest. Be assertive but considerate of others.

If you find that you are involved in conflict situations more frequently than most other individuals, a personal inventory is appropriate. Questions you should ask yourself might include the following:

- Do I have good relationships with most of my coworkers?
- How do I manage stress in other situations?
- Do I have the proper balance between work and relaxation?

- Do I feel competent in this situation?
- Do I hold personal biases that are interfering with my interactions with others?
- What else is going on in my life?

If after completing this inventory you find there are areas that give you concern, then they can be addressed in an appropriate manner. Clearly, if you are experiencing high levels of stress in any area of life, you may find yourself more easily in conflict with others and less able to manage that conflict effectively. Therefore, if there is a lack of opportunity for relaxation in your life, you can adjust your schedule so that you maximize the time you spend on things that result in leisure and rest. If you feel less than competent regarding the expectations of the job you do, some continuing education, reading, or research may be helpful. Seeking and working with a mentor may also bring positive results. If relationships with other coworkers or in your private life are lacking, seeking the help of a qualified counselor may be the best approach.

Key Concepts

- Change is inevitable in today's health care environment. Individuals tend to resist change, and leaders must become familiar with the steps that will facilitate the change process.
- A number of theories of change have been developed. Many of them describe processes to facilitate change, including helping others see the need for change, involving those who will be affected by the change in the process, and stabilizing the change once it is in place.
- Three major strategies for change include the empirical–rational strategy, the power–coercive strategy, and the normative–reeducative strategy. Each one might be the appropriate strategy to use in a particular situation.
- Changes that occur most often are led by a change agent who may come from within the organization or might be hired from outside to assist with the change. Sometimes groups or teams can serve as change agents.
- A number of activities facilitate change. Good communications is primary. In addition the environment where change is to occur should be assessed, thinking and planning need to occur, the change is then implemented, and the process evaluated. Finally the change must be standardized and refined in order for it to persist.
- You will experience change as a new employee. You can make the process more positive by learning all that you can about the anticipated changes, understanding the benefits, asking appropriate questions of the right individuals, and expressing any concerns you may have respectfully and to the right people.
- Conflict occurs in all aspects of our lives. Conflict can be intrapersonal, interpersonal, intergroup, or organizational.
- Filley (1975) has identified three possible outcomes of conflict: the lose-lose outcome, in which both parties leave the situation feeling defeated; the win-lose outcome, in which one party wins and the other loses; and the win-win outcome, in which both parties have positive feelings about the end results.
- Strategies for dealing with conflict include withdrawing or avoiding the conflict; smoothing, suppressing or accommodating to the conflict; forcing, fighting, or

competing; negotiating or compromising; and problem solving or collaborating. There is a proper time and circumstance for the use of each strategy.

- Conflict can have positive aspects. It can provide an impetus for change, it can energize individuals, it can help persons in different roles understand one another better, and it can facilitate communication.

- If you find yourself in conflict more than is desirable, a self-inventory can be helpful. Asking yourself a variety of questions may help identify the actions you will want to take.

Relevant Web Sites

Change:

Kurt Lewin Institute homepage:

  www.psy.vu.nl/fpp.php/research/psychology/kurt_lewin_institute/

The Learning Organizations: *http://leeds-faculty.colorado.edu/larsenk/learnorg.html*

Massachusetts Institute of Technology: *http://web.mit.edu/hr/oed/learn/change*

Maurer & Associates Consulting Firm: *www.beyondresistance.com/htm/9resource.html*

Nickols, Fred. Distance Consulting: *http://home.att.net/~nickols/change.htm*

Performance Management Company: *www.squarewheels.com*

Conflict:

Bacal & Associates Consulting: *http://conflict911.com/guestconflict/resolveconflict.htm*

Center for Effective Leadership:

  www.ccl.org/leadership/enewsletter/2005/APRissue.aspx?pageId=583

Conservation Technology Information Center:

  www.2.ctic.purdue.edu/KYW/Brochures/ManageConflict.html

University of Colorado Conflict Research Consortium: *http://conflict.colorado.edu*

References

Abrahamson, E. (2004). *Change without pain*. Boston: Harvard Business School Publishing.

Asprec, E. (1975). The process of change. *Supervisor Nurse, 6,* 15–24.

Benne, K. D., Bennis, G., & Chin, R. (1976). Planned change in America. In W. G. Bennis, K. D. Benne, R. Chin, & K. E. Corey (Eds.), *The planning of change*. New York: Holt, Rinehart and Winston.

Buchanan, D., & Badham, R. (1999). Politics and organizational change: The lived experience. *Human Relations, 52*(5), 609–629.

Carr, D. K., Hard, K. J., & Trahant, W. J. (1996). *Managing the change process*. New York: McGraw Hill.

Dove, M. A. (1998). Conflict: process and resolution. *Nursing Management, 29*(4), 30–32.

Filley, A. (1975). *Interpersonal Conflict Resolution*. Glenview, IL: Scott, Foresman.

Johnson, S. (1998). *Who moved my cheese?* New York: G. P. Putnam's Sons.

Kritek, P. B. (2001). Some reflections on conflict resolution in nursing: The implications of negotiating at an uneven table. In

J. M. Dochterman & H. K. Grace, *Current issues in nursing* (6th ed.) (pp. 473–478). St. Louis, MO: Mosby.

Lewin, K. (1951). *Field theory in social service: Selected theoretical papers*. New York: Harper Brothers.

Lippitt, R., Watson, J., & Westley, B. (1958). *The dynamics of planned change*. New York: Harcourt, Brace & World.

Perlman, D., & Takacs, G. J. (1990). The ten stages of change. *Nursing management, 212*(4), 33–38.

Quinn, R. E., Spreitzer, G. M., & Brown, M. V. (June 2000). Changing others through changing ourselves. *Journal of Management Inquiry, 9*(2), 147–165.

Rogers, E., & Shoemaker, F. (1971). *Communication of innovations: A cross cultural approach*. New York: Free Press.

Senge, P. M. (1990). *The fifth discipline: The art and practice of the learning organization*. New York: Doubleday.

Smith, D. K. (1996). *Taking charge of change: Ten principles for managing people and performance*. Menlo Park: Addison-Wesley.

Thomas, J. M., & Bennis, W. G. (1972). *The management of change and conflict*. Baltimore: Penguin.

U N I T   V

Career Opportunities and Professional Growth

As you approach graduation from your nursing program you will be thinking about employment opportunities. The final unit in this textbook is devoted to topics designed to assist you to move into the world of employment as a registered nurse.

Chapter 15 focuses on your beginning job search. Information is provided about the competencies needed for the wide variety of opportunities available to nurses today. The various career opportunities in nursing are outlined as well as the expectations of employers. Then there are helpful strategies in seeking that special first job. Information about writing résumés, composing letters of application, and composing letters following up on interviews are included. Interviewing strategies, including dress, deportment, and your role in the process are emphasized. The goal is to support you in attaining your desired career start.

Once in the workplace, managing the stresses this environment generates is important. Chapter 16 discusses reality shock and burnout and provides strategies to help you deal with these phenomena. In addition, exploration of topics addressing workplace safety and coping with the realities of the work world, including workplace violence, discrimination, and harassment, will assist you to function effectively as a registered nurse in the work environment.

Making Professional Goals a Reality

LEARNING OUTCOMES

After completing this chapter, you should be able to:

1. Describe a variety of employment opportunities available to nurses today and the educational requirements of each.
2. Explain the competencies needed by the new graduate as outlined by the job analysis study that is the basis for the National Council Licensure Examination (NCLEX).
3. Analyze the eight common expectations employers have of new graduates

and relate them to your own background and education.
4. Develop a list of your personal short- and long-term career goals.
5. Develop a personal résumé and sample letters of application, follow-up, and resignation.
6. Describe aspects to consider when preparing for an interview.
7. Formulate possible responses to an employment interview.

KEY TERMS

Competency	Long-term goals	Proficiency
Cover letter	Short-term goals	Résumé
Criticality		

When you graduate, one of your first goals will be obtaining employment as a registered nurse (RN). You probably look forward to practicing in the nursing role you have spent so long attaining. You may even envision the perfect nursing position and have thought no further ahead than this first job. For other new graduates, the desire for a job is initially general, rather than specific, in view of student loans to be repaid and the desire to move into a lifestyle different from that of the student.

Unlike graduates of the hospital programs of the past, you will have spent fewer hours working in the patient care setting. Although some new graduates have worked as unlicensed assistive staff or practical (vocational) nurses during their education, for others' contact with health care settings may have been as students rather than as employees. You may not have experienced all of the many settings in which RNs are employed. You may have questions regarding employer expectations and your own role as an RN.

In the past, the expectations of most new graduates were simple, but a nursing career is now much more complex. In this chapter, we try to assist you as you survey the RN job market and plan for a successful approach to obtaining that important first position.

EMPLOYMENT OPPORTUNITIES TODAY

The nursing shortage (discussed in Chapter 6) has resulted in unfilled nursing positions in many health care agencies. Thus, as a new graduate, you will find yourself in high demand as an employee. However, know that high demand does not mean that you have unlimited choices. In many institutions, current employees are given the choice of moving into vacant positions before a new employee is sought for that position. And remember that hospitals operate 24 hours a day, 7 days a week. Often new graduates are offered positions on less preferred shifts. Further, not all positions are suitable for entry-level nurses because many demand greater expertise or specialized education. For example, the travel nurse who moves from facility to facility needs experience in one system as a solid foundation for moving easily into new settings. Thus, you may find it most productive to consider a range of positions you would like or to examine whether your most desired position would best be obtained by starting in a different position and moving to the desired position after becoming more experienced.

Most new graduates choose to begin their careers in structured health care settings that offer support for the novice in making the adjustment to the RN role. According to a U.S. study, approximately 65% of all RNs are employed in acute care hospitals ("Projected supply, demand, and shortages of registered nurses: 2000–2020," 2002). According to a National Council of State Boards of Nursing study (NCSBN, 2002), this percentage is higher for newly graduated RNs. This may result from the fact that many of the noninstitutional positions require expertise and independent functioning. It also may be that new graduates seek these positions for the orientations and mentoring available.

In its trend studies, initiated in January 1998, the NCSBN identified changes over time in the work environments, employment characteristics, and job activities of newly licensed nurses. The most recent publication includes the data from the 2002 survey (NCSBN, 2002). According to the study, the majority of newly licensed nurses work in hospitals. Very few reported working in community-based facilities and long-term care. Of those responding, 39.8% worked in medical/surgical and 30.9% in critical care settings. Only 10.5% worked in nursing homes, and an even smaller percentage—6.2%—reported working in pediatrics. This shows an increase in those employed in critical care and nursing homes and a decrease in those employed in pediatrics compared to the 1999 study. When reporting the types of clients for whom they care, newly licensed nurses most frequently identified acutely ill clients, clients with stable chronic conditions, clients with unstable chronic conditions, and clients at end-of-life who were between the ages of 31 to 64 years. Of those working a regular shift, 38.6% reported working day shift and 38% evening shift, leaving 23.4% on the night shift. Rotating shifts are less common, with 10.6% reporting that they work rotating shifts.

The growth of autonomy for the RN has been even more marked outside the hospital setting than in it. Community health nurses have always operated much more independently than hospital nurses. Many positions in the community require a baccalaureate degree or specialized educational programs. Although these settings once required that new graduates have experience in a structured setting before beginning practice in such an independent setting, the shortage has caused some employers to begin recruiting new graduates. New graduates in these settings need to be assertive in obtaining the necessary support to make the transition into the role.

The number of positions for RNs in many settings other than those involved in providing direct client care also has grown. Health care–oriented businesses, such as insurance companies and medical equipment supply companies, have found that it is often easier to teach nurses about business than to teach business people about health care. As a result, nurses are being employed in what some individuals see as non-nursing positions. Others argue that these, too, should be considered nursing positions, because the expertise that makes the individual successful is nursing expertise. Although experienced nurses usually hold these positions, moving into such positions may be a part of a career plan of the new graduate.

The number of men in nursing, which remained relatively small for many years, is beginning to grow as society reassesses its attitude toward labeling jobs as women's or men's work. In 2004 the number of men in nursing was estimated at 5.7%—up from 5.4% in 2000 (U.S. Bureau of Health Professions, 2004). This same survey showed that more men begin their education in associate degree nursing (ADN) programs than in other types of programs. Men have been attracted by the career opportunities and improving the economic picture of nursing.

The economic position of the nurse has improved for several reasons. One reason is the extension of laws governing fair labor practices to nonprofit institutions and the advent of collective bargaining (see Chapter 11). Another major reason is the nursing shortage that occurred the 1980s. The demand for nurses rose faster than the supply, and employers began increasing salaries and benefits to attract nurses. This trend was especially notable in urban communities.

Although wages have increased substantially since the 1980s, the 2002 survey of RNs concluded that inflation accounts for most of the increase. Real wages in terms of purchasing power have risen only slightly (Spratley, Johnson, Sochalski, Fritz, & Spencer, 2002). Nurses have expressed concern that high wages quoted in some settings often reflect large amounts of overtime pay, and thus increased stress on the job.

All these factors bring you, as a new graduate, into a world of uncertainty, but one also filled with opportunity and promise. The nursing shortage is acute. Now you must determine your place in this world. We encourage you to look forward to the positive contribution that you can make to patients and to nursing practice.

Critical Thinking Activity

Obtain the Sunday classified advertising section of a local newspaper. Count the advertisements for RNs. How many employers are represented? Think of the health care agencies in the community. Does this represent most of them, some of them, or only a few of the potential employers of nurses? Of those listed, how many specify background or experience beyond that which a new graduate would have? How many specify the shift or work schedule? If wages are noted, what is the range of wages quoted? Reflect on your own expectations for employment after graduation. How do your expectations compare with what you find in these advertisements?

COMPETENCIES OF THE NEW GRADUATE

Recently you may have heard the term **competency** used a great deal, especially as it applied to you as a student. Competency, as used here, refers to the ability of the person to effectively and safely perform specified nursing skills, including the application of critical thinking skills. Some have differentiated competency, which is an entry-level expectation, and **proficiency**, which is expected of the experienced nurse (Fig. 15-1).

Competencies Identified by Nursing Organizations

A number of nursing organizations have developed statements regarding the competencies expected of the new graduate. Chief among these organizations is the NCSBN.

National Council of State Boards of Nursing Competencies

The most definitive statements on the competencies needed by the newly licensed practical nurse (PN) and the RN have been developed by the NCSBN based on its job analysis studies, which serve as the basis for the NCLEX-RN and NCLEX-PN.

In these studies, activities reported by a stratified random sample of newly licensed, entry-level nurses were examined. Both the frequency of the nursing activities and their criticality were studied. **Criticality** refers to activities that cannot be delayed or omitted without creating a "substantial risk of unnecessary complications, impairment of function, or serious distress to clients" (NCSBN, 2002). The last published RN study was completed in 2002; the results of that study supported the continuation of the current test plan and passing score (NCSBN, 2002). The most recent PN study was completed in 2003 (NCSBN, 2003).

DON'T WORRY, I KNOW EXACTLY WHAT I'M DOING! ...I THINK!

FIGURE 15-1 New graduates are expected to know both their own abilities and when to seek appropriate help.

Activities expected of newly licensed RNs that led the list for criticality included the following:

- Use appropriate infection-control measures
- Report significant changes in the client's condition
- Perform cardiopulmonary resuscitation
- Perform the Heimlich maneuver/abdominal thrust
- Provide emergency care for a wound disruption
- Recognize the occurrence of hemorrhage
- Manage a medical emergency until a physician arrives
- Implement measures to prevent circulatory complications (eg, embolus, shock, hemorrhage)
- Respond to symptoms of fetal distress

Activities were studied further in terms of the frequency with which they were expected of newly licensed RNs. In all settings, nurses were expected to perform these duties:

- Coordinate care through working with others on the health care team and supervising delivery of care by assistive personnel
- Preserve the quality of care through such activities as advocating for needed changes in care, documenting errors or problems, and intervening in situations involving unsafe or inadequate care
- Maintain the safety of the client as exemplified by verifying, identifying, and reporting unsafe equipment, and following infection-control guidelines
- Prepare clients and families for care that is to be done, including procedures and treatments, and help them to understand expected outcomes
- Carry out procedures in a safe, effective manner

Physiologic and psychosocial integrity were supported by many individual nursing actions. Some, such as assessing vital signs, seemed almost universal. Others, such as monitoring for side effects of radiation therapy, were needed in a minority of settings. Allowing clients to talk about their concerns and assisting them to communicate effectively were almost universal activities.

Nursing process continues to be a strong expectation for RNs. In the 2002 study, newly licensed RNs indicated that they spent 19% of their time on assessment and evaluation activities. Other activities that were a large part of their roles included managing medications, working with the health care team, and performing administrative duties. They spent 16% of their time in medication-related activities. Working within the health care team involved 14% of their time. While only 10% reported having a primarily administrative position (these were largely in long-term care), 29.9% of the respondents reported having some administrative responsibilities (Smith & Crawford, 2003).

National League for Nursing Competencies

In addition to the NCSBN, other organizations have explored the issue of competencies of new nursing graduates. The various educational councils that were previously a part of the National League for Nursing (NLN) structure developed statements regarding competencies of new graduates. In 1978, the Council of Baccalaureate and Higher Degree programs of the NLN published a statement of the *Characteristics of Baccalaureate Education in Nursing*, which included competencies of the graduate (NLN, 1978). These were later revised in 1986 and published in 1987 (NLN, 1987). The first set of outcomes of competencies for the associate degree graduate were described in a 1978 document prepared by the Council of Associate Degree Programs (CADP) of the NLN (NLN, 1978). In 1990, the CADP approved a revised set of competencies for the associate degree graduate. This clarification of the role of the associate degree graduate as provider of care, manager of care, and member of the profession continues to guide the development of many ADN curricula (NLN, 1990). In 1999, the CADP appointed a Task Force on Educational Outcomes of ADN Programs. This task force identified a list of areas of competency. These included professional behavior, communication, assessment, clinical decision making, caring interventions, teaching and learning, collaboration, and managing care (NLN Council of Associate Degree Programs Task Force on Educational Outcomes of ADN Programs, 1999). These competencies have never received the attention garnered by the 1990 document, perhaps because people had adapted to the three roles spelled out in the earlier publication and found them to be useful.

Competencies Expressed by Other Groups

The American Association of Colleges of Nursing developed a document titled *Essentials of Baccalaureate Education for Professional Nursing* (1998), which includes expected competencies. Additionally, some states have developed statements of competencies for graduates of the nursing programs in those states. This often has been part of a process to improve articulation between programs at different levels.

Similarities and patterns have emerged from all of these statements. The outline of theoretic knowledge and functioning regarding the nursing process seems to be the most consistent. The most divergent opinions seem to be in the area of specific skill or task competency.

Employers' Expectations Regarding Competencies

Employers often ask for further clarification of competence. Have these graduates only the necessary theoretic knowledge of the skill? Have they actually performed the skill? If so, was it in a practice laboratory only, or was it in a client care situation? Does competence mean that the new graduate can function independently, or will some supervision still be needed?

Further complicating the picture is the confusion surrounding competencies of the graduates of the three types of nursing education programs that prepare individuals for RN licensure: the hospital-based diploma program, the ADN program, and the baccalaureate degree program. Although statements by several organizations have distinguished among levels of functioning, many employers do not differentiate expectations. Some employers state that new graduates from different types of programs have not clearly demonstrated differences in competencies. This has created confusion in the minds of nurses, employers, and the public over the role of the RN prepared in each type of educational program.

What is expected of the new graduate varies across health care agencies and geographic areas. Expectations are affected by factors in the community, such as whether there are nursing programs in that community and whether new graduates come from one or from many different schools. The acuity of the client care load and the types of services offered by an agency also may affect expectations. The Joint Commission has a criterion requiring that accredited institutions monitor and ensure the competence of their staff. This requires that an institution identify expected competencies for staff and then design an assessment method. As institutions move to comply with this standard, most direct their initial efforts toward technical skills because these are more easily identified and assessed. Other competencies will be more difficult to assess.

Based on the NCSBN job analysis studies, some general patterns of expectations can be seen:

1. **Possess the necessary theoretic background for safe client care and for decision-making.** For example, the new graduate should understand the signs and symptoms of an insulin reaction, recognize the reaction when it occurs, and know what nursing actions to take. The new graduate must know when an emergency or complication occurs and secure medical help for the client. Many employers believe that new graduates today are very competent in their theoretic foundations for practice.

2. **Use the nursing process in a systematic way.** This includes assessment, analysis, planning, intervention, and evaluation. As noted previously, a large percentage of the new graduates' time is spent in activities they would describe as using the steps of the nursing process. New graduates should be able to develop plans of care and follow plans, such as care pathways, that have been developed by the agency.

3. **Recognize own abilities and limitations.** To provide safe care, the nurse must identify when a situation requires greater expertise or knowledge and when assistance is needed. Employers may be able to assist if nurses ask for help and direction, but cannot accept the risk to clients created by nurses who do not know or accept their own limitations.

4. **Use communication skills effectively with clients and coworkers.** In every setting, there are clients and families who are anxious, depressed, suffering loss, angry, or experiencing other emotional distress. The nurse is expected to respond appropriately to these individuals and to facilitate their coping and adaptation. Effective communication skills are essential to the functioning of the entire interdisciplinary health care team. Often, the nurse is expected to help coordinate the work of others, and this cannot be done without effective communication skills.

5. **Work effectively with assistive personnel, delegating and supervising nursing care tasks in an appropriate manner.** In most settings, assistive personnel are a part of the nursing team. The RN, and in some instances the PN, is expected to identify which nursing activities can be delegated and do so in a way that contributes to appropriate patient care outcomes.

6. **Understand the importance of accurate and complete documentation.** Employers generally recognize that the new graduate must be given time to learn the documentation system used in the facility. However, the new graduate is expected to recognize the need for recording data. It is anticipated that the nurse will keep accurate, grammatically correct, and legible records that provide the necessary legal documentation of care.

7. **Possess proficiency in the basic technical nursing skills.** This is an area in which a wide variety of expectations may be present. In most settings, proficiency in the basic skills required to support activities of daily living is expected. These skills include transferring, giving baths, and performing general hygienic measures. In some settings, nurses will carry out these tasks, whereas in others they will direct or teach others, such as nursing assistants or family members, to do them. In either case, proficiency is essential to evaluating the care provided. The technical skills or tasks that are reserved for the RN represent the area of widest diversity in the identification of essential skills.

The settings in which nurses practice are wide-ranging, and technical skills may be needed in one setting but not in another. Some facilities provide extensive orientation programs in which every skill is checked before the new graduate is allowed to proceed independently. Other employers expect the new graduate to perform the skill if able, and be checked off as required, or to ask for help if unable to function independently. Often, employers are flexible in their expectations, so that it may be acceptable if an individual seems to have competency in a reasonable percentage of the skills required by that agency. Further development of skill competency will be supported by the institution. Other employers have a list of skills in which competency is mandatory at the time of hire, although speed may not be expected. Also, there may be a difference between what the employer would wish and what the employer will accept.

In addition to these professional responsibilities performed as a nurse, employers also speak of their concern for worker-related competencies they want to see in all health care workers. These include the following:

1. **Understand and have a commitment to a work ethic.** This means that the employee will take the responsibility of the job seriously and will be on time, take only the allowed coffee and lunch breaks, and will not take sick days unless truly ill. It also means that the new graduate recognizes that nurses may be needed 24 hours a day, 365 days a year, and that this may require sacrifices of personal convenience, including working evening shifts or on holidays.
2. **Function with acceptable speed.** This is another area in which expectations differ greatly. Most employers state that they expect the new graduate will be slower; however, they may vary in how much slowness is acceptable and how soon they feel that nursing actions should become more time efficient. Generally, an orientation period is planned—although, with the pressures on health care agencies, this often has been shortened considerably. An acceptable speed of function is reflected by the ability to carry out a usual RN assignment within a shift. Thus, if the usual client assignment for an RN is the care of four to six moderately ill clients, the new graduate is expected to accomplish this by the end of the orientation period.

Critical Thinking Activity

Compare your nursing program outcomes with the new graduate expectations. How are they similar, how different? What is the difference in the language used to describe competencies? Translate or interpret the language of your school outcomes to the language found in the NCSBN information.

PERSONAL CAREER GOALS

In caring for clients, you are involved in the process of goal setting. Many nurses recognize the value of this in client care but never transfer the concept to their personal lives. Nursing as a profession offers many career options. Without carefully setting goals, your professional growth may be impeded.

Focusing Your Goals

You may want to focus on a broad area of clinical competency, such as pediatric nursing, or on a more restricted area, such as neonatal care. Clinical areas available for concentrated effort become more varied as health care becomes more complex. Most of these areas offer certification to individuals who possess the expertise and pass the examinations. Many individuals focus their careers on particular client populations without ever seeking formal certification in that field. A person might take a critical care nursing course and work in critical care nursing without being certified. However, there may be advantages in terms of salary and recognition to holding specialty certification.

Additional education and certification is available in emergency care, coronary care, neurologic and neurosurgical nursing, and many other clinical fields. Nurses specialize in aerospace nursing, enterostomal therapy, and respiratory care, as well as operating room nursing and postanesthesia care. Opportunities for additional education and certification in most of these clinical specialties are available for any experienced RN, although some require that the individual have a bachelor's degree in nursing.

Some specialty positions are in the primary care field, such as the woman's health care specialist, the family nurse practitioner, and the pediatric nurse practitioner. These advanced practice specialties require a master's degree for certification. Although some educational programs preparing advanced practice nurses require the bachelor's degree in nursing for entry, many will accept an individual with an ADN and a bachelor's degree in another field.

Another approach may be to focus your goals on the setting in which care is delivered, such as acute, long-term, or community care. As health care needs expand, these separate realms of care delivery all demand more specialized knowledge. Even within the individual area of focus, differences are present. For example, within the community are ambulatory care settings, public health nursing agencies, occupational health nursing departments, and day care facilities.

Another way of focusing your goals is according to functional categories. Although nurses are initially thought of as direct care providers, they are also needed in many other positions. For example, there is need for those who would move into supervisory and administrative capacities, those who teach, and those who conduct nursing research. Additional education supports the ability to advance into these fields. Nursing also lends itself to writing, community service, and even political involvement.

You may decide to set your goals in relation to all three foci. That is, you might identify a clinical area, care setting, and functional category.

Setting Your Goals

The first step in setting personal career goals is a thorough self assessment. Determine how your abilities and competencies correspond to your own expectations and to those of employers. Other factors to explore are your likes and dislikes and the situations or types of work you particularly enjoyed as a student. Also, recognize the area in which you were most comfortable. Were there areas in which you or your instructor felt that you were an above-average student? Consider your health and personal characteristics in relation to types of work. Do you have physical restrictions? Do you prefer working independently or with others? How do you respond to close supervision or to freedom in the job setting? Do you prefer a work environment that is relatively predictable, or do you thrive in a situation that changes frequently? Do you work well with long-term goals and a few immediate reinforcements, or do you need to see results quickly? Another factor to consider is your own geographic mobility: Would you be willing to move or travel as part of a job? Both your personal responsibilities and preferences operate in this arena.

As you plan ahead, examine many of the options offered by nursing. What types of jobs and opportunities are open to you? What education and personal abilities are needed in these areas? Are you interested? Does the education you have meet the educational requirements? Are avenues for additional education available to you? All of these considerations are important as you plan for the future. Career goals need to be both short- and long-term. They will help you to plan your future constructively. This does not mean that goals are static. Just as client goals must be realistic, personal, and flexible, so must your own goals.

Short-term goals encompass what you want to accomplish this month and this year. What do you want to do and what do you want to be in the immediate future? For example, you might decide that your short-term goal is to have 2 years of solid experience in a busy metropolitan hospital.

Long-term goals represent where you want to be in your profession 5 or more years from now. A long-term goal may be to work in a small, remote community in which you will have the opportunity to function autonomously.

■■ COMMUNICATION IN *ACTION*
■■

Planning for Short- and Long-Term Goals

John Wilson and Richard Martin were both in the final term of their bachelor's degree program. They were making plans about job application. John said, "I am not sure what to do. I really want to work in public health, but a lot of people have been telling me that I have to have a couple of years of basic med-surg before even considering that and public health is more of a long-term goal. What do you think?" Richard replied, "I am not sure about that. My goal is intensive care, and a year of general med-surg seems good to me. I think I need to get my assessment skills and my organizational abilities firm before I take on intensive care. I have already begun applying with that in mind. However, I don't think you should just put your goal for public health aside. I remember my clinical instructor in public health told us that the necessary 2 years of med-surg was an old-fashioned myth." John responded, "Wow—I had not heard that perspective. Maybe I should check it out with the public health department before I make a decision. Thanks for the input."

Although both long- and short-term goals will be revised as your life evolves, they guide you in making day-to-day decisions more effectively. In today's world of rapid health care change, you may need to keep your goals somewhat broad and flexible. Be ready to consider alternative goals and a variety of pathways to one goal. These approaches will be of value as you enter a system in transition (Fig. 15-2).

Critical Thinking Activity

Write out your short- and long-term professional goals, with a brief plan on how you can achieve these goals. Think critically about the obstacles you will need to overcome to reach these goals. How will you deal with the obstacles?

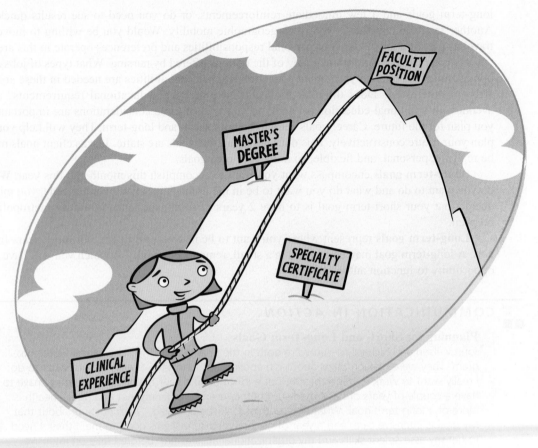

FIGURE 15-2   Clearly visualizing goals helps you to achieve them.

Maintaining and Enhancing Your Competence

Included in your goal setting should be an approach to maintaining and enhancing your competence. Every nurse has an obligation to society to maintain competence and continue practicing high-quality, safe care. Continuing education may occur through learning on the job, reading professional publications, or attending on-line or in-person classes. There are on-line courses, programmed instruction computer programs, and examinations related to journal articles. For example, Medscape for Nurses has on-line articles and associated quizzes and provides continuing education certificates (*www.medscape.com*). Registration for Medscape is free. Any of these avenues may be appropriate, depending on the circumstances. Some nurses may want to advance through specialty or higher education.

MAKING GOALS REALITY

Philosophic questions regarding goals must be resolved by practical approaches. As a new graduate, your first goal simply may be to get a job in nursing. Some new graduates, who recognize that there is a severe nursing shortage, assume that there is no need to put effort into making a positive impression on employers. After all, the employer will be glad to have any RN. Although this may be true in some circumstances, keep in mind that you are not applying only for an entry-level job. If you have identified a specific clinical area in which you wish to work, a specific employer you prefer, or a long-term goal that requires moving from one position to another, then you need to do those things that will obtain your preferred position, not just any position. Additionally, when applying for your first job you may also be making an impression that will affect later promotions or requests for educational opportunities. Those who interview you for an entry-level position may make decisions about future job assignments. The impression you make initially will carry over into other situations.

Whatever the situation, you are more likely to realize your goals if you are prepared to present yourself in the best possible way to a prospective employer. Many of you have held different jobs in the community as students and as adults. You may be familiar with and competent in the job search process. Others have never applied for the kind of job that truly could be considered the beginning of a career. Employers and prospective employees may hold different expectations in such a situation.

Identifying Potential Employers

To begin your job search effectively, you need to identify potential employers. You might begin your review with those more familiar to you and gradually move outward in an ever-widening circle to identify others.

A good place to begin is with the clinical sites where you had experiences as a student. You know these agencies and are somewhat familiar with the type of care provided. You may already be oriented to many of their policies and procedures. Your prior association with these agencies may provide you with ready access to their hiring procedures. If you worked as an employee in a health care setting before graduation, you may be given preference in hiring. This is one reason for seeking health care employment during your nursing education process.

Job fairs for health care employers are becoming more common. Each employer participating sets up a booth or table to provide information on job openings in its agency. An individual looking for employment may explore a variety of employers, learning about job openings, benefits, and opportunities in a brief time without the difficulty of searching out each employer. The employer may see many potential employees in a focused period. Thus, job fairs benefit both employers and potential employees. Job fairs may be held in the community, attracting experienced health care workers as well as students and new graduates. Some colleges arrange job fairs on campus. Nursing programs or nursing student clubs also may arrange job fairs.

A prominent source of potential jobs is the Internet. Many government job openings are posted on-line. An on-line search may reveal the names of nursing employers in your area as well as those at other locations of interest to you. If you do not have personal on-line access, use the computers at your local library. Using a search engine, look for "employment opportunities," "jobs," or "careers" combined with the term "nursing." Some on-line service providers have additional support services for a job search that might include career guidance (for a fee) or sample documents such as résumés and letters of application. Some examples of free sites specific to nursing are *allnurses.com*, *NursingJobs.org*, and *hospitaljobsonline.com*. Some general job sites such as Monster, Careerbuilder, and Hot Jobs may also list nursing positions.

Major nursing journals have sections in the back pages devoted to advertisements. Some of these advertise nursing positions. Sometimes an entire issue is devoted to a specific geographic area. This provides the ability to do a quick overview of possible employers. Your nursing program may receive advertising magazines that are designed to present job opportunities for new graduates. These magazines provide a few articles about relevant job search topics, such as interviewing, as well as advertisements from health care agencies. These advertisements present information on the agency itself and how to contact it for an application.

Another source of potential jobs is the classified section of the local newspaper. There you are more likely to find single jobs in small facilities, as well as general recruitment announcements from larger facilities. However, just because an agency fails to advertise does not mean it will not be hiring any employees. Advertising is expensive and may not result in the desired outcome. Therefore, some health care agencies do not advertise and rely on those who independently seek them out as potential employers.

Letter of Inquiry or Application

Writing a letter of inquiry is an excellent way to approach many prospective employers (Display 15-1). This letter is often termed a **cover letter** because it is sent with your résumé. You can present yourself positively through a well-written letter. In addition, a letter may be dealt with at the recipient's convenience, whereas a telephone call may interrupt a busy schedule. There are fewer chances for misunderstanding if your request is in writing and if you receive a written reply.

Before you write your letter, make sure you have information about the prospective employer. What kind of facility is this? What types of clients does it serve, and what special services does it offer? It makes a poor impression to write to a prospective employer stating that your goal is to work in pediatrics when that facility does not provide any pediatric services. Many agencies maintain a Web site with information regarding their mission, goals, and services. You might also obtain this information by calling the human resources department of the facility or by contacting a public information office. In a small agency, you may simply speak with a receptionist or secretary. If you call for information, be honest and straightforward in explaining that you are considering applying for employment and would like information about the agency before making that decision. The cover letter is sent to the nurse recruiter (if the agency has one) or to the human resources department. If you are not sure to whom to address your letter, check the agency's Web site or ask when you call to inquire about the agency itself.

Another part of your advance planning is identifying how you will focus your letter on your special qualifications and what you want to highlight. Focus on the skills or accomplishments related to the position you want. Your letter should be no more than one page in length, but should present all essential information. Introduce yourself and your purpose for writing in the first paragraph so that the reader immediately understands why you are writing. You may want to state briefly your reasons for applying for a position with this particular employer. The more specific the reasons, the better the impression you are likely to make.

Use the body of the letter to briefly highlight your qualifications for the position. This should not be a simple recitation of what is in your résumé, but should either present the information in a

Maribeth Wilson
3428 1st Ave. N.
Seattle, WA 98103
(206) 274-5978
e-mail: maribethw@email.com

January 30, 2007

Joyce Montgall, R.N.
Nurse Recruiter
Seattle General Medical Center
321 Heath Blvd.
Seattle, WA 98101

Dear Ms. Montgall:

Enclosed please find a copy of my résumé, along with my application to Seattle General Medical Center's New Graduate Residency Program. I will graduate from Shoreline Community College's associate degree nursing program on May 28. I expect to acquire my registered nurse license by the end of June. I am extremely interested in a medical-surgical nursing position within your upcoming residency program.

I believe that I would bring many strengths to a new graduate position. I have worked here at Seattle General as a nursing assistant for the past year, and my experience has given me an excellent foundation in understanding the philosophy and mission of the Medical Center. During this time I have been assigned to several different units, including 4 West and 4 Center, where new graduate positions are available. The nurses at Seattle General have been generous in their mentoring and have helped me to increase my understanding of the patients' conditions. They have been supportive as I developed increased problem-solving and decision-making skills.

Within my nursing student educational experience, I have had the privilege of working in a wide variety of health care institutions throughout the city. From these experiences I would bring an understanding of the community standards of care as well as a unique appreciation of the position of Seattle General in the health care community.

I hope that I will be selected for an interview and look forward to hearing from you. My phone number, e-mail address, and home address are at the top of this letter. If I do not hear from you within the next two weeks, I will contact your office to ascertain the status of my application.

Sincerely,

Maribeth Wilson

Maribeth Wilson

slightly different light or add pertinent detail that is not in the résumé. If you are responding to an advertisement, touch on each of the qualifications listed in the advertisement. You might include personal qualities that would make you an effective employee in the position, such as interest in learning and skill in teamwork. Relate your skills and abilities to the needs of this particular agency. If your health care experience is limited, point out skills you have gained from other jobs that would be useful in nursing. These might be interpersonal skills, management skills, or adaptability.

In the final paragraph, make a summary statement indicating why you want to work for this employer and ask for an appointment for an interview. Be sure to indicate the times you are available and how and where you can be contacted if the employer so wishes. It also is wise to indicate that you will contact the person to whom the letter is addressed to request an appointment. This allows you to maintain some initiative in the process. Thank the person for considering your application, and close.

Another point to remember is that the letter's appearance and its content both represent you. You will be judged on spelling, grammar, clarity, and neatness, in addition to content. Be cautious about relying on the spell-checking function on your computer. An incorrect word may pass the spell-check but be clearly seen as an error by the careful reader. Your letter of application should be written in standard business format on plain white or off-white business paper. Make it brief and clear. Ask a friend or family member to check your first draft if you have any questions about its correctness.

EXAMPLE

Seeking Information Regarding a Potential Employer

Joseph Williams will be graduating from a basic nursing program in 3 months. He has decided he would be interested in applying to a hospital in the state capital. He wants to move to a larger community and be in an institution where research is being conducted, advanced technology is used, and nurses have a voice in the institution. Through a Web search using the name of the city and "hospitals," he obtains a list of hospitals. He saves the search for future access and begins linking to each of the hospitals. On the hospital sites, he reads the mission statement and any other general information about the hospital. He reviews the services that they describe and narrows his exploration to those that mention research. He notes that one hospital prominently displays that it has achieved designation as a Magnet Hospital. He links to the human resources page to gather information about applying for a job in each institution that interests him. In some institutions a link to a nurse recruiter is found prominently displayed, but in others there is no indication of a specific nurse recruiter. He decides to start his personal contacts with the nurse recruiter at the Magnet Hospital.

Critical Thinking Activity

Identify an area of the country and type of nursing position that interests you. Using the various Internet resources, learn about job availability, salaries, and working conditions for at least three employers in that area. Determine which of the three would be of most interest to you and provide a brief rationale for why you would choose that employer.

Preparing an Effective Résumé

A **résumé** is a brief overview of your qualifications for a position. Its purpose is to present you in the most positive light to be considered for the position in which you are interested and to provide the employer with a way to identify quickly whether you have the basic qualifications for a position. Résumés are used primarily to screen applicants for interviewing; therefore, you will want to make an impression that is good enough to result in an interview. You will want to include your résumé with your initial letter. In addition, have copies of your résumé to take with you to any interview or appointment. You may want to leave a copy of your résumé with a unit manager at the end of an interview because your original résumé may be retained in the human resources office. Résumés may be posted on-line by job search sites. If posting on-line, check on the privacy policies of the site. Use care in what you place on an on-line résumé for your own safety. Often you will not include personally identifying information, but rather a code from the job site.

Appearance

The appearance of your résumé is important because it initially presents your image to the prospective employer. You want its appearance to reflect a competent, professional image. It is not necessary to have a professionally produced résumé. Nursing employers, when asked, have indicated that it neither adds to nor detracts from their impression to read a résumé that has been produced by some professional printing method. The important point is that it be a somewhat formal, standard, informative document that is neat and without errors.

Your résumé should be on standard-sized (8.5" × 11"), white or off-white, good-quality paper so that it is easy to handle, file, and read. A résumé that is individually printed (or reproduced well enough so that it appears to be) usually will be received more positively than an obvious photocopy. You will find it valuable to create a résumé and save it to a disk. In this way, you will be able to revise it easily, and you may even be able to tailor it to an individual job situation. In addition to the capabilities of standard word processing software (which usually include résumé templates), there are inexpensive software programs especially designed to facilitate the production of a well-organized and formatted résumé.

To achieve legibility, use sufficient margins (usually 1"), spacing, indentation, bullets and even line separators to separate different sections and topics. You might want to underline or italicize related items or bold print or highlight important items to draw swift attention. A résumé looks better when the content is evenly balanced on a page. Dense paragraphs do not attract the reader, but lists and topics do. When an employer is reviewing many such documents, anything that facilitates review and makes you stand out is an advantage. Ask individuals you trust to review the appearance of your résumé and identify those areas that first caught their attention. This helps you to evaluate its appearance.

If your résumé will be sent or posted on-line, consider how that will affect the appearance. Special fonts or nonstandard résumé programs may not transfer effectively into the on-line environment. A job site will provide directions for a posted résumé. If your résumé is to be sent as an attachment to an e-mail, then it should be composed in a common word processing program such as Microsoft Word. You might check with the receiving human resources department as to its preference for format. Some may ask for a plain text file.

Display 15-2   Questions to Help You Plan a Résumé

1. What educational institutions have you attended? Dates? Degrees or certificates?
2. What credentials do you have that might be useful in a nursing employment setting?
3. What jobs have you held that you want to highlight? Were any of them health care related?
4. What specific skills did you apply in your workplace that would be transferable to nursing?
5. What skills, abilities, or personal characteristics do you want to draw the employer's attention to?
6. Have you had volunteer or community experiences that demonstrate positive personal attributes?
7. Have you had any awards or recognition that identify your positive abilities or attributes?

Content

The content of your résumé is critical. When you are beginning the preparation of a résumé, first assemble the information that you want to include in some way. Display 15-2 provides some questions you can ask yourself to begin a list of information that you want to include on your résumé. Making such a list before beginning the process of actually formatting a résumé helps you to take an organized approach and not forget to include important information. If you will be submitting a résumé on-line, this process should include identifying specific key words that you want to include within the résumé. Often employers search on-line résumés using key words that pertain to the type of position they have available or specific skills and abilities that are needed in the position. If your résumé does not contain these key words, it will not be identified as relevant to the employer.

A standard résumé always begins with your name, address, and telephone number (including area code). If you will be moving, indicate the date the move will be effective and provide an alternate method of contacting you after that date. A permanently settled relative or friend who would be willing to forward your mail is appropriate. Employers are not permitted to ask about age, race, religion, marital status, and dependents (and in some jurisdictions, sexual orientation), and you do not need to include this information. An e-mail address is helpful to employers. However, if your e-mail address is an informal phrase such as "studmuffin2" or "prettygirl," plan to set up a separate e-mail address for business use. This can be done for no cost through one of several Internet mail providers such as Gmail, Yahoo, Juno, or Hotmail. Use a simple derivation from your name that gives you a more professional appearance.

Objective. Many résumés include a personal goal or objective. This is helpful to a recruiter or human resources department that considers many different occupations within the agency. The objective immediately alerts the reader to the type of position being sought. This may include both a short-term goal such as "employment as a beginning registered nurse" and a longer-term goal such as "with eventual move to employment in coronary care." Be sure that your goal is realistic and does not imply that you are not really interested in a beginning-level position. If you state that your goal is to work in an emergency room and you do not have the experience for this kind of position, your application usually will be discarded. If you state that you want to work in maternity nursing and the only position available is in medical-surgical nursing, you may not be considered for the medical-surgical position that you would have accepted although it was not your first choice. You may wish to write an objective that is tailored to a specific employer or job announcement. When you are more experienced, you may want to make your objective more specific to a particular department or role.

Credentials. Include information regarding your licensure and other credentials. Indicate the date your license will be effective and whether you have a temporary permit to work as a nurse. Your nursing license or permit number should be listed after you have it. If you do not have a license at the time you are preparing your résumé, you may choose to include information about when you expect to have your license in your letter of application.

Education. Educational background should form a separate section and cover your nursing education and any specialized courses or postgraduate work you have completed. It is appropriate to note any college-level work. Do not include high school information. In each group of information, list the most recent items first.

Employment History. Work experience is of critical importance, and you should provide a meaningful employment history. If using a traditional format, for each job you held include employer, address (city and state are sufficient), dates employed, position, and duties. List the most recent employer first and follow with the remaining information in reverse chronological order. The prospective employer will be especially interested in a previous nursing assistant position or any other position that demonstrates your knowledge of or experience in some area of health care or the assumption of responsibility. Other positions also may be important if you are clearly able to identify skills used in those settings that are transferable to nursing.

If you have had only one or two part-time jobs during your educational program, it would be appropriate to include them in detail. However, if during your educational program you held 15 part-time jobs, it is appropriate to list significant ones that offered valuable experience. In one line, it is acceptable to write, "Various part-time jobs to finance schooling: clerk and waitress. Individual names provided on request." Include the overall dates for this period.

Focus on accomplishments and use active verbs to describe skills. Words such as supervised, designed, managed, developed, analyzed, coordinated, documented, planned, delegated, created, completed, and operated give life to your résumé and create interest in the reader. If you were part of a team that accomplished a significant project or task, you might indicate that. However, be careful not to take personal credit for team accomplishments. See the accompanying display for a list of active verbs you might use in describing your skills and abilities (Display 15-3). If you are responding to a specific job announcement, be sure that your résumé reflects the education and skills that are noted.

To keep your résumé on one page, consider how you might most effectively present employment history. In a skill-focused résumé, you can emphasize the responsibilities you had within positions rather than each specific position. These might come from other jobs or life experience. See Display 15-4 for an example of a skill-focused résumé. You might also highlight specific experiences in an area that especially relates to the position for which you are applying. For example, you might have had a senior leadership practicum on an orthopedic unit—this would be particularly relevant to an application for a nursing position in orthopedics. If you had a practicum in the facility or agency to which you are applying, indicate this in some way. Your familiarity with its policies and procedures will be a valuable asset. If you attended any special

Display 15-3   Power Verbs for Résumés

- Use of verbs without subjects will be more concise and space conserving.
- Use of active, not passive, voice, such as "advanced to" rather than "was promoted to," "earned" rather than "was given," indicates a person who does things rather than receives them.
- Use of "-ed" or "-ing" as verb endings can both be effective.

accompanied	demonstrated	generated	mastered	prompted
achieved	designed	governed	mediated	proposed
acquired	detailed	graduated	motivated	proved
activated	determined			provided
administered	developed	headed	negotiated	
advanced to	devised		nominated	reconciled
advised	diagnosed	identified		reduced
analyzed	directed	implemented	obtained	regulated
arranged	discovered	improved	officiated	related
assembled	displayed	improvised	operated	reorganized
assessed	doubled	increased	ordered	reported
assisted		induced	organized	represented
	earned	influenced	originated	researched
balanced	educated	informed	overcame	
budgeted	employed	initiated		satisfied
	enacted	innovated	participated	secured
clarified	encouraged	inspired	perceived	served
composed	engineered	installed	perfected	simplified
conceived	established	instructed	performed	solved
concluded	evaluated	insured	piloted	structured
conducted	executed	integrated	pioneered	succeeded
constructed	exhibited	intensified	placed	supervised
consulted	expanded	interviewed	planned	
controlled		invented	prepared	trained
converted	facilitated		presided	transferred
coordinated	financed	led	processed	transformed
counseled	formalized	located	procured	unified
created	formed		produced	
	formulated	maintained	progressed	verified
decided	founded	managed	promoted	won
delegated		marketed		wrote

workshops, include those in a separate section. Information included in this part of the résumé can be used to demonstrate your ability to meet deadlines, produce good work, and relate to people in ambiguous situations. Use numbers when possible to describe achievements. For example, if you previously worked evenings in a long-term care facility as an LPN, you might state, "Supervised five nursing assistants" or "Administered all medications to 30 patients per shift." Be sure to include language proficiency if you are fluent in more than English. Computer literacy is also a valuable skill.

Display 15-4   Skill-Focused Résumé of a Recent Graduate

Sarah Mitchell

5714 31st Ave. N., Seattle, WA 98117 • (206) 733-8934 • e-mail: *sarahmit@email.com*

Objective

An entry-level registered nurse position in an acute care hospital.

Experience

2005-present   Seattle General Medical Center   Seattle, WA

Patient Care Technician, Medical-Surgical Units

- Provide basic care and ADLs with attention to psychosocial needs for acutely ill medical-surgical patients. Assist RN with procedures and carry out delegated duties.
- Work collaboratively with nursing team, assuring prompt response to patient needs.
- Effectively manage time to support seven patients on evening shift.
- Document care on computerized system, maintaining accuracy and confidentiality.

2003–2005   Health Choice Urgent Care Center   Seattle, WA

Nursing Technician, Urgent Care Clinic

- Interviewed clients, took vital signs, initiated documentation, and prioritized care for urgently ill and injured adults and children.
- Under RN supervision, performed assessments, dressing changes, ECGs, nebulizer treatments, and hospital admission processes.
- Attended to psychosocial needs of family and others accompanying a sick or injured individual.

2001–2003   First United Bank   Lynnwood, WA

Bank Teller

- Maintained excellent customer service by following detailed bank policies and procedures.
- Utilized a variety of computerized systems to assure accurate and detailed documentation of all activities.
- Incorporated information from employee training classes into job skills to assure up-to-date function.

Education

2005–2007   Shoreline Community College, Seattle, WA

AAAS Nursing, to be awarded June, 2007

Display 15-5   Chronological Position-focused Résumé of a Recent Graduate

Joseph M. Sanchez
1298 Avenida Diaz
La Quinta, CA 92252
(619) 524-4321

Objective:
A beginning Registered Nurse position that will provide the opportunity for professional development and advancement toward critical care nursing.

Skills:
- Work effectively in a multicultural environment
- Communicate in a positive, supportive way with coworkers, clients, and families
- Bilingual Spanish/English
- Strong work ethic and experience in working multiple shifts/floating positions
- Excellent critical thinking and problem solving developed in a wide variety of occupations as well as in the nursing context

Education:
College of the Desert, Palm Desert, CA

> Management practicum, Desert Health Center 5-West: Working with RN preceptor, demonstrated RN level skills in managing care of a module of five acutely ill patients. Delegated care appropriately to nursing assistant. Facilitated interdisciplinary communication.

Associate in Science in Nursing, June 2007

Experience:
Manor Care Center, Palm Desert, CA

Nursing Assistant, Certified: 2001–Present
- Maintained function and dignity of dependent elderly adults by providing direct care, strong inter-personal relationships, and effective collaboration with nursing and allied health.
- Earned promotion to position of mentor for new hires and team leader for a group of nursing assistants. Facilitated team performance to accomplish assigned responsibilities.

Northrup Corporation, Los Angeles, CA

Machinist: 1990–2001
- Performed precision skills with accuracy and attention to detail.
- Followed precise written protocols and procedures to ensure quality.
- Led a team in a program of total quality management within our department.

Awards:
- College of the Desert Merit Scholar 2006
- Golden Acorn Award for Leadership in Parent Involvement, Cactus Valley Elementary School PTA, La Quinta, CA

You may choose a more position-focused résumé and not include details of all your previous positions separately. For individuals who are older and have an extensive employment history, a résumé focused on types of positions with related skills rather than a chronologic list of employers is often the most effective. List a position such as LPN and include responsibilities and skills for all employers followed by a simple list of employers. This keeps the résumé from becoming repetitive as the same information is presented for each employer. See Display 15-5 for an example of a chronological position-focused employment section.

Additional Experience. Volunteer or community work and awards and honors form two sections when you have these experiences. You also might want to add a section for special skills such as computer familiarity or experience with special types of equipment. Choose the items you list under volunteer and community work carefully. If you are older, the fact that you were student body president in high school would probably be considered irrelevant. However, if you went from high school directly into a nursing program, this information could be important in demonstrating your leadership ability. If you are an older student, your leadership participation in a community organization, such being president of the Parent–Teacher Association might be significant to an employer. If you are applying for a position in pediatrics, various volunteer activities working with children might be relevant.

Employers are interested in skills you would bring to the job that require decision making and the exercise of good judgment both in volunteer work and in past work experience (Fig. 15-3). In

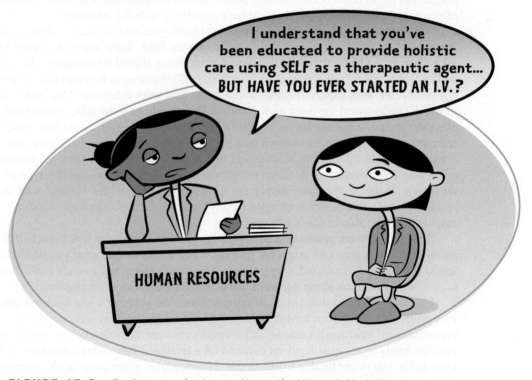

FIGURE 15-3   Employers are often interested in specific skills needed in their setting.

some instances, you may want to list briefly the skills or abilities gained from a particular volunteer activity just as you would for employment. For example, if you worked as a volunteer for a Planned Parenthood clinic, you might specify that your duties included individual client counseling in relation to family planning methods. Simply stating that you were a volunteer would not communicate the level of responsibility you assumed. This is an area that you might want to individualize to target the particular skills you think are important to the position for which you are applying. For example, you might use your volunteer experience to demonstrate past success in the skill of organization, managing or coordinating people and events, and effectively delegating responsibilities. It also might be used to highlight public relations skills: the ability to write, work within or control a budget, prioritize multiple tasks, or cope with deadlines. If you have served as the coach of a Little League baseball team or a soccer team, or as a Girl or Boy Scout leader, focus on your ability to direct, coach, and teach others.

List awards, honors, and professional associations (such as the National Student Nurses' Association) that would demonstrate your competence, professional involvement, or leadership ability. This provides an opportunity to show responsibility in directing the activities of others, public speaking, and, perhaps, motivating people. You may omit this section if you feel that you have nothing pertinent to enter.

Personal References. References are typed on a separate page and given to the prospective employer or copied onto an application form, if they are requested. Be selective in choosing the people you list as references. Consider people who know you, would be able to speak positively of you to a future employer, and would have credibility with the employer.

A primary reference should be an instructor from your basic educational program. This person would be able to affirm your ability in the nursing field. Some agencies request two instructor references, so be prepared for that. Another reference should be someone who has employed you and who can describe your work habits and effectiveness as an employee. If you have had any health care work experience, this would be the best work reference. Also look at the position in which you assumed the most responsibility. This should be reasonably recent (within the past 10 years). Again, some employers ask for two work references. You should have available, as one reference, someone who has known you personally for a relatively long time and who could attest to your ability to relate with others and to such attributes as personal integrity. Not all employers are interested in personal references. Some agencies indicate the type of references they want. If this is the case, supply the names of references that comply with the agency's request. Include full names with titles (if any), addresses, and telephone numbers, so that the employer will be able to contact the references easily.

Seek the person's permission before giving his or her name as a reference. When seeking permission to use someone as a work reference, you might outline what you would like the person to emphasize if contacted—for example: "If you are contacted, I would particularly like you to provide information about my work habits and effectiveness as an employee."

Employers express differences of opinion about the value of a standardized letter of reference addressed "To Whom It May Concern." Some employers may consider this a useful initial presentation of your qualifications. Other employers want the reference to address the specific position needs or the qualifications outlined on a reference form. One advantage of the general letter is that you might be able to obtain this reference from a part-time faculty member or supervisor who may no longer be employed by the institution. If you do obtain this type of letter, be sure to preserve the original carefully (perhaps in a clear, plastic page protector) to show to a potential employer; you then would provide a good-quality photocopy for the employer to place in your file. Even when an employer accepts this as an initial reference, your references probably will be personally contacted as well.

Critical Thinking Activity

Create an effective résumé and samples of letters to employers that present you as a positive addition to their staff. Base these letters on specific nursing positions you have learned about in a search of possible employers.

Completing An Application

Whether the application is on-line or completed in a print format, there are similarities. First, be sure that you fill in all the information requested. It is never appropriate to simply write on the application form "see résumé" and leave the sections blank or to simply leave out requested information for an on-line application. Information often will be entered into a database, and the employer wants it in a standardized format. The failure to follow directions accurately is a poor reflection on your skills and abilities. If the application must be completed onsite, bring all needed information with you, including information about references and names, addresses, and dates for past employers. If it is an on-line application, you may need to complete it at one time and then submit it. Sometimes it is beneficial to print out the on-line form to be certain you have the information before starting it on the computer.

Successful Interviewing

The interview should be a two-way conversation in which you will gain as well as give information. Typically, employers have three major concerns for which they seek answers in the interview: they want to know whether you have the required knowledge and skills to do the job, whether you possess an attitude toward the job and the organization that is compatible with what they are seeking, and whether your personality and style will fit with the image the organization wishes to put forth. They are going to be interested in what you can do for them and, at this point, are often more interested in what you can do than in your opinions. They may be especially interested in your problem-solving and critical thinking skills. When planning for an employment interview, consider your appearance, your attitude and approach, and what the content of the interview will be.

Learning About Your Potential Employer

Once you know that you have gained an interview with a potential employer, learn as much about that specific position and the organization as you can. This can be done a number of ways. Review information you received when you were searching for organizations to which you would apply. Look again at information on its Web site if one exists. Be sure you have information regarding the organization's mission statement and other public pronouncements. Look especially for information on the various types of health care service the institution provides. If possible, contact current employees. Check local newspapers for information regarding the facility.

Preparing Your Questions for the Interviewer

Think through the situation before going to the interview and outline information that you want to obtain and questions that you want answered. It is helpful to write out your questions so that they are clearly stated, and so that you do not forget items while in the tense atmosphere that often exists in an interview situation for example "How and when will I learn of your decision?"

Time spent reflecting on your personal views in advance will be valuable for the interview. Remember that an interview is a chance to sell yourself to an employer, a chance to present yourself as a valuable addition to their nursing staff, and an opportunity to determine how you will fit into that work setting. A question such as "Please tell me about the educational opportunities that would be available to me," indicates an interest in learning.

Dressing for the Interview

You need to make a conscious decision about the impression you want to create through your attire. Your personal appearance and demeanor are likely to evoke some response from the interviewer. Although some may wish that appearances had no effect on the opinions of others, remember that, in reality, appearance often does make a significant difference.

Consider what you would like the interviewer's response to be and choose your attire with that in mind. This means that what you wear when applying for one type of job might be inappropriate when applying for another type of job. In most instances, such as applying for a position at a hospital, you would wear businesslike clothing, such as dress pants or skirt and shirt or blouse or sweater, or a suit or dress. Being neat and well groomed contributes to a businesslike atmosphere. If you were applying for a position in a walk-in health care clinic that offered services to persons who are uncomfortable in a traditional environment, it might be appropriate to wear more casual clothing, such as that worn by the workers at the clinic. Avoid fads and extremes. Appropriate casual clothing does not include attire with a bare midriff, shorts, athletic attire, body piercing jewelry other than the earlobe, or pants with holes in the legs. Wear regular shoes, not flip-flops. Avoid the use of strong cologne or perfume. Most interviewers indicate that being more businesslike in dress is never a mistake, while being too casual is a frequent mistake.

In all instances, your hair should be clean and neatly styled. Although wild colors and elaborate styles may be popular in some circles, they may be looked on unfavorably in a professional interview. Do not chew gum while in the interview. If you smoke, avoid smoking immediately before the interview so that the odor of smoke is not apparent on your clothes or person.

Things to Take With You

Take several copies of your résumé with you to the interview. You may want to refer to it or you may find it appropriate to leave a copy with someone. In addition, be prepared with the names, addresses, and telephone numbers of all references, as well as your Social Security number. If you have already received your nursing license, take that with you. Take along a black pen to fill out any forms, and a note pad with your questions listed and a place to make personal notes of important information obtained during the interview. You might want to purchase a special job interview hard-backed folder that will hold materials in a pocket on one side, has a notepad on the other, has a place for a pen, and will be a surface upon which you can write. You do not want to infringe on an interviewer's space by using that person's desk to take notes. Having all the information and supplies you need with you can increase your self-confidence if you have forms to fill out or if questions about statements on your résumé arise during the interview.

Arriving at the Interview

Plan to arrive at an interview early. This gives you time to check your appearance and focus your thoughts. When you arrive at an interview, be sensitive to the problems and concerns of the interviewer. If it is apparent that unplanned events are demanding the interviewer's attention, state that you are aware of the difficulty and ask whether it would be more convenient if you made another appointment. Your sensitivity to the interviewer's cues is evidence of your sensitivity to clients' cues.

Your manner during the interview is important also. It has been said that a first impression is made in the initial 10 seconds of contact. Although the employer expects an applicant to be nervous, he or she will be interested in whether your nervousness makes you unable to respond appropriately. Follow common rules of courtesy. Greet your interviewer with a smile and firm handshake and establish eye contact and maintain it throughout the interview. Making and maintaining eye contact communicates confidence and honesty—two important characteristics employers value. Wait to be asked to sit down before you take a chair. Do not put anything of yours on the interviewer's desk other than your résumé. Avoid any distracting mannerisms, such as chewing gum or fussing with your hair, face, or clothes. Nervousness often causes people to fidget, bounce their feet, or drum their fingers; be careful to avoid these behaviors. Sit up straight, as slouching communicates a message of disinterest. If you carry a cell phone, turn it off before the interview. Be serious when appropriate, but do not forget to smile and be pleasant. The interviewer is also thinking of your impact on clients, visitors, and other staff members.

Anticipating Interview Questions

When you prepare your responses, try to anticipate possible questions from the interviewer. To do this, you must know the role of the person conducting the interview. In large agencies, your first interview might be with a human resources department employee, not a nursing department representative. If you are successful at this stage, you might be recommended for an interview in the nursing department.

Role-playing an interview situation with a friend or relative may help you to feel more confident in your responses. Another technique is to visualize the interview situation in your mind and mentally rehearse responses to questions.

An interview usually covers a wide variety of subjects. The interviewer may direct the flow of topics or may encourage you to bring up the ones that concern you during the process. Some interviewers focus on asking questions about your past experiences and your future plans. Others focus their questions on specific accomplishments and problems encountered in your past nursing experiences. Presenting hypothetical problems for you to consider and asking you to provide appropriate nursing responses is common. You may find it helpful to use your nursing process approach to any situation presented. Specifically state, "I would need to begin by assessing . . . ." Talk about clearly identifying the problem (analysis of data) and planning for action. Don't neglect to indicate that you would evaluate the effectiveness of your actions. See Display 15-6 for a list of questions you might reflect on as you prepare.

In most instances, be sure to answer questions that are asked, rather than skirting them. However, if the interviewer asks a question that is illegal or inappropriate, such as a question regarding age or marital status, you might want to redirect the question to address what appears to be the concern of the interviewer. For example, in response to a question about your age, you might say, "Perhaps you believe that I appear to be young and inexperienced. I want

Display 15-6   Questions to Help You Prepare for a Job Interview

Philosophy
- What is your philosophy of nursing?
- Is there a nursing theorist that you use as a basis for your nursing practice?
- What do you believe is the most central concept to support excellence in nursing?

Personal Goals and Planning
- Where do you see yourself in 1 year? 5 years? 10 years?
- Have you developed any professional goals? If so, would you share those with me?
- Why do you want to work here?
- What plans do you have for continuing education in nursing?
- What do you see as your weakest area in nursing?
- What do you see as your strengths in nursing?

Your Experiences
- What experience in your nursing education did you find the most rewarding? Why?
- What experience in your nursing education did you like the least? Why?
- In what kind of settings did you have an opportunity to work as a nursing student?
- What other job experiences have you had? What skill did you develop there that will be useful in nursing?

Problem Solving
- Identify a problem in patient care that you encountered as a student and explain how you solved that problem.
- Describe a difficult patient with whom you worked. Include why you found that patient difficult and how you managed the situation.
- Identify a situation in which you were involved in a conflict and describe how you handled that situation. If you had to do it over again, what would you do differently?
- Explain how you would use the nursing process in patient care.
- A problem may be presented to you for your solution. Plan ahead to approach it in a systematic manner.

Technical Skills
- What technical nursing skills do you feel comfortable peforming?
- What skills will you require assistance with?
- What do you do when you encounter a technical skill you have not performed before?

The Employment Setting
- In what type of unit do you wish to work?
- Why do you want to work here?
- Why do you think we should hire you for this position?

to assure you that I have demonstrated my maturity and responsibility both in my nursing education and in my position with [name of employer]." In response to a question about marital status or children, you could reply, "Perhaps you are concerned about how long I plan to stay in my first position? I want to assure you that whatever my personal situation, professionally, I am looking for a position in an organization where I can be a long-term employee and plan for advancement within the organization." Avoid simple yes or no answers, but try to describe or explain to give a more complete picture of yourself.

Some interviews are conducted by a group of interviewers. This might include a person from nursing administration, a unit manager, and a staff development nurse. For an applicant to sit across the table from three to five individuals can be intimidating. You will need to look around the group, being sure to make eye contact with each individual. Make sure that you understand the role of each person present. You might actually write down individual names and roles on your notepad. This would allow you to direct a question to a specific individual or to use an individual's name when replying to a question. If you use a name, be sure to address them formally as "Mr.," "Ms." (if marital status of a woman is not known), "Miss," or "Mrs." rather than by first name. If they want you to use another form of address, they will let you know. While replying to the person who asks the question, glance at others as you make your point. Be sure that you do not ignore any individual, even if one of the interviewers does not seem to ask questions or to be as active in the process as the others. Interviews of this type are often longer than interviews with one person.

Some interviewers are less skilled than others; in these situations the questions may seem less focused and more vague. You may sometimes feel at a loss as to exactly what is being asked. Before proceeding, seek clarification, but be careful that your manner of asking for clarification does not offend the interviewer. In this situation, you may have to take the initiative to be sure that you have an opportunity to present your strengths and skills. Don't hesitate to elaborate on questions to more effectively present yourself.

■■ COMMUNICATION IN *ACTION*
■■

Clarifying Questions in an Interview
Cheryl Layton, a new graduate, interviewed for a nursing position. She found that she did not understand many of the interviewer's questions and decided to use clarifying questions and statements throughout the interview. When there was a rather unclear question about communicating with others, she asked, "Would you give me an example of the type of situation you were thinking about?" Another clarifying approach she used was to state clearly what she perceived to be the central question before continuing: "Let me clarify. You would like me to identify a situation in which I believe I responded effectively to a problem. Is that correct?" Still another clarifying response she used was, "If I understand correctly, your unit will be switching to computerized charting, and you are interested in my experience with computerized documentation. Is that right?" In this way, she indicated interest and attention to accuracy but did not challenge or offend the interviewer.

Almost all interviews provide an opportunity for the interviewee to ask questions before the interview is terminated. Applicants who focus initial attention on the issues of wages and benefits may be viewed as more concerned about themselves than about nursing. Therefore, if you are asked to present questions, ask professional questions first. Make sure your questions are appropriate for the interviewer. In the human resources department, you might ask about the overall mission and philosophy of the organization, its organizational structure, and how authority and accountability are determined. You might also ask, "Do you have any questions about my résumé? Are there other details I can provide?" With a nursing interviewer, demonstrate that you are concerned about how nursing care is given and by whom, where responsibility and authority for nursing care decisions lie, the philosophy underlying care, the availability of continuing education, and where you would be expected to fit into the facility's overall picture. For example, you might ask, "Can you outline for me the responsibilities of this position?" or "What type of individuals do well in this type of position?"

Then be sure to cover such topics as hours, schedules, pay scales, and benefits. Before you leave, be sure to ask when you can expect to know the results of your interview and how you can follow-up. State clearly that you are interested in the position and hope to be hired (if that is true). An important reason for not getting a position is the failure to clearly state that you want to work there.

If you are unfamiliar with the interview process, you might benefit from reading books on the topic. Reading several different books will give you a variety of viewpoints and might provide you with strategies that are comfortable for you.

■■ COMMUNICATION IN *ACTION*
■

Replying Professionally to an Interview
Rosa Quintana had been interviewing for a position in a new graduate residency program in which she would really like to be a participant. The interviewer said, "Well that concludes my questions, do you have any questions for me?" Rosa responded, "I prepared some questions before I came. Some of those were already answered. However, I would like to hear more about the shared governance system you briefly mentioned on your Web site. Exactly what types of issues are addressed through shared governance and how might I, as a newly hired new graduate, participate in shared governance?" In this reply, Rosa demonstrated her pre-planning and organization as well as her understanding of organizational function. After hearing the response to this question, Rosa then said, "Thank you so much for that information. It really confirms that I would really like to work here. I do hope to be chosen to enter this new graduate residency. What are the next steps I can take to learn about my status in the selection process?"

Telephone and On-line Interviews

Because interviews are costly to an employer, telephone and on-line interviews may be conducted and an in-person interview only scheduled for individuals in whom the organization is interested in employing. Do not mistake these telephone or on-line interviews for unimportant or casual conversations. Plan for them in the same way that you would for an in-person interview. Prepare and have all your materials at hand. You will want to be professional and businesslike in this context also. The one advantage is that you do not need to worry about your appearance.

Follow-up Strategies

Always follow up after your initial inquiry. If you were granted an interview, follow up with a letter. If you did not obtain an interview, you should continue to contact the potential employer at intervals to learn of other job opportunities and to indicate that you still seek a position. When a new position opens, employers do not necessarily go back through previous employment files. They are more likely to interview a person who appears to be currently searching for a position than one who was searching several months previously. They will assume that you have found desirable employment.

After your interview, write a brief thank-you letter to the person who interviewed you. If a group interviewed you, direct the letter to the person who seemed to be in charge. In that letter, thank the individual for the time and attention to your questions and concerns. Restate any agreement you feel was reached. For example, write, "I understand that I am to call your office next week to learn whether I have been scheduled for an interview with the maternity unit manager." Close your letter with a positive comment about the organization. Even if you are not offered a job or do not choose to work at that facility, you are leaving a positive impression. You can never tell when that will be important to you in the future (Display 15-7).

Display 15-7   Interview Follow-up Letter

Maribeth Wilson
3428 1st Ave. N.
Seattle, WA 98103
(206) 274-5978
e-mail: maribethw@email.com

February 9, 2007

Joyce Montgall, R.N.
Nurse Recruiter
Seattle General Medical Center
321 Heath Blvd.
Seattle, WA 98101

Dear Ms. Montgall:

I want to thank you for meeting with me today to discuss your new nursing graduate residency program at Seattle General. I am particularly interested in the medical-surgical positions available on 4 West and 4 Center, although I am certainly willing to consider another unit.

My educational background, clinical experience, and commitment to excellent patient care appear to make me an ideal match with Seattle General. In addition, I feel very "at home" in the Seattle General environment, having worked there as a nursing assistant for the last year.

Again, I hope that you will consider me for one of the medical-surgical positions in the June graduate program. I am available to meet with any of the unit managers, which I understand is the next step in your hiring process. I can be contacted at the above telephone number or by e-mail. I do have an answering machine and would promptly return your call if I were not there to receive it. If I have not heard from you within two weeks, I will check with your office regarding the status of my application.

Thank you again for your time and consideration.

Sincerely,

Maribeth Wilson

Maribeth Wilson

Do not let this letter be your last contact with that potential employer. Call back as agreed. Even if you do not get a position at this time, you might ask that your application be kept on file because you are still interested in employment with that particular agency. You might then continue to call back every month or so to find out if any other positions are available.

EXAMPLE

Following Up After an Interview

A student in her last term of a nursing program interviewed for a position in a new graduate residency program of a major medical center. She was disappointed when she called to follow up and was told that she had not been selected. The nurse recruiter assured her that she was a good candidate but that they had just had more applicants than they could place. After thanking the recruiter for notifying her, she asked if she could call back every couple of weeks to see if any new opportunities were available. She emphasized how much she would like to work at this medical center. She kept in contact with the recruiter as she widened her job search. Four weeks after she had been told that she was not selected, she called the nurse recruiter. The nurse recruiter told her, "I am so glad you called. One of the new graduates selected for the program has decided to move back to her hometown. We will have a place for you after all. Can you come in today or tomorrow to complete the paperwork?" Continuing her contact in a professional manner was a successful strategy.

Setting up your own record-keeping system often enhances managing a job search. Maintain a record of when you contacted an agency, in what manner (letter or telephone call), interviews—including the interviewer's name and the content of the interview—and dates and times of any follow-up letters or calls. Have a place to record your own notes or impressions. This will enable you to keep track of details when you manage an extensive job search. By keeping this type of record, you will not forget to call an agency to recheck on job availability, or mistakenly send an inquiry letter and résumé twice to the same agency.

Resignation

When you decide to leave a nursing position, it is important that you provide the employer with an appropriate amount of time to seek a replacement. The more responsible your position, the more time the employer will need. For a staff nursing position, strive to provide a month's notice, unless an urgent matter requires that less notice be given. Notice of resignation should be in a letter that is directed to the manager of your department. Copies should be sent to other supervisory people, such as the chief nursing officer.

The letter of resignation is important in concluding your relationship with the employer on a cordial and positive basis. The feelings left behind when you resign will influence letters of recommendation and future opportunities for employment with that agency. Give a reason for your resignation and the exact date when it will be effective. If you have accrued vacation or holiday time and want to take the time off or be paid for it, clearly state that. Comment about positive factors in the employment setting and acknowledge those who have provided special support or assistance in your growth.

If you are resigning because of problems in the work setting, you may find it wiser to address those in person, separate from your letter of resignation, and in a manner that will not affect future recommendations. However you address problems, do so in a clear, factual, unemotional way. Avoid attacking anyone personally and do not make broad, sweeping negative comments. Try to make any written statement a clear and reasonable presentation of your position as a professional (Display 15-8). Remember that the nursing community is not large and a career path

---

Display 15-8   Letter of Resignation

1546 Avenida Escuela
Palm Desert, CA 76321
February 14, 2007

Marvin Short, R.N., Unit Manager
Transitional Care Unit
Desert Hospital
509 Desert Highway
Palm Desert, CA 76320

Dear Marvin:

It is with mixed feelings that I am submitting my resignation to be effective March 23.
I will be moving to Oregon and returning to school full time beginning spring quarter.

My two years here at Desert Hospital have been an excellent foundation for my future
career. The nurses were supportive of me as a new graduate and have always encouraged
me to think of my career as a lifetime opportunity for growth.

The last day I plan to work will be at the end of this pay period. My understanding is that
my unused vacation and holiday pay will be included in my final paycheck.

Thank you again for all of your help.

Sincerely,

John Webster

John Webster, R.N.

cc: Maria Gonzales, Vice President for Patient Care Services

---

may bring you back to this agency or may bring these individuals to a place where you work. Try
always to leave with appropriate professional relationships intact.

Key Concepts

- Developing a successful career pathway involves setting personal short- and long-term
  goals and developing a plan for maintaining and enhancing your own competence.
- Throughout the history of nursing, employment patterns have changed, moving from a
  focus on the home and the community in the first part of this century to a focus on acute
  care institutions.
- In today's health care world, the percentage of nurses employed in hospital inpatient
  settings, while still high, is diminishing as more outpatient, home care, long-term care,
  and community settings are established for the delivery of care.

- Competencies needed by the newly licensed RN can be categorized by criticality and by frequency.
- Employers have expectations in eight basic areas: theoretic knowledge for safe practice and decision making; ability to use the nursing process; self awareness; communication skills; understanding the importance of documentation; commitment to a work ethic; proficiency in specified technical skills; and speed of functioning.
- To obtain a nursing position, you will need to identify potential employers, develop a professional résumé, write appropriate letters to employers, and interview effectively using both in-person and on-line strategies.
- Successful interviewing involves learning about the organization, dressing appropriately, arriving a bit early, being self-confident, maintaining eye contact throughout the interview, and remaining attentive.
- To make the best impression, interview questions should be answered directly and clearly. The use of clarifying statements and questions may help to assure that you are providing needed data, while specific details rather than generalities in your response are often received more favorably. Approaching problem-solving questions using the nursing process provides a pattern for effective response.
- Following up after the interview has been completed includes sending a note of thanks to the key decision makers, and checking back to learn of decisions about the position, and maintaining contact with the institution if not selected and you still would like a position there.
- When resigning from a position, communicating your plans to the head of the department with a sufficient time interval to allow the organization to find a replacement to fill your position leaves a professional impression and may result in a more positive reference.

References

American Association of Colleges of Nursing. (1998). *The essentials of baccalaureate nursing education for professional nursing practice.* Washington, DC: Author.

National Council of State Boards of Nursing. (2002). *2002 practice analysis of newly licensed registered nurses in the U.S.* [On-line]. *www.ncsbn.org/testing/testingservicesresearch_9481CE11545F46E09E98C2AD1B246367.htm.* Accessed January 21, 2006.

National Council of State Boards of Nursing. (2003). Linking the NCLEX-PN National Licensure Examination to Practice. Chicago: Author.

National League for Nursing. (1978). *Competencies of the Associate Degree Graduate on Entry Into Practice.* Publication No. 23-1731. Council for Associate Degree Programs. New York: Author.

National League for Nursing. (1987). *Characteristics of baccalaureate education in nursing.* Publication No. 15-1758, Council of Baccalaureate and Higher Degrees. New York: Author.

National League for Nursing. (1990). *Educational outcomes of associate degree nursing programs: Roles and competencies.* Publication No. 23-2348. New York: Author.

National League for Nursing Council of Associate Degree Programs Task Force on Educational Outcomes of ADN Programs. (1999). *Educational competencies for graduates of associate degree programs.* New York: Author.

Projected supply, demand, and shortages of registered nurses: 2000–2020. (2002). U.S. Department of Health and Human Services, Health Resources and Services Administration, Bureau of Health Professions, National Center for Health Workforce Analysis. [On-line]. *http://bhpr.hrsa.gov/healthworkforce/rnproject/report.htm.* Accessed October 18, 2002.

Smith, J., & Crawford, L. (2003). *2002 RN practice analysis: Linking the NCLEX-RN® examination to practice, executive summary.* Chicago: National Council of State Boards of Nursing. [On-line]. *www.ncsbn.org/resources/publications.asp.* Accessed January 28, 2006.

Spratley, E., Johnson, A., Sochalski, J., Fritz, M., & Spencer, W. (2002). Findings from the national sample survey of registered nurses. The Department of Health and Human Services, Bureau of Health Professions. [On-line]. *http://bhpr.hrsa.gov/ healthworkforce/rnsurvey/rnss1.htm#T1.* Accessed January 16, 2006.

U.S. Bureau of Health Professions. (2004). *The registered nurse population: National sample survey of the registered nurse population: Preliminary findings*. [On-line]. *http://bhpr.hrsa. gov/ healthworkforce/reports/rnpopulation/preliminaryfindings. htm*. Accessed May 13, 2006.

Spetz, J., Rickles, J., Chapman, S., & Herrera, C. W. (2008). Identifying and eliminating survey of registered nurses. The Department of Health and Human Services: Bureau of Health Professions, Division of Nursing. Retrieved from http://bhpr.hrsa.gov/ healthworkforce/rnsurvey04/default.htm

The National Health Workforce (2008). Explanatory notes on National Sample Survey of Registered Nurses. Retrieved from http://bhpr.hrsa.gov/ healthworkforce/

16

Facing the Challenges of Today's Workplace

LEARNING OUTCOMES

After completing this chapter, you should be able to:

1. Compare the roles identified in the ranking of novice to expert to the various expectations of employers regarding new graduates.
2. Construct strategies to prevent or alleviate reality shock.
3. Analyze your own values and life situation and identify your personal potential for burnout.
4. Adapt personal stress management techniques to control your work stress.
5. Describe the physical hazards in the workplace and identify strategies to protect yourself from them.
6. Discuss how nursing has been affected by racial, ethnic, and sex discrimination.
7. Explain appropriate techniques to manage sexual harassment in the workplace.
8. Discuss ways to respond effectively to verbal abuse in the workplace.
9. Describe approaches to managing physical violence in the health care workplace.

KEY TERMS

Burnout	Mentee	Quality assurance report
Coaches	Mentor	Reality shock
Discrimination	Novice to expert	Sentinal event
Ergonomics	Occupational hazard	Sexual harassment
Incident report	Preceptor	Stereotypes

For many of you, graduating from a nursing program and becoming a registered nurse (RN) is the realization of a long-cherished goal. You have put a great deal of effort into preparing for this status, and now it is here! What you have viewed as an ideal state, freed from financial pressures that you felt as a student, liberated from the tyranny of examinations, may prove to be quite different from what you expected. Let us consider some of the problems that may emerge as you make this transition from student to professional.

⚙ MOVING FROM "NOVICE TO EXPERT"

The path from **novice to expert** is a challenging one. Benner's (1984) work in this area has provided a basis for an understanding of and research into this process. She related this path to the Dreyfus Model of Skill Acquisition that was first published in 1980 (Dreyfus & Dreyfus, 1980), in which the individual moves from novice to advanced beginner to competent to proficient to expert. Table 16-1 presents characteristics of these skill levels.

Throughout this progression, Benner identified exemplars of nurses performing in six roles:

1. The helping role
2. The teaching–coaching function
3. The diagnostic and monitoring function
4. Effective management of rapidly changing situations
5. Administering and monitoring therapeutic interventions and regimens
6. Monitoring and ensuring the quality of health care practices and organizational and work-role competencies.

The helping role encompasses planning and implementing all the basic nursing skills used to assist patients. The teaching-coaching function pertains to teaching the patient and family to manage their own health status and adaptations in living. The diagnostic and monitoring role relates to assessment and evaluation of the patient's health status and various needs. Responding to changing situations is rooted in critical thinking and a comprehensive knowledge base. While all of these roles differ between the novice and the expert category, it is in this role that outsiders often more clearly see the differences between the novice and expert nurse. Administering and monitoring the therapeutic interventions and regimens relates to the medical plan of

TABLE 16-1	BENNER'S LEVELS OF FUNCTION
LEVEL	**CHARACTERISTICS**
1. Novice	No experience of the situations. Have context-free rules to guide behavior. Relatively inflexible.
2. Advanced Beginner	Marginally acceptable performance. Have some experiences with real situations. Can identify "aspects of the situation" (p. 22). May formulate principles or guidelines for action.
3. Competent	Begins to see current situation in terms of long range goals. Is able to prioritize among patients and base actions on conscious deliberate planning. May still lack speed and flexibility.
4. Proficient	Perceives situations as wholes rather than as a collection of parts. This perception is not thought out but is unconscious. Experience has given this nurse a "web of perspectives" (p. 28). Responds to nuances of the situation using maxims.
5. Expert	Has an intuitive grasp of the whole situation and does not rely on rules, guidelines, or maxims. Focuses immediately on the most critical elements of the situation. May have difficulty articulating the thought processes that resulted in decisions.

Benner, P. (1984). *From novice to expert: Excellence and power in clinical nursing practice.* Upper Saddle River, NJ: Prentice Hall.

care. The final role is the leadership and management role that all nurses must perform. All must be concerned about quality improvement and ensuring the best health care practices for the patient.

Through interviews with nurses, Benner described the depth of nursing skills and abilities found in the expert nurse. This expertise is forged over time and results from personal experience and personal knowing. One of the challenges for beginning nurses is pressure to function as an expert without this background of growth.

As you look for a first nursing position, learn about the mechanisms the employer has in place to facilitate your transition to the RN role. Is there an orientation program specially designed for new graduates? Will you have an individually assigned preceptor or mentor for support? How long will you be given support before being expected to function independently? If you feel you need more time to be independent, will the employer accommodate this need? As a new graduate, will you be expected to float to different units, or will you be helped to become competent in one area before being asked to go to another? Is there assistance with and support for continuing education for nurses? As you answer these questions, you will begin to develop a broader picture of the employer and be able to evaluate whether this job is a fit for your personal journey from novice to expert.

Critical Thinking Activity

Examine your own background and experience in light of the characteristics noted in Benner's levels of skill. In your analysis, identify areas where you might exhibit a particular level of skill. What do you believe is the general level of skill expected of the new graduate?

REALITY SHOCK

One problem confronted by the new graduate is the seeming impossibility of delivering quality care within the constraints of the system as it exists. You may feel powerless to effect any changes and be depressed over your lack of effectiveness in the situation. Marlene Kramer (1979) was the first to call the feelings that result from such a situation **reality shock**. She noted that the new graduate often experiences considerable psychological stress and that this may exacerbate the problem. The person undergoing such stress is less able to perceive the entire situation and to solve problems effectively (Fig. 16-1).

Causes of Reality Shock

With all of the uncertain expectations and demands, the new graduate often feels caught in the middle. As a student, you may think that you are expected to learn a tremendous amount in an alarmingly short time. The expectations may seem high and in some ways unrealistic.

Then, as a new graduate suddenly thrust into the real world, you may feel unsure of yourself without the security of the instructor's availability and the support of your fellow students. You may think that your education program did not adequately prepare you for what is expected of you. On one hand, you are expected to function like a nurse who has 10 years of experience, but on the other hand, your new ideas may not be considered because you have so little experience.

FIGURE 16-1   Some new graduates are disillusioned by the working conditions that they find on their first job.

You may become frustrated because you do not have time to provide the same type of care you gave as a student. For example, you may not have adequate time to deal with a client's psychosocial problems or teaching needs.

As a student, you are taught that the good nurse never gives a medication without understanding its actions and side effects, and that evaluating the effectiveness of the drug is essential. As a staff nurse, you may find that the priority is getting the medications passed correctly and on time, and that there is little or no time to look up 15 new drugs. As for evaluation, that becomes a dream. How can you evaluate the subtle effects of a medication in the 2 minutes spent passing the medication to a client you do not know? The individually and meticulously planned care that was so important to you as a student may become a luxury when you are a graduate. Often the focus is on accomplishing the required tasks in the time allotted, and it is efficiency in tasks that may earn praise from a supervisor.

Bradby (1990) suggested that reality shock is part of the passage from novice to experienced nurse. She suggests that it be treated as a normal transitional process, with a focus on the growth that can occur. This can best occur if you understand what is happening and are prepared to address the problem.

Effects of Reality Shock

The person experiencing reality shock may feel discouraged and depressed over the conditions of work. There may be anger toward the system, and this may result in diffused anger that erupts over situations that in other circumstances might be met with a calm demeanor.

In an attempt to cope, some push themselves to the limit, trying to provide ideal care and criticizing the system. This may result in their being labeled nonconformists and troublemakers. Still others give up their values and standards for care and reject ideals as impossibly unrealistic expectations that cannot be fulfilled in the real world. These persons simply mesh with the current framework and become part of the system. When reality shock occurs, some nurses begin to job hop or return to school, searching for the perfect place to practice perfect nursing as it was learned. Others become disillusioned and leave nursing altogether (Kramer, 1979).

Finding Solutions for Reality Shock

There is an alternative to these nonproductive coping methods. It is possible to create a role for yourself that blends the ideal with the possible—one in which you do not give up ideals but see them as goals toward which you will move, however slowly. To do this, you need to be realistically prepared for the demands of the real world.

Self-Appraisal

One way of meeting the challenge is to assess yourself as you approach the end of your education program. Evaluate your own competencies in relationship to the common expectations of employers of new graduates that were discussed in Chapter 15:

1. Theoretic knowledge for safe practice
2. Use of the nursing process
3. Self-awareness
4. Communication skill
5. Delegation
6. Documentation
7. Skill proficiency
8. Work ethic
9. Speed of functioning
10. Interpersonal skills and cultural sensitivity

Evaluating Employers Carefully

Gain information about what the employers in your particular community expect from new graduates. Do this by talking with experienced nurses, meeting with faculty, and contacting recent graduates who are currently employed. Try to get specific information. If you have a nursing student organization, setting up a forum for speakers from various agencies might be one avenue to gaining this insight. Once you apply for a position, you could explore this issue in an employment interview.

When you are selecting a place of employment, there are many factors to consider. While the specific position is important to you, there are aspects of the overall setting that will make a great deal of difference to your success. You are not as likely to experience severe stress if the employment setting is a good match for you. Review the information in Chapter 15 regarding investigating the practice environment for nursing. The professional practice environment makes a difference in the problems of reality shock and of burnout, which we will discuss.

Some hospitals attempt to help new graduates deal with reality shock by making orientation programs more comprehensive and by providing an experienced nurse to work as a preceptor to the new graduate. Nurse internships or residencies in some settings have been created to provide a planned and organized transition time during which the new graduate participates in a formal program, including classes, seminars, and rotations to various units of the hospital. In some settings, the new graduate is required to be more self directed in identifying needs and the ways that those might be met within the constraints of the system.

Some hospitals provide an opportunity for nursing students to work during the summer before the last year of their basic program to become familiar with the hospital and the nursing role. In this type of program, the nursing student may be employed as a nursing assistant but participate in a planned program that introduces the role of the RN. In other instances, nursing students work as nursing assistants, and the orientation to the nursing role in the agency depends on the initiative the individual takes. You may wish to inquire whether hospitals in your area have developed any of these or other programs to assist you when you are a new graduate.

Comparing Your Skills to Expectations

After you have done a self-appraisal and gained information about prospective employers, analyze your own ability to function in accordance with an employer's expectations. If you identify any shortcomings, try to remedy them before graduation. If you identify a lack in certain technical skills, register for extra time in the nursing practice laboratory to increase your proficiency. You could even time yourself and work to increase speed as well as skill. Consult with your clinical instructor to arrange for experiences that would help you gain increased competence, especially in procedures with which you have had little experience. Having met an objective is far different from skillfully and efficiently carrying out a procedure. If you recognize that you consistently have difficulty functioning within a time frame, you might obtain employment in a hospital or other health care facility while still in school; this will give you more experience in organizing work within the time limits that the employer sees as reasonable. If you perform well, it also may lead to a job offer upon graduation.

When confronted with areas of practice in your work environment that you would like to see changed, weigh the importance of an issue. Use your energies wisely. The "politics of the possible" is important. Learn how the system in which you are employed functions and how to use that system for effective change (see Chapter 14). You are important to nursing, so it is important that you neither burn yourself out nor abandon the quest for higher-quality nursing care. You should be able to continue to work toward improving nursing and bringing it closer to its ideals (see Chapter 14 for more information about change).

Critical Thinking Activity

With a group of nursing students, develop personal strategies for managing reality shock. Discuss your rationale for any strategy you propose.

Mentors, Preceptors, and Coaches

A **mentor** is an individual who actively supports the development and growth of another person (referred to as the **mentee** or **protégé**.) Within a professional field, the mentor is usually an experienced professional who develops a supportive relationship with someone with less experience in the profession and provides advice and emotional support for that person. While the mentor may provide some direct assistance in learning the specific skills of the nursing role, more important, the mentor provides help in learning how to work effectively within the system. The mentor is a role model of effective practice. The mentor also may provide guidance in professional development and career suggestions. Sometimes the mentor is in a position to assist the mentee in navigating the organization's informal system of rules and expectations (see Chapter 11) and in applying for advancement.

Mentor–mentee relationships typically begin when an experienced senior nurse takes an interest in a nurse with beginning experience who is pursuing a similar professional pathway as the senior nurse. It often works best when it occurs spontaneously as a relationship develops between a junior and a senior employee within an organization. It is important that the mentor can assist the protégé with career and personal development and provide personal support, acceptance, and counseling—qualities not seen in preceptor or coaching relationships. In this way, the mentor sponsors the mentee and often facilitates that person's influence within the organization by helping to establish networks and organizational know-how. Plans for the development of the mentee need to be developed and reviewed with periodic feedback and debriefing sessions. Typically this relationship extends over a period of 5 to 10 years and serves as an avenue for the development of leaders in nursing (Restifo & Yoder, 2004).

A good mentor is a seasoned member of the organization and an experienced practitioner. A model employee, this individual has a positive attitude and a caring approach toward others, communicates effectively, listens well, and enjoys working with less experienced professionals. As might be expected, they are usually intelligent, hardworking, and busy people (Restifo & Yoder, 2004).

Mentor–mentee relationships change over time and may become more collegial. As you progress in your career, you may need a new mentor in a new setting or in regard to a new field of practice. This role is not to be confused with that of a preceptor or a coach.

In nursing, many new graduates are assigned to a **preceptor** as part of their orientation process. A preceptor is an officially assigned role in which an experienced and capable employee assists with the orientation and development of a new employee. Some of you may have experience with preceptors as part of your educational program. The preceptor usually has responsibility for evaluating the work of the preceptee. A preceptor may or may not become a mentor. Some preceptors may see the role as primarily one of supervising, teaching, and evaluating in relationship to the specific job and do not see it as a broader role of encouraging professional development. Some preceptors develop personal relationships with new nurses. They act in ways described as mentoring.

If you are fortunate enough to have a preceptor who becomes your mentor, you will have additional support and guidance from the beginning of your career. If your individual preceptor does not view the role that way, then you may wish to develop relationships with other experienced nurses who might provide a mentoring relationship.

Coaches operate somewhere between preceptors and mentors and help the less experienced nurse master more advanced skills and understand the politics of the organization. But coaches lack the long-term commitment to the mentee involved in mentorship.

Peer Support Groups

As you plan for your first job, you can examine the psychological challenges to be met. Understanding that you are not alone in your feelings of frustration is often helpful. It may be useful to form a peer support group of new graduates who meet regularly to discuss problems and concerns and seek solutions jointly. You also can gain valuable reinforcement from other nurses in your work setting. Many have dealt successfully with the problems you face and are able to provide support and help. Finding a specific mentor in your work site will assist you as you grow in your profession.

A peer support group is usually composed of new nurses at a particular facility and is often initiated by the new nurses themselves. The group meets regularly to share its experiences, offer support and advice, and help all the individuals to recognize that others are also experiencing stress during this time.

Some peer support groups are composed of individuals from a single graduating class who may be working in different settings. Although their settings differ, many of the individuals' concerns surrounding transition are alike, and their relationships with their educational program have created a bond that makes the group able to function effectively.

Personal Stress Management

Recognizing your own response to stress and identifying your personal stress management strategies will be significant. As a nursing student, you experienced stressful times and coped successfully or you would not have graduated. Remind yourself of your own successful coping and draw on the strategies you found successful in the past. As is always the case, personal health needs to be a part of those strategies. Attend to your diet, rest, and activity plan. Maintain time for family and friends in order to have balance in life. Life should never be all work.

BURNOUT

Burnout is a form of chronic stress related to one's job. Burnout can occur to individuals in any occupation, and articles regarding burnout appear in the professional literature for almost all the helping or supporting professions.

This problem arises after you have been in practice for a period of time. It can be identified by feelings of hopelessness and powerlessness, and is accompanied by a decreased ability to function both on the job and in personal life. Burnout occurs more frequently in nurses who work in particularly stressful areas of nursing, such as critical care, oncology, or burn units. Some writers explore burnout as "compassion fatigue," relating it to the high stress of managing personal feelings in the face of overwhelming crises experienced by others. Burnout also occurs when staffing is inadequate or interpersonal relationships are strained. The downsizing of nursing staff and the rapid changes in the health care environment have contributed to burnout in some settings.

Symptoms of Burnout

Symptoms of burnout include both physical changes and psychological distress. The items found in the Maslach Burnout Inventory (Maslach & Jackson, 1986) provide an overview of symptoms that may occur in burnout. These include exhaustion and fatigue, frequent colds, headaches, backaches, and insomnia. There may be changes in disposition, such as being quick to anger or exhibiting all emotions excessively. Individuals experience a decreased ability to solve problems and make decisions as burnout progresses. This frequently results in an unwillingness to face change and a tendency to block new ideas. There may be feelings of guilt, anger, and depression because one cannot meet the expectations for doing a "perfect job." Burnout begins gradually

> ### Display 16-1   Are You Experiencing Burnout?
>
> 1. Do you find yourself dreading going to work in the morning?
> 2. Are you regularly experiencing fatigue and low energy levels at your job?
> 3. Are you easily bored with your job?
> 4. Do work activities you once found enjoyable now feel like drudgery?
> 5. Are you depressed on your day off thinking about going back to work and the coming week?
> 6. Have you become more cynical or bitter about your job, your boss, or the company? Do you find yourself easily annoyed or irritated by your coworkers?
> 7. Are nonwork relationships (marital, family, friendships) affected by your work feelings?
> 8. Do you find yourself envious of individuals who are happy in their work?
> 9. Do you now care less than you used to about doing a "good job" at work?
>
> Adapted from Canuff, A. (n.d.). American Counseling Association. *www.workplaceblues.com*

and is more effectively managed early in its onset. Canuff (n.d.) provides a list of questions found in Display 16-1 to assess yourself for early symptoms of burnout.

In response to these feelings, some nurses quit their jobs and move on to other settings that may be outside the nursing profession. Others remain in their jobs but develop a personal shell that tends to separate them from real contact with clients and coworkers; they may become cynical about the possibility of anyone doing a good job and may function at a minimal level. A few become increasingly unable to function and find themselves in jeopardy of losing their positions.

Causes of Burnout

Many causes of burnout have been discussed in the literature. Prominent among them is the conflict between ideals and reality. Just as this is a problem for the new graduate, it is also a problem for the experienced nurse. In trying to achieve the ideal, nurses drive harder and become critical of the environment and of themselves. These nurses believe they are responsible for all things to all people and often take on more responsibility, thus increasing their own stress level.

Another cause of burnout is the high level of stress that results from practicing nursing in areas that have high mortality rates. Continually investing oneself in clients who die can take a tremendous toll on personal resources. In addition, the demand for optimal functioning is constant.

Inadequately staffed institutions also may place great stress on nurses. The clients are in need of care, the nurse has the skills to provide the care, and yet the clients do not receive good care. The nurse typically tries to accomplish more, putting in overtime, skipping breaks and lunch, and running throughout the shift. Despite this effort, there is little job satisfaction because the things that are left undone or that are not done well seem to be more apparent than all the good that is accomplished.

Preventing Burnout

As an individual nurse, you can take actions to prevent burnout. These are the same general actions that are designed to control stress in any aspect of life. Paying attention to your own physical health is an important preventive measure; this includes maintaining a balanced program of rest, nutrition, and exercise. Another important point is not to subject yourself to excessive changes over short periods of time, because changes increase stress. You may decide, for example, not to relocate your living setting (apartment or house) at the same time you change to a different shift. A period of wind-down or decompression after work will help you to avoid carrying the stress of the workplace into your private life; this period may involve physical exercise, reading, meditation, or any different activity. This may seem like a daydream to individuals who are working full-time, have responsibility for children, and perhaps also for aging parents. Yet, it is important that some personally rewarding activity be incorporated into the daily routine. The activity you choose should not create more demands and increase stress. An important resource is someone who is willing to listen while you express your feelings and talk about your problems. Sometimes this is a family member or personal friend, but it may be more appropriate for this to be a coworker or counselor. The Web site *www.workplaceblues.com* has many suggestions for managing stress that occurs at work.

Rotating out of a high-stress area, such as a burn unit or pediatric oncology, before you begin to experience burnout may allow you to rebuild resources and return to the job with enthusiasm. This can be done only if there is no stigma or blame attached to the need to rotate and if other nurses are available for replacement. In client care areas that are known to be stressful, it is helpful to have a counselor available for nurses. Consulting with this counselor should be viewed by the staff as a positive step and not as an admission of some lack or fault. The counselor needs to be someone who understands the setting and who has the skills to assist people in coping with stress.

■■■ COMMUNICATION IN *ACTION*
■■

Acting to Prevent Burnout

Linda Wilson returned to employment after maternity leave when her baby was 3 months old. A new critical care unit was being opened in the hospital and she eagerly accepted the invitation to work there. However, after 2 months on the 3 PM to 11 PM shift, she found she was burning out, due in part to understaffing, lots of overtime, and the critical nature of the patients for whom she cared. With the demands of the baby, she seldom got more than 4–5 hours sleep. She approached the supervisor of the unit and asked for an appointment to meet with him prior to beginning her shift. During their meeting Linda explained, "I am very appreciative of the opportunity to work in this unit. However, I think it was not the right time in my life to undertake such a challenge. With the demands of a new baby at home, I just do not have the energy this position demands. I get home late, often have trouble going to sleep, and the baby wakens early. I would like to request a transfer to a less intensive work unit." The supervisor was supportive of Linda and her request and agreed to follow through on the request for transfer.

In this communication, Linda did not blame others for the situation in which she found herself. She was honest and forthright in her explanations, and clear in her request.

Display 16-2　The Art of Nursing

- Informed caring
- Thoughtful doing
- Lifelong learning

Lindeman, C. (1999). The art of nursing. *Creative Nursing, 5*(3), 3–4.

Another strategy is to focus on those positive aspects of nursing that drew you to it initially. Much is being written about cognitively reframing situations and settings to focus on those parts that are positive and affirming. The art of nursing reflects that positive view of nursing (Display 16-2). Lindeman (1999) suggests that the art of nursing is composed of three central aspects. The first, informed caring, refers to behaviors that make a difference for patients: attending to what patients say, analyzing and synthesizing information, and acting as an advocate for patient and family. The second aspect is thoughtful doing. She characterizes nursing practice as a "continuous, interactive, unbroken spectrum of thought and action" (p. 3). The third aspect is lifelong learning. Lifelong learning is an essential foundation for the informed caring and thoughtful doing that are the first two components. Looking at the art of nursing and focusing your energy and attention on this may help you surmount the everyday pressures you encounter.

The most effective prevention of burnout is an institution-wide stress-reduction effort to prevent burnout involving the nursing staff, supervisory personnel, the hospital administration, and other health care workers. The most important objective seems to be bringing burnout into the open and acknowledging the existence of the problems. This alone helps the individual nurse move away from the feelings of separation and alienation that often accompany burnout. Whatever the problems, they seem less frightening if they are defined as normal and if the individual nurse does not see him- or herself as the only person not performing as the perfect nurse. Investigate the resources that a prospective employer has to assist nurses in preventing burnout.

Another approach may be initiated by individual nurses but requires the cooperation of the institution; this includes establishing group discussions during which nurses can share feelings and specific concerns in an accepting atmosphere. This sharing may lead to concrete plans to reduce the stress created by the setting. For example, if one source of stress is conflicting orders between two sets of physicians involved in care, a plan might be developed whereby the nurses no longer take responsibility for the conflict but refer the problem to some authority within the medical hierarchy. This type of resolution is possible only when the whole health care team addresses the problem of burnout. However, it also requires that nurses give up trying to control everything for which they feel responsible.

Giving nurses more control over their own practice often decreases stress. Although more control is limited by the constraints of the setting, it could involve flexible scheduling, volunteering for specific assignments, and participating in committees that determine policies and procedures.

Critical Thinking Activity

Compare burnout with the stress response you have studied in relation to client care. Compare the strategies that you have taught clients with those suggested for preventing burnout. Discuss these with a classmate and see how many similarities you have.

PATIENT SAFETY INITIATIVES

As a new graduate you will be expected to be an effective and knowledgeable participant in working toward a safer health care environment.

Identifying the Safety Problem

In 2000, the Institute of Medicine (IOM) released its groundbreaking report *To Err is Human: Building a Safer Healthcare System* (Kohn, Corrigan, & Donaldson, 2000). The data presented caught the attention of the general public as well as that of health care providers. According to studies the committee reviewed, medical errors in the United States cause an estimated 44,000 deaths each year making it the 8th leading cause of death in the United States. Some studies would indicate that the mortality from medical errors is actually more than that (Kohn et al., 2000, p. 1). In addition to lives lost, the economic cost of these errors is staggering, amounting to between $17 billion and $29 billion annually (Kohn et al., 2000, p. 2).

However, the report did not stop with identifying the problem. It also provided an analysis of the multiple causes underlying the safety problem. The report noted that the system is not a coordinated system at all, but rather is fragmented. Areas of care have been traditionally isolated from one another with ineffective communication between various specialties and agencies as the patient moves from provider to provider. Neither patients nor payers (insurance companies, Medicare, Medicaid, and health maintenance organizations) have been aware of the safety concerns or, if aware, have not identified their responsibility to create change.

The third part of the report focused on suggestions for change. One of the major emphases was that individuals not become the scapegoats of the system. When problems are systemic, individuals become powerless to make changes independently. The report contained three recommendations for action. The first recommendation centered on changing the legal environment in which people are so anxious about lawsuits that they cover up rather than correct problems. The second recommendation suggested initiating a system response to error that includes analysis of root causes and changes in the system. The third recommendation was to change the institutional response from addressing a concern only after an error has occurred to being proactive in identifying potential errors. In response to this report, all regulatory agencies and health care providers began examining what they should do to achieve the aims of the IOM report.

The Joint Commission Safety Emphasis

To address concerns about errors in health care, The Joint Commission (formerly known as The Joint Commission on the Accreditation of Healthcare Organizations [JCAHO]) established Patient Safety Goals for each year beginning in 2002. Agencies that were accredited by The Joint Commission were encouraged to begin targeting high-incidence preventable safety problems, such as falls, misread physician orders, and communication errors. An example is The Joint Commission requirement that each institution adopt procedures designed to eliminate instances of wrong patient, wrong site surgeries.

The Joint Commission requires that accredited institutions investigate and report all **sentinel events**.

A sentinel event is an unexpected occurrence involving death or serious physical or psychological injury, or the risk thereof. Serious injury specifically includes loss of limb or function. The phrase, "or the risk thereof" includes any process variation for which a recurrence would carry a significant chance of a serious adverse outcome. Serious adverse outcome is defined as instances of error that have the potential for serious harm or death to the client (The Joint Commission, 2005).

Each year, The Joint Commission has re-examined its safety goals and revised them by deleting those that have been largely achieved and adding new safety goals. Its emphasis is to move toward a culture of safety. These patient safety goals are available on-line at *www.jointcommission.org*.

Federal Safety Legislation

Almost immediately after the IOM report was released, federal legislation was introduced in relationship to patient safety. Although bills were submitted in the House of Representatives and Senate each year, it was not until 2005 that the Patient Safety and Quality Improvement Act was finally passed by both legislative bodies and signed into law by President Bush (Patient Safety and Quality Improvement Act, 2005). This law provided protection for individually identifiable health care data that might be used in assessing safety concerns, provided for the certification of patient safety organizations, set up a plan for a network of patient safety databases that could be used for research and development without fear of disclosure of data about individual agencies, and established mechanisms to provide technical assistance to facilitate work on patient safety data.

Quality Improvement and Safety

The Joint Commission has defined quality assessment and quality improvement (QI) as "ongoing activities designed to objectively and systematically evaluate the quality of patient/resident care and services, pursue opportunities to improve patient/resident care and services, and resolve identified problems" (The Joint Commission, 2003). As part of their commitment to safety, individual institutions have expanded their use of QI processes to give a special emphasis to issues related to safety. Employees are encouraged to identify possible safety concerns and refer them for management through a variety of process improvement strategies. Most organizations have adopted the approach advocated by the IOM and worked to eliminate the culture of blame that formerly surrounded the issues of errors and safety. Data from the IOM clearly showed that a punitive environment actually increases the potential for safety problems.

EXAMPLE

A Punitive Environment Compromises Safety
In the past, it was not uncommon for institutions to have punitive approaches to any errors. XYZ nursing home had a policy that employment was terminated after the third medication error. In that facility, the turnover of licensed practical nurses and RNs was extremely high and many problems were identified on its state survey. Meanwhile, the

nurses passing medications were overworked, the facility had a shortage of licensed staff, and the systems for managing medications were confusing. The rate of errors did not decrease. The failure to recognize that a harsh and punitive attitude toward staff members was a part of its problem made it impossible for it to improve safety.

Fortunately the majority of health care employers have moved beyond punitive approaches and recognize that those entering the health professions in general are motivated to achieve patient well-being and anxious to increase safety. By instituting QI programs in which individuals feel empowered to identify safety issues and participate in efforts to increase safety, safety for all patients is enhanced.

Individual Provider Involvement

As an individual working in health care, you are greatly affected by the attitudes toward patient safety that exist in the workplace. Part of your role as an RN includes your recognition of responsibility for the safety of all patients. It is not enough to make sure that you are personally careful. You need to look at systems and processes to identify areas that need to be studied and changed to be safer. An example is the storage locations for look-alike or sound-alike emergency drugs. In an emergency, look-alike drugs may be mistakenly confused and administered. While as an individual nurse you might focus on more careful reading of the label, addressing the system concern toward moving the storage areas would protect all patients.

In light of these concerns, another pitfall for the nurse is the attempt to become faster and more efficient by omitting some of the safeguards that the institution has put in place because they are time-consuming. These short-cuts, sometimes referred to as work-arounds, may even be shown to you by more experienced nurses who have not recognized the effect of their actions. If safety precautions are too burdensome, the correct approach is to address this through the QI process. Omitting safety features puts the patient in jeopardy.

 COMMUNICATION IN *ACTION*

Refusing to Adopt a Work-Around

Joyce Means had recently begun working as a new RN on 7-Center. Her regular preceptor was out sick, and she was working with Melody, another nurse on the unit. As she was beginning to prepare her 9:00 AM medications from the automated machine, Melody said, "Oh, you know you will never get everything done if you go in and out of that machine every time you turn around. When the drawer opens for 9:00 AM, I just take out stuff for other times during the day, put them in a little container and put them in the cupboard right here with the patient's name. It saves tons of time." Joyce replied, "I guess I'll just have to learn to be faster at the machine, because I wouldn't be comfortable doing that. The safeguards in the machine help me to not make mistakes, and I really appreciate that. I think it is safer for my patients, too."

An Inappropriate Work-Around

In Mercy Hospital, all medications are dispensed from the pharmacy for the individual patient. The computer system used by the pharmacy has information on appropriate dosages, allergies, and incompatibilities, and provides a warning to the pharmacist if the order does not conform to safe practice. A patient was admitted with an acute problem. The physician ordered a medication. The nurse noted that this was a medication that another patient was also taking and that there was a dose available in that patient's drawer. She decided that treatment could be initiated more quickly if she gave the available medication and replaced it when the medication for the new patient arrived from the pharmacy. Her intent was to improve the speed of responding to the patient's problem. Her actions circumvented the safeguards that included a pharmacist's double check of dosages, drug interactions, allergies, and other factors that could affect safety that had been built into the system. This really endangered the patient rather than increasing therapeutic effectiveness. While this might not cause a problem in an individual situation, it sets in place a practice that increases the risks to patients overall.

WORKPLACE SAFETY AND HEALTH FOR NURSES

Nurses have expressed concern regarding safety in the working environment for many years. Employees have a right to expect their employers to provide the safest working environment possible. Some hospitals employ an occupational health nurse to examine the working environment, and use employment practices to promote health and safety on the job. Nurses themselves, however, often have been lax in recognizing on-the-job hazards and acting for self-protection; this can be likened to the response of those who continue to smoke despite their knowledge of the health hazards of smoking, or those who fail to wear seatbelts even though statistics show fewer fatalities in automobile accidents when seatbelts are worn. Some people continue to do those things that they know are detrimental to their health and well-being. Unfortunately, nurses are no exception. Personal awareness is the first step in attempting to control this growing problem.

Infection as an Occupational Hazard

Transmission of infection is a major concern when caring for infected clients. The presence of resistant organisms causes extra concern and makes treatment difficult. All hospitals have an infection-control officer, usually an RN, who has the expertise to guide the staff in planning appropriate infection-control procedures. Staff in other settings may not have access to such an expert.

The hidden danger for nurses lies in those clients who have not been diagnosed as having an infection and for whom specific infection-control measures have therefore not been prescribed. Universal precautions have been mandated by the Occupational Safety and Health Administration (OSHA) for use with clients in all settings to protect staff members from blood-borne pathogens. These precautions prevent the spread of HIV, hepatitis B, and other such blood-borne pathogens. Nurses who have frequent contact with blood and blood products, and those engaged in intravenous (IV) therapy, have a special risk for exposure to hepatitis B. OSHA has developed standards that require employers to pay for hepatitis B immunization for those employees with significant exposure to blood and body fluids that can transmit blood-borne organisms.

AIDS has created a re-evaluation of all approaches to infection control and of health care workers' obligations to provide care for those with communicable diseases. AIDS remains a serious concern for all health care workers. One of the first employer actions toward preventing AIDS and other blood-borne diseases was the provision of sharps containers wherever needles were used. Another important employer responsibility is the provision of a supply of gloves and protective eyewear for employee use. OSHA mandates these measures as part of universal precautions. However, not all cases of transmission of blood-borne pathogens can be prevented by universal precautions. Needlestick injuries—especially those with large-bore needles (eg, bone-marrow aspiration needles)—continue to be the most frequent transmission source. Wearing gloves does not prevent these injuries (Fig. 16-2).

More attention is now being given to designing needles and other sharp devices in ways that prevent needlestick injuries. For example, a needle with a protective plastic housing is available for injections. Even if these needles are not handled properly, they are unlikely to injure the individual. Needleless IV connections are also available. Syringes are available that have a protective cover into which the needle retracts immediately after use. To participate knowledgeably in decisions regarding needle systems and devices, nurses need to seek information about what devices are available. OSHA does mandate that health care facilities have in place a plan to reduce the risk of needlestick injuries through using safe devices. The American Nursing Association (ANA) has been active in workplace advocacy related to needlestick injuries and supports a Web site devoted to this topic (*http://needlestick.org*).

FIGURE 16-2 Needlestick injuries are a major concern in all health care environments.

Blood-borne pathogens are not the only pathogens of concern in the health care environment. The Standard Precautions recommended by the Centers for Disease Control and Prevention (Garner, 1996), often referred to as Body Substance Precautions, are used in almost all settings, but they are not required by OSHA. These precautions protect clients and staff members from infections that might be transmitted by any body substance. When these Standard Precautions were being formulated, OSHA indicated that regulations would likely be changed from the current requirement for Universal Precautions to a requirement for the more extensive Standard Precautions. Because of the antiregulatory stance of Congress, OSHA did not proceed with formulating specific new requirements for employers. There is, however, an OSHA regulation, called the "general duty clause," that requires that employers protect workers from known workplace hazards. Because the infection hazards of all moist body substances are well-documented, employers have recognized that they are liable to action under this clause if they do not provide the means to carry out Standard Precautions.

The incidence of tuberculosis (TB) is again on the rise, with drug-resistant strains of the organism appearing. Although rooms with special ventilation and special masks that are impervious to the TB organism are available, individuals with the disease may be in contact with health care providers long before they are clearly diagnosed. Should nurses in high-risk areas, such as the emergency room, wear special masks during all client contact, or is this unrealistic? These are important questions to consider. New guidelines for the prevention of the spread of TB were released in 2005 (Jensen, Lambert, Iademarco, & Ridzon, 2005).

Although the details of infection control are beyond the scope of this text, we remind you that you hold the key to protecting yourself in many ways. Health care workers often become lax in their attention to the use of gloves or eye protection because these measures are inconvenient. It is your responsibility to use the very best techniques for self-protection, including diligent attention to hand hygiene. Nurses must assume responsibility for their own protection by conscientiously carrying out appropriate measures at all times. Employers must be held accountable for providing the supplies and environment to make this possible.

Hazardous Chemical Agents

Anesthetic gases can increase the risk of fetal malformation and spontaneous abortion in pregnant women who are exposed to them on a regular basis. Standards exist for waste-gas retrieval systems and the allowable level of these gases in the air. Nurses working in operating rooms should seek information on the subject and expect hospitals to provide a safe work environment.

Chemotherapeutic agents used in the treatment of cancer are extremely toxic, and nurses who work in settings where such agents are prepared and administered should seek additional education regarding their administration, not only in relation to the client's safety but also in relation to personal safety. The employer is responsible for providing the equipment needed to maintain safety when handling these agents. In many settings, protocols now require the routine use of personal protective equipment when handling chemotherapeutic agents.

Contact with many medications, especially antibiotics, during preparation and administration may cause the nurse to develop sensitivity. This can create transitory problems (eg, a hand rash), and may be a threat if treatment for a serious infection is compromised later. Other medications are absorbed through the skin and may produce an undesirable effect. Nurses must take responsibility for their own safety regarding these agents. Nurses who understand these hazards handle all drugs with discretion and are careful not to expose themselves to these agents.

■■ COMMUNICATION IN *ACTION*
■■

Speaking up Regarding Unsafe Practice

Jose Morales, RN, worked in the medication administration area side-by-side with another RN. He noted that the RN spiked an antibiotic bag, hung the bag on a hanger, and proceeded to open the tubing to clear air but got fluid from the bag on the counter. Jose spoke up, "Hey, John, I don't mean to be overly critical, but I am concerned about antibiotics getting spilled around here. That contributes to the development of resistant organisms that are a danger to us as well as patients. Besides, you and I might get sensitized to that stuff. I learned a technique for backfilling from the primary bag so that there is never a danger of spilling. Are you familiar with that technique? I would be glad to show you."

Cleaning agents and disinfectants used in the hospital also may be hazardous if used improperly. Employers are now required by OSHA to maintain a list of all chemicals used in the work environment, along with information on their possible effects and the appropriate treatment if individuals are accidentally exposed to them. If you work with these agents, seek out this information, found in the Material Safety Data Sheets, and be sure that you handle chemicals correctly.

Ergonomic Hazards in the Workplace

Ergonomics is the science of fitting a job to one's physical characteristics in order to enhance safety, efficiency, and well-being. When the job does not conform to one's physical characteristics, musculoskeletal stress and injuries may occur. Patient handling and transfer require the movement of a weight load beyond that which most human bodies are designed to manage. In addition, the health care setting often requires that patient movement and transfer be done in awkward positions and inadequate spaces. Thus, musculoskeletal disorders (MSD) are a common occupational hazard.

In analysis of health care work settings, nursing personnel had an incidence of 8.8 injuries per 100 employees in hospital settings and 13.5 per 100 in nursing home settings. Health care settings are one of the top 10 occupations for work-related MSDs (Bureau of Labor Statistics, 2002). Older nurses may be at even higher risk, with evidence that 25% of older nurses reported a job-related injury in the past 5 years, while 33% reported a job-related health problem within that time frame (Letvak, 2005).

In November of 2000, OSHA established ergonomic standards that addressed back injuries in the health care workplace. These were to take effect in January 2001. Although these standards had been in preparation for 10 years, Congress disapproved the standards in March 2001 and included language that ensured that OSHA could not address the ergonomics issue through new regulation for at least 6 years.

Voluntary efforts by employers have been developed in some settings. Some institutions provide instruction in lifting, transfer, posture, body mechanics, and other back-saving strategies to help prevent injury. None of these strategies can protect an individual from repetitive stress injury from lifting more than is appropriate. Further, a patient is, by definition, unstable when being helped, and a sudden move or change in the patient can have a devastating effect on the caregiver. Mechanical lifting devices provide a means of moving clients without danger to staff members. More types of lifting devices are now available, and more employers are open to purchasing equipment to prevent these costly injuries.

The ANA, in cooperation with Johnson & Johnson, has spearheaded a nationwide campaign titled "Handle With Care," aimed at safe patient transfer (ANA, 2004). In its materials, the ANA emphasizes that that there is no safe way for caregivers to lift and transfer dependent patients. They advocate a no-lift policy, the use of mechanical devices for lifting, and the use of lift teams when lifting is essential. In its brochure, background statistics are highlighted to emphasize the importance of the problem, and specific suggestions for lifting strategies and approaches are provided (ANA, 2004). The ANA is also active in supporting the efforts of state constituent organizations to work for the enactment of safe patient handling state legislation. In 2005, the state of Texas became the first to sign into law an act focused on safe patient handling. It requires employers to study the problem and seek safer patient handling strategies, and empowers individuals to refuse to perform actions that might be injurious to themselves (ANA, 2005). Additional states have passed safe patient handling legislation since that time.

An ergonomic concern that is growing for nurses relates to the computer work stations. Those who work at computer work stations for long periods of time are subject to back, neck, wrist, and hand strain. While most nurses do not spend long periods of time at the computer, this is changing as nurses work in telephone care while sitting at computers and even spend long periods documenting care. When one individual uses the same computer station throughout the work day, that station can be adapted to the individual. However, in most nursing settings, the computer station is used by many people. Adjustability of the screen, keyboard, chair, and armrests becomes important in order to provide each person using it with an ergonomically safe work station. In many settings, computer work stations were added to an existing desk area. This may or may not serve the users well. Be alert to the problems that may occur; help yourself by maintaining correct posture and using the adjustments available; report concerns to the appropriate manager.

Be aware of the potential for musculoskeletal injury and examine your work habits. Some nurses feel that they must accomplish certain tasks even if the necessary assistance is not available, and therefore carry out actions of danger to themselves. Nurses need to continue to work toward safer workplaces for all health care providers. They must learn to be assertive regarding their own safety (Fig. 16-3).

Critical Thinking Activity

Research the occupational health program offered by a local employer of nurses. Evaluate that program in relation to health hazards in the workplace of which you are aware.

Workers' Compensation

If you believe that you have a work-related injury or illness, follow the policies and procedures prescribed by your facility or by state regulation. This includes reporting the injury as soon as possible after it happens. In most institutions, this is done on an **incident report** or **quality assurance report**. A common error is to delay reporting in the belief that you should report

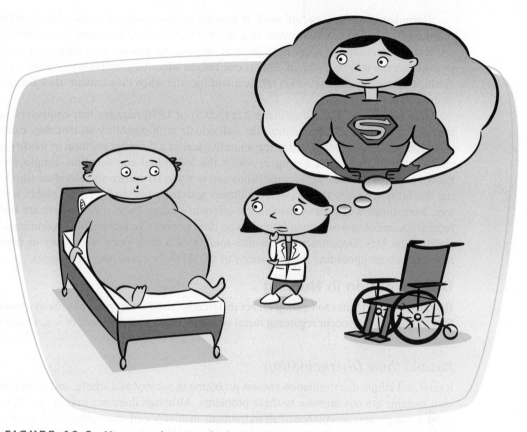

FIGURE 16-3   Nurses must become active in protecting themselves from musculoskeletal injuries.

something only if you know it will be serious or require medical care. By the time you know this, it may be much more difficult to prove that the problem was work related.

Employers may seek to have workers' compensation claims disallowed to limit their financial liability. Because back injuries are the most common work-related injuries, and often have no clear objective evidence of damage even when pain is present, stigma frequently is attached to those who have back injuries. HIV and hepatitis B are transmitted through needlestick injuries, but they are also transmitted through other unsafe behaviors. These factors may underlie attempts by an employer to disallow claims for care and time lost from work due to these work-related illnesses or injuries. Prompt, thorough reporting is essential to future claims.

Have any injury assessed by an appropriate health care provider. If your agency has an occupational health nurse, you may be required to be seen by that individual for initial screening. One concern is whether you may receive care from the provider of your choice or whether you must receive care from a designated provider. This varies based on the regulations governing work-related injury and illness in your state. Ask this question of your employer and then research it through your state workers' compensation office. If the laws allow the employer or a state agency to designate the provider and you go to another of your choice, you may not be reimbursed for expenses incurred.

Compensation for time off work is another concern when a work-related problem occurs; you usually are required to use your sick leave, but additional time may be available through the workers' compensation program. In general, these programs do not match your working salary, so your income will be lessened. This is one reason why many individuals choose to have private disability insurance that provides replacement income when they cannot work because of illness or disability.

The Americans With Disabilities Act (ADA) of 1990 requires that employers seek ways to provide reasonable accommodation for individuals with disability so that they can continue to work. This might include transferring an individual to a different position or modifying the work environment to provide a setting in which the individual can function. Employers have been known to refuse to make accommodations and to try to terminate an individual who has an ongoing disability. Those with work-related illness and disability do have legal rights within the system. Sometimes it requires considerable effort to sustain those rights. There are both state and federal resources to assist an individual who does not receive reasonable accommodation for disability. The U.S. Department of Justice maintains a Web page with links to many different resources about upholding the provisions of the ADA (*www.usdoj.gov/crt/ada*).

Discrimination in Nursing

Discrimination relates to treating others differently based on **stereotypes** about groups of people. Discrimination may occur regarding racial or ethnic background, gender or sex, sexual orientation, and/or age.

Racial/Ethnic Discrimination

Racial and ethnic discrimination remain problems in society as a whole, and unfortunately health care systems are not immune to these problems. Although there are indications that nurses have moved into greater acceptance of all individuals in advance of some other portions of society, concerns about discrimination remain. Historically, the American Association of Colored Graduate Nurses united with the ANA in 1952, before the general civil rights movement in the United States. There have always been prominent nurses of color, such as the past president of the ANA (Beverly Malone), former president of the National League for Nursing (Rhetaugh Dumas), and past president of Sigma Theta Tau (May Wykle), who are all African-American women who have been leaders for all of nursing throughout their long and distinguished careers. They are just three of the many ethnic/racial minority nurses who have made significant contributions to nursing.

However, the number of minorities in nursing does not reflect the number of minorities in the general population. Spratley and colleagues (2000) reported that 12.3% of nurses represent minority groups. This contrasts with a general population that has approximately 25% racial/ethnic minorities (U.S. Census Bureau, 2000). This difference may stem from many causes, but is of concern because a workforce that reflects the population is more likely to meet the health care needs of that population in a culturally sensitive manner. Some of the root causes of the lower participation of minorities in nursing have to do with access to education, support for high career goals, economic status, the image of nursing, institutionalized racism, and other general societal problems.

A survey of minority nurses published by the ANA indicated that many believe they have been adversely affected by discrimination in the nursing profession. Some concerns cited were the perception that others questioned their capabilities and that they were passed over for promotions.

To combat these issues, several organizations for ethnic nurses have joined together to create the National Coalition of Ethnic Minority Nurses Associations (Bessent, 2002).

Nurses are challenged to examine this situation and be a part of the solution. All of us need to recognize and welcome diversity in the nursing profession. We need to acknowledge that a diversity of views and life experiences will enrich nursing as a profession and support excellence in patient care. When we see discrimination occur, whether in education or in the workplace, we each need to speak up as agents for change. The National Student Nurses' Association has supported a program called Breakthrough to Nursing, in which nursing students mentor minority individuals in nursing education. These efforts and similar ones help nursing to move forward as a profession that welcomes and provides opportunities for all.

Discrimination Against Men

Men in nursing also have expressed concern about discrimination. Their concern is not monetary, but is related to being allowed to practice in all areas of nursing and being accepted within the profession. As reported by Nelson and Belcher (2006), this is not an issue of the past; men still continue to feel discriminated against while in nursing school as well as after graduation. Some report having been called names such as "jerk" or "idiot" and having been denied promotion due to their gender.

Anti-male sexism of nurses in the United States was brought to the forefront by the research of Kus (1985), who pointed out that society stereotypes men just as feminists have criticized that it stereotypes women. He made a strong case for the importance of nurses examining the stereotypes they hold about men. Stereotypes narrow our thinking and interfere with people being able to develop to their fullest potential. It is important for women in nursing to examine their own behavior and identify whether they have been guilty of perpetuating outmoded stereotypes of the nurse and supporting a type of discrimination toward men that they would fight to eliminate for women.

Stereotyping also contributes to the low percentage of men in the nursing profession. Although gradually moving slightly up, men still make up only 5% to 6% of nurses. The survey of men in nursing conducted by *Nursing2005* revealed that 40% sometimes felt awkward or defensive in telling others that they were nurses due to the stereotypes that the public holds in regard to men in nursing (Hart, 2005).

In some facilities or areas, men are not allowed to care for women clients, or if they are allowed to care for women, restrictions are placed on them in terms of obtaining consent for care from each client. Those who support the limitations on the practice of men in nursing state that it is a matter of providing for the modesty and privacy of female clients. The argument is made that clients do not have free choice of a nurse but, rather, are assigned a nurse for care, and therefore restrictions are appropriate.

In an interview, Luther Christman, PhD, RN, discussed the discrimination that he encountered throughout a long and prestigious career in nursing. His career began with his graduation from a hospital-based diploma program in 1939 and extended through doctoral studies and a joint position as dean of Rush University and vice-president of nursing for Rush-Presbyterian-St. Luke's Medical Center in Chicago. He identified overt acts that excluded him from positions and covert acts that tried to undermine his influence. He identified this as being an issue of power and control just as is sex discrimination against women (Sullivan, 2002).

Those who oppose limitations on the practice of men in nursing state that, as a professional, a nurse (whether a man or woman) should always consider the privacy and modesty of a client of either gender. This can be done without excluding anyone from providing care in any area. By careful assessment, the nurse can determine the true needs of the client and plan for appropriate avenues to deliver that care. Further, the point has been made that male physicians have not been excluded from any branch of medicine and this has not created problems. The client does not always choose physicians, either. Resident physicians are assigned, referrals are made to specialty physicians, and many group plans designate a physician to provide care. Female nurses care for male clients in all situations. This has been accepted because women are seen in a nurturing, mothering role that the public associates with nursing.

The American Assembly for Men in Nursing provides a forum for the concerns of men in nursing and those who are concerned about the problems of sex discrimination. This organization seeks to educate people and opposes any limitations on opportunities available to men. A specialty journal for men titled *Men in Nursing* has begun publication. Further information can be found on its Web site *http://aamn.org/*.

Critical Thinking Activity

Review the advertisements for nursing positions in three current journals and analyze them for gender bias.

Harassment

Harassment and violence are often discussed together because they are both rooted in the same issues of the abuse of power. "Violence isn't limited to the kinds of incidents that make headlines. It includes a range of behavior from verbal abuse, threats, and unwanted sexual advances to physical assault and at the extreme, homicide" (ANA, 1994).

Sexual harassment is grouped into two sets of behavior. The first is the creation of a hostile work environment through behavior of a sexual nature. This type of sexual harassment may take the form of comments about an individual's body, persistent unwanted attempts to initiate a personal relationship, the ongoing use of suggestive or obscene language, unwanted touching, or direct sexual advances. Another type of sexual harassment is called "quid pro quo." This involves the explicit granting of job-related benefits (working conditions, salary, privileges, or even simply the benefit of remaining employed) in return for sexual favors (Roberts & Mann, n.d.).

Both men and women may be the objects of sexual harassment. Because nurses are involved with personal care of individuals of the opposite sex, there is sometimes the unspoken assumption that nurses will not be offended by sexual comments, jokes, or innuendo.

Sexual harassment was the subject of a position paper by the ANA (1993), as nurses began to voice their concerns about its presence in nursing. This position paper provided background on the costs of the problem and identified areas of redress for nurses who were subjected to sexual harassment.

Harassers in the health care workplace may be clients, coworkers, or physicians. According to Kaye (1996) and Williams (1995), most harassers in the health care workplace are physicians; this follows the general data showing that sexual harassment is a demonstration of personal power over others. Traditionally, physicians have had the most power in health care environments. While recognizing the problem, it is important not to stereotype physicians, because the majority of physicians are professional and appropriate in their relationships.

Individuals should take steps to stop sexual harassment by giving clear, direct verbal messages indicating that the behavior in question is unwanted, unpleasant, and must stop. Sometimes this action alone stops inappropriate behavior. If clear, direct messages are not successful, the individual then should report the matter in writing to an immediate supervisor. Any individual who believes that he or she has been the victim of sexual harassment should keep personal records of the behavior and of all attempts to stop the behavior in question. Most organizations and agencies have an individual designated to deal with issues related to sexual harassment. If you encounter problem behavior, discuss your concerns with this person. If you belong to a collective bargaining group, that group can serve as a resource to assist you. In some instances, it may be necessary to seek independent legal counsel to force resolution of the problem.

Employers are legally and ethically responsible for having clear policies that prohibit sexual harassment, and for providing an appropriate work environment. If an employer fails to respond appropriately, the employer may be legally liable. These policies should be publicized so that everyone is aware of them. The courts support the responsibility of the employer to maintain a work environment free of sexual harassment (Equal Employment Opportunity Commission, 2006).

Unfortunately, some employers do not respond appropriately to sexual harassment. In a survey by *NurseWeek* and the American Organization of Nurse Executive, nurses reported that sexual harassment is still present in the health care workplace. Sossin reported an example of an individual who reported repeated sexual harassment and the employer did not respond (Sossin, 2003).

■■ COMMUNICATION IN *ACTION*
■■

A Clear Message About Sexual Harassment

Jean Wilson, RN, was new to the medical center where she worked. While sitting at the desk by herself in the evening, a male resident physician sat down beside her. He draped his arm around her shoulders, put his face close to hers and said, "Hi there, sweetie! How's it going for the prettiest nurse on 3-Southwest?" Jean was taken aback and very uncomfortable. She immediately stood and said, "We are virtual strangers. I don't like your touching me in that way or calling me 'Sweetie.' It is inappropriate. Don't do that again." He then said, "Hey, hey—don't get so upset. I was just being friendly." She replied, "We're not friends, we are colleagues, and that does not include touching me and calling me names like 'Sweetie.' " He muttered to himself and walked away. Jean felt nervous but glad she had stood her ground.

Verbal Abuse

Verbal abuse also occurs in health care settings. In efforts to increase retention of nurses, hospitals have begun asking why nurses leave specific hospitals and nursing altogether. An important factor is the extent to which nurses see themselves as disrespected and verbally abused in the workplace. In a study conducted by Rosenstein and reported in the *American Journal of Nursing* (2002), nurses were asked to categorize the types of disruptive behavior they either witnessed or experienced. Most frequently cited were yelling or raised voices, disrespect, condescension, berating colleagues, berating patients, and use of abusive language. Verbal abuse may also be referred to as violence and bullying (Leiper, 2005).

In the past, these behaviors often were tolerated from physicians because other health professionals knew that they did not have the power to change them. Bruder (2001) speaks of this as the "elephant in the dining room" of health care. Everyone knows it's there, but no one addresses it directly. This type of disrespectful behavior has been identified by the IOM report as contributing to errors in health care. The person who fears being the subject of verbal abuse may delay communicating about a problem. The person who feels free to be disrespectful of a colleague may carry that disrespect into ignoring concerns about the patient (Kohn et al., 2000).

Not all verbal abuse is vertical, moving from more powerful to less powerful. Some verbal abuse is horizontal—nurses verbally abusing one another, saying things to one another that would be clearly inappropriate if said to a patient. This may include intimidation, bullying, scapegoating, blaming, and sabotaging (Leiper, 2005). Verbal abuse may also come from patients who become demanding.

Why does verbal abuse continue? There are many theories regarding the exercise of power, oppressed group behavior, low self-esteem, and others (Leiper, 2005). The bottom line must be that regardless of why it happens, verbal abuse must be stopped.

Bruder (2001) suggests the following general strategies to establish a more equitable workplace initially. Nurses must assess themselves and identify their own feelings about self-worth. They must recognize their own potential for verbal abuse toward others and deal ethically with one another. He further suggests that nurses start with expecting respect in the use of names. If physicians call nurses by their first names, then nurses should call physicians by their first names. If physicians insist on being called "Dr. X," then nurses should be addressed as "Nurse X" or "Ms. X." This helps to diminish the power differential.

Specific actions a nurse should take regarding verbal abuse are similar to those suggested above for sexual harassment. Familiarize yourself with your employer's policies; there may be policies regarding reporting mechanisms. Leiper (2005) suggests that the cycle can be stopped by refusing to be a victim. She suggests getting help from the employer. Immediately report any cases of abuse to your supervisor. Making a plan and taking action are essential. The aggressor should be confronted and formal written complaints filed as appropriate. Legal action may be needed. Keep good personal records with details of the incident, the time, the circumstances, and a listing of any witnesses. Nurses need not remain powerless regarding situations of workplace abuse.

Nurses must work together to not succumb to intimidation. Some hospitals have initiated what they are calling a code white, which is a signal for others to come and be observers when an individual begins any type of verbal abuse. This verbal abuse might consist of insults, a personal attack, a temper tantrum, or a tirade. These people are witnesses and provide emotional support to the recipient of abuse. Administrators and other physicians must also learn not to turn their backs to abuse occurring in the environment. They have both ethical and legal (in the case of administrators) responsibilities for the workplace.

Violence in the Workplace

Most nursing students think of hospitals as places where victims of violence are helped. Rarely do they think of themselves as potential victims of violence in their own workplace. According to OSHA, two thirds of nonfatal workplace assaults happen in health and social services facilities.

The majority of these are assaults by clients on nursing staff, and more occur in psychiatric mental health settings than in other settings. Assaults on staff members by visitors and outsiders also occur; most of these take place in emergency rooms. Health care workplace violence is not confined to industrialized societies. The World Health Organization (WHO) has identified violence as a worldwide problem that threatens the effective delivery of health care (WHO, 2002). In the United States, violence is also very costly. While the average cost for an injury in terms of lost time and medical treatment was $5,719, costs can go higher than $100,000 for those with permanent injuries. In addition to monetary costs, there are costs in terms of psychological damage and loss of individuals to the profession of nursing (Worthington, 2002). Not included in these estimates were less severe injuries, injuries to patients or property, and the long-term physical and psychological costs of trauma.

OSHA has issued guidelines for use by facilities trying to establish a safer workplace. These are not enforceable rules but may represent what is termed the "General Duty" clause in the OSHA Act. The guidelines call for clear programs designed to protect workers. These programs would include an assessment and analysis of the workplace for hazards and a plan for prevention of problems.

One form of prevention is to train employees in the management of hostile and violent behavior. Ways of identifying hostile and assaultive clients should be developed so that staff can be warned to take extra personal safety precautions. The Crisis Prevention Institute (CPI) has developed a comprehensive training program called "Nonviolent Crisis Intervention" that is used in many settings (CPI, 2006).

Other important environmental safeguards include the use of such devices as metal detectors, panic buttons, and bulletproof glass, where appropriate. Adequate staff to manage potentially violent behavior is of particular concern in psychiatric/mental health settings. The addition of security personnel is important in some environments. There should be an attitude throughout the institution of zero tolerance for abusive or assaultive behavior.

In addition to preventing and managing problem situations, there should be clear guidelines for reporting both verbal and physical abuse and following through on all complaints. Health care institutions should work with law enforcement professionals when abusive or assaultive behavior occurs to ensure that legal procedures are carried out correctly.

Those who report incidents should receive support and assistance and be assured that there will be no reprisals or blaming. Some nurses have been reluctant to report verbal and physical abuse or assault because of personal and institutional beliefs that health care employees should be able to handle these behaviors independently. Another common belief in health care environments is that all behavior has meaning for the individual and that employees should accept inappropriate behaviors on the part of clients. Social constraints and adverse consequences related to inappropriate behavior are a valuable ally in redirecting the behaviors of those who are cognitively impaired, mentally ill, or developmentally delayed. Nurses need support from their work environments in accessing these avenues to protect themselves.

Critical Thinking Activity

Formulate an appropriate response to experiencing verbal abuse in the workplace. Include specific statements you would use and each step you would take if the verbal abuse occurred again.

Key Concepts

- The process of moving from novice to expert has been divided into five stages: novice, advanced beginner, competent, proficient, and expert.
- Reality shock occurs when an idealistic new graduate enters the real world of practice and has difficulty with the expectations and demands found there. You can prepare for the stress created by this transition through attending to your own expectations and developing personal strategies for coping including self-appraisal; evaluating employers; seeking mentors, preceptors, or coaches; joining a peer support group; and using personal stress management strategies.
- Burnout is a stress response experienced by nurses and others who work in occupations that make many emotional demands. Burnout may be alleviated by planned actions. In some instances it may be necessary to change job settings when stress accumulates.
- Concerns about patient safety were highlighted by the Institute of Medicine report. Initiatives to improve patient safety have originated with The Joint Commission, the Patient Safety and Quality Improvement Act of 2005, quality improvement activities of health care agencies, and the efforts of individual health care providers.
- Occupational safety and health are special concerns for nurses because of the infectious nature of the illnesses with which they come in contact, the toxicity of some chemicals in the nursing environment, and the potential for musculoskeletal injury and violence.
- Nurses who experience a work-related injury must carefully follow all relevant rules and regulations for reporting the injury, completing appropriate forms, and seeking care to ensure that they receive assistance for any medical care and lost wages.
- Nurses may see discrimination in the workplace manifested as racial/ethnic discrimination, wage discrimination against women, and job opportunity discrimination against men.
- Sexual harassment in the workplace is illegal. Understanding how to defend oneself against sexual harassment provides a greater feeling of personal power and control in the situation.
- Verbal abuse contributes to patient safety concerns as well as to an aversive workplace where individuals decide to leave nursing. Administrative authorities should act to stop verbal abuse, but nurses working collectively can also act to decrease the impact of verbal abuse.
- Violence in the workplace is found in health care settings as well as the rest of society. Nurses working individually and collectively can develop strategies to combat this serious concern.

Relevant Web Sites

American Assembly for Men in Nursing: *http://aamn.org*
American Nurses Association (ANA): *http://nursingworld.org*
American Nurses Association (ANA), Occupational Health and Safety Issues:
   http://nursingworld.org/dlwa/osh/index.htm
American Nurses Association (ANA) Position Statement: Sexual Harassment:
   http://nursingworld.org/readroom/position/workplac/wkharass.htm

American Nurses Association (ANA) RN No Harm/Pollution Prevention: *http://nursing world.org/rnnoharm*

American Nurses Association (ANA) and Nursing World Online Health and Safety Survey (2001): *http://nursingworld.org/surveys/hssurvey.htm*

Americans with Disabilities Act Information: *www.usdoj.gov/crt/ada*

Bureau of Labor Statistics, U.S. Dept of Labor, Occupational Outlook Handbook: *www.bls.gov/oco/ocos083.htm*

Crisis Prevention Institute: *www.crisisprevention.com*

Institute of Medicine Report (IOM): *To Err is Human*: *www.iom.edu/?id ± 12735*

The Joint Commission: *www.jointcommission.org*

Nurse Advocate: Nurses and Workplace Violence: *www.nurseadvocate.org*

Occupational Safety and Health Administration: *www.osha.gov*

Safety and Health in Nursing Homes: *www.osha.gov/SLTC/nursinghome*

U.S. Department of Justice: Americans With Disabilities: *www.usdoj.gov/crt/ada*

Workplace problems: *www.workplaceblues.com*

References

American Nurses Association. (1993). Position Statement: Sexual Harassment. [On-line]. *http://nursingworld.org/readroom/position/workplac/wkharass.htm*. Accessed May 28, 2006.

American Nurses Association. (1994). Workplace violence: Can you close the door on it? [Brochure]. [On-line]. *http://nursing world.org/dlwa/osh/wp5.htm*. Accessed October, 12, 2002.

American Nurses Association. (2004). *Handle with care*. [On-line]. *http://nursingworld.org/handlewithcare/hwc.pdf*. Accessed January 26, 2006.

American Nurses Association. (2005). Texas passes safe patient lifting law for hospitals, nursing homes. (News release). [On-line]. *http://nursingworld.org/handlewithcare/txleg.htm*. Accessed January 26, 2006.

Benner, P. (1984). *From novice to expert: Excellence and power in clinical nursing practice*. Commemorative edition (2001). Upper Saddle River, NJ: Prentice Hall.

Bessent, H. (2002). *Minority nurses in the new century*. Washington, DC: American Nurses Association Publishing.

Bradby, M. (1990). Status passage into nursing: Another view of the process of socialization into nursing. *Journal of Advanced Nursing, 15*(10), 1220–1225.

Bruder, P. (2001, fall). Verbal abuse of female nurses: An American medical form of gender apartheid? *Hospital Topics, 4*(79), 30–34.

Bureau of Labor Statistics. (2002, December 19). *Survey of occupational injuries and illnesses, 2001*. U.S. Department of Labor. [On-line]. *www.bls.gov/iif/home.htm*. Accessed January 22, 2006.

Canuff, A. J. (n.d.) Recognizing Job Burnout, American Counseling Association. [On-line]. *www.workplaceblues.com/mental_health/recognizing.asp*. Accessed June 1, 2006.

Crisis Prevention Institute. (2006). Nonviolent Crisis Intervention. [On-line]. *www.crisisprevention.com/program/nci.html*. Accessed June 1, 2006.

Dreyfus, S. E., & Dreyfus, H. L. (1980). A five-stage model of the mental activities involved in directed skill acquisition. Unpublished report supported by the Air Force Office of Scientific Research (AFSC), USAF (Contract F49620-79-C-0063), University of California at Berkeley, 1980 (as reported in P. Benner [1984], *From Novice to Expert*, Upper Saddle River, NJ: Prentice Hall.

Equal Employment Opportunity Commission. (2006). Sexual Harassment. [On-line]. *www.eeoc.gov/types/sexual_harassment.html*. Accessed May 29, 2006.

Garner, J. (1996). Guidelines for isolation precautions in hospitals. *Infection Control and Hospital Epidemiology. 17*, 53–80.

Hart, K. A. (2005) What do men in nursing really think? *Nursing 2005, 35*(11), 46–48.

Jensen P. A., Lambert, L. A., Iademarco, M. F., & Ridzon, R. (2005). Guidelines for Preventing the Transmission of Mycobacterium tuberculosis in Health-Care Settings, MMWR Recommendations and Reports. December 30, 2005, 54(RR17), 1–141. [On-line]. *www.cdc.gov/mmwr/preview/mmwrhtml/rr5417a1.htm*. Accessed January 25, 2006.

Joint Commission for the Accreditation of Healthcare Organizations. (2003). *Comprehensive accreditation manual for hospitals: The official handbook*. Chicago: Author.

Joint Commission on the Accreditation of Health Care Organizations. JCAHO (2005). Sentinel Event Policy and Procedures Updated: June 2005. [On-line]. *www.jointcommission.org/JointCommission*. Accessed June 1, 2006.

Kaye. J. (1996). Sexual harassment and hostile environments in the perioperative area. *Journal of the Association of Perioperative Registered Nurses, 63*(2), 443–446, 448–449.

Kohn, L. T., Corrigan, J. M., & Donaldson, M. S. (Eds.) (2000). *To Err Is Human: Building a Safer Health System.* Committee on Quality of Health Care in America, Institute of Medicine, Washington, DC: National Academy Press. [On-line]. *http://darwin. nap.edu/books/0309068371/html.* Accessed January 23, 2006.

Kramer, M. (1979). *Reality shock.* St. Louis, MO: CV Mosby.

Kus, R. J. (1985). Stages of coming out: An ethnographic approach. *Western Journal of Nursing Research, 7*(2), 177–194.

Leiper, J. (2005). Nurse against nurse: How to stop horizontal violence. *Nursing2005, 33*(3), 44–45.

Letvak S. (2005, March–April). Health and safety of older nurses. *Nursing Outlook, 53*(2), 66–72.

Lindeman, C. (1999). The art of nursing. *Creative Nursing, 5*(3), 3–4.

Maslach, C., & Jackson, S. E. (1986). *Maslach Burnout Inventory manual* (2nd ed.). Palo Alto, CA: Consulting Psychologists Press.

Nelson, R., & Belcher, D. (2006). Men in nursing: Still too few. *American Journal of Nursing, 106*(2), 25–26.

Neuhs, H. P. (1994). Sexual harassment: A concern for nursing administrators. *Journal of Nursing Administration, 24*(5), 47–52.

Patient Safety and Quality Improvement Act. (2005). [On-line]. *www.govtrack.us/congress/bill.xpd?bill ± s109-544.* Accessed January 24, 2006.

Restifo, V., & Yoder, L. H. (2004). Partnership: Making the Most of Mentoring. *NurseWeek–Mountain Edition, 5*(7), 30–33.

Roberts, B. S., & Mann, R. A. (n.d.). Sexual Harassment In The Workplace: A Primer. [On-line]. *www3.uakron.edu/lawrev/ robert1.html.* Accessed May 28, 2006.

Rosenstein, A. H. (2002). Nurse–physician relationships: Impact on nurse satisfaction and retention, *American Journal of Nursing, 102*(6), 26–34.

Sossin, J. (2003, February 28). Indecent Proposal. *Nurseweek.* [On-line]. *www.nurseweek.com/news/features/03-02/discrimination. asp.* Accessed May 29, 2006.

Spratley, E., Johnson, A., Sochalski, J., Fritz, M., & Spencer, W. (2000). *The registered nurse population: Findings from the National Sample Survey of Registered Nurses.* The Department of Health and Human Services: Health Resources and Services Administration. [On-line]. *http://bhpr.hrsa.gov/healthworkforce/ rnsurvey/rnss1.htm.* Accessed May, 26, 2006.

Sullivan, E. (2002). In a women's world. *Reflections on Nursing Leadership, 28*(3), 10–17.

U.S. Census Bureau. (2000). Fact Sheet 2000 Census Demographic Profile Highlights. [On-line]. *http://factfinder. census.gov.* Accessed May 29, 2006.

Williams, M. (1995). The prevalence and impact of violence and sexual harassment of registered nurses in the workplace. *Chart, 92*(4), 5–6.

World Health Organization. (2002). *New research shows workplace violence threatens health services.* [On-line]. *www.who. int/inf/en/pr-2002-37.html.* Accessed October 12, 2002.

Worthington, K. (2002). Violence in the health care workplace. *American Journal of Nursing, 100*(11). [On-line]. *http://nursing world.org/AJN/2000/nov/Issues.htm.* Accessed October 12, 2002.

Commonly Used Acronyms

AACN	American Association of Colleges of Nursing
AAN	American Academy of Nursing
ABNS	American Board of Nursing Specialties
ACNM	American College of Nurse Midwives
AONE	American Organization of Nurse Executives
ADA	Americans with Disabilities Act
ADEA	Age Discrimination and Employment Act
ADL	Activity of daily living
ADN	Associate Degree Nursing
AFL/CIO	American Federation of Labor/Congress of Industrial Organizations
AHA	American Hospital Association
AHCPR	Agency for Health Care Policy and Research* (now the AHRQ)
AHRQ	Agency for Health Care Research and Quality (formerly the Agency for Health Care Policy and Research—AHCPR)
AMA	American Medical Association
ANA	American Nurses Association
ANA-PAC	American Nurses Association Political Action Committee
ANCC	American Nurses' Credentialing Center
ANF	American Nurses Foundation
APIC	Association for Professionals in Infection Control
APN	Advanced practice nurse
BC	Board certified
CADP**	Council of Associate Degree Programs of the NLN
CAI	Computer-assisted instruction
CAM	Complementary and alternative medicine
CAT	Computer adaptive testing
CBHDP**	Council of Baccalaureate and Higher Degree Programs
CBO	Competency-based orientation
CCNE	Commission on Collegiate Nursing Education (related to American Association of Colleges of Nursing)
CDC	Centers for Disease Control and Prevention
CDPN**	Council of Diploma Programs in Nursing
CE	Continuing education
CEU	Continuing education unit
CGFNS	Committee on Graduates of Foreign Nursing Schools

CHAP	Community Health Accreditation Program
CINAHL	Cumulative Index to Nursing and Allied Health Literature
CMS	Centers for Medicare & Medicaid Services
CNA	Canadian Nurses Association
CNA	Certified nursing assistant
CNL	Clinical nurse leader
CNM	Certified nurse-midwife
CNPE •	Congress on Nursing Practice and Economics
CNS	Clinical nurse specialist
COE	Computerized order entry
CPNP**	Council of Practical Nursing Programs
CPT	Current procedural terminology
CQI	Continuous quality improvement
CRNA	Certified registered nurse anesthetist
DNP	Doctor of nursing practice
DNR	Do not resuscitate
DNS	Doctor of science in nursing
DOE	Department of Education
DOE	Department of Energy
DPH	Doctor of public health
DRG	Diagnosis-related group
EBP	Evidence-based practice
EEOC	Equal Employment Opportunity Commission
EdD	Doctor of education
EI	Emotional intelligence
EPO	Exclusive Provider Organization
FCC	Federal Communications Commission
FDA	Food and Drug Administration
FTE	Full-time equivalent
GDP	Gross domestic product
HCFA*	Health Care Finance Administration (see CMS)
HEDIS	Health Plan Employer Data and Information Set
HGP	Human Genome Project
HHCC	Home Health Care Classifications
HHS	Department of Health and Human Services
HIPAA	Health Insurance Portability and Accountability Act
HMO	Health maintenance organization
ICD-9 CM	International Classification of Diseases Version 9
ICN	International Council of Nurses
ICNPP	International Classification for Nursing Practice Project
IOM	Institute of Medicine
IPA	Independent Practice Association
ISP	Internet service provider
IVF	In vitro fertilization

JCAHO*	Joint Commission on Accreditation of Healthcare Organizations (now known as The Joint Commission)
MASH	Mobile Army Surgical Hospital
MBO	Management by objectives
MCO	Managed care organizations
MDS	Minimum data set
MOTTEP	National Minority Organ and Tissue Transplant Education Program
MSN	Master's of science in nursing
MT	Medical technologist
NAC	Nursing assistant–certified
NACEP	National Aide Competency Evaluation Program
NACNEP	National Advisory Council on Nurse Education & Practice
NANDA*	North American Nursing Diagnosis Association
NANDA–I	North American Nursing Diagnosis Association–International
NAPNES	National Association for Practical Nurse Education and Service
NCCAM	National Center for Complementary and Alternative Medicine
NCH	Nursing care hours
NCLEX–PN	National Council Licensing Examination for Practical Nursing
NCLEX–RN	National Council Licensing Examination for Registered Nursing
NCNIP	National Commission Nursing Implementation Project
NCQA	National Committee for Quality Assurance
NCSBN	National Council of State Boards of Nursing
ND	Doctorate in nursing
NFLPN	National Federation of Licensed Practical Nurses
NFSNO*	National Federation for Specialty Nursing Organizations (now part of Nursing Organizations Alliance)
NIC	Nursing Interventions Classifications
NIDSEC	National Information and Data Set Evaluation Center
NIH	National Institutes of Health
NINR	National Institute of Nursing Research
NIOSH	National Institute of Occupational Safety and Health
NLM	National Library of Medicine
NLN	National League for Nursing
NLNAC	National League for Nursing Accrediting Commission (related to the National League for Nursing)
NLRA	National Labor Relations Act
NLRB	National Labor Relations Board
NMDS	Nursing minimum data set
NOADN	National Organization for Associate Degree Nursing
NOC	Nursing Outcomes Classification
NP	Nurse practitioner
NSNA	National Student Nurse Association
N-STAT	Nurses Strategic Action Team
OASIS	Outcomes and Assessment Information Set

OBRA	Omnibus Budget Reconciliation Act
OSHA	Occupational Health and Safety Administration
PA	Physician assistant
PAC	Political action committee
PAS	Physician-assisted suicide
PCP	Primary care provider
PGD	Pre-implantation genetic diagnosis
PhD	Doctor of philosophy
PNDS	Perioperative Nursing Data Set
POLST	Physician Orders for Life-Sustaining Treatments
PPO	Preferred provider organization
PPS	Prospective payment system
PSDA	Patient Self-Determination Act
PSRO	Professional Standards Review Organizations
QA	Quality assurance
QAI	Quality assessment and improvement
QI	Quality indicator
RAP	Resident Assessment Protocols
ROP	Regional Occupation Programs
RUG	Resource utilization group
SEIU	Service Employees International Union
SNF	Skilled nursing facility
SNOMED-RT	Systematized Nomenclature of Medicine–Reference Terminology
UAN	United American Nurses
UAP	Unlicensed assistive personnel
UMAP	Unlicensed Medication Administration Personnel
UNOS	United Network for Organ Sharing
WHO	World Health Organization

*Indicates that the title has changed
**Indicates that the organization is no longer active

Index

Page numbers followed by d *indicate displays; those followed by* f *indicate figures; those followed by* t *indicate tables.*